Food Service Manual

for Health Care Institutions

1994 Edition

Brenda A. Byers, M.S., R.D., L.D., Carol W. Shanklin, Ph.D., R.D., and Linda C. Hoover, Ph.D., R.D.

AHA books are published by American Hospital Publishing, Inc., an American Hospital Association company

The views expressed in this publication are strictly those of the authors and do not necessarily represent official positions of the American Hospital Association.

Library of Congress Cataloging-in-Publication Data

Food service manual for health care institutions /
Brenda A. Byers, Carol W. Shanklin, and Linda C. Hoover. —
1994 ed.
    p.   cm.
Rev. ed. of: Food service manual for health care
institutions / Ruby P. Puckett, Bonnie B. Miller. 1988 ed.
©1988.
    Includes bibliographical references and index.
    ISBN 1-55648-114-4
    1. Hospitals—Food service. I. Shanklin, Carol W. II.
Hoover, Linda C. III. Puckett, Ruby P. Food service manual
for health care institutions. IV. Title
    [DNLM: 1. Food Service, Hospital.   WX 168 B9925f 1994]
RA975.5.D5P83   1994
642'.5—dc20
DNLM/DLC
for Library of Congress   94-7495
                                                                       CIP

Catalog no. 046172

©1994 by American Hospital Publishing, Inc.,
an American Hospital Association company

Printed in the USA

Text set in Sabon
7M—03/94—0368

Audrey Kaufman, Acquisitions/Development Editor
Lee Benaka, Production Editor
Marcia Bottoms, Books Division Assistant Director
Peggy DuMais, Production Coordinator
Luke Smith, Cover Designer
Brian Schenk, Books Division Director

Contents

List of Figures

List of Tables

About the Authors

Brenda A. Byers, M.S., R.D., L.D., is director of nutrition and food services at All Saints Health System, in Fort Worth, Texas. Ms. Byers has 11 years of experience in food service operations management and 5 years of experience as department director, as well as having served as a staff dietitian.

Linda C. Hoover, Ph.D., R.D., is an assistant professor in the Department of Education, Nutrition, and Restaurant/Hotel Management, College of Human Sciences, at Texas Tech University, in Lubbock. Previously, Dr. Hoover served as a faculty member, specializing in food service systems management, at Texas Woman's University, in Denton, and Texas Christian University, in Fort Worth. Her operational experience includes working as associate director of food service and as director of materials management at Methodist Hospitals of Dallas.

Carol W. Shanklin, Ph.D., R.D., is the director of the graduate program in the Department of Hotel, Restaurant, Institution Management and Dietetics at Kansas State University, in Manhattan. Dr. Shanklin teaches and conducts research in food service and hospitality management. Prior to joining the faculty at Kansas State University, she worked at Texas Woman's University, in Denton, and served as a productivity consultant for a major medical center in Dallas. Dr. Shanklin is active in The American Dietetic Association and has authored and coauthored several articles in professional journals.

Preface

Individuals seeking a career in health care food service management will experience increasing challenges and opportunities. Effective management in a rapidly changing environment requires continuous learning and planning based on the internal and external environment. Many factors have been identified that influence both the internal and external environment of the health care food service department. Government interest in health care reform will result in increased regulations with which managers and organizations must comply. The changing demographics of the population will affect both the demands of customers and the needs and abilities of the work force. Increased emphasis on health and wellness will provide additional opportunities for nutrition education and will impact meal planning, production, and service. Advances in technology will continue to influence the life expectancy of the population and the costs and methods of delivering health care and food service. Managers will be challenged to effectively use technological advances.

☐ Scope of the Text

The latest edition of the *Food Service Manual for Health Care Institutions* is designed for use by students and/or managers and supervisors of health care food service. Whether students are preparing for careers in food service management or clinical nutrition, this manual will contribute to an understanding of food service operations. Managers and supervisors in health care operations will find the information and suggested forms, formulas, policies, and techniques valuable in managing limited resources.

Past editions of this manual were designed to provide information for successful management of daily operations. The newest edition continues to provide practical operational information and to emphasize application of the managerial functions of planning, organizing, leading, and controlling. The text, while extensive, cannot answer all of the questions or concerns of those managing health care food service. Notations are made throughout the text of suggested companion resources that can be used to supplement the information in this manual.

☐ Content of the New Text

The first part of the manual is designed to provide information needed for management of the nutrition and food service department. The introductory chapter identifies issues relevant to health care reform with an emphasis on the rapidly changing environment surrounding health care food service. The issues identified in chapter 1 are discussed throughout the text. In addition to traditional hospital food service, the delivery of services to skilled nursing units, rehabilitation units, extended care centers, home care, and outpatients is presented.

Chapter 2 discusses participative leadership, managing for change, and employee involvement through teamwork. Marketing is examined in chapter 3, which includes details for conducting and acting on market research. Although quality issues are highlighted throughout the text, chapter 4 discusses continuous quality improvement, quality control, and customer satisfaction. The planning chapter has been expanded to include information on developing a departmental business plan. The chapter on human resources has been revised to include issues related to cultural diversity, literacy, shifting work-force demographics, and the Americans with Disabilities Act and the Family Leave Act. In the previous edition, communication consisted of a section of a chapter, but the topic has now been expanded to a full chapter with additional information on developing presentations and writing effective justifications and proposals. A separate chapter is included on the use of management information systems. The discussion of financial accountability has been expanded to a full chapter with details of analyzing financial statements and the application of financial indicators and cost control strategies. Both the organization chapter and the nutrition management chapter have been revised.

Part two of the manual outlines specific information necessary for operation of the food service department. A complete chapter is included on the environment and encompasses relevant legislation and regulation applicable to food service and issues related to water quality, energy utilization, and waste. The separate chapter on sanitation includes information on microbiological hazards and emerging pathogens, application of sanitary food handling, and HACCP guidelines. The safety chapter provides information on the latest OSHA guidelines, including hazardous materials and material safety data sheets. Newly revised chapters in this section include: menu planning, product selection, purchasing, food production, meal service, and facility design and equipment selection.

Acknowledgments

The authors wish to acknowledge the following individuals who provided valuable assistance in obtaining resources for the authors and technical assistance: Norma Sanchez, Allison Penka, and Carol Perlmutter, graduate students in the Department of Hotel, Restaurant, Institution Management, and Dietetics at Kansas State University; Dana Lloyd and Kimberly Mays in the Department of Nutrition and Food Services at All Saints Hospital in Fort Worth, Texas; Steve Morse, Ph.D., and Rita Pohlmeier in the Department of Restaurant, Hotel, and Institutional Management at Texas Tech University; and Eva Mutai, a graduate student at Texas Tech.

On a personal note, the authors wish to thank their families for the support and encouragement that provided an atmosphere conducive to completing this manual: Johnny, Diana, and James Byers; Robin and Emily Hoover; and Larry and Chris Shanklin.

Overview
of Current Issues

□ Introduction

In the remaining years of the 1990s, health care will be met with increased public awareness associated with the cost of, and equal access to, high-quality care. The percentage of the national budget spent on health care is still rising at an alarming rate and will require persistent emphasis on cost-effective management. Past cost-control efforts include rightsizing by staff reductions, flattening of management levels, and multidepartment management, as well as heightened productivity and participation in purchasing groups. Changes occurring within health care will be affected by the economy and by business and industry trends. In addition to their impact on health care cost, these trends will affect methods of operation, especially as those methods relate to quality, customer satisfaction, and management style.

Hospitals of the future will experience increases in patient age and acuity level and a continued population shift from inpatients to outpatients. Responses to these changes have caused hospitals to add extended care services such as rehabilitation units, skilled nursing units, and behavioral health centers to increase inpatient census. Hospital-owned home care services now extend services for patients after discharge while they increase revenues. Once the primary health care facility, hospitals now face competition from a growing number of alternative health care facilities. These competitors will include nursing homes, adult day care centers, retirement centers with acute care facilities, freestanding outpatient clinics, and independent home care agencies.

The period 1983 through 1992 was marked by emphasis on cost containment, staff reductions, increased productivity, group purchasing, and service expansion designed to generate revenue. Nutrition and food service managers will witness a shift in the provision of services for patients or clients between now and the year 2000. In addition to the continued cost containment requirements of the past 10 years, managers must contend effectively with increased government intervention, a less literate and more culturally diverse work force, a focus on customer satisfaction, participation in continuous quality improvement, more emphasis on nutrition awareness, and advances in technology.

This chapter reviews four key areas that will continue to direct health care nutrition and food service: the political environment, work force issues, a customer-oriented focus, and new trends in technology. The information reviewed here will be applied in subsequent chapters, specifically as it relates to and is affected directly by the above-mentioned trends and issues.

☐ Political Issues

The future direction of health care will be influenced by politics and government intervention, as a direct result of increased public awareness and demands. As one of his first official acts, President Bill Clinton, a proponent of managed competition coupled with a global budget mechanism to ensure cost containment, established a task force on health care and its related costs. Regulation of the health care industry is likely to continue, even intensify, while access to care becomes a concern of politicians and consumers alike. Health care food service departments will feel the impact of the political environment as it shapes and regulates the way service is delivered. In addition to regulation, managers will see the effects of more emphasis on environmental safety while they struggle to provide accurate nutrition information to the consumer.

Regulation and Legislation

The nature of this text precludes a comprehensive discussion of legislation as it pertains to health care nutrition and food service delivery. Even so, legislative impact and subsequent regulations must be taken into account when food service directors plan the direction of their departments. This section briefly reviews various government and private-sector regulations that affect food service delivery. In addition to those covered, the 12-week family leave legislation (Family and Medical Leave Act of 1993) should be scrutinized closely to determine what—if any—modifications are required on work methods and staffing patterns.

Medicare and Medicaid

The regulations that currently have the greatest effect on health care are those dictated by Medicare and Medicaid, the largest managed care providers in the United States. Reimbursement rates for services have been set by Medicare and embraced by other managed care systems. Although most food service managers recognize their responsibility for providing a high-quality and safe food delivery system, Medicare regulations will continue to ensure these entitlements for the consumer. Medicare regulation affects the nutrition services offered, those services for which a fee is charged, and the quality of care delivered through meal service. Emphasis is on adherence to medically approved diets, written prescriptions, and service of wholesome food.

Omnibus Budget Reconciliation Act of 1987 (OBRA)

Food service departments that serve hospital extended care units and long-term care facilities also must comply with the Medicare and Medicaid Requirements for Long Term Care Facilities. These requirements, finalized on September 26, 1992, implement the nursing home reform amendments enacted by the Omnibus Budget Reconciliation Act of 1987 (OBRA '87), as published by the Health Care Financing Administration. It is estimated that nearly 50 percent of the OBRA regulations relate directly or indirectly to the nutrition and food service department. The OBRA standards pertain to dignity and independence in dining, initial and annual nutrition assessments, nutrition care plans, and participation of the dietitian in family conferences. Discussion of how to maintain compliance with these regulations is covered in chapters 9 and 20.

Joint Commission on Accreditation of Healthcare Organizations (JCAHO)

Medicare and Medicaid regulations are government imposed, but some facilities choose to further their compliance efforts by following standards set by independent organizations. One such organization is the Joint Commission on Accreditation of Healthcare Organizations (JCAHO). Standards set by the JCAHO are similar to those set by Medicare; however, JCAHO surveys tend to place more emphasis on the systems, processes, and procedures that influence quality of patient care and outcomes. More recently, publications by the JCAHO report that future emphasis will be on education and training of patient and family; orientation, training, and education of staff; leadership roles of directors; and approaches and methods of quality improvement. Because JCAHO guidelines are updated and published annually, they must be reviewed annually to ensure compliance.

Americans with Disabilities Act (ADA)

In addition to significantly influencing operations, legislation will continue to dictate employment practices. As the labor force shrinks and alternative labor sources are explored, Americans with disabilities are one solution to some of the problems associated with inadequate staffing. Furthermore, ensuring equal employment opportunities for this segment of the population is mandated by federal law. On July 26, 1990, President Bush signed the Americans with Disabilities Act (ADA). The act mandated employers with 25 or more employees to comply by July 26, 1992, and for employers with 15 to 24 employees to comply by July 26, 1994. The full impact of the ADA has yet to be seen for employers in general, or for health care food service specifically. The ADA will affect both the selection of employees and the service of meals to consumers. Reasonable accommodations will have to be made for both groups. Further explanation of the ADA is found in chapters 8 and 20.

Health Care Affordability

Given the alarming rate of increase in health care costs and in an aging population, alternative health care options will be necessary. More than 14 percent of the gross domestic product was spent on health care in 1992. Due to the cost of caring for those with AIDS, this figure is estimated to reach $15.2 billion in 1995, up from $10.3 billion in 1992. The American Hospital Association (AHA) is calling for hospital leaders to become active in reforming the health care delivery system. Specifically, the AHA model calls for health care organizations to integrate care and collaborate to form networks at the community level. Community networking would prevent duplication of services and thereby lower cost. Through assessment of community needs and consolidation of services, access to care also can be expanded to the uninsured. More health care institutions will move toward a seamless delivery of service and evolve into acute care facilities, with extended care, home care, and ambulatory care facilities becoming majority caregivers.

Extended Care Facilities

The concept of seamless delivery of care is demonstrated by hospital-based, long-term care beds, with patients being moved to skilled nursing beds or rehabilitation units designed to assist them in becoming self-sufficient. Moving from the higher-cost acute care setting benefits the patient, the hospital, and the payer. Meals and menus will continue to increase in complexity and diversity to meet the needs of inpatients in skilled nursing units and rehabilitation units. Although hospitals will continue to convert unused beds to long-term care beds, most growth in long-term care will occur in outside facilities. For example, by the year 2000 a growth rate of 2.4 percent is projected for nursing homes and 2.7 percent for other elder care facilities. Extended care facilities are becoming more innovative in meeting their patients' mealtime needs. Many such facilities now provide selective menus; others have experimented with wait service and restaurant-style menus (that is, a number of selections per category per meal). Providing meals that meet the required nutrition modifications for elderly patients is becoming easier with the use of general diets that are lower in fat, sodium, and sugar, and with the increased number of products on the market that meet texture adjustment needs.

Home Care Service

Although patient length of stay varies from one institution to another and from one geographic region to another, the national average was reported by the American Hospital Association to be 7.17 days in 1991. The average *length of stay* is affected by the high acuity level

3

of patients. The high acuity level of patients identifies a need for extended care after discharge. Home care is one type of extended care that can positively influence the cost of health care, allowing for shorter hospital stays while ensuring that the patient is cared for in a familiar setting. Furthermore, readmissions have been shown to decrease as a result of team-managed home care. Advances in technology allow more services to be performed in the home, including infusion therapy (such as total parenteral nutrition). Home care will offer bigger challenges for home delivery of meals, as will the continuing decline in funding for elderly meal programs.

Ambulatory Care

Ambulatory care is expected to show significant growth throughout the 1990s. Increases in outpatient procedures between 1987 and 1992 more than offset inpatient declines, resulting in a net increase in adjusted admissions. Between 1981 and 1991, surgical procedures in ambulatory care settings increased nationwide from 18.5 percent to 52.3 percent. Technological advancements and reimbursement trends will continue to support the shift from inpatient services to outpatient services.

Even though hospital food service departments continue to encounter declines in the number of inpatient meal demands, they will likely experience an increase in the number of nonpatient meals prepared. For example, as outpatient procedures increase, food service departments will serve more visitors and family members who accompany patients, as well as employees associated with ambulatory care.

Case Management and Patient-Focused Care

The goals of case management and patient-focused (or patient-centered) care are to improve patient care and satisfaction, decrease cost of delivery, and improve access to health care. Patient-centered care is a more sophisticated extension of case management, but both are designed to use critical pathways or standardized care paths that specify a "road map" for the care team and are specific to individual diagnosis. The standards of care or critical paths, developed with input from all team members, are based on the best demonstrated practice within the facility. Comparing the standards and paths with those at other organizations can help further quality improvement efforts. The patient-focused care model utilizes a case manager or coordinator who is assigned to the patient upon admission and is responsible for monitoring the patient's progress throughout the hospital stay.

Patient-centered care eliminates traditional departmental lines, opting instead for health care teams that focus on patients with related conditions. To realize this type of care, a change in employee attitudes and structural changes to patient care units are necessary. Changes in these units will affect the nutrition and food service department as well as clinical caregivers. In models across the nation, food service workers are cross-trained to deliver meals and assist patients with their other needs. Some models assimilate jobs previously done by food service staff, housekeeping staff, and nurses aides into new positions, such as the multiskilled patient care employee.

Access to Service and Care

In addition to health care affordability, health care access has become a national priority in public calls for health care reform. The number of underinsured or uninsured persons will continue to rise as unemployment increases. Indigent care will continue to be a major issue as society's demographics change and the number of individuals living at or below the poverty level rises. Access to care will be coupled with equal quality for all, meaning that a uniform standard of care will continue to be a regulatory focus. The question confronting health care reform advocates is: Will universal access apply only to basic services or to all services? Some health care institutions have begun to meet the need of the indigent through mobile clinics designed to deliver basic health services. Caring for these individuals will likely require participation from nutrition and food service personnel through provision of either meals or clinical services such as nutritional assessment and counseling.

Access to care will be connected to questions on ethical decision making. Because today's health care system is ill equipped to provide equal care to the entire population, reforms must address what services should have universal access, versus those limited to individuals capable of paying. This question, raised by the state government in Oregon, was met with mixed reviews. Whereas the general population may recognize the restrictions of providing complete care for all, the context changes when the choice must be made for an individual or his or her loved one.

Accountability and Ethics

Government intervention and regulation have placed new emphasis on institutional accountability as it relates to physician recruiting. Once able to recruit physicians with income guarantees and low-interest loans, hospitals now must use their physician manpower plans and development plans to assess and document their requirement for additional physicians. Demand cannot be based on the institution's need alone but must be supported by hard evidence of community need. In addition to recruitment accountability, hospitals are confronted with questions related to joint ventures between physicians and hospitals. Usually, these joint ventures have been entered into for freestanding laboratories and diagnostic centers. A federal ban now prohibits physicians from referring patients to joint venture facilities where referral is a condition of investment.

Ethics play a role for nutrition and food service managers in their decisions regarding meal delivery and clinical care. For example, purchasers of food and supplies must avoid suppliers whose offer of favors or gifts would place them in a compromising purchasing position. Further discussion on ethics related to food procurement is presented in chapter 17. As part of the health care team, registered dietitians (RDs) must give input regarding the delivery of nutrition services to terminally ill patients. Some ethical issues dealing with nutrition management will be addressed by state-specific advance directives signed when patients are admitted. These advance directives, which reflect the patient's wishes, will help physicians and other caregivers in their decisions about the course of treatment.

Environmental Trends

Despite inroads on the amount of waste sent to landfills, more effort is needed. In 1990, the Environmental Protection Agency (EPA) reported that the amount of waste being sent to landfills had decreased to 67 percent, down from 80 percent in 1988. Even so, Americans generate more waste than ever before. The 4.3 pounds generated *per individual* in 1990 is expected to reach 4.4 pounds by 1995. If this rate of growth continues, many landfills will be closed by the end of the decade. Health care and food service, both separately and together, have been targets in the environmental controversy. Waste management efforts in all areas of health care should consider three agendas: reducing the quantity of waste, reusing as many materials or items as possible, and recycling used materials. The increase in environment regulation and public concern will force health care institutions to take innovative measures in handling medical waste, which includes many hazardous products as well as infectious waste that usually is incinerated.

Many food service opportunities exist to decrease waste and to implement recycling systems. For example, waste reduction can be accomplished by using individualized reusable coffee mugs and soft drink cups and eliminating or limiting disposable tableware. Recycling of office paper, glass, steel and aluminum cans, and corrugated paper is another waste-reduction effort.

Many health care organizations have found a way to simultaneously decrease landfill waste and help those less fortunate. For example, programs designed to feed the hungry are operated in a number of metropolitan areas. Food products prepared by health care food service departments are picked up by volunteers and distributed to organizations that distribute the food to homeless or low-income individuals. These programs have an added advantage in that the food service manager can measure and monitor food waste so as to improve preparation forecasts. An in-depth look at the environment and the responsibility of health care food service managers is presented in chapter 12.

Food Labeling and Nutrition Claims

On December 2, 1992, the Food and Drug Administration (FDA) announced food-labeling regulations in conjunction with the Nutrition Labeling and Education Act of 1990. Both the number of foods covered and the amount of information required on labels have increased. The purpose of this legislation and ensuing regulation is to provide the consumer with more reliable and informative material. As of May 1994, all processed foods regulated by the FDA must be appropriately labeled, and labels must include standardized serving sizes, grams of saturated fat, and fiber content. The percentage of daily values will provide the percentage of fat, saturated fat, cholesterol, sodium, carbohydrate, and fiber contributed by a single serving based on a 2,000-calorie daily diet. The new guidelines will allow seven nutrient or disease-specific relationship claims and provide more detailed ingredient listings.

An exemption to providing nutrition labels has been made for food served for immediate consumption, unless health claims are made. This exemption applies to restaurants and health care food service facilities. However, if health claims are made, facilities would have to meet the specific guidelines for the nutrient and the food be verified by a minimum of three chemical analyses. For example, a claim that a product is low cholesterol would require that the product have three verification analyses that proved it is at least 30 percent lower than the original product.

☐ Work Force Issues

As the year 2000 approaches, total growth of the work force will be less than 1 percent a year, representing the slowest growth since the 1930s. The Bureau of Labor Statistics (BLS) reports that entry-level workers are declining nationwide, with a 10 percent drop predicted between 1988 and 2000. Despite the shrinking work force, institutional food service jobs are predicted to increase 34 percent by the year 2005 — demand for chefs and cooks is expected to be the highest. Because of the increased numbers of dual-income families and women in the work force, and due to the aging of baby boomers, demand for service workers has grown. Health care food service managers will have to compete with other service industries for the dwindling labor resources. A reduction in workers coupled with an increased need for food service workers will require higher pay scales, which will negatively affect budget and cost-control efforts.

Not only has the labor market diminished, the demographics have changed: The work force of the next decade will be older, more culturally diverse, and include more women. The decrease in number of teenage workers and the increase in number of workers above age 50 will change the face of the average employee. As mentioned earlier, the full impact of the Americans with Disabilities Act has yet to be felt but is expected to be tied closely with aging of the population, escalation of AIDS, and worker shortage. The decreasing literacy rate among the nation's workers will continue to be an area of focus. A shrinking labor pool will necessitate identifying employees as customers and focusing on their needs. Specifics on managing, recruiting, and retaining tomorrow's work force are outlined in chapters 2 and 8.

Cultural Diversity of the Work Force

Cultural diversity in the nation is reflected by the growing number of minority workers. The BLS expects this trend to continue, with white, non-Hispanic workers projected to decline from 79 percent of the labor force in 1990 to 73 percent by 2000. Whereas this portion of the labor pool is expected to contract, all other groups are expected to expand, with the most rapid expansion predicted for Hispanics, who by the end of the decade will represent 11.1 percent of the labor pool.

Cultural diversity of the work force will be experienced to some degree by managers nationwide but will vary regionally. For instance, the African-American population is centered primarily in the South and Southeast, whereas Hispanics are located in the Southwest, West, Florida, and the Chicago metropolitan area. Native Americans are concentrated in Alaska, the Southwest, and the Plains states, but Asian Americans most likely live in the West, with concentration in Hawaii and California.

Along with gains in cultural diversity will come the necessity for managers to recognize opportunities to draw on differences that enhance quality and service. In addition, these differences must be understood so as to provide compatible leadership that can create career ladders and encourage minorities in entry-level health care positions to access the system for further development. Health care nutrition and food service departments will represent one of these entry points where training will become more of a priority. Employee socialization and retention will be specific concerns for the food service director of the 1990s and beyond.

The number of younger women (age 25 to 29) entering the work force continues to increase but at a substantially lower rate than prior to 1985. A slower economy and an escalation in the number of births for this age group are cited by the BLS as rationale for the slowdown. The lower number of total workers during the 1990s will make this group of women a valuable recruiting option. However, it will be necessary to provide them with the needed incentives—benefits, flexible schedules, job sharing, maternity leave, and child care centers—for returning to work.

Age of the Work Force

Working teenagers (16 to 19 year olds), a traditional food service complement, have declined in number due to the low birthrate that marked the 1970s. This decline in the work force is expected to reverse in 1995 and significantly increase by the year 2005. Despite the swell in this age group to a projected 8.8 million in 2005, their number in the labor pool still will be 1.2 million below the 1979 level.

The average age of the work force in the year 2000 is predicted to be 39 years. Middle-age (40 and older) workers are expected to remain the dominant age group during the remainder of the 1990s. The aging of the work force has been attributed to maturing of the baby boomers, lower birthrates, and an increase in life expectancy. The shrinking pool of available workers in the 1990s and the growing number of older workers will necessitate their selection as alternative labor. Today's older worker is healthier and can work longer than the same-age worker of a few decades ago.

Having knowledge of the average worker's age and the diversity of the labor force will help food service managers make the changes needed to attract and retain employees. The value system of the majority of the work force during the 1990s will be based on worker individuality, maximum amount and control of free time away from work, and participation in how work is accomplished. These values will require the nutrition and food service manager to be flexible with schedules including total hours worked, workdays, and responsibilities.

Infectious Disease in the Workplace

Closely tied to the Americans with Disabilities Act will be the treatment of employees with AIDS in the workplace. In terms of knives and other tools and equipment that could cause cuts, certain risks are involved with kitchen employees who test HIV positive. Closely tied to AIDS—and perhaps more important to food service managers—will be the near-epidemic number of tuberculosis cases currently identified. Because TB is an airborne infection that is highly contagious, food service managers will have to diligently ensure annual employee physicals.

Literacy and the Work Force

Approximately 2.5 million Americans who are illiterate are expected to enter the work force each year; many will be attracted to the service industry, specifically food service. Of approximately 74 percent of Americans who finish high school, only two-thirds will have adequate skills for employment. With the predictions of future labor shortages, quality of education and on-the-job training will become increasingly important employment considerations. On-the-job training, once limited to specific job skills, will have to go a step further to provide basic reading and writing skills. Partnerships between educational institutions and health care organizations will be in demand to improve the knowledge base of the fewer number of entry-level employees available for food service work. Some organizations now include basic literacy courses as part of the health care employee training program intended to provide service areas with needed staff.

Employee as Customer

The leaders of today and tomorrow will have to consider employees not only as a resource but also as a valuable asset to be empowered, trained, and properly motivated. Although expert predictions that the demands of tomorrow's work force will be linked to autonomy, more time off, and their being included in decisions affecting their work may hold some truth, differing employee value systems must be considered as a factor in this scenario. Value systems vary from one individual to another based on age, culture, and past experiences.

Viewing the employee as a customer can be effectively demonstrated through scheduling. Flexible scheduling based on the desires and needs of the work force is not necessarily new. However, not all food service managers have felt the need to be accommodating. Part-time and occasional staff can be utilized to provide adequate coverage while maintaining flexible scheduling for staff. Occasional staff may consist of full-time mothers who wish to earn extra income, older workers who wish to remain active without jeopardizing their retirement income, or disabled workers who may be unable to work full-time hours. Over the past few years, 32-hour schedules have become commonplace in many health care institutions, allowing full-time benefits with an extra day off for personal activities. Food service managers might learn by observing schedule patterns from other health care departments. Over a number of years, a shortage of professionals created the demand for flexible, imaginative scheduling to provide adequate coverage, and no method of coverage should be dismissed without being given adequate consideration.

If not settled by government within the next few years, medical coverage in this country will remain a primary concern for low-income workers. Benefits are not limited to health insurance and may even include paid time off, freedom to design work areas, on-site child care, elder care, maternity leave, and time off to care for an ailing family member, to name a few.

Compensation will continue to be a priority concern for health care food service employees, traditionally among the lowest-paid positions. Compensation will be a focus for employees deciding which jobs to pursue. Specifically, cooks and chefs can expect income gains due to higher demand for their technical expertise.

☐ Customer-Oriented Focus

The views and demands of customers affect their choices and have a tremendous impact on the health care delivery system. To determine customer wants and needs, customers must first be identified. Seven customer groups can be identified: patients, family and visitors, physicians, employees, volunteers, vendors, and payers. Of these, the immediate future will find seniors, their children—the baby boomers—and women to have the most influence in the purchase of health care services. The customer concept is relatively new to health care providers and may be somewhat disconcerting in that it depicts the delivery of health care as a business, an outlook that many of today's health care leaders believe necessary for survival.

The trend of identifying and meeting customer needs will likely intensify. Added services intended to increase satisfaction eventually become expected, so that further service-expansion attempts must be made continuously to ensure customer satisfaction. This phenomenon encourages the philosophies of continuous quality improvement and total quality management, discussed in chapter 4. Frontline employees will become more important in providing customer satisfaction because they are the ones who represent the organization or department. Identifying customers and what they want will be accomplished through market research and its application, discussed in chapter 3.

Value in the Quality–Cost Equation

To provide value, quality must be delivered while maintaining cost parameters. Customers' demands for quality from their perspective have provided the stimulus for customer satisfaction programs in health care. These programs span the continuum from simple customer service guidelines to detailed continuous quality improvement programs. All have the essential objective of improving quality and customer satisfaction in an effort to improve outcomes and increase utilization. Whereas customer satisfaction programs emphasize service delivery, continuous quality improvement programs provide a mechanism for in-depth enhancement of systems, processes, and methods of delivery.

Nutrition and food service departments have many opportunities to provide full quality and satisfaction to customers. Three distinct opportunities related to the food service component are the product, the service or delivery of the product, and the nutritional value of the product. In addition to these food service opportunities, many more exist in the delivery of clinical nutrition care. Each of these opportunities for quality enhancement must be evaluated in the customer service or quality improvement process selected.

Programs and services continue to evolve with the purpose of generating revenue for nutrition and food service departments, but they are now developed with a dual focus on customer satisfaction. Approaches to patient meal service include menu enhancement, nontraditional offerings such as room service, and home meal delivery after discharge. Cafeterias continue to be the primary type of service in health care facilities, although many have added restaurants, 24-hour coffee shops, and cooperative vending. Vending operations may be managed by hiring an outside contractor, by leasing machines and managing the operations in house (cooperative vending), or by purchasing machines for independent operation. Branding is another concept adopted by some health care food service departments to improve satisfaction for a variety of customer groups, either through inclusion of products in the existing service areas or with fast-food franchises opening on-site. *Branding* is defined as the use of a nationally known labeled product for sale in the current food service area or the inclusion of an entire operation (for example, McDonald's in a hospital lobby). More detailed application of quality and customer satisfaction is found in chapter 4, and branding information is presented in chapter 20.

Nutrition Awareness

Today's consumers have an increased awareness of nutrition and the effect diet can have on their health. Nutrition information collected through research efforts is no longer the exclusive domain of professionals who pass this information on to their patients. Consumers are bombarded at every turn with reports on the latest nutrition research through television, newspapers, magazines, and numerous books and pamphlets. Although intended to educate the consumer, this information is often conflicting and not easily interpreted for application to daily dietary intake. Because informed consumers are not always wiser consumers, attempts must be made to meet their perceived needs if customer satisfaction is the goal.

Heightened nutrition awareness is closely linked with an increased emphasis on fitness. Yesterday's fitness fad is today's life-style for many consumers of health care and nutrition and food service. Even so, people continue to indulge their appetites, especially when dining out. According to the 1992 Tastes of America Survey, despite the concern with healthy eating, examples of dietary conflict can be observed when diners order salads but still eat the french fries, or wash down dessert with a diet drink. Consumers more often are opting for grilled chicken over fried chicken but in 1992 still ordered fried chicken 68.5 percent of the time, compared to 48.5 percent of the time for selecting grilled or broiled chicken. Other dietary changes disclosed in the 1992 survey include consumption of more decaffeinated coffee and diet soft drinks and more frozen yogurt instead of traditional desserts. Consciousness has been raised; the next step will be application of the knowledge. Nutrition and food service managers must consider these perceptions and realities in menu planning and service delivery (see chapter 15).

Increased nutrition awareness and health education will prove beneficial for the patient who desires to participate actively in his or her care. This trend may be one answer to lowering the cost of delivering health care while improving customer satisfaction. In contrast, the large number of less knowledgeable persons living at or below the poverty level will be further disadvantaged by the continued economic dual tiering of society and the growth of a minority immigrant population. The upward trend of poverty will negatively influence the number of individuals at nutritional risk in communities and further validate the role of nutrition awareness.

Demographic Changes

Three primary demographic changes will affect the delivery of nutrition and food services in health care: an aging population, more women as decision makers, and cultural diversity. The aging population will create two consumer subgroups, each having specific health care needs. As mentioned previously, the baby boomers are the middle-agers of the 1990s. By the year 2000, only 25 percent of the total population will comprise the second subgroup, pre-middle-agers (those between ages 35 and 49). Their health care needs will continue to center on preventive medicine, fitness, nutrition, and well-child checkups. In addition, this age group will become the primary caregivers for the majority segment—the elderly. (The elderly are sometimes classified as either "young elderly," ages 65 to 74, or "older elderly," ages 75 and over.)

The Aging Population

The aging population, or graying of America, will increase the acuity level of patients, increase the number of patients at nutrition risk, and provide care to more older patients than at any other time in history. The fastest-growing population segment includes those over age 50, who will represent 28 percent of the population by the year 2000. By 2010, the U.S. Census Bureau projects that 21 million Americans will be between the ages of 65 and 74, a 15 percent increase over 1989. This shift will foster extensive growth in extended care facilities, including nursing homes, adult day care centers, and retirement centers. In addition to the increased growth in these freestanding facilities, a larger number of hospitals will include skilled nursing units and rehabilitation units. In addition to caring for the elderly once they become ill, health care organizations must proactively design preventive care programs to evaluate the health needs of older persons and provide appropriate education. Evaluation will include individualized screens for nutrition risk and guidelines for improving nutrition status related to illness prevention and treatment.

Women as Primary Decision Makers

Women are the primary decision makers in health care delivery choices and want more involvement in matters dealing with their health and that of their families. Centers and specific departments that consider their unique needs will continue to influence the delivery of care. Interest in women's health concerns also will be evidenced by increased research in this area. As the average life expectancy continues to increase, women will face more responsibility in caring for parents and other extended family members as well as their immediate families. This fact, together with the expanding number of women entering the work force, will further emphasize customer satisfaction from the perspective of women. As health care decision makers, women will influence the balance between high-touch and high-technology aspects of care.

In addition to those nutrition and food service demands already mentioned—affordability, continuity of care, equal access, and so forth—the growing number of working women will expect convenience. Food choices for this group will be influenced by the makeup of the family unit, and many experts in nutrition and food service predict that children will become the new "gatekeepers" of the food supply. Convenience becomes a key element in this scenario as the demands of female consumers provide opportunities for health care food service managers. For example, the cafeteria can be extended to offer take-out services, bakery products, and quick prepackaged kid meals.

Cultural Diversity in Menus

The effects of cultural diversity on food service are prominently reflected in menus enhanced with ethnic dishes. Some operators call for a return to more basic, home-style "American" food choices, but the question arises as to what that means. For example, one of the most popular foods in America is pizza, followed closely by Mexican and Oriental food selections. These cuisines have become American menu staples. In planning menus, food service managers should consider the population to be served. Demographics vary by region in regard to age and cultural diversity and should be evaluated prior to making menu selections. Although menus may return to basics in the coming decade and reflect lighter fare, the signature items of various cultures will find a place. Application of this and other information pertinent to menu planning is found in chapter 15.

☐ Technology Trends

The 1980s were marked by pronounced growth in technology. The area that underwent the most rapid growth was information services. In general, health care has been slow to implement computerization, especially in food service. Many hospitals today, however, have chief information officers who coordinate computer systems planning and implementation. In addition to information technology, medical technology has significantly changed the delivery of health care. Both diagnostic advances and treatment technology have improved patient outcomes while placing extreme financial burdens on health care organizations. Because of heavy diagnostic and clinical advances, many nutrition and food service departments have been left out of the capital expenditure cycle or have spent more time justifying equipment needs. However, this does not mean that advances have not been made in food service technology that are significant and important to the delivery of cost-effective, high-quality food service.

Information Systems

Information systems will continue to dominate the technological front in the coming decade. Information systems in health care organizations over the past decade have been primarily in the area of financial, accounting, and human resource management. This emphasis will continue and become more refined in assisting management with making budget-related decisions.

Current emphasis is on design and implementation of a universal electronic data interchange system for processing health care claims. This system will necessitate development of a common language for hospitals, the federal government, and insurers, along with standardization of core financial information. Most hospital billing departments will not find it easy to accommodate a common language or method, due to lack of integration in computer systems and the large volume of services billed. This type of common claims processing will make it increasingly necessary for hospitals to improve their current computer systems.

Medical professionals have been slower to embrace the clinical information systems introduced to the market. Some of this reluctance may be tied to the fact that these persons had no prior introduction to computer technology. As the technology becomes more commonplace, future professionals will have greater access and comfort levels. Future clinical information systems will tie diagnostic testing results directly to the nurses station or the physician's office, a linkage that will allow quick review and action on test results and facilitate improved patient care. *Bedside charting,* a term used more and more frequently in discussions of patient care, and the computerized medical record will improve information flow, thereby assisting with reimbursement.

Information systems also are important in the food service department, where management control systems are numerous and their applications vary considerably. Systems may include software packages designed to manage information from procurement, standardized recipes, inventory control, and point-of-sale information. Many vendors or distributors offer food service operators a direct computer link to warehouses for the purpose of placing orders and accessing information regarding purchase history. Food service inventory systems range from department-specific personal computers and software to mainframe systems designed for the organization. Entering information into inventory is done either manually or through the use of a scanner. Scanners function by reading label information with a handheld device, which is then uploaded to a personal computer or mainframe terminal.

Still other software programs include nutrition analysis and additional clinical applications. As it becomes increasingly important to evaluate past and current information to make the best decisions for tomorrow, advanced information systems will become more significant. The use of computer systems may not decrease staff needs, but in today's environment they are necessary to manage the increasing amount of information needed by managers to run their departments effectively. Computer software should be purchased based on individual needs. What works for a hospital department may not work for a nursing home. Detailed discussion of management information systems is covered in chapter 10.

Medical Technology

The delivery of high-quality health care will continue to rely on technology, the increased cost of which tends to affect health care faster than other businesses. This cost dynamic is due to rapid changes in technology that can be linked to equipment obsolescence over a short time period, acquisition or replacement costs, and the effects of competition among facilities. Some technological advances have been able to reduce labor needs, but more have required new or higher skill levels. A more demanding skill requirement has led to specialization within departments or fields, making it difficult to utilize staff for a variety of tasks. Technology also can be effective not only in diagnostics but in treatment to lower costs and decrease the length of stay. Technology has been responsible for decreasing patient admissions and for increasing utilization of outpatient services. More general surgery is being performed as laparoscopic surgery, which is occurring in the outpatient setting.

Another type of medical technology with widespread impact on health care involves pharmaceuticals. The number of new medications entering the marketplace yearly is staggering. The rapid pace of development creates new problems for the Food and Drug Administration (FDA) and for the public in that a number of medications have been recalled after their extended use was found to cause side effects not predicted in trials prior to FDA approval. In view of the AIDS crisis, for instance, demands for rapid approval and release of pharmaceuticals are not likely to decrease.

Food Technology

This section briefly describes four developments in food technology that food service operators should become familiar with. These are sous vide, biotechnology, irradiation, and fat replacement.

The sous vide process, developed and perfected in Europe, uses freshly prepared foods that are processed with low-temperature cooking and vacuum-sealed in individual pouches. The process presented some problems with bacterial growth during the 1980s, but perfection of the slow-cooking method to achieve pasteurization and improved packaging have made it a safe, viable option for food service operators. This technology is proving to be the least controversial and most widely accepted by both food service professionals and customers. Because many of the products prepared and preserved with low-temperature cooking and vacuum sealing are considered gourmet in nature, food service managers can expand and improve menu options for patients and other customer groups.

Biotechnology is creating the taste of the future. In this form of genetic engineering, a gene foreign to a product is spliced or added to its DNA to enhance or inhibit qualities of the original product. This bioengineering technology is being used to improve the current food supply; for example, vegetables and fruits are engineered to resist spoilage, increase variety, improve nutritional content, enhance resistance to disease and freezing, and provide a longer shelf life. The major reason for pursuing these genetically altered products is to decrease the amount of chemicals used during growing; by altering certain genes, the plants can be made resistant to insects.

In May 1992, the Food and Drug Administration decided that these bioengineered foods would not require special labels or testing before being sent to market. The National Food Processors Association (NFPA) announced prior to the FDA ruling that, in its view, no new regulation was necessary for foods produced through biotechnology. Groups opposing the FDA guidelines include the Center for Science in the Public Interest, the Environmental Defense Fund, and the National Wildlife Federation. Since the FDA decision, many—including a number of chefs—have publicly renounced bioengineered foods. It is not clear whether this disapproval mirrors sentiments of the general public or is limited to this group. Nutrition and food service managers should follow development on this topic so as to make informed buying decisions.

Although it has been approved for food since the 1960s, irradiation is a technological breakthrough affecting current food supplies. Irradiation is used to destroy salmonella bacteria in chicken and to increase the shelf life of produce. Consumer acceptance of this process will dictate the extent of its use in the future. If 1992 sales of irradiated produce are an indication of consumer acceptance, however, food service departments will see more on the market.

After years of research and development, fat replacers or substitutes are beginning to obtain FDA approval. Fat substitutes are classified by the core ingredient used in their production and are carbohydrate, protein, or fat based. Carbohydrate-based fat substitutes are made from dextrins, modified food starches, polydextrose, and gums. Many generic forms of these fats have been approved for use in baking but are not heat stable enough for use in frying. The most common protein-based fat substitute is Simplesse®, produced by the NutraSweet Company and approved by the FDA in February 1990 for use in frozen desserts. Because protein is not an effective heat conductor, Simplesse cannot be used in frying but can be used at high temperatures, for example, in cheese melted on pizza. The most widely known fat-based replacement is Olestra®, produced by Procter and Gamble. As of this writing, a petition is pending before the FDA requesting approval to use Olestra in specific food items. Olestra is heat stable and will likely be used in frying if its use is approved. There is some concern that fat substitutes will not decrease the desire for fatty foods and may in fact increase overall fat consumption, similar to the effect sugar substitutes have had on sugar consumption.

13

Food Service Equipment

Advances in equipment should be considered annually when making capital equipment plans. Equipment needs vary from one institution to another and depend on the types of food purchased, the production methods used, staffing, and the menu. Recent advances in food service equipment include cook–chill units, microwaves, and smaller versions of existing equipment. Cook–chill has been used in Europe since the 1960s but was not in widespread use in the United States until 20 years later. Its use is important in institutional food service, as operators strive to serve high-quality products assisted by a dwindling labor force. Food is prepared using standard cooking methods and then chilled rapidly in a blast chiller for later use. Some managers have also advocated the use of blast chillers to ensure safe cooling of bulk products prior to storage so as to prevent spoilage. Cook–chill can be used with standard production techniques, where food is prepared for one day's service, placed in serving pans and chilled, and then used to plate meals cold for rethermalization. Cook–chill systems also can be complex, requiring the purchase of other equipment such as cook tanks, specially designed pumps, and rethermalization units.

Many smaller versions of ovens and other equipment on the market were developed in response to limitations on space and the desire of some operators to use equipment in the customer's view. Other operators have installed preparation equipment—for example, a pizza oven—in full view of their customers. Microwaves, once used for boiling water or reheating foods, are finding their way into preparation areas of many food service departments. Microwaves can be utilized to rethermalize the many frozen products on the market and are excellent for preparation of vegetables.

Another equipment advancement is robotics, computerized units that assist with repetitive motions, such as placing items on patient trays. By the year 2000, technology will be available to fully automate many kitchen and service activities. Equipment designs no doubt will consider changes in tomorrow's labor force. Instructions must be clear and understandable to workers whose abilities to read English may be limited, and knobs or switches must be designed for physically challenged individuals.

☐ Summary

This chapter analyzed the current and projected external environment for health care food service. The external environment includes trends and issues arising from the government, businesses and industries, health care institutions, work force demographics, customer needs and demographics, and technology affecting the delivery of service. Many of these elements are evolving constantly and will continue to direct the operation of health care nutrition and food service departments.

As the environment changes, food service managers should modify the goals, objectives, and operation of their departments. Many trends discussed in this chapter will have a direct effect on how other information in the text should be applied to individual departments and will be noted in the relevant chapters.

By anticipating trends, successful managers will plan their department operations with a vision—both the department's and the facility's—of tomorrow. This is accomplished through conducting an internal and external environmental analysis and applying the information to organizing and planning functions, topics discussed fully in chapter 5.

☐ Bibliography

American Hospital Association: adjusted admissions hit new high in 1991. *Hospitals* 66(21):14–15, Nov. 5, 1992.

Americans with Disabilities Act of 1990, Selected Regulations. Chicago: Commerce Clearing House, 1991.

Anthony, W. P. *Management: Competencies and Incompetencies.* Reading, MA: Addison-Wesley, 1981.

Barlett, M. Foodservice market. *Restaurants and Institutions* 100(1):20–23, Jan. 10, 1990.

Baum, D. L. The three r's: reducing, reusing & recycling. *Southern Hospitals* 58(4):21, July–Aug. 1992.

Bernstein, C. Robots to run foodservice. *Restaurants and Institutions* 102(19):20, Aug. 12, 1992.

Bloch, J. W. How ethical is our behavior? *Food Management* 27(8):27–29, Aug. 1992.

Bomar, F. Keep the patient happy. *Southern Hospitals* 58(4):20, July–Aug. 1992.

Cohen, M., King, P., and Sherer, M. Letting the gene out of the bottle & other notions for the future. *Food Management* 27(10):115–17, Oct. 1992.

Cross, E. W. Implementing the Americans with Disabilities Act. *Journal of The American Dietetic Association* 93(3):273–75, Mar. 1993.

Derr, D. D. Food processing technology. *Food & Nutrition News* 65(1):5–6, Jan.–Feb. 1993.

Didomenico, P. The next great food fight. *Restaurants USA* 12(4):13–16, Apr. 1992.

Durocher, J. Cook–chill systems. *Restaurant Business* 91(10):154–56, July 1, 1992.

Durocher, J. Scrubbing bubbles. *Restaurant Business* 91(17):188, Nov. 20, 1992.

DVA to study financial impact of home care. *Hospitals* 66(24):44, Dec. 20, 1992.

Foodservice industry 2000, current issue report. Chicago: National Restaurant Association, 1988.

Friedman, E. Rationing healthcare: crisis and courage. *Healthcare Forum Journal* 34(6):12–15, Nov.–Dec. 1991.

Gatty, B., and Blalock, C. Bioengineered foods, stronger FDA? label delay, milk in schools. *Food Management* 27(8):36, Aug. 1992.

George, C. S., Jr. *Supervisor in Action: The Art of Managing Others.* Reston, VA: Reston, 1981.

Goddard, R. W. Workforce 2000. *Personnel Journal* 68(2):65, Feb. 1989.

Grayson, M. A. News at deadline: Washington outlook. *Hospitals* 67(2):8, Jan. 20, 1993.

Griffin, R. W. *Management.* 2nd ed. Boston: Houghton Mifflin, 1987.

Hagland, M. Experts agree on this: it was a banner year for health care polls. *Hospitals* 66(24):32–33, Dec. 20, 1992.

Haight, G. Managing diversity. *Across the Board* 22(8):27, Mar. 1990.

Haimann, T., and Hilgert, R. *Supervison Concepts and Practices of Management.* 3rd ed. Cincinnati: South-Western, 1982.

Hard, R. Inching toward EDI: experts look at obstacles. *Hospitals* 66(24):42–43, Dec. 20, 1992.

Hard, R. More hospitals move toward bedside systems. *Hospitals* 66(19):72–74, Oct. 5, 1992.

Hudnall, M. J., Connor, S. L., and Connor, W. E. Position of the American Dietetic Association: fat replacements. *Journal of The American Dietetic Association* 91(10):1285–88, Oct. 1991.

Hudson, T. New test: Hanlester decision clamps down on MD ventures. *Hospitals* 66(14):24–26, July 20, 1992.

Hull, K. Employment of full-time staff outpaces part-time growth. *Hospitals* 66(21):44–46, Nov. 5, 1992.

An introduction to sous vide technology. *Hospital Food Service* 25(6):3–4, Nov.–Dec. 1992.

Kaszuba, J., and Antoni, S. Managing volunteers in foodservice. *Food Service Management* 27(11):50, Nov. 1, 1992.

Keogh, K. The changing face of the American culture. *Chef,* Jan. 1993, pp. 23–24.

King, P. Recycling & source reduction. *Food Management* 28(1):54–60, Jan. 1993.

Koontz, H., O'Donnell, C., and Weihrich, H. *Management.* 7th ed. New York City: McGraw-Hill, 1980.

Koska, M. T. JCAHO introduces three new areas of survey concentration. *Hospitals* 66(19):62–66, Oct. 5, 1992.

Koska, M. T. The new medical staff development planning: hospitals link plans to community benefits. *Hospitals* 66(20):26–30, Oct. 20, 1992.

Longenecker, J., and Pringle, C. *Management.* 5th ed. Columbus, OH: Charles E. Merrill, 1981.

Lumsdon, K. Smart moves. *Hospitals* 66(20):18–19, Oct. 20, 1992.

Megginson, L., Mosley, D., and Pietri, P., Jr. *Management: Concepts and Applications.* New York City: Harper and Row, 1986.

Merritt, R. J. Dietary compensation for fat reduction and fat substitutes. *Nutrition & the M.D.* 19(3):1–3, Mar. 1993.

Monsen, E. R. Final food labeling regulations. *Journal of The American Dietetic Association* 93(2):146–48, Feb. 1993.

Mosley, D., Megginson, L., and Pietri, P., Jr. *Supervisory Management: The Art of Working with and through People.* Cincinnati: South-Western, 1985.

Pintell, K. G. Complying with OBRA. *Food Management* 28(1):40, Jan. 1993.

Roberts, J. Managing cultural diversity in the workplace. *Southern Hospitals* 58(4):19,28, July–Aug. 1992.

Scanlon, B., and Keyes, B. *Management and Organization Behavior.* 2nd ed. New York City: John Wiley and Sons, 1983.

Stephenson, S., and Chaudhry, R. Small kitchens, big ideas. *Restaurants and Institutions* 103(1):115–20, Jan. 1, 1993.

Troup, N., and Rushing, S. Working smarter with patient-focused care. *Southern Hospitals* 58(4):13, 14, 27, July–Aug. 1992.

Vaughn, A. New label format. *Chef,* Jan. 1993, p. 71.

Vaughn, A. D. The chef's role in a changing culture. *Chef,* Jan. 1993, pp. 22–23.

Wagel, W. H. Make their day—the non-cash way! *Personnel* 41(4):87, May 1990.

Weinstein, J. Restrooms are the biggest obstacle for restaurants. *Restaurants and Institutions* 102(25):108, Oct. 21, 1992.

Part One

Management of the Food Service Department

Leadership: Managing for Change

☐ Introduction

The traditional role of nutrition and food service director or manager has expanded into a more complex role, due in part to the trends described in chapter 1. The political environment calls for a manager who is fiscally responsible, knows regulatory requirements, and understands how food service department functions affect the facility. The manager also must have a heightened awareness of work force issues, customer needs, technological implications, and continuous quality improvement systems.

Management—the process of achieving a common goal through group effort by planning, organizing, leading, and controlling an organization's human, physical, and financial resources and by considering all information relevant to accessing those resources—requires increased emphasis on the leadership function. This is particularly true in light of the work force trends identified in chapter 1 (cultural diversity, an older labor force, reduced literacy and skill levels, for example). Although managing implies controlling the activities of others, leadership is characterized by ability to influence individuals to participate in decision making and willingness to assume responsibility for job accomplishment. Employee involvement is essential to service improvement, whether employees participate as department team members or on cross-functional teams within the facility.

This chapter will identify behaviors, traits, and skills that characterize an effective leader and how they can be applied in various situations to guide employees and manage the food service department. Practical application of these three components will be explored within the context of creating a participative work environment that motivates and empowers employees.

☐ Leadership Style

Leadership style is defined by the behaviors, traits, and skills a manager exhibits over time in influencing the work of others so as to accomplish common goals for the department. Leadership style can be better understood by exploring certain theories on behavior and reviewing situational theories that link management behavior to work factors. In other words, an individual employee's unique level of job task development within the work environment may derive from or respond to a particular leadership style.

Behavior Theories of Effective Leadership

Theories on effective leadership styles have evolved from early research that focused on analyzing personality traits of individuals who demonstrated leadership ability. Studies conducted prior to World War II identified traits such as intelligence, self-confidence, and physical attractiveness as—not surprisingly—being desirable. These studies, however, were unable to isolate a single trait that could *predict* leadership ability. Research since World War II has focused more on *behaviors* as indicators for identifying what creates an effective leader.

Using the behavioral approach, leadership styles have been defined or categorized using a variety of terms. Perhaps the most familiar categories (or terminologies) are *autocratic, democratic,* and *laissez-faire* approaches. Another classification uses terms such as *directive, supportive, participative,* and *achievement* as descriptors. Work conducted by Robert R. Blake and Jane S. Mouton in the late 1970s grouped behaviors into five categories to identify leadership styles:

- *Task management* describes a behavior that exhibits little concern for employees and emphasizes production activities. This leader delegates very little authority and is autocratic in dealings with subordinates.
- *Country-club management* is demonstrated by the manager whose primary interest is in keeping employees happy and satisfied in their work. The work environment is very permissive, and pressure of any kind is avoided.
- *Middle-of-the-road management* characterizes the style of a manager who seems to focus on tasks *and* employees. However, decision making is marked by compromise and ambivalence, with constant fluctuation between opposing viewpoints.
- *Impoverished management* describes the management behavior of one who provides virtually no leadership to subordinates, with all productivity attributable to the employees' own initiative.
- *Team management* is demonstrated by the manager who shows a high level of concern for both people and productivity. Unlike middle-of-the-road management, however, this behavior emphasizes the importance of mutual trust, understanding, and common objectives.

These leadership behaviors, and their variations, will be revisited throughout this book as necessary.

Situational Leadership

Theories on situational leadership attempt to identify basic factors in the work environment that determine appropriate leadership behavior. One such theory, called the *contingency theory,* suggests that effective leadership behavior is based on three factors: the organization's task, the relationship between the leader and other members of the organization, and the leader's power base within the organization. The contingency theory assumes that a leader is either task oriented or people oriented and that he or she cannot change leadership styles to suit the work situation. Therefore, the work situation must be changed to suit the leader's style.

Numerous other theories dispute the contingency theory, saying it is the leader, not the work environment, who must be flexible in situational leadership. One such theory was proposed by Victor H. Vroom and Philip W. Yetton in 1973. According to the *Vroom–Yetton theory,* leaders can change their approach, but the only flexibility exhibited in situational leadership is the degree to which leaders allow subordinates to participate in decision making for the organization. The *path–goal theory* states that the leader's behavior should change to correspond to employee characteristics and the work environment.

A situational theory that assumes a leader can be flexible in exhibiting the degree of control, concern for productivity and employees, structure provided, and risk taken in decision making is defined in *Effective Behavior in Organizations,* by Cohen, Fink, Gadon,

Willits, and Josefowitz. The authors define leadership style using five distinct dimensions and arguing that a leader may respond or exhibit behavior at various points along the dimensions depending on the situation. These five dimensions (called herein the *five-dimension theory*) help describe how a leader might carry out various functions and may be applied directly to food service department functions.

1. *Retaining control versus sharing control.* The degree of control retained or shared is apparent based on who makes decisions (manager or employees), how decisions are made (with or without employee input), whether information is shared with staff, and the amount and nature of work delegated.
2. *High task-concern versus low task-concern.* This dimension relates to the emphasis placed on the quality and quantity of production or output. A food service manager, for example, may place high or low emphasis on employee productivity. Although for financial reasons a high level of task concern may be desirable, it need not occur to the exclusion of concern for clients or workers.
3. *High person-concern versus low person-concern.* Concern for individuals—consumers or staff—considers the effect of actions or changes on department morale.
4. *Explicit versus implicit expectations (degree of structure provided).* This dimension is determined by how clearly and in how much detail tasks are identified; the number of written policies; and the form of communication, whether written or verbal.
5. *Cautious versus venturous decision making.* The level of risk involved in decision making, the manager's level of visibility within the organization, and how willing the manager is to push the outer limits characterize this dimension of leadership style.

The situational leadership models discussed so far provide the basis for work presented by Kenneth Blanchard, Patricia Zigarmi, and Drea Zigarmi in their book *Leadership and the One Minute Manager.* The four styles defined by Blanchard and associates, which are progressive and can be applied by management personnel at all levels, are directing, coaching, supporting, and delegating. Each style serves to create and nurture a participative work environment. It is understood that managers will develop a leadership style that is preferable and most compatible with their individual makeup, but it is also desirable that the style be appropriate for dealing with a variety of employees and situations. Ultimately, complex situations and/or employees with mixed skill levels will necessitate the use of more than one leadership style.

The four styles identified by Blanchard and associates depend on the situation and the developmental levels of employees. Employees who are new to the department or perhaps performing a job for the first time will need a leader whose approach is *directive,* that is, he or she provides specific instructions and close supervision until the task is completed. As the employee becomes more comfortable with the department (or job), the manager will need to move toward *coaching,* the second leadership style. The coaching leader will continue to be directive and provide close supervision but will explain decisions, encourage progress, and ask for suggestions or input from the employee. Coaching as a positive approach to improving performance will be discussed in chapter 8 on human resource management.

The third style, *supportive* leadership, is exercised with an employee who has knowledge concerning the tasks he or she is assigned but may still lack confidence in his or her abilities. A supportive leader shares responsibility for the task and decision making with the employee while helping to accomplish it. The fourth leadership style recognizes an employee who is highly motivated, knowledgeable about the job, and is ready for full *delegation* from the manager. A delegating leadership style allows the manager to turn over responsibility for both decision making and problem solving to the employee. The leader whose employees are capable of taking on this responsibility should remember that delegation is not abdication but a sharing of responsibility. Employees will continue to need the leader's guidance to ensure task completion. Further discussion on delegation can be found in chapter 5 on planning and decision making.

Again, depending on the employee's developmental level and the situation, more than one style can be used with the same employee. For example, an employee responsible for tray preparation, meal delivery, and cleanup may have varying levels of expertise in these areas. Whereas total delegation may be appropriate for meal preparation and cleanup, tasks related to meal service may require more of a directing or coaching role.

☐ The Leader as Manager

If leadership style is defined by characteristic behaviors and traits in various situations, then management applies these items in the planning, organizing, staffing, and controlling of resources to achieve goals. In this context, leading, rather than being part of what defines management, dictates how management is carried out. In other words, good managers place more emphasis on leadership and apply what they know and learn to the daily and long-term management of their departments.

Leadership Characteristics for Effective Management

Based on the leadership theories discussed above, what attributes will the successful health care food service manager need in the future? Current literature and expert opinion lean toward two general categories: (1) technical expertise and knowledge and (2) interpersonal skills that promote a participative, enabling environment for employees. The common denominator between the two is flexibility, the essential ingredient for dealing with the rapid change that will permeate health care food service throughout the 1990s. As identified in chapter 1, external environmental changes will alter both work methodology and those who perform the work. Flexibility allows the food service manager to plan, organize, and lead according to the dictates of the work situation and employee diversity. Flexibility in leadership style also helps employees deal with change. Addressing the effects of change is presented in chapter 5. The two key attributes, technical proficiency and interpersonal skills, are discussed below.

Technical Expertise and Knowledge

Technical proficiency uses the knowledge, tools, and techniques of a particular profession or job. A leader's technical skills include ability to use administrative knowledge and tools to carry out basic management functions (described later in the chapter). They also include ability to develop and implement standards and/or policies and procedures; to process paperwork in an orderly manner; to manage the work of the unit or department with the resources allocated; and to coordinate work and elicit the cooperation of employees and others within the organization. Administrative skills are used most often by top-level managers and least often by first-line supervisors. Managers on all levels are responsible for processing paperwork, whereas the responsibility for implementing standards falls primarily on the first-line supervisor.

Technical skills are used frequently by first-line supervisors who have daily contact with employees and must spend a large portion of their time training, evaluating performance, and answering task-related questions. First-line supervisors in smaller organizations may be expected to perform tasks that in larger organizations are assigned to nonmanagerial employees; or they may be expected to act as lead workers on employee teams. Evaluation of technical skills should be one consideration given to employees who show supervisory potential. Although technical skills are important, however, an employee highly skilled in task performance but lacking the administrative and interpersonal skills required by the position may not be a good candidate for a supervisory position. At the same time, the otherwise competent manager who lacks technical skills may be less than successful if the position requires monitoring the performance of production-level employees. Put simply, both are needed.

Effective leaders must view development for themselves, for their employees, and for the organization as a continuous process. Technical knowledge for food service managers, for example, may be enhanced through trade shows, which provide information on the latest equipment, supplies, and food items. Continuing or higher education classes and professional organization meetings also may provide an ongoing flow of information to manage the department effectively. Future demands will include technical expertise and knowledge in the following areas:

- Environmental protection rules
- The political environment
- Marketing and customer satisfaction
- Continuous quality improvement
- Work redesign and productivity
- Innovative cost containment measures
- Food consumption patterns
- Food and equipment technology
- Human resource trends

This knowledge will be important to establishing the strategic direction for the department that is in tune with the vision of the larger organization.

Interpersonal Skills

An effective leader will rely on basic interpersonal skills—communication, empathy, understanding, ethical conduct, and motivation—to influence the behavior of others in a positive manner so as to ensure peak performance. The higher the level of management, the less emphasis is placed on technical skills and the more emphasis is placed on interpersonal skills. Middle-level managers spend about 50 percent of their time applying their interpersonal skills. These skills also depend on the manager's awareness of the various beliefs, needs, and attitudes of group members and of their perceptions of themselves, their work, and the organization. Some would argue that it is these interpersonal skills that truly make the difference between effective and ineffective leadership.

Interpersonal skills are important to managerial success in the food service department because they promote harmony among food service workers and try to fit the needs of individual workers into the operating requirements of the department. They also enable the food service director to develop a network of positive relationships with administrators and other hospital staff members (as well as with other health care workers, physicians, patients, and vendors). Without such relationships, few managers would meet their own professional goals or fulfill the organization's objectives.

Successful leaders must prove their authenticity to employees, that is, that they are persons of character and integrity. Employees need to know that their manager can be trusted and that they consistently will be treated fairly. A manager who remains above reproach will win the staff's respect and dedication. Department leaders must enforce rules that protect the safety and security of employees and customers. Employees will come to know the leader's values through his or her actions and interactions with others. The behavior exhibited by a manager when interfacing with employees, peers, and vendors says more about his or her leadership style than does any verbal rhetoric.

An effective leader consistently follows two practices: promoting an environment or culture that fosters learning, innovation, and risk taking; and believing that employees are the most important resource in the department and treating them accordingly. In this nurturing environment a manager has an open-door policy to ensure that employee needs are met, and he or she most likely will find employees doing things right and will offer praise accordingly.

Effective communication is perhaps one of the most important interpersonal skills, helping to instill in employees the department's vision and departmental objectives as well as being attuned to their needs and providing performance feedback. Identifying how the department fits into the organization's vision—and clearly articulating this to employees—is a necessary characteristic of an effective leader. Chapter 7 identifies effective communication skills.

23

The Manager's Role

Current and future managers must view their role in light of changes and trends that dictate the need for strong leadership. The application of leadership can be seen in the traditional roles of management as described in the theory developed by Henry Mintzberg. The three roles identified in the Mintzberg model are interpersonal, informational, and decisional.

The *interpersonal* role involves building and maintaining contacts and relationships with a variety of people both inside and outside the department. This role requires the manager to act as a symbolic figurehead representing the department; to function as a liaison with others outside the department; and to provide supervision in hiring, training, and motivating employees. The importance of interpersonal skills for the leader–manager were discussed in the subsection on leadership characteristics for effective management. As the demands for quality, customer satisfaction, and employee empowerment continue to evolve, a manager's interpersonal skills will take on added importance.

The *informational* role requires the manager to monitor operations through data collection and analysis, to disseminate information to employees and others, and to act as a spokesperson outside the department. The manager's informational role can be defined in terms of effective communication as outlined in chapter 7. The manager must keep up to date on events by attending organizational and professional meetings, reading current literature, and networking. The manager must then disseminate relevant information to other department members, acting as the department spokesperson/information conduit and negotiator who "sells" or persuades others to buy into plans for additional resources or policy changes that affect patients and coworkers. In this spokesperson role, the manager keeps others up to date on changes within the department.

The *decisional* role requires the manager to be innovative, to handle conflict and problem resolution, and to allocate resources. The innovative manager must identify and interpret trends so as to anticipate and plan for future service opportunities and improvements. He or she must proactively seek new business or program possibilities and discover new approaches to effective problem solving. Conflict management occurs at all levels of management, and frontline supervisors will be required to deal decisively with disruptions that can arise daily in the health care environment. In general, the higher the level of management, the less time is spent in dealing with conflict.

Because the decision-making role also involves the allocation of resources, a manager must set priorities for departmental functions and how resources—from department personnel to food and equipment, time, information, and money—are used. Decision-making responsibilities can be closely controlled by the manager or shared with supervisors and frontline employees, depending on the matter being decided and on the leadership style. Decision making is discussed as it relates to individuals, teams, and a participative work environment later in this chapter and in chapter 5.

These three management roles are interdependent. For example, the manager can gather outside information by using interpersonal skills and then use decision-making skills in applying the information to determine how work is planned and executed within the department. The roles of management as outlined in this section need not be the sole responsibility of the manager. In fact, it is through sharing of these roles and responsibility that a participative work environment is created and fostered.

Health care food service department managers must fulfill their roles within the context of providing food and nutrition services to the organization's clients. To accomplish this goal, they must use specific functions of management—planning, organizing, staffing, leading, and controlling—to ensure that the department's resources are used efficiently and effectively.

Levels of Management

The number of management levels in a food service department depends on many factors including number of employees, hours of operation, complexity and scope of service, and the department's organizational structure. In smaller organizations, where there are fewer employees and limited hours of operation, only two levels of management, department director and supervisors or lead employees, may be needed. Most medium- to large-sized food service departments have at least three levels of management: top level (director), middle level (managers), and first line (supervisors).

The scope of service can influence both the number of management positions and the number of levels. A department responsible only for feeding patients or residents will have fewer management personnel and levels than one responsible for feeding patients and nonpatients. If additional services are provided (for example, catering, vending service, coffee shops, child care, extended care, bakery operations, physician dining facilities), more management levels may be needed, such as a director, assistant directors, managers, and supervisors. Added meals means additional preparation and service requirements and, consequently, more employees.

Traditionally, levels of management have been differentiated using the functional–hierarchical organizational structure shown in figure 2-1. This structure, developed in the late 19th century and supported by the "scientific management" theory of Frederick Taylor, is based on a rigid chain of command and layers of management with varying levels of authority and responsibility. Total authority and control in this model rest with management. Using the functional–hierarchical structure, organizations assign different levels of management by virtue of the responsibilities and authority needed to fulfill them. In this context, *responsibility* is a manager's obligation to perform certain tasks or duties, and *authority* is his or her power to allocate specific resources in the performance of those tasks or duties. For example, a hospital's CEO has more responsibility for overall operation of the hospital and therefore more authority to direct the use of hospital resources than does the food service director.

Other management structures used by health care organizations to foster teamwork and employee empowerment are matrix design, product line management, and team-based organizational design. These models create an organizational structure that shares responsibility and authority to move decision making to the lowest possible level in the organization. They also make it possible to have fewer layers of management by virtue of shared responsibility and authority. Organizational structure is discussed in more detail in chapter 6.

All levels of management have one thing in common: All managers must use leadership skills to plan, organize, coordinate, and control the resources for which they are responsible. Food service directors must develop departmental plans that are based on the goals, vision, mission, and objectives of the institution. Middle managers also must guide and monitor the performance of their departments.

Figure 2-1. Levels of Hospital Management

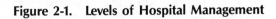

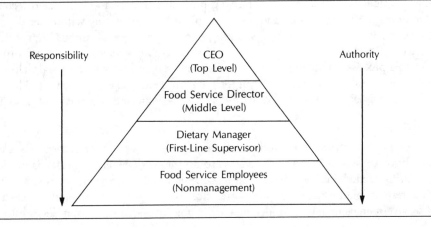

The scope of first-line managers is narrower, but they too must plan, coordinate, and control the daily activities (for example, efficient operation of the tray line in the food preparation area) of employees they supervise. Again, the more participative the work environment, the more the functions of management are shared among various levels of management.

Basic Functions of Management

Coordinating the work of individuals, teams, or a department requires managers in any organization and at any level to perform four basic managerial functions: planning, organizing, leading, and controlling. These four functions are interrelated, and the extent to which the manager exercises them depends on the complexity of the problems or issues in question and on the manager's level within the organization. For example, although top- and middle-level managers typically spend more time on planning and control functions, participative work environments bid managers at all levels to provide input and be accountable for carrying out the work of the organization. All management levels contribute to the organizing function, which defines the scope of jobs and determines staffing requirements. As mentioned earlier in this chapter, the function of leading places increased demands on all levels of managers in influencing work completion by employees. The next four subsections take a closer look at each of these basic functions of management.

Planning

Through planning, the future course of an organization or group is determined. The planning function helps set goals and objectives and define policies and procedures to achieve them. Planning is a continuous process of reviewing information, weighing alternatives, making decisions about those alternatives, and devising strategies to make the best use of available resources. Information reviewed includes trends and issues in the external environment and long-range plans for the organization.

Most organizations engage in two types of planning, operational and strategic, each of which is defined by the time span covered by the plan. For example, when developing short-range plans for day-to-day operations, the food service manager engages in *operational planning*. These short-range plans generally are based on existing facilities and markets. *Strategic planning*, on the other hand, emphasizes long-range issues and new opportunities related to the organization's mission and objectives. A third type of planning, called *performance planning*, is built on individual employee potential, contribution, and achievement. Planning is discussed further in chapter 5.

As already noted, planning occurs at every level of management. Top-level management in a hospital—for instance, the CEO—must work with other decision makers within the organization to develop the hospital's vision and strategic plan, which will guide overall activities and changes in the institution for a long period—five years or more. One element in the strategic plan might be to add a skilled nursing unit. In turn, the food service director would need to develop specific policies and operating plans for cooperating with other departments to deliver meals and nutrition services, taking into consideration Omnibus Budget Reconciliation Act (OBRA) regulations. First-line food service managers also would need to participate in this process, for example, if it appears necessary to restructure meal delivery times to ensure that meals are delivered within the guidelines established for the unit. The planning function establishes the general picture of what is to be done and how it is to be accomplished.

Organizing

The organizing function involves defining fine points of job specifications and determining how work is to be grouped, who is to do the work, what authority is needed, how much staff is needed, and how work will be accomplished by using what resources. Whether they are responsible for the whole department or for a smaller unit such as the cafeteria, all food service managers must consider how their objectives can be broken down into specific tasks and assignments and how these assignments can best relate to one another in terms of authority, responsibility, and communication of information. Managers must then decide which tasks to accomplish personally and which ones to delegate. It is vital that the authority needed to make use of appropriate resources be delegated along with the responsibility. Finally, the organizing function also includes the task of staffing the positions identified. Recruiting, interviewing, hiring, orienting, and training and developing new employees are major parts of most managers' responsibilities. The human resource, or personnel, department may assist managers in some or all of these staffing responsibilities.

Leading

Leading requires managers to use their interpersonal skills to influence individuals and teams, and to communicate information and instructions. Individuals and teams must be motivated to accept and strive to meet departmental and organizational objectives as established through the planning and organizing functions. Effective leading requires the manager to understand how to motivate employees to achieve individual goals and how to coordinate the work and interactions of employee groups.

Controlling

Exercising control ensures that actual outcomes are consistent with the planned outcomes specified by the goals and objectives. Because goals and objectives should be accomplished with the most effective and efficient use of resources, control is essential. It is the medium by which accountability—for instance, adherence to time lines, resource use, and quality of outcomes—is ensured. Ensuring control involves several actions:

- Establishing standards of performance or outcome and communicating them to the persons who must meet those standards
- Devising systems for measuring performance, either by monitoring the work process or by examining the work product
- Comparing performance measures to the standards set
- Adjusting performance as necessary by first determining why it does not meet established standards

☐ Participative Management

Creating a work environment in which employees are not only allowed but openly encouraged to participate in job-related decisions takes dedication and persistence on the part of all management levels. The reason for creating such an environment is to be positioned to respond to changing demographics and demands of the work force, increased emphasis on customer satisfaction, and the demands for continuous quality improvement.

Participative management has positive effects for both the organization and employees. Because employees are closer to the customer, they can more readily identify and meet customers' needs. Employees empowered to act instantly to satisfy customers win customer dedication and return business for the organization and gain a feeling of self-worth and further incentive to complete their jobs. These feelings motivate employees, improve the quality of their work life, and increase their level of commitment to the department and to the organization. Another benefit to promoting employee autonomy is that the organization gains from employees' knowledge and experience, in turn giving them a sense of ownership in the work process.

Creation of Participative Culture

Organizational culture (and therefore departmental culture) is identified by how things get done. As is true for other social units, a facility's cultural climate (or personality) is determined by the accepted norms, values, and beliefs demonstrated through the behaviors and relationships of its management and employees in various situations. It influences how employees view and perform their jobs, how they work with colleagues, and how they look at their institution's future. The internal culture is a blend of the following components:

- The external environment (that is, the larger community) in which the organization exists
- The employee selection process
- Execution of managerial functions
- Accepted behaviors within the organization
- Organizational structure and processes
- The removal of deviate members (unsatisfactory workers)

Creating a participative environment requires a change in the views, beliefs, and behaviors of managers and employees. These changes in turn influence how things get done and, eventually, the culture (or "feel") of the organization.

A culture inventory, or audit (often conducted by consultants), may help an organization assess its current culture by asking employees to define their ideal culture. For example, questioning employees about how free they feel to do their jobs, whether they feel comfortable approaching their supervisors, to what extent they regard the customer as being important to the organization, whether they feel that reward and recognition are linked to satisfying the customer, and so on can disclose much about the organizational climate. Once audit results have been tabulated, analysis of the information can uncover areas in which change is needed to support continuous quality improvement. Audit results should be shared with staff and an action plan created to define how the ideal pro-CQI culture can be achieved. More is detailed on culture as it relates to quality in chapter 4.

Management Responsibilities in a Participative Culture

To establish a participative work setting that enables employees and strengthens their commitment, managers must assume a number of responsibilities. Some key tasks are listed below:

- Training and developing employees to their highest potential
- Sharing decision-making authority
- Building a team mind-set
- Compensating and rewarding employee achievement
- Removing obstacles to employee advancement
- Communicating effectively

These responsibilities, summarized in the following subsections, will require greater emphasis on the managerial function of leading.

Training and Development

Managers must assess employee development levels so as to appropriately match capabilities to work situations. One key to ensuring a participative culture is to provide the right mix of information, power, and incentive that will positively influence departmental performance.

A positive work environment is fueled by development of employee potential. This is accomplished through new employee orientation; continuing education and in-service training; cross-training across jobs and across department lines; skill enhancement programs, both inside and outside the organization; and daily coaching from managers. In addition, successful empowerment ensures that roles, interrelationships, job duties, and performance expectations are clearly defined up front for new employees. Further discussion on the manager's training responsibility can be found in chapter 8.

Shared Decision Making

As mentioned earlier, shared power and decision-making authority between managers and employees enables employees to influence their day-to-day work life, which enhances job ownership and commitment. Therefore, when job descriptions are written or revised, when work processes are designed or reviewed, or when procedures are changed, employees should be polled for their input. This can be done by means of questionnaires that disclose how the work *is* done, suggestion forms for how the job *should be* done, or group meetings where managers and employees brainstorm new methods. Brainstorming is an idea- and information-sharing session at which everyone is allowed to give input without being judged. Shared authority can be applied in employee performance appraisals, at which employees can participate in rating the quality and quantity of their work and in setting goals to improve or enhance their performance. Empowerment is discussed further in a later subsection.

Team Building

Participative management appreciates the benefits of having employees work in teams to influence quality improvement, customer satisfaction, and job performance. Managers must be part of the team, not above it, providing the information and training needed to foster team success. Once employees become accustomed to working in groups to influence job design or to solve problems, they will be capable of meeting with less input or guidance from the manager. This does not mean the manager should abdicate responsibility for ensuring that meeting time is scheduled, that recommendations are considered fully, and that resources are available to implement team recommendations.

Compensation and Rewards

Employee incentives, either formal (compensation) or informal (rewards), are key to nurturing a participative work environment. *Formal rewards* encompass pay policies, employee benefits, and career paths, all of which usually are set up and administered by the human resource department. Some organizations have implemented formal employee profit-sharing and gain-sharing programs. *Informal rewards* can include anything from verbal praise and positive feedback for a job well done to outside training programs or celebrations (at the work site or elsewhere) upon reaching a specific goal or goals. Team and group performance should be rewarded as well as individual performance. It should be remembered that in a participative environment improvement and innovation cannot take place without mistakes. Employees should be rewarded for effort and initiative even if the desired outcome is not reached. Tolerance of minor "failures" and mistakes will encourage employees to try again without fear of being punished or losing their job.

Obstacle Removal

In a participative environment, the department manager must anticipate potential obstacles to employee advancement and seek to remove them. For example, policies and procedures that prevent employees from making appropriate decisions to satisfy customers may jeopardize employee morale, the customer base, and productivity. Appropriate decisions are those that fall within an employee's job scope and capabilities. Although policies and procedures provide adequate structure, efficiency, and safety of operations, procedure overload can make for avoidable delay while stifling employee spirit. Another obstacle is the employee who refuses to participate or support team efforts. It is the manager's responsibility to identify such persons, coach them toward involvement, or apply the established disciplinary steps to remove them. Other obstacles include budget constraints, productivity and labor demands, unrealistic demands and expectations from other departments, lack of understanding and/or cooperation from other organization members, insufficient employee knowledge or expertise, and time constraints for meetings and problem solving.

Communication

Effective communication in a participative work climate includes (among other methods) conducting meetings for the purposes of identifying strategic plans for the organization and updating employees on the status of organizational goals. Employees also should be informed of how department goals fit into the larger organization's vision, how the employees contribute to accomplishing department goals, and what future planning efforts will include. Good communication in a participative setting moves in two directions—"downward" from managers and "upward" from employees—which means that managers must sharpen their listening skills. Chapter 7 is devoted to skillful use of communication techniques.

By bridging communication gaps with other departments, managers will become more aware of conditions faced by others in the organization. This way, they can sensitize their staff and improve relations throughout the facility. By opening communication across departmental lines, managers learn what is considered politically correct in the organization's cultural climate, thereby better protecting their staff against uncomfortable situations.

Employee Involvement

A participative or high-involvement manager understands the values and beliefs that motivate employee involvement through empowerment. This section will explore theories on motivation and their application in a collaborative work environment. Also, the levels of empowerment and its application to health care food service will be described.

Motivating Employees

Motivation is the process by which individuals are stimulated to act on their innermost needs, desires, and drives. Motivation is a repetitive, circular process: An individual's *needs* cause him or her to behave in a way that *fulfills,* or promises to fulfill, those needs. Once needs have been met (either partially or fully), the individual feels *satisfaction.* The feeling of satisfaction reinforces the need, and the need–fulfillment–satisfaction cycle of motivation is repeated.

One of the most important managerial responsibilities is to motivate employees to work toward organizational and departmental goals and objectives. To accomplish this task, the manager must find a way to make those aims fit each employee's needs. Of course, motivation is only part of work performance—individual ability and the work environment also bear on performance level. In other words, employees need to know how to do their work well (ability); they need to want to do their work well (motivation); and they need adequate equipment, supplies, facilities, and authority to do their work well (environment). Absence of any one of these three factors will jeopardize performance.

Compensation (money) and benefits programs are the most tangible means for motivating and rewarding employees for their work. (Compensation and benefits are discussed in chapter 8.) However, it is questionable how well money and benefits alone motivate employees to performance levels beyond the minimum required to accomplish the work at hand. Compensation and benefits are extrinsic motivators, having limited long-term effect. In fact, employees generally rate four things above salary—appreciation for work done, a sense of "being in on things," help with personal problems, and job security.

More theories about worker motivation have been proposed than can be described within the scope of this manual on food service management. It may be useful, however, to explain basic theories that have influenced modern management practices. The flagship theories can be divided into three categories: content theories, process theories, and reinforcement theory.

Content Theories of Motivation

Content theories of motivation focus on specific factors that influence an individual to behave in a certain way. These factors are related to the individual's basic biological needs and immediate environment.

One proponent of content theory was Abraham H. Maslow, a psychologist who developed a theory known as the *hierarchy of needs,* discussed in his book *Motivation and Personality* (1954). As shown in figure 2-2, Maslow believed that certain needs (for example, physiological and safety needs) are more basic (or primary) than other higher (or secondary)

Figure 2-2. Maslow's Hierarchy of Needs

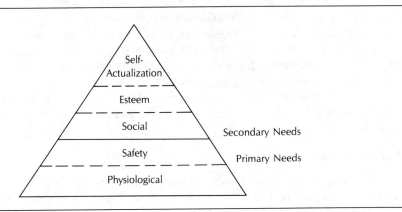

needs (for example, esteem). Maslow concluded that a person's primary needs will affect his or her behavior before any secondary needs have a chance to affect that person's actions. Once the primary needs have been fulfilled, however, they no longer operate as strong motivators, and the drive to fulfill needs farther up in the hierarchy begins to dominate the person's behavior.

According to Maslow, a work environment that allows employees to meet their physiological and safety needs will succeed, for employees will be motivated to better performance than in an environment that ignores their basic needs. The influence of Maslow's theory on modern management practices partially explains the reasoning behind the fair wage and salary practices in most of today's organizations. Maslow's influence also can be seen in medical and life insurance benefits, safety standards, and retirement plans.

Most food service directors do not directly control the compensation and benefits offered to their employees (see chapter 8). Food service directors, however, can reward good performance with promotions and regular salary increases. They also can make sure that their departments are pleasant and safe places in which to work and, by exercising fair and professional management, can ensure employees of reasonably secure prospects for future employment.

Another content theory that is influential in the development of modern management practices is Frederick Herzberg's *two-factor theory* of motivation, based on studies he conducted during the 1950s. He concluded that two sets of factors (which he called hygiene factors and motivation factors) influence employee attitudes and behavior. *Hygiene factors* include such things as personnel policies, job security, and salary and benefits. Herzberg believed that hygiene factors can prevent job dissatisfaction if employees perceive them to be adequate and fair, but that these factors cannot increase motivation levels or job satisfaction. *Motivation factors* include responsibility, recognition, achievement, advancement, and other elements related to job content. Herzberg believed that these motivation factors are the conditions under which employee performance is motivated. In other words, giving additional responsibility or recognition for a job provides motivation.

Herzberg emphasized that managers need to work simultaneously on hygiene and motivation factors to foster a positively motivated work force. This theory has important application in the operation of a food service department and should be considered during the process of job design, job enrichment, or job enlargement because motivation factors may influence the level of employee productivity in new positions.

Process Theories of Motivation

Whereas content theories focus on the *why* of behavior, process theories focus on *how* motivation occurs. Process theories look at motivation from the point at which an individual's behavior is energized, through the behavior choices he or she makes to the quality of the effort.

Among the body of process theories, *expectancy theory* proposes that motivation begins with a desire for something, such as more recognition on the job, higher pay, or a stronger feeling of accomplishment. An individual would then consider whether the effort to do a certain job (performance) could be expected to achieve his or her goal.

Expectancy theory can help managers understand motivation on an employee-by-employee basis because it takes individual differences among employees into account in a way that content theories do not. For example, Herzberg's theory suggests that job enlargement would increase the level of motivation in all individuals. Expectancy theory admits that not all individuals are willing or even able to accept job enlargement as a likely means for achieving what they want.

Reinforcement Theory of Motivation

Originally, reinforcement theory was based on the behavior of animals under experimental conditions. Rat performance in mazes, for example, tested the psychological theory of reinforcement. B. F. Skinner and other psychologists, however, have demonstrated how the theory can be applied to human behavior. Basically, reinforcement theory assumes that behavior that brings positive results probably will be repeated, whereas behavior that has negative results probably will not.

Four basic elements are at work in the theory. *Positive reinforcement* strengthens a specific behavior because the result of the behavior is desirable to the individual. *Avoidance* strengthens a specific behavior because the result allows the individual to escape an undesirable result. *Punishment* weakens a specific behavior because the result is undesirable to the individual. *Extinction* weakens a specific behavior because no desirable result is provided by the behavior.

For example, a food service director who praises an employee for preparing an especially attractive casserole provides positive reinforcement, and the employee is likely to repeat the work behavior. But for an employee who is careful to wash his or her hands after handling uncooked meat because of past counseling for violating hand-washing procedures, *avoidance* is at work; that is, the employee behaves in a certain way to avoid another counseling session.

Managers often use punishment to reduce the likelihood that employees will repeat inappropriate behavior. However, this approach (for example, punishing food service employees for breaking rules or missing work) can lead to anger and resentment among employees. When practical, reinforcing proper behavior through praise and reward should be used in place of punishment.

A food service director might use extinction to discourage inappropriate behavior that was rewarded in the past. Suppose that an employee who habitually engages in horseplay in the department was rewarded in the past when the previous director or other managers joined in the laughter at the employee's antics. The director could discourage the behavior by ignoring it instead of rewarding or punishing it.

Application of Motivational Theories

No one theory of motivation is completely relevant to every work situation or to every employee. Managers with effective leadership qualities are sensitive to employee differences, but they also recognize that each of the theories has some application to their ability to motivate employees. General motivation guidelines suggested by these theories are summarized below.

- Reinforce desired performance by providing formal rewards (fair salaries, benefits, and opportunities for advancement).
- Design jobs that are interesting and challenging as defined by each employee's skills.
- When an employee's performance falls short of expectations, praise positive aspects of the performance and suggest specific improvements without threats or punishment.
- Recognize and reinforce improvements through praise and other rewards.
- Make employees feel important by encouraging, helping, and supporting them in their work.

- Allow employees to set their own goals within the limits of the department's objectives and the organization's goals.
- Provide a work environment that is responsive to employee needs.
- Treat employees as the unique individuals they are by learning their names, interests, and concerns.
- Show trust in employees by delegating responsibilities to them and by emphasizing their contribution to the organization.
- Keep employees fully informed about policies, procedures, and organizational changes that affect their jobs.
- Protect employee privacy and confidential information as prescribed by law.
- Encourage employees to participate in planning department activities and solving work-related problems.

Motivating employees is a challenging responsibility, for each employee is unique, bringing different needs, desires, and perceptions to the work situation. Good managers help pave the way for employees to realize their full potential, becoming satisfied and proud contributors to their organization. To help all employees reach this state, managers must provide them with opportunities to participate, to gain self-esteem through greater responsibility, and to achieve a real sense of accomplishment.

Empowering Employees

Employee empowerment, best defined as self-management accomplished through intrinsic motivation, is a positive outcome of a participative work environment created by a flexible situational leadership style. When employees choose responsibility for becoming involved and managers commit to encouraging that involvement, employee empowerment is under way. This manager–employee relationship is developed through communicating information, providing knowledge through training, sharing decision-making power, providing rewards and recognition, creating a team atmosphere, and delegating meaningful work. The remainder of this subsection will focus on the varying levels of empowerment and when it is appropriate to apply these levels.

Levels of Empowerment

David Bowen and Edward Lawler define three levels of employee empowerment: suggestion involvement, job involvement, and high involvement. Each level has a place in food service operations where employee empowerment is a priority. All three can provide a road map for the manager seeking to change a tightly controlled work environment into a highly participative one.

With *suggestion involvement,* employees are encouraged to contribute ideas through formal suggestion systems, but there is little change in how day-to-day work is accomplished. Or, employees are encouraged to make recommendations for change, but management usually retains power to decide whether the recommendations are implemented. Suggestion involvement, then, is closely related to a control model of management. Managers may use suggestion involvement as the first step to leading employees to high (or full) involvement, or they may decide that this level is appropriate for their department based on the organizational culture. Suggestion involvement may be appropriate to certain tasks or situations, whereas job involvement or high involvement is better suited to others.

Job involvement takes a large step up from the typical control model. At this level employees are involved in job design (how to do their work), they exercise a larger variety of skills, get more feedback on how the work is proceeding, and are responsible for an identifiable piece of work. This level of involvement offers more employee enrichment, which in turn leads to higher motivation, commitment, and quality of work. It is at the job involvement level that many organizations begin team emphasis. Teams will be especially important in health care food service because no one individual will be responsible for customer contact from beginning to end. The complex nature of the work and service delivery will make it necessary to increase emphasis on job completion through teamwork. It is also at this level of involvement in employee empowerment that training becomes more important. With more demand for employee involvement, managers must ensure that workers have the knowledge and skills to make decisions effectively. Finally, managers at the job involvement level become more supportive and less directive in their situational leadership approach.

High involvement derives from employees' keen sense of how they do their jobs, how their group or team performs, and how successfully the organization performs as a whole. This level of involvement thrives in a culture that promotes employee empowerment and participative management, where information on the organization's business performance is shared; skill development in teamwork, problem solving, and business operations is offered; and employee participation in job-related decisions is promoted. Managers at this level must be highly competent in participatory management and team-building, coaching, training, and delegation skills. High-involvement empowerment strategies also can be more costly in terms of additional time taken in hiring employees and in their training and development.

Application of Empowerment to Food Service

Is it appropriate in every situation to empower food service employees to make decisions? Probably not. Recall that policies and procedures are established to provide consistent and safe service. For example, it is unwise to authorize employees on the patient trayline to make substitutions, which might compromise patients' nutrition needs or food preferences. Using another example, a standard greeting for answering the phone or addressing customers in the cafeteria lines promotes an image of continuity and corporate identity. Management judgment and discretion come into play when application of empowerment versus strict procedural adherence is at issue.

Individual differences in value systems and belief systems must be taken into account when making empowerment application decisions. For those employees whose cultural comfort zone is more amenable to structure and management-based decisions, tasks requiring strict adherence to procedural protocol will be more readily completed. Regardless of whether employees require more control than autonomy (or vice versa), they should be selected for positions that allow them to utilize their skills to maximum potential.

Roadblocks to Participative Management

Participative management and employee empowerment are not always accomplished easily, and roadblocks may lie ahead if the organization is unsupportive of an empowered work force. Although it may be difficult for managers or employees to exert influence outside their department without commitment to participative management from the top, managers can begin with suggestion involvement, encouraging employee input on how things are done within their department.

Employee skepticism may present another roadblock to participative management if employees doubt management's sincerity to welcome their input in decision making and job completion. Skepticism can be due to employees' past experiences with the current organization or a previous one. For example, employees whose participation and input were solicited in the past but consistently overruled may doubt the manager's seriousness. Longtime employees who have seen programs, processes, and managers come and go may feel this is just another empty effort. For employees who view the manager as being lazy or abdicating responsibilities, this may be the thought at first glance, but a manager who continues to encourage and support them will eventually win their allegiance.

A third obstacle to participative management may be the employees' level of development. Without adequate training and information, employees are incapable of providing input. The manager must be responsible for employee education so as to ensure success while providing constant feedback and praise. Again, not all employees desire autonomy on the job or opportunity for input.

If cultural differences provide a stumbling block to empowerment, managers must recognize this opportunity and find a way to utilize the differences. Chapter 8 further discusses the issue of cultural differences.

Fear of failure or job insecurity can hamper employee involvement. Fear that the manager is "setting me up to fail so I can be fired" may be unfounded, but it is up to the manager to reassure the employee. This can be done by starting at the basic level and allowing the employee to offer suggestions, but taking the ultimate responsibility for the decision until the employee is trusting enough to move beyond this level.

Managers themselves can be obstacles to a participative work environment. Those who "grew up" (that is, developed their management styles) in nonparticipative environments may face some of the same fears their employees do in trying to change to participatory management. They may not be willing to give up the power and authority that come with their position, feeling that they worked hard for it and that by sharing it they somehow admit their inadequacy. It may also appear to some managers that by sharing their power and authority, they—and therefore their jobs—become devalued. It may be difficult for some managers to give up responsibility and authority because they need to be in control and to know what's going on. Being responsible and knowledgeable is possible in a participative environment if the manager is a member of the overall team. The manager who simply may not have the skills and information necessary to be a participative leader will have to defer to the organization's responsibility for making this knowledge available.

☐ Summary

Emphasis on customer satisfaction, continuous quality improvement, and increased demands from employees for participation will place more demand on managers to become effective leaders. A practical approach to leadership can be established using the styles identified by Kenneth Blanchard—directing, coaching, supporting, and delegating. Each style requires the leader to be flexible in the application of his or her style based on an employee's developmental level and the task's complexity.

An effective leader is flexible and possesses both technical expertise and interpersonal skills. Application of these skills is important to accomplishing the management functions of planning, organizing, leading, and controlling. Interpersonal skills are extremely important to creating and nurturing a participative work environment that enables employees and allows them to be active in decision making. A manager who advocates a participative setting will possess skills for communicating effectively, training, coaching, sharing decision making, team building, providing rewards and recognition, delegating work, removing obstacles, and bridging gaps with other departments.

Providing a collaborative environment for employees will stimulate their feelings of self-worth and inspire a commitment to the organization. Empowerment can be simplistic and allow only suggestion involvement, or be more complex and allow for involvement with job design and completion and decision making. Creating a participative work environment takes time and requires change on the part of managers and employees. It is an evolutionary process that can suffer setbacks due to obstacles. These roadblocks can be overcome with understanding and persistence on the part of employees and managers.

Benefits of a participative work environment accrue to employee and organization alike. When allowed to influence their work life, employees develop a higher level of self-esteem and job satisfaction. Organizations gain from employee loyalty and enhancements in customer service, productivity, and quality.

☐ Bibliography

American Hospital Association. *Productivity and Performance Management in Health Care Institutions.* Chicago: American Hospital Publishing, 1989.

Blake, R. R., and Mouton, J. S. *The New Management Grid.* Houston: Gulf, 1978.

Blanchard, K., Zigarmi, P., and Zigarmi, D. *Leadership and the One Minute Manager.* New York City: William Morrow & Company, 1985.

Bowen, D. E., and Lawler, E. E. The empowerment of service workers: what, why, how, and when. *Sloan Management Review* (33)3:31–39, Spring 1992.

Cohen, A. R., Fink, S. L., Gadon, H., Willits, R. D., and Josefowitz, N. *Effective Behavior in Organizations.* 4th ed. Homewood, IL: Irwin, 1988.

Davison, G. Becoming a manager. *Harvard Business School Bulletin,* Apr. 4, 1992, pp. 6–7.

Dougherty, D. A. Are you a manager or a leader? *Hospital Food & Nutrition Focus* 7(8):4–5, Apr. 1991.

Dougherty, D. A. Employee empowerment: a management responsibility. *Hospital Food & Nutrition Focus* 8(5):6–7, Jan. 1992.

Dougherty, D. A. Knowing your employees: beyond demographics. *Hospital Food & Nutrition Focus* 7(11):4–7, July 1991.

Dubnicki, C., and Williams, J. B. Getting peak performance in the knowledge-based organization. *Healthcare Forum Journal* 34(1):32–36, Jan.–Feb. 1991.

Flannery, T. P., and Williams, J. B. Management culture & process. *Healthcare Forum Journal* 33(4):52–57, July–Aug. 1990.

Flower, J. Don't wait for the crisis. *Healthcare Forum Journal* 34(6):28–34, Nov.–Dec. 1991.

Freedman, D. H. Is management still a science? *Harvard Business Review* 70(6):26–38, Nov.–Dec. 1992.

Gibson, J. L., Ivancevich, J. M., and Donnelly, J. H., Jr. *Organizations' Behavior Structure Processes.* 7th ed. Homewood, IL: Irwin, 1991.

Grayson, M. A. CEO's in the 1990s. *Hospitals* 67(2):32–35, Jan. 20, 1993.

Hamilton, J. Toppling the power of the pyramid. *Hospitals* 67(1):39–41, Jan. 5, 1993.

Herzberg, F. One more time: how do you motivate employees? *Harvard Business Review,* Jan.–Feb. 1968.

Hogue, M. A. How to develop a creative and self-motivated work team. *Hospital Food & Nutrition Focus* 6(5):1–4, Jan. 1990.

Kazemek, E. A. Interactive leadership gaining sway in the 1990s. *Healthcare Financial Management* 45(6):16, 1991.

Lawler, E. E., and Mohrman, S. A. High-involvement management. *Personnel* 66(4):26–31, Apr. 1989.

Leebov, W., and Scott, G. *Health Care Managers in Transition.* San Francisco: Jossey-Bass, 1990.

Lombardi, D. N. *Progressive Health Care Management Strategies.* Chicago: American Hospital Publishing, 1992.

Maslow, A. H. *Motivation and Personality.* New York City: Harper and Row, 1954.

Metzger, N. Making employees feel that they "make a difference." *Health Care Supervisor* 7(3):1–7, Apr. 1989.

Mintzberg, H. *The Nature of Managerial Work.* New York City: Harper & Row, 1973.

Pagonis, W. G. The work of the leader. *Harvard Business Review* 70(6):118–26, Nov.–Dec. 1992.

Reihle, H. The foodservice manager in the year 2000. *Restaurants USA* 12(2):36–37, Feb. 1992.

Schuller, R. S. *Personnel and Human Resource Management.* 3rd ed. St. Paul: West Publishing Company, 1987.

Vroom, V. H., and Yetton, P. W. *Leadership and Decision Making.* Pittsburgh: University of Pittsburgh Press, 1973.

Chapter 3

Marketing

☐ Introduction

In the past, health care providers managed operations with little concern for environmental pressures and changes in the marketplace. However, given that health care technology has expanded and that the percentage of the gross national product spent on health care has increased, the health care system now must change its approach to be more consistent with other sectors. It is no longer immune to the complexities and uncertainties of its environment.

A number of uncontrollable pressures within the health care environment (discussed in chapter 1) make health care delivery today increasingly more turbulent and stressful. These pressures have forced providers to learn and implement new skills to make their operations more cost-effective while maintaining quality standards. Primary among these responses has been the implementation of marketing, which has long been used in other consumer-oriented fields.

Marketing is often confused with sales, advertising, and public relations. In fact, these activities are part of marketing. To produce targeted results, not only must marketing become a way of doing business in the health care operation, it must become a function of management. In the health care context, marketing is oriented to the consumer, as opposed to sales or the product.

To apply to the health care field, *marketing* must be defined as the process of profiling what customers want or need and then developing and providing products and services that meet the profile. Because many different health care options currently exist, and because changes in health care delivery will continue, providers must design services with the opinions and perceptions of their customers in mind. Therefore, health care nutrition and food service departments are becoming increasingly—and more overtly—important in facilities' overall marketing strategies.

This chapter will introduce key marketing concepts, including services marketing, the difference between goods and services, types of markets, market and basis for segmentation, target markets, and marketing mix. These concepts then will be applied to devising a cyclical, five-phase marketing management model based on the following elements:

1. Information (maintaining records; collecting, analyzing, and interpreting data)
2. Planning (operational and strategic planning, the planning process, documentation and components of the marketing plan)

3. Implementation (dealing with change, employee training, advertising and promotion)
4. Evaluation (monitoring and measuring marketing outcome)
5. Feedback (reporting successes and/or failures and returning to the information phase)

☐ Key Marketing Concepts

Although relatively new to the health care field, marketing is a discipline of sophisticated and proven theories, techniques, and concepts. Although a complete discussion of these areas is beyond the scope of this book, it is critical that health care food service managers be familiar with at least three of the concepts: services marketing, markets and segmentation, and marketing mix.

Services Marketing

Since the early 1980s, the service sector of the nation's economy has grown at an astounding rate. According to the Bureau of the Census, this sector, of which the health care field is a member, accounts for more than 50 percent of both the gross domestic product and consumer expenditures. Despite the importance of the service sector, only recently has services marketing been differentiated from goods marketing. Marketing techniques originally developed to sell goods are not always appropriate for selling services.

Goods versus Services

Prior to examining services marketing, the distinction between goods and services must be understood. Goods may be objects, devices, or things; when goods are purchased, something tangible is acquired for possession. Services, on the other hand, are mostly intangible; a service is an activity performed for the benefit of the purchaser. A service transaction often is accomplished on a personal basis and usually does not result in ownership (possession) of a physical (or tangible) item. A service is created by its provider—for example, a facility that employs a meal hostess to deliver patient trays or a chef to carve roasted meat on the cafeteria line is a service provider.

Most health care food service operations probably deliver a combination of goods *and* services. In such operations, acquisition of food and supplies, preparation and service of meals, and cleanup afterward is performed for patients by food service employees. Hence, health care food service is considered an industry—a service industry—even though tangibles (food and equipment) are involved.

Characteristics of Services

Although service industries themselves are quite heterogeneous (ranging from barber shops to health care operations), certain generalizations can be made about the characteristics of services. The most important of these characteristics are intangibility, simultaneous production and consumption, less uniformity and standardization, and absence of inventories.

Intangibility

Services provided by health care food service operations are *consumed* but not *possessed*. What is being bought is a performance of an activity rendered by a food service employee or group of employees for the benefit of the customer. Generally, the provision of services is a people-intensive process. To the patient, the meal hostess's delivery of the breakfast tray is as much a part of the meal as the tangible portion—the food.

Simultaneous Production and Consumption

Goods are generally produced, sold, and then consumed, with much emphasis placed on distributing goods at the "right place" and at the "right time." Services are produced and consumed simultaneously, meaning that the service provider is often physically present while consumption takes place: The clinical dietitian produces an educational service while (at the same time) the patient consumes it. Because a dialogue occurs between customer and service provider, the manner in which services are delivered becomes important. How food service employees conduct themselves in the presence of a customer can influence future business. Figure 3-1 shows production and consumption of goods versus services over time.

Less Uniformity and Standardization

Because people are involved on both the production and consumption sides, services are less uniform and standardized than are goods. With extensive involvement of people, a degree of variability in the outcome is introduced. Whereas a patient may expect his or her favorite breakfast cereal always to taste the same, two different meal hostesses could do an effective but different job in delivering the breakfast tray to the patient.

Absence of Inventories

In most service settings, some levels of inventory must be maintained, as is the case with food and supplies in food service departments. However, some resources cannot be stored for future sale and thus are considered perishable. A sale is lost (perished) when a hospital guest finds the wait time in the hospital restaurant to be too long, and it cannot be recovered. Despite surges in demand, service organizations also experience slack periods. Because of this variability in demand, service operations are often concerned with how to manage demand. For example, the above-described hospital restaurant with long wait times might feature special offers during low periods of demand in an attempt to manage demand more effectively.

Markets and Segmentation

To maximize the success of a health care food service operation, its manager must be able to identify the potential market for the operation's goods and services. A market is simply a group of individuals or organizations that might want the good or service being offered for sale.

Types of Markets

If the buyer is the individual who will use the product to satisfy personal needs, the buyer is part of the consumer market. When a product is purchased for business purposes, the buyer

Figure 3-1. Production and Consumption of Goods versus Services

Production of Goods	Selling of Goods	Consumption of Goods

Assembly of Services
Selling of Services
Consumption of Services

Time

Note: Shaded boxes indicate the points at which buyers and sellers interact. For services, each point can influence buyer satisfaction and must be addressed by the operation's marketing program.

is part of the organizational market. Different marketing strategies must be used when dealing with consumer versus organizational markets. Clearly, many health care food service operations market not only to individual consumers but also to organizations. Marketing nutrition counseling services to an individual on an outpatient basis, then, probably would require a different approach from that used to market the same services on a contract basis to a nearby nursing home.

Segmentation

Most managers find it necessary to further divide consumer and organizational markets into smaller, more homogeneous submarkets. This process, referred to as market segmentation, recognizes that all buyers are not alike. Appropriately implemented, market segmentation can be one of the health care food service manager's most powerful marketing tools.

Basis for Segmentation

Almost any buyer characteristic may be used as a basis for segmenting markets into submarkets. Common characteristics used to define segments of consumer markets include geographic, demographic, psychographic, and behavioral dimensions of buyers.

Geographic Dimension

Geographic segmentation is a logical segmentation characteristic in that it is based on the assumption that consumers' wants and needs vary depending on where they live. Most health care operations provide services in a specific geographic area, called a service area. Basic statistics about the service area's population and health care needs should be analyzed by the operation's management staff, including food service. This could prove beneficial when reviewing existing services and when considering new ventures. For instance, when menus are developed or revised, the menu planner must consider the regional food and beverage preferences of potential customers.

Demographic Dimension

Most health care operations segment their markets according to the diagnosis of the patient. Other demographic characteristics, such as age, sex, family size, income, stage in the family life cycle, ethnicity, religion, and nationality, are segmentation variables that have long been popular bases for determining market segments in the health care industry. The health care services, including food and nutrition services, used by an individual are highly associated with demographic variables. These variables have a major impact on most of the functional units of the food service operation. When a health care operation serves certain diagnostic segments, patient menus must be developed for those segments (for example, fat-controlled menus for cardiac patients and diabetic menus for diabetic patients). Likewise, the age of the patients served must be considered. The specific impact of selected demographic variables on menu planning and meal service are described in chapters 15 and 20, respectively.

Psychographic Dimension

Because individuals within the same demographic group do not always exhibit the same buying behaviors, other dimensions must be considered. One of these, psychographic segmentation, divides buyers into groups based on social class, lifestyle, or personality characteristics. Lifestyle is an important factor because it is a strong predictor of future health care consumption. Likewise, it has an impact on the types of food and beverages desired by the food service operation's customers, both patients and nonpatients. In the lifestyle category, health-conscious consumer segments would typically select menu choices with lower fat, sugar, and sodium than regular menu items.

Behavioral Dimension

Behavioral segmentation focuses on the knowledge, attitude, use, or response by consumers to actual services. A number of factors can be analyzed when attempting to segment the market according to this dimension. Factors applicable to the health care food service operation include the benefit sought by the consumer in terms of quality, service, and value; consumer usage rate (that is, how often the consumer will use the operation's services); and the consumer's general attitude toward the operation's products.

Target Markets

Based on the dimensions described above, a number of market segments could be created from the health care food service operation's consumer market. It might be tempting to create a rather large collection of goods and services to meet the wants and needs of each segment. However, most marketers agree that to market to everyone is to market to no one. Therefore, it is necessary for food service managers to choose a few meaningful segments and concentrate efforts on satisfying those selected submarkets. A market segment toward which the organization directs its marketing efforts is called the target market. Most often in a health care operation, this selection process is not left entirely to the discretion of food service managers. They may be involved in identifying target markets, but final decision as to where efforts are concentrated will be made by the facility as a whole.

Marketing Mix

A successful health care food service operation focuses on the wants and needs of its customers and markets the operation's products efficiently. To accomplish this objective, food service management must adjust specific elements of its operation as necessary so that its products will appeal to potential customers. Those elements over which an operation has control so as to influence salability of its products are called the marketing mix. (See figure 3-2.)

Traditionally, elements of the marketing mix considered common among all businesses and industries include product, place, promotion, and price. A fifth element that must be included for most service sector businesses, including health care food service, is public image. When considering a specific type of business or industry, this list can be customized. Each element is essential to ensuring that the health care food service positions its products optimally to meet the wants and needs of its customers.

Product

The health care food service product is a combination of goods and services that are unique to food service and that meet the wants and needs of targeted customers. Of several factors that influence how acceptable a product is to customers, quality is a key measure. Quality is discussed in chapter 4, but the main point here is that food service managers can adjust quality to meet customer expectations. Other adjustable product characteristics include

Figure 3-2. Health Care Food Service Marketing Mix

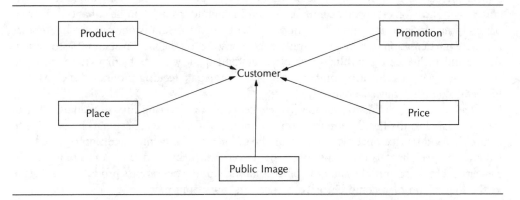

labeling (such as naming the employee cafeteria or cafeteria products in inviting and interesting ways) and packaging (how goods and services are combined to affect sales). Closely related to packaging is accommodation. For instance, when the food service operation joins forces (combines) with the health care operation as a whole to provide an elegant dinner for new parents, the product has been qualitatively adjusted, resulting in a special accommodation.

Place

Health care food service products are offered for sale in a specific place. The location and method of distribution must be convenient and attractive to customers. Because the typical operation serves a variety of patients and nonpatients, multiple locations for food service facilities may be a major marketing consideration. Sales may be enhanced by implementing new methods of distribution, such as offering take-out services. Physical characteristics of place—shape, size, and certainly the facility's decor—are important to the marketing effort.

Promotion

Promotion includes those methods by which the operation makes potential customers aware of its products. Many forms of communication take place between the operation and its potential customers. Advertising and sales promotion facilitate customization of the message and image conveyed to groups identified as potential customers (for example, visitors). As an example, table tents can be used in hospital coffee shops to describe a new food item and therefore promote its sale to coffee shop patrons who might not normally purchase such an item. Most food service managers know that word-of-mouth communication by satisfied customers can have a positive effect on sales. For example, the popularity of a Sunday brunch for hospital visitors could increase significantly from the endorsement of satisfied customers.

Price

A price must be established that reconciles value of the product to the customer with value of the exchange to the food service operation. Prior to purchase, price is one of the few indicators of quality. Unfortunately, it also may be one of the least reliable quality indicators because a variety of variables, some related to quality and some not, are used to establish prices. Accurate cost information is critical to effective pricing. When establishing product prices, food service managers must consider not only their costs but other factors, key among which are the demand of consumers for products and the prices charged by competitors for comparable products. Because the cost, demand, and competition variables differ from one geographic region to another, price variations for similar products are often noted.

Public Image

Public image, or how service sector businesses are viewed by current and potential customers, affects the salability of services. A food service facility's reputation among customers and potential customers, peers, community, and the public at large can be enhanced. Participation in nutrition-related interviews in print or broadcast media is one approach. Another might be participation in annual tasting events sponsored by the local restaurant association. Both could influence the public's perception of food quality at the facility. Responding to community needs by donating prepared foods to congregate feeding programs, such as soup kitchens, could be viewed positively.

The preceding discussion on the five elements of a marketing mix gives only a broad look as related to the health care food service industry. For these concepts to be of value to a specific food service operation, they must be tailored to the facility and implemented systematically (see chapter 15). This might be accomplished by means of a customized self-evaluation checklist. Initial evaluation of the salability of the operation's products could serve as the foundation of a comprehensive, structured marketing plan.

☐ The Marketing Management Model

Successful marketing of health care food service products is a challenging task, unachievable without managerial involvement and a systematic approach. The marketing management process is a sequence of steps designed to ensure that the right decisions are made to sell an organization's goods and services effectively. In many health care organizations, the coordination of this process is centralized in a functional unit of at least department standing. Regardless of whether this is the case or not, the food service manager, along with the other operational managers, should be actively involved in this process. Their level of participation will depend on the complexity of the marketing unit. Although market research may be conducted by the organization's marketing unit, the food service manager should be involved in translating resulting information into new ventures and services.

Numerous models depict the marketing management process, and the following discussion extracts those minimum essential elements that make up a tried-and-true marketing management continuum. A review of marketing management models reveals that they differ primarily in the number of elements around which they are organized. Elements may range from as few as three to as many as ten. The model in this discussion uses five: information, planning, implementation, evaluation, and feedback. These elements are best described as cyclical, with each element—or phase—evolving from the previous one (see figure 3-3). *Feedback* is composed of the processes that enable information to flow from the evaluation element back to the information element.

Phase 1: Information

Sound information makes for sound decision making. Thus, marketing information, provided either by routine record keeping or as a result of market research, is extremely valuable to the marketing management process. Especially in light of today's health care environment, it is imperative that organizational and departmental managers, including food service, develop effective and efficient marketing information systems to get the precise information required for sound and timely decision making.

A marketing information system is a set of ongoing organized procedures, personnel, and equipment that collects, sorts, analyzes, stores, and retrieves information for use by marketing decision makers. According to Philip Kotler and Roberta N. Clarke, the marketing information system is composed of four subsystems: internal records, marketing intelligence, research, and analytical marketing.

Internal Records

Probably the most well-established subsystem of the information element is made up of internal records, routine data sources generated many times during the course of day-to-day operations. The data generally focus on issues of cost, inventory, dollar sales, volume of services, and other recurrent data that are routinely collected. From these records, the food service manager can develop basic statistics such as number of meals by diet type, average customer check in the employee cafeteria, and restaurant seat turnover.

Figure 3-3. Marketing Management Model

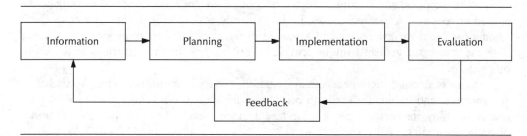

The internal records should be evaluated routinely to determine where problems might exist. The goal is to design a resource network that meets the food service manager's information needs cost-effectively. Ability to use these statistics to support future decision making can be greatly enhanced if the data are computerized, as detailed in chapter 10.

Marketing Intelligence

Environmental intelligence describes a network of procedures and sources that provide managers with information about the organization's external marketing environment. This subsystem yields valuable information from a routine scan of relevant articles from magazines and journals and from outside parties, such as suppliers. A particularly effective method for gathering this type of information is to hire "mystery shoppers" for the purpose of purchasing and evaluating services from the operation and to compare them with those purchased from competing food service operations. This provides information about the types of service offered, prices charged by competitors, and staff performance in the manager's own and similar operations.

Research

Market research, the systematic assembly of data that use statistical technology to analyze the potential sales success of a good or service, is a highly developed field of study. Because market research provides information on the basis of which business decisions will be made, it must be conducted carefully to ensure that the results reflect the situation accurately. It also can be costly. Unless a food service manager has the training to carry out market research, it is wise to enlist the services of the facility's marketing department or hire a consultant. Regardless of who conducts the research, the food service manager should monitor its progress to ensure that appropriate methods are carried out in the proper sequence. A recommended sequence is to define the problem, collect the data, analyze the data, and interpret the research findings.

Step 1: Define the Problem

The problem must be defined in enough detail so that subsequent steps in the research process can be planned and carried out based on reality of purpose. Problems that might be defined include:

- Whether opportunities exist for off-premises catering services
- Why competitors are gaining a bigger share of the outpatient weight loss business
- Whether implementation of a take-out bakery counter would be profitable
- What promotional activities would have a positive effect on demand in a hospital's restaurant during slack periods

Step 2: Collect the Data

Data collection involves determining what data are needed, what collection method(s) will be used, and the actual collection of data. After the problem has been defined clearly, researchers must review already-existing departmental and hospital data. Because implementation of new promotional activities in the hospital restaurant might require expenditures for equipment, supplies, and training, the food service manager might want to investigate the cost-effectiveness of various techniques. In this case, past sales records (including average check amount) and seat turnover would be reviewed in terms of previous promotions. Interviews with the restaurant waitstaff might provide additional insight into customer reactions to promotions.

The next step is review of secondary data, or previously published data. A number of governmental and public agencies can provide valuable data, but with regard to a hospital restaurant study, the best sources of secondary data most likely are found in the publications of trade and professional associations.

If secondary data fail to yield the documentation required, researchers must turn to primary data. Normally, collecting primary data is accomplished by relying on a predetermined research design that uses an observational, survey, or experimental approach. Each design involves standardized techniques so that data will be valid and reliable. In considering which promotional techniques to implement in the hospital restaurant, for example, researchers might use the observational method by recording reactions of customers to various promotional techniques. As an alternative, a customer survey questionnaire could be utilized to determine what techniques to consider. The effectiveness of the techniques could be evaluated by means of the experimental design by determining the effect of each technique on sales in the hospital restaurant.

Step 3: Analyze the Data

Once data have been collected, they must be analyzed. If valid and reliable, data can be tested statistically to measure relationships among the data. The appropriate statistical testing would help the food service manager determine the relative effectiveness of two or more promotional techniques—for example, whether a table tent or cafeteria signage would introduce a new menu item with better results.

Step 4: Interpret the Research Findings

Following data analysis, study results should be interpreted and recommendations made. At this point, the food service manager would decide which promotional technique(s) to implement in the restaurant. Study results should be documented in report form for the benefit of future studies.

Market research techniques can be highly technical and, if not conducted carefully, could result in flawed information on which decisions are made. Food service managers might find this an appropriate topic to include in their personal continuing education plans. A less formal technique includes development and completion of a marketing mix checklist, discussed earlier in the chapter. Other informal, qualitative market research tools that can provide valuable information about an operation's products, customers, and competition are focus groups and SWOT (strengths, weaknesses, opportunities, and threats) analyses.

Analytical Marketing

The fourth subsystem, called analytical marketing, comprises a set of advanced techniques for analyzing data. Usually it incorporates statistical, spreadsheet, and data-base software systems. Large organizations use analytical marketing extensively because it focuses on diagnosing relationships within a set of data, determining statistical reliability, and using mathematical models to predict outcome. Because it is highly technical, this technique generally is not used in smaller organizations or at the departmental level. The information generated from this subsystem flows into phase 2, planning, and is used for decision-making purposes.

Phase 2: Planning

Planning, the second phase in the marketing management cycle, usually occurs at two levels in a health care organization. Planning at the organizational level, called *corporate marketing,* focuses on organizational objectives, management's view of mission, and resource allocation for the organization as a whole. At the departmental level, the planning process may be as focused as arranging for implementation of promotional activities in the restaurant or as broad as developing a three-year departmental marketing plan. Regardless of its scope, the planning process should be driven by the information collected in phase 1 of the cycle. The planning process results in marketing goals and programs to be implemented.

The Planning Process

Each phase (and all its components) of the marketing management cycle must be aimed at satisfying customers' wants and needs. Therefore, most health care operations satisfy three requirements before adopting a specific model for their planning process. These requirements are discussed in the following subsections.

Identify and Evaluate Opportunities and Threats

At the outset of the planning process, the health care operation's mission statement and objectives established for the plan's time span should be reviewed. Next, the food service manager should review the market information system to identify marketplace opportunities that are consistent with the organization's objectives. This activity, called a *marketing opportunity analysis,* apprises managers not only of benefits associated with specific opportunities but also potential problems. Marketing opportunity analysis pays close attention to the environment in which the health care organization and food service facility operate. It identifies competitor facilities and compares their strengths and weaknesses with those of the food service operation. Such analysis allows the food service manager to select opportunities that are best suited to the operation. At the same time, effort should be made to correct weaknesses disclosed by the analysis.

Marketing opportunity analysis should be conducted by the food service manager when considering projects such as expanding existing catering services to off-premises events. Even though the market information system may indicate that this is a likely opportunity, careful analysis should be made prior to further action.

Analyze Market Segments and Select Target Markets

The results of opportunity analysis leads to decisions about where marketing efforts will be directed. It is important to stress that the health care food service manager must identify specific markets from all the possible market segments. To accomplish this, the market segments should be analyzed carefully to determine which ones are likely to have heavy users of the services and which hold little potential or present unreasonable risk. Specific targeting can improve revenue and may help control costs.

Referring back to the catering expansion example, based on the principles of segmenting and targeting markets, the food service manager must determine the focus for the proposed project. Operational characteristics necessary to support the venture for each segment under consideration must be explored. Examples of operational characteristics include hours of operation, the number of employees to consider, the addition of new employees, and cost-effectiveness of the venture. If the most promising market appears to be current hospital employees, a possible outcome of this analysis would be to design the off-premises business primarily for this segment.

Plan and Develop a Marketing Mix

The third requirement in the planning process is to construct the marketing mix, discussed earlier in this chapter. The main objective here is to manipulate the characteristics of product, place, promotion, price, and public image so that the wants and needs of target markets can be satisfied and the desired outcome of the marketing project can be achieved.

For the off-premises catering project, the existing marketing mix of the on-premises catering program can serve as the basis. For example, the product element (food) must be analyzed to determine service characteristics to be offered by the off-premises facility. Specifically, menu offerings, hours of service, and methods of service would be considered. Simply by offering the services off-premises changes the place element of the mix. The remaining elements of promotion, price, and public image would require analysis and revision as well.

The Marketing Plan

All details resulting from the planning process should be documented in a working document called a *marketing plan.* The marketing plan identifies a systematic, structured program of action to be undertaken over a specified period (for example, one year) to achieve targeted financial results. Simply stated, the marketing plan provides the details necessary to achieve the stated goals.

Many health care operations specify a format for the marketing plan. Otherwise, the food service manager should adopt a format similar to that suggested in the book *Marketing for Health Care Organizations,* written by Philip Kotler and Roberta N. Clarke. Format components for the plan are:

- *Executive summary:* The plan's main goals and recommendations are summarized so that readers can determine areas of major emphasis. The summary also facilitates plan evaluation.
- *Marketing opportunity analysis:* Results of the marketing opportunity analysis are provided, along with background information, forecasts, and assumptions. This section also should include a comparison of the operation's strengths and weaknesses with those of its competitors.
- *Goals and objectives:* Measurable goals and objectives for the food service department and its projects must be specified. Generally, these must be related to overall organizational goals for the coming period (as specified).
- *Marketing strategy:* The food service marketing strategy consists of a coordinated set of decisions about target markets and the marketing mix that will be developed to appeal to these markets.
- *Action plans:* Action plans turn the marketing strategy into a specific set of actions required to achieve the operation's goals and objectives. A table is an appropriate format for an action plan because it can include a time line, which enables the reader to determine when various activities will be initiated and completed (see figure 3-4).
- *Budgets:* The proposals recommended in the marketing plan must be supported by resources. A budget that shows projected revenues and expenses related to marketing activities must be provided.
- *Controls:* This section describes controls that will be used to monitor the plan's progress. For example, by arranging goals and budgets by appropriate time periods (usually monthly or quarterly), the health care operation's management can review results periodically.

Phase 3: Implementation

Implementation of the marketing management process begins once actions are taken to initiate the marketing plan. These actions include organizing and coordinating procedures, people,

Figure 3-4. Sample Action Plan

Action Plan		
Topic: Off-premise catering		
Strategy: Distribute brochure promoting off-premise catering to supervisory and managerial staff		
Action	**Completion Date**	**Person Responsible (Coordinated by)**
Establish format for brochure.	September 15	M. Bloom
Identify possible photographs and topics for copy.	September 22	T. Warren
Take photographs.	September 30	Contracted out (T. Warren)
Write copy.	October 5	T. Hardy
Design layout of brochure.	October 12	T. Warren
Approve layout, copy, and photographs.	October 19	M. Bloom
Obtain mailing labels.	October 26	L. Williams
Print brochures.	October 26	Contracted out (T. Warren)
Mail brochures.	November 6	L. Williams

resources, and tasks. For instance, prior to introducing a new menu, a number of operational procedures must be developed and/or changed. To ensure that all necessary ingredients are available for the proposed menu items, new vendors may need to be located, and new purchasing contracts may need to be signed. The food storage, inventory, and requisition systems will require revision to incorporate new ingredients. Production records such as recipes and production schedules will have to be developed to support the new menu.

In preparation for the introduction of new products, the responsibilities for preparing and serving food items on the new menu must be assigned. As a result, employee training may be required. Modification of physical facilities, such as new equipment or storage facilities, may be necessary. Advertising and promoting the new menu by means of signage, merchandising, and personal selling are important implementation activities that the manager will need to oversee both prior to and during the actual introduction of a new menu.

Although it may sound pretty simple, implementation is only the beginning. Managers must monitor the process continually by means of techniques such as sales analysis, operating ratios (food cost to revenue), and customer comments. All procedures as specified in the marketing plan must be reviewed and operations altered as necessary to ensure success. Without the proper implementation and effective monitoring procedures, even the best marketing plan will fail.

Phase 4: Evaluation

Results of the marketing effort must be measured and evaluated to determine whether the plan objectives have been achieved. A variety of qualitative, quantitative, and financial analysis methods can help make this determination. For example, recall the promotional technique of special offers during low-demand periods in the hospital restaurant (discussed under "Absence of Inventories" earlier in this chapter). Sales analyses should be conducted to show whether dollar sales increased during those slack periods. If sales did increase, the food service manager would then compare the actual increase to the increase forecast. Customer counts during hours of operation must also be monitored to see whether volume objectives were reached.

Sometimes a comprehensive review and appraisal of the marketing effort can be beneficial. Called a *marketing audit,* this activity evaluates an operation's marketing environment within the framework of operations organizationwide. Because the marketing audit must be conducted systematically and impartially to produce valid results, it may be necessary to contract an outside consultant to perform it in order to ensure an unbiased analysis of the operation's strengths and weaknesses.

Phase 5: Feedback

As demonstrated in this chapter, the marketing management process is not linear but cyclical in nature. Therefore, at the end of the evaluation phase, information about the programs presented in the marketing plan should flow back to the information phase. Feedback is composed of a wide variety of techniques designed to facilitate this process. For instance, the implications of a status report could be discussed in a management staff meeting. Feedback information on successes and failures identified by this process could provide valuable input and create new marketing opportunities. This feature of cyclicity acknowledges the dynamic nature of health care food service operations and allows for adjustments in response to ongoing competitive and environmental changes. Implementing new strategies and ventures can be both frightening and exciting for the food service manager. Using this five-phase model can help the manager design programs for almost any situation that may arise.

☐ Summary

All too often, health care food service managers try to advertise, promote, and sell goods and services without giving adequate thought to marketing. In times of intense competition and rapid change in this environment, a thorough understanding of marketing principles and techniques maximizes service to customers and revenues for the operation and its parent organization.

This chapter covered several key marketing concepts the food service manager must grasp in order to design, plan, and implement effective marketing programs. Ideally, these concepts should be implemented within the context of the five-phase marketing management model presented.

Finally, managers should assess their operations continuously for opportunities to apply marketing principles and techniques. The marketing orientation is critical in these times because of the pressure to satisfy increasingly complex and sophisticated wants and needs of health care food service customers.

☐ Bibliography

Axler, B. H. *Foodservice: A Managerial Approach.* Lexington, MA: D. C. Heath, 1979.

Berry, L. L. Services marketing is different. In: P. Kotler and K. K. Cox, editors. *Marketing Management and Strategy: A Reader.* Englewood Cliffs, NJ: Prentice-Hall, 1988.

Bureau of the Census. *Statistical Abstract of the United States, 1993.* 113rd ed. Washington, DC: U.S. Department of Commerce, Economic and Statistics Administration, 1993.

Chaudhry, R. Whining and dining. *Restaurants & Institutions* 102(17):12–22, July 1992.

Dodd, J. L. President's page: the fifth p. *Journal of The American Dietetic Association* 92(5):616–17, May 1992.

Helm, K. K., and Rose, J. C. *The Competitive Edge: Marketing Strategies for the Registered Dietitian.* Chicago: American Dietetic Association, 1986.

Johnson, J. Survey: many CEOs overlook PR staff's role in strategic planning. *Hospitals* 66(17):34–42, Sept. 1992.

Kotler, P., and Clarke, R. N. *Marketing for Health Care Organizations.* Englewood Cliffs, NJ: Prentice-Hall, 1987.

Marketing skills in the 1990s: practical steps for promoting dietetics professionals. *Journal of The American Dietetic Association* 90(1):37–39, Jan. 1990.

National Restaurant Association 1993 foodservice industry forecast. *Restaurants USA* 12(11):13–36, Dec. 1992.

Nelson, C. W. Patient satisfaction surveys: an opportunity for total quality improvement. *Hospital & Health Services Administration* 35(3):409–23, Fall 1990.

Parry, M., and Parry, A. E. Strategy and marketing tactics in non-profit hospitals. *Health Care Management Review* 17(1):51–62, Winter 1992.

Powers, T. *Marketing Hospitality.* New York City: John Wiley & Sons, 1990.

Reid, R. D. *Hospitality Marketing Management.* 2nd ed. New York City: Van Nostrand Reinhold, 1989.

Spears, M. C. *Foodservice Organizations: A Managerial and Systems Approach.* 2nd ed. New York City: Macmillan Publishing, 1991.

Zikmund, W. *Exploring Marketing Research.* Chicago: Dryden Press, 1989.

Zikmund, W., and D'Amico, M. *Marketing.* New York City: John Wiley & Sons, 1989.

Chapter 4

Quality Management

☐ Introduction

A primary responsibility of nutrition and food service managers is to help ensure the highest quality of patient care through provision of high-quality food products and service to all consumers. The trends mentioned in chapter 1 have caused renewed interest in health care quality management—in particular, health care reform issues, an expanding body of regulations, a shrinking and changing labor force, increased customer demands, and computer technology.

Health care organizations have become value driven, stressing quality as well as cost containment. *Value* is defined here as the relationship between quality and cost, or a focus on delivering the highest quality at the lowest possible cost. A value-driven approach requires more emphasis on quality of care and service with cost containment becoming the added benefit of delivering high quality.

This chapter will provide a brief background of quality in general industry and in health care, with emphasis on requirements established by the Joint Commission on Accreditation of Healthcare Organizations (JCAHO). Specific characteristics of organizational culture that are supportive of continuous quality improvement (CQI) are presented, together with a description of the infrastructure necessary for CQI program implementation. The chapter also will give guidelines for developing a CQI plan that ensures service quality, quality control, and quality assessment related to clinical care. Finally, various quality-enhancing techniques and devices applicable to the nutrition and food service department are offered.

☐ The Development of Quality in Health Care

Health care reform has forced administrators to transform their view of quality as an intangible to a view that recognizes it as an identifiable, measurable, and improvable entity. Although responsibility for quality was once delegated to a single department, managers now recognize quality improvement as the responsibility of each individual in the organization. Quality improvement is seen as a long-term proactive (rather than retrospective) strategy to improve patient care and satisfaction, increase utilization, strengthen productivity, and enhance cost-effectiveness throughout the organization.

51

General History of Quality Management

In the 1930s, Walter A. Shewhart provided a scientific foundation for quality control measurement in industry and manufacturing. He believed efforts should focus on identifying and correcting problems during the manufacture of products rather than on correcting the final product. Shewhart is credited with designing the plan-do-check-act (PDCA) cycle shown in figure 4-1.

Subsequently, W. Edwards Deming, who provided statistical quality control teaching to engineers and inspectors during World War II, expanded the PDCA cycle, defining each of the four quadrants in Shewhart's model and providing specific suggestions to foster improvement (see figure 4-2). Deming also is credited with the use of statistical process control tools that are the foundation of total quality management (TQM). In the handbook *An Executive's Pocket Guide to QI/TQM Terminology,* TQM is defined as "a continuous quality improvement management system, directed from the top, empowering employees and focused on systemic, not individual employee problems."

In 1951, in his *Quality Control Handbook,* Joseph Juran introduced the dimension of economics to quality by categorizing the costs of quality as "avoidable" and "unavoidable." According to Juran, avoidable costs are associated with defects and product failures, scrapped materials, labor hours for rework and repair, complaint processing, and losses resulting from unhappy customers. Unavoidable costs, he explains, are associated with prevention, inspection, sampling, sorting, and other quality control initiatives. Juran's work provided managers with objective measures for deciding how much to invest in quality improvement.

According to Garvin (1988), Armand Feigenbaum expanded manufacturing quality control in 1956 by proposing a total quality control system, adding product development, vendor selection, and customer service to the existing quality system. Feigenbaum supported reliability engineering designed to prevent defects and to emphasize attention to quality throughout the design process.

Another well-known name in the quality movement is Philip Crosby, who focused on management expectations and human relations. Crosby believed in getting the job done correctly the first time—or zero defects. Zero defects was achieved through training, communicating quality results, goal setting, and personal feedback.

Figure 4-1. Shewhart's PDCA Cycle for Process Improvement

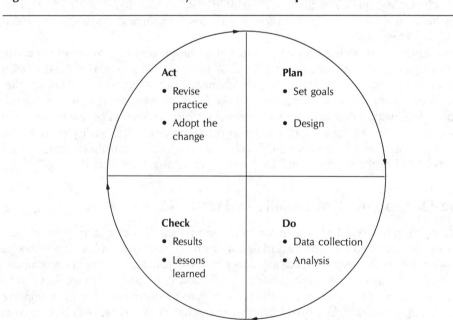

Figure 4-2. Deming's PDCA Cycle

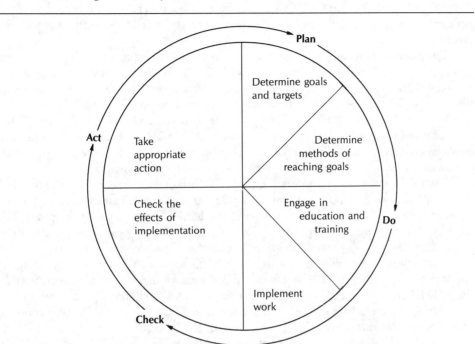

History of JCAHO's Influence on Health Care Quality

Until the late 1980s, the quality process in health care institutions was designed to meet the demands of outside regulations or guidelines. For nutrition and food service departments, reviews have come from the Health Care Financing Administration (HCFA) and the Joint Commission on Accreditation of Healthcare Organizations (JCAHO). The HCFA is responsible for reviewing organizations that serve patients who receive Medicare funds. The JCAHO reviews are educational and must be requested by the facility being surveyed.

The JCAHO has been instrumental in establishing quality guidelines for most health care institutions. Quality assessment (QA), a measure of the quality of clinical care provided to patients, reviews individual practitioner performance and identifies problems. Once viewed as primarily the responsibility of the quality assessment department, QA was often felt to be punitive in nature.

Another component of health care food service quality programs is quality control (QC). Quality control, which works in tandem with quality assessment, is designed to measure the effectiveness of equipment and the quality of products received and served. Maintaining an active QC process is essential for meeting JCAHO and other regulatory standards. Frequently, QC problems have an effect on the quality and appropriateness of care the patient receives.

The JCAHO's accreditation process works this way: An institution asks to be surveyed against a set of standards identified as essential factors that result in safe, effective, high-quality patient care. The standards cover all areas of hospital operations, including hospital and medical staff organizations, environmental safety and security, departmental procedures, and, most important, quality considerations. On the basis of an on-site survey, the JCAHO awards three-year accreditation. It may deny accreditation based on noncompliance to established standards. About three-fourths of the hospitals in the United States have been accredited by the JCAHO.

The Move to CQI in Health Care

The term *continuous quality improvement (CQI)* has been selected by many to identify their quality initiatives. For the purpose of this text, *CQI* will be defined as "the base theory that quality can be improved on a continuous, or never-ending basis," a definition taken from *An Executive's Pocket Guide to QI/TQM Terminology*. The concept of CQI is based on the principle that poor quality is the result of poorly functioning or poorly structured processes that can be improved.

The individual credited with moving continuous quality improvement from the manufacturing arena to health care is Donald Berwick, M.D. Dr. Berwick was co-designer of the National Demonstration Project on Quality Improvement in Healthcare, which was designed using the TQM approach. The project was led by the Harvard Community Health Plan in Boston in the late 1980s and ended in 1991. The demonstration project included 21 health care organizations, many of which have become leaders in TQM. This demonstration project has been credited with beginning the shift that brought more than 60 percent of the health care organizations in this country to continuous quality improvement.

The CQI concept was first introduced in the *JCAHO Accreditation Manual for Healthcare* in 1992. The JCAHO's position is that 95 percent of an organization's problems can be solved through process improvement, and the JCAHO encouraged all hospitals to have some type of CQI process in place by 1994. The remaining 5 percent of problems should be handled through traditional quality assessment and peer review.

With release of the 1994 standards, the JCAHO had renamed the "Quality Assessment and Improvement" chapter as "Organizational Performance Improvement." Representatives for the JCAHO advise hospitals to learn the concepts of CQI without abandoning traditional monitoring and evaluation of QA. This advice means that traditional QA will continue to play a major role in accreditation standards with the JCAHO.

The JCAHO allows that a number of different approaches lead to CQI and that it endorses no one method. However, elements of CQI have been incorporated into the standards for accreditation as follows:

- The key role that leaders (individually and collectively) play in enabling the assessment and improvement of performance
- The fact that most problems/opportunities for improvement derive from process weaknesses, not from individual incompetence
- The need for careful coordination of work across departments and professional groups
- The importance of seeking judgments about quality from patients and other "customers" and using such judgments to identify areas for improvement
- The importance of carefully setting priorities for improvement
- The need for both systematic improvement of the performance of important functions and maintenance of the stability of these functions

Another standard introduced in 1992 addresses education of health care executives in regard to quality improvement. The standard requires facilities to demonstrate that the executive team has acquired education in the approaches and methods of quality improvement. A plan must be in place to demonstrate how the organization will meet quality improvement standards for:

- Setting priorities for quality improvement activities
- Allocating resources for improvement activities
- Training staff members regarding quality improvement
- Fostering better communication and coordination of quality improvement activities
- Determining how the effectiveness of their contributions to quality improvement is analyzed

☐ Meeting JCAHO Standards

The JCAHO releases its *Accreditation Manual for Hospitals* (AMH) once a year. A rating scale of 1 to 5 with NA for not applicable is used to help the institution and the JCAHO surveyor determine the degree of compliance with the standards for each department. An asterisk beside an item in the manual indicates that the item is a key factor in the accreditation process and must be addressed with policies, procedures, and programs.

It is extremely important for an organization routinely surveyed by the JCAHO to obtain a new AMH annually to ensure continued compliance. Some of the changes proposed for 1994 and 1995 have specific impact on nutrition and food service departments and are discussed in the following sections.

Standards Affecting Nutrition and Food Services

In 1993, the JCAHO began to revise the AMH and its standards along process rather than departmental lines with the intent to develop a more concise and practical manual focused on quality of patient care. The manual is divided into three sections: patient care functions, organizational functions, and essential structural components. The 1994 manual contains leftover standards in a fourth section. These standards will be incorporated into the main three chapters by 1995.

In section 4, a dietetic chapter contains specific departmental standards. In addition, standards related to patient and staff education and director leadership are found in chapters dealing with patient and family education, human resource management, and leadership, respectively. In 1995, the JCAHO will move the remaining standards in the chapter titled "Dietetic Services" to the section on patient care functions and change the title to "Nutritional Care."

Standards Related to Patient Care Functions

The chapter titled "Patient and Family Education" includes standards to measure how well organizations provide education to patients, family members, and other caregivers. Topics include safe and effective use of medication; safe and effective use of medical equipment; and drug–food interactions and modified diets, and when to obtain further treatment if needed. The objective of these standards is to ensure that patients are informed sufficiently so as to support their care when they leave the hospital. All discharge instructions must be documented in the medical record and provided to the organization or individual responsible for the patient's continuing care. It is important to note that the JCAHO does not specify which health care practitioner is responsible for providing this education, which leaves a great deal of latitude. Dietitians must work with their organizations to ensure that the appropriate individuals are assigned to provide nutrition education and information on drug–food interactions and modified diets.

In regard to parenteral nutrition, the section on nonsurgical treatment is important to nutrition and food service departments. The proposed standard reads as follows:

> When parenteral nutrition services are provided, mechanisms are designed, implemented, and maintained that address:
>
> - The determination of the therapeutic requirement for parenteral nutrition, based on the patient assessment
> - Initial and ongoing medication orders for parenteral nutrition
> - Preparation and dispensing
> - Administration including implication for patient care
> - Assessment of the parenteral nutrition's effects on the patient

The chapter on patient assessment, also included in the section on patient care functions, states: "All patients who present to the organization for care or treatment are assessed by qualified individuals . . . ongoing throughout the patient's contact with the organization." Although determining the need for assessment of the patient's nutrition status is highlighted in this standard, the term *qualified individual* is not clearly defined and is left to the organization.

55

Standards Related to Organizational Functions

The human resource management chapter includes staff training and education that emphasizes preparing employees for their jobs and maintaining professional competence. Coordinated educational efforts must include information on at least the following topics:

- Organization and department mission, governance, and policies and procedures
- Employee's job description
- Performance expectations
- Plant, technology, and safety management of the organization and the individual employee's role in safety responsibilities (including material safety data sheets)
- The organization's infection control program and the employee's individual role in preventing infections
- The organization's quality assessment and improvement process and the individual employee's role in these activities

Continuing education for employees to maintain knowledge and skill must be provided along specific guidelines, including the patient population served (for example, age), the type and nature of care delivered, and needs of individual staff members. Individual needs are obtained from QA and CQI information, as well as performance reviews, peer review, and safety and infection control activities. Continuing education also is based on advances in technology, health care management, and health care science. Nutrition and food service managers must ensure adequate training and provide documentation of equipment use, infection control, and the prevention of contamination related to food handling. Details of these items are presented in chapters 13 and 14.

The JCAHO standards for dietetic services previously contained requirements for food service directors. These standards are now in the combined chapter on leadership, under organizational functions. The chapter, created to establish uniform expectations for performance of all directors within the institution, outlined specific duties:

- Integration of the department/services into the functions of the organization
- Coordination of the department with other departments
- Development and implementation of policies and procedures that guide and support the provision of services
- Recommendation of sufficient number of qualified and competent persons to provide care/service
- Determination of the qualifications and competence of staff members who provide patient care services
- Assessment and improvement of the quality of care provided by the department
- Maintenance of quality control programs
- Orientation, in-service training, and continuing education of all persons in the department
- Recommendations for needed resources such as space, training, personnel, expertise, or financial support

☐ Creating a Continuous Quality Improvement Culture

To create a culture that fosters CQI, an organization or department must adhere to the principles for creating a participative culture as described in chapter 2. Culture, identified as the way things get done in an organization, influences not only how employees view and perform their jobs and how they work with colleagues, it also influences how they view their customers and how they view quality.

Principles That Drive a CQI Culture

Continuous quality improvement requires integration of quality and change management methods, practices, concepts, and beliefs into the organization's current culture. Adopting any

CQI process means integrating focus on quality into all aspects of the organization, making it everyone's priority. Three principles are essential to establishing a CQI culture:

1. Leadership and commitment from the top
2. Customer orientation and focus
3. Involvement of the total organization in improving quality for customer satisfaction

Leadership and Commitment from the Top

Ideally, an organizational culture that promotes continuous quality improvement has commitment from top leadership, including the board and other management staff. Chief executive officers interviewed by *Hospitals* magazine in June 1992 spent an average of 17 percent of their workweek time directing or reviewing their organization's CQI efforts. It is this type of commitment from upper leadership that is necessary to sustain CQI. Leaders in CQI organizations recognize the need for employee participation and team building. Their role consists of coaching, teaching, facilitating, and empowering.

Creating a CQI environment takes structure, planning, training, trust, patience, rewarding positive change, and, most important, time. Developing a CQI culture can take 5 to 10 years, which is not surprising considering the complexity of most health care organizations. For suggestions on creating a participative environment that empowers employees and fosters teamwork, see chapters 2 and 6.

Gauging commitment from the top may include assembling leadership profiles of all managers and their leadership philosophies and practices. Once the profiles are completed and assessed, training sessions can be developed to address specific areas and move managers toward participative leadership. Some of these areas may include team building, change management, coaching for quality-oriented performance, and developing a customer orientation. Starting at the management level prior to introducing CQI to the entire organization is important; without top-level commitment and support, employees will become frustrated in their attempts to practice CQI.

Leadership commitment must be ongoing, even after implementation of employee CQI practices. Employees will need time to attend scheduled team meetings and carry out improvement plans. Nutrition and food service managers may find it difficult to encourage employee involvement without first leading a few teams as success models. Management is responsible for providing structure by ensuring that all employees participate in training sessions and understand their role in achieving customer satisfaction.

Customer Orientation and Focus

A customer-focused organization recognizes the need to identify and exceed customer expectations. An organization focused on quality improvement recognizes that the purpose of improvement is to provide the best service at the lowest possible cost and that without this value-driven goal customer orientation is futile. Potential customers—individual patients, physicians, and/or managed care organizations—have choices when it comes to selecting health care. Often these choices may conflict. For example, patients may want some say in the health care facility they use and the physician they see. To remain competitive, organizations must seek to be provider of choice for all of these customer groups.

Customers are more likely to take their business elsewhere because of poor service than for any other reason. Changing patronage due to unsatisfactory service is more common than changing due to unsatisfactory quality or cost of the product. Research has shown that customers will even pay more for products if they *perceive* the service to be of excellent quality.

In health care, a customer orientation often has focused only on external customers (patients, for example). However, internal customers include nurses, physicians, laboratory technicians, nurses aides, and a number of other health care professionals. This is especially important to food service managers, who must understand the needs of internal customers and balance them with those of external customers. For example, nurses can influence how patients and their families perceive product service and quality. If nurses are dissatisfied when calling for patient tray service, or if they find the cafeteria service to be inferior, they can affect how the department's service is interpreted by patients and physicians.

An effective technique for helping employees develop a customer focus is to have them meet as a group to identify their customers. Then "customer-focused" posters can be designed and displayed throughout the department as a reminder to new and veteran employees.

Organizationwide Involvement

Although having a quality assurance department staffed by experts is necessary, it is equally important that employees not rely solely on one department to be responsible for quality for the entire organization. Through training programs and management support, organization-wide involvement on the part of each employee can be enhanced. Once employees are trained in teamwork and the tools of quality improvement, they should be encouraged to participate in teams. With this training and support comes accountability. Often employees are reluctant to participate without understanding the importance of their roles. Accountability and employees' value to the organization are conveyed by including guidelines in general duties and responsibilities in job descriptions. Performance appraisal criteria can be set that reward employees for concentrating on customer satisfaction, working in teams, and improving processes.

Characteristics of a CQI Culture

Health care organizations that embrace CQI have been found to have certain cultural characteristics in common. The remainder of this section describes 13 of these characteristics, which are summarized in table 4-1.

Table 4-1. Cultural Traits Shared by CQI Organizations

Characteristic	Summary
Quality definition	Knowing what quality "looks like" in an organization (for example, a statement on how to greet customers)
Business strategy	Business plan incorporating strategies for quality goals and objectives, along with written plans for meeting them
Communication	Two-way flow between employees and leaders
Supplier partnerships	Organization–vendor commitment to provide best value at lowest possible cost
Error-free attitude	Mind-set to "do it right the *first* time—*every* time"
Fact-based management versus result-based management	Process orientation versus outcome (quantity) orientation; long-term effects versus short-term results
Employee empowerment	Employee autonomy, involvement, ownership of work process
Physician involvement	Improved quality of practice patterns through multidisciplinary teamwork, critical paths, physician liaisons
Training and retraining	Continuing education through hands-on learning, cross-functional training, development of in-house expertise, for example
Problem solving through teamwork	Inter- and intradepartmental evaluation, decision making, prioritizing; some accountability to QC
Work process focus	Realization that processes account for 85–95% of problems and that individuals *may or may not* account for remaining 5–15%
Innovation and risk taking	Employee freedom to be creative and experiment without fear of reprisal or job loss
Reward and recognition	Social (verbal congratulations), tangible (success celebrations), symbolic (plaques or pins), acknowledgment for effort and accomplishment

Quality Definition

Each organization, and each of its departments, has defined "what quality looks like" for its products and services. The definition provides a baseline for meeting or exceeding customer expectations for quality. The quality definition is subject to change in tandem with changes in customer population. Once developed (or revised), the quality definition is shared with all employees. Defining quality allows for measurement of whether service provision meets expectations. A quality definition must be accompanied by a policy of how service will be delivered. How quality is defined in food service is addressed fully in the subsection on customer service and satisfaction later in this chapter.

Quality as a Business Strategy

Having incorporated quality as a long-term business strategy, CQI organizations set organizational goals and objectives and require departments to design a plan for meeting and exceeding those objectives. Food service department managers are required to have a written plan for monitoring, measuring, and improving quality. The quality plan should be integrated with the department business plan (see chapter 5).

Communication

Employees in a CQI culture are clear about what direction the organization is taking and are able to articulate both the organization's vision and their department's quality definition. Communication from upper leadership is critical to ensuring continuous improvement because as goals and objectives change, staff members must be informed. Top-level leaders also must convey information on the organization's successes, including its financial status.

Remember, communication also should flow from the bottom up. Employees must feel free to express concerns and to give managers their input on what changes are needed for improvement. Employee-generated communication is a must for quality improvement teams and for interdepartmental teams.

One method for communicating the plan, quality definition, and reporting requirements is an employee handbook or manual that includes a list of trainer–facilitators, references to assist with teamwork and measurement, and forms for reporting and monitoring team activities. A loose-leaf binder should be used so that material can be added to reflect CQI changes. Communication is discussed further in chapter 7.

Supplier Partnerships

A customer orientation requires health care organizations to focus on supplier partnerships from two aspects: the health care organization as a supplier and as a customer. It is important to develop strong relationships with vendors and with purchasing groups that buy their services. As suppliers, health care institutions must prove their ability to offer the best possible care at the lowest cost.

Institutions must develop strong relationships with supply companies so that value becomes more than simply the best price. Quality must become a factor of the product purchased and of the service rendered in delivering that product. Long-term relationships between purchaser and supplier should serve to ensure loyalty on both sides and improved quality and cost savings for all concerned.

The caliber of service offered by food service vendors in turn affects the level of quality and service provided to the department's customers. Before awarding bids or selecting a primary vendor, food service managers must assess vendor flexibility and willingness to understand and meet the needs of the organization's customers. Today, more food vendors practice CQI and customer service and therefore understand that in order to remain competitive and retain business, they must be customer responsive and willing to make adjustments. Food service managers should meet with vendors routinely to share information from their customers or determine other ways to communicate needs. Improvements in products and packaging and the development of new products are possible if suppliers listen and respond to customer needs.

Employees can be key individuals in these supplier partnerships. For example, taste panels can allow employees to sample and compare products prior to making purchasing decisions. Not only will this involve employees and educate them about the product served, taste panels will disclose information regarding product cost. As an added benefit for managers, less time is spent reviewing products, leaving more time to promote employee involvement.

Error-Free Attitude

Organizations must move from a focus on quantity to a focus on quality of work done, thus encouraging an error-free attitude. This includes setting goals for continuously improving results rather than setting productivity/volume thresholds. A *threshold* is the level, pattern, or trend in data that would trigger intensive evaluation. Instead of a single focus on work standards and productivity levels, employee time must be evaluated from a value-added standpoint: Does a few extra minutes spent with a patient or other customer outweigh the cost of completing every task in the allotted time frame? Rather than only viewing a job as completed if it is done "in time," the focus must include the percentage error rate for all tasks completed. That is, if the job is not done right, is it worth doing? In a true CQI environment, employees instead of supervisors are encouraged to inspect the quality of their work.

Creating an environment driven by an error-free attitude also means working proactively to encourage systems by which everyone knows how to reduce variation and eliminate errors. In a proactive culture, employees will seek to avoid mistakes before they happen or at least to prevent their recurrence. A proactive culture asks: Why did this event occur? and determines how it can be corrected or prevented in the future. For example, if a hostess delivered a patient's tray that contained a wrong menu item, she would attempt to determine how the mistake occurred in addition to obtaining the correct item for the patient.

Management by Fact versus Management by Result

Management by fact requires everyone in the organization to understand and regularly use standard tools to measure and improve quality. Later in this chapter, measurement, data collection, and analysis tools will be described. Continuous improvement does not stop at measuring whether the desired outcome was achieved but goes deeper to question whether the intervention was appropriate and whether appropriate skills and level of competence were applied. To do this, managers must have accurate facts about the processes and systems used so as to assist in determining the need for change. These facts provide information about customers and their needs and help determine where processes fall short of achieving satisfaction.

Management by fact is not to be confused with management by result. Management by result, a tradition in American industry, pays little or no attention to the *process* that leads to end results. This type of management is concerned primarily with final outcome and is based on numerical goals. Too frequently, employees and supervisors find ways to meet these short-term numerical goals but at the expense of improving the process for the long term.

Management by result perpetuates short-term thinking that looks for what is accomplished today versus what serves to meet future needs. This type of thinking has caused many health care workers to disagree with the JCAHO and others who use outcome indicators. An *indicator* is a measure whose deviation from accepted standards of care signals the existence of a potential problem with quality. However, outcome indicators can identify areas of concern with a process, so that the process can then be charted and analyzed for improvement needs. Management by fact, then, allows managers to create the best possible results while monitoring the systems and processes involved.

Employee Empowerment

Pro-CQI organizations recognize that the employee closest to the customer knows the customer best. As noted in chapter 2, empowered employees are free to use their creativity to design improvements. Managers must view employees as wanting to do their best and must provide the leadership necessary to assist them.

Establishing expectations for employee involvement starts at a basic level and grows with experience, for example, requiring involvement on at least one quality improvement team for the first year. Accountability should be based on involvement, not necessarily on accomplishment, so that initially, at least, it is more important to help employees feel comfortable working in teams. Another expectation measure for employee involvement is to require cafeteria servers or cashiers to ask a specified number of customers questions regarding wait time, adequacy of menu variety, or their suggestions for menu items. To ensure that the questions asked are consistent and to provide documentation, a standard questionnaire can be developed. Employees also can be responsible for passing out comment cards; for submitting suggestions for improvements or for processes that need analysis; or for brainstorming and then prioritizing a list of processes or customer issues that teams can work on. In the last example, a list of projects can be posted, and employees can sign up to participate in their areas of interest.

Physician Involvement

Physician involvement is critical to long-term culture changes and quality improvement. Health care organizations are unique in that the physician, a major player in the care of the primary customer, is an individual outside of operations. Physician practice patterns are influenced by physicians' trust in operational systems within facilities. For example, if it is difficult to get laboratory results for a simple and inexpensive test, the physician may order a more complex and expensive test, creating a costly pattern of practice that does not improve patient care.

Physician involvement, then, can strengthen multidisciplinary teams. For example, physician involvement is essential in developing critical paths. *Critical paths,* suggested as a means to decrease variation in patient outcome, are standardized specifications for care of the typical patient in the typical situation. They cannot improve quality if they are not interfaced with the hospital's systems. Critical paths (discussed later in the chapter) are designed to reflect the best method of care and must have systems and processes that support them.

Some organizations involve physicians early in the decision-making and implementation phases of CQI. Medical staff participation can be enhanced by including a physician liaison on the quality council (QC) (discussed in the following section) who can assist with coordinating physician participation on quality improvement teams. This individual also can coordinate activities between consultants and management, help establish goals, and assist with data collection and analysis. Key benefits to having a physician liaison are that he or she can be an advocate and a source of expertise for the medical staff. Finally, the liaison can maintain clear communication between the medical staff and the organization while assisting with education of medical staff members regarding hospital improvements and the need for changes in their practice patterns.

Training and Retraining

Organizations committed to CQI recognize that training is an ongoing process and that continuous training is the basis for success. Continued education can be done in a number of ways, but memorization of philosophy and methods alone is not one of them. Learning can be done in a hands-on manner or simulated to bring the activity to life. Both methods allow the participant to learn by doing in a reality-based context. Some of the best learning occurs in small groups where everyone is allowed to participate in applying the techniques learned.

For any CQI initiative to succeed, employees must receive training in the process, methods, and tools used by the institution. Training consultants can be contracted, but to sustain the process and be cost-effective, it is wise to create in-house experts. This can be accomplished with "cascade" training or "train-the-trainer" sessions. With this type of training, a number of managers and/or employees are trained (perhaps by consultants) and they in turn train others in the organization. Thus, those trained become trainers and facilitators for the CQI process.

The role of trainer–facilitators will depend on the CQI process selected. They might conduct overview sessions to familiarize all employees in the organization with CQI, or they might provide guidance to teams and their leaders. As an added benefit, managers involved as trainers further develop their coaching skills, essential for participative management and employee empowerment. This technique provides increased job satisfaction among managers, allowing them to break out of their daily departmental role while enhancing their view of the organization as process oriented across departmental lines.

The trainer–facilitator role becomes increasingly important to cross-functional teams, which often need neutral leadership that can downplay turf battles and lend insight on hospital operations. Specific areas to address in facilitator training include:

- Skills in group dynamics
- Roles and behaviors in meetings
- Interpersonal skills
- The stages of team development (see chapter 6)
- Use of CQI tools for data collection, analysis, and decision making

Trainer–facilitators can provide team members with "just-in-time" training in statistical process or control tools (charts, graphs, diagrams, and the like). This training allows more employees to become involved initially with only the information they need to start the process. As their need for more information grows, trainers can provide it.

Problem Solving through Teamwork

One of the principles of CQI is involving the entire organization in improving quality. This is best accomplished through intradepartmental or interdepartmental teams. Intradepartmental teams usually focus on processes or service areas within one department (sometimes as related to one other department, which acts as a "customer"). Interdepartmental, or cross-functional, teams are formed when a process needs to be evaluated and spans two or more departments.

Intradepartmental teams usually identify the project or process to be worked on. This may be done during an initial meeting of a team created to identify customer needs, or it may be done as a department task. As mentioned earlier, processes and problems can be listed, prioritized, and then posted so that employees can volunteer. Accountability for actions of intradepartmental teams lies with the department manager and the team leader, although team members should have some understanding and "ownership" of the process being studied. The team leader is generally selected by the team or may be appointed by a manager based on the knowledge of an individual. An intradepartmental team can have up to 10 members and usually will include a supervisor. Once they become experienced with CQI, employees can form teams and meet without a supervisor. However, it should be made clear that the progress, actions, and outcomes of the team must be shared with the department manager. Team meetings can take anywhere from 30 minutes up to one hour per week. The life span of intradepartmental teams can vary from short term to indefinite, depending on how productive they are in identifying and addressing CQI issues. Implementation of the team recommendations will be department based and will occur based on complexity. For example, if a team's goal was to decrease the amount of time it takes for a patient to receive a late tray, the action plan may include steps to shorten the time between receiving the order and preparing the tray. All of these steps would occur inside the department.

Interdepartmental (cross-functional) teams are selected based on input and priority level established by the QC, to which they are accountable. Membership (commonly limited to eight members) should be representative of each functional area involved in the process under investigation and should include department managers and supervisors. The team's life span depends on the complexity of the process under investigation and of the recommendations to be implemented. Generally, the team will have to meet for more than one hour per week. The QC should monitor the performance of cross-functional teams to determine whether politics or turf battles might compromise final recommendations. As a rule, the "owners" of the process under study are accountable for implementation of recommendations, with assistance from team members and the QC.

Generally speaking, CQI teams, whether intradepartmental or cross-functional, consist of a team facilitator, team leader, and team members. The facilitator is responsible for providing training and information about the process under study, suggesting tools for problem solving or measurement, providing feedback and support, ensuring equal participation, and, if necessary, mediating and resolving conflicts. A facilitator may not be necessary for every process improvement. For example, an intradepartmental team whose leader has had prior experience in teamwork and understands the fundamentals of process improvement may not need a facilitator.

The leader of a CQI team is responsible for guiding the team to resolution through achieving the desired objectives or problem resolution. Conducting team meetings, providing direction and focus to the team, and keeping the group on track and on time are some of the leader's responsibilities. (It may be necessary to appoint a team member to be a timekeeper to ensure efficient use of time.) The leader also is responsible for conveying the team's need for resources, recommendations, and other concerns to the QC or to management. Documentation and reporting of team activity and progress is an important function of the team leader. A sample team documentation form is shown in figure 4-3.

As already shown, team members should be vested with some sense of ownership in, and knowledge of, the process or problem being investigated. Members provide ideas and different perspectives through their active participation. They must agree to adhere to meeting ground rules, to support the leader, and to support implementation of the recommendations agreed on by the team. Assignments must be performed on time to ensure smooth progress during team meetings. More information for conducting team meetings is provided in chapter 7.

Work Process Focus

Organizations successful in creating a CQI culture understand that processes, not individuals, create inefficiencies or problems. A process is a sequence of events or tasks performed to reach a desired outcome. For example, a patient's receipt of his or her late tray is the outcome of the late tray process, composed of a number of steps from receipt of an order by the food service department to delivery of the tray to the patient. Productivity is improved when unnecessary steps in a process are eliminated or when steps can be combined. Although some processes can be improved by making minor adjustments, others must be replaced or redesigned entirely. Quality management experts estimate that 85 to 95 percent of all problems within an organization are caused by work processes and systems, leaving only 5 to 15 percent that are controlled (not necessarily caused) by individuals. Viewing related tasks as processes provides employees with a broader view of how work is accomplished. This type of thinking allows them to understand that quality of output (outcome) is affected by quality of input (process or system).

Innovation and Risk Taking

Testing the unknown and trying unproven solutions and ideas is another characteristic of a CQI culture. An environment that encourages innovation and experimentation leads to creative thinking on the part of all workers. Once employees are assured that they can take reasonable chances to improve care or service without fear of punishment for failure, more ideas will be tested. Thus, creativity among all department members can be nurtured, rather than depending on the experiences and ideas of a few.

Reward and Recognition

Without properly recognizing and rewarding employees and managers who are successful with CQI initiatives, it will be difficult to sustain their long-term commitment. Rewards and recognition may be social, tangible, or symbolic. Congratulations to a team from the

Figure 4-3. Team Documentation Form

Action Planning Worksheet

Leader:

Team members:

Issue:

Customer:

Satisfier:

Quality requirement:

Action plan:	Responsible person:

Measurements:

Resources needed:

Source: Reprinted with permission of All Saints Health Systems, Fort Worth, TX.

manager or upper leadership is a type of social reward. Celebrations, such as fairs where teams are encouraged to display the work and results of their efforts, are more tangible. Plaques, pins, or ribbons are examples of symbolic reward and recognition for involvement as well as for success. Positive reinforcement is crucial to sustaining long-term empowerment and assisting with success. It is important that the reward and recognition be genuine. Some CQI proponents caution that team-of-the-month awards or other such distinctions may prove counterproductive to the CQI process because they honor only one group among many and create negative competition and possible resentment among those who did not "win." However, these types of programs have also been advocated to establish friendly competition, which leads to larger numbers of staff members becoming involved in the organizational culture.

☐ Role of the Quality Council in CQI Infrastructure

The infrastructure for CQI is the foundation on which it is implemented, that is, the vision for the organization. To create a cultural change, the organization's leadership must send a strong message to emphasize the importance of quality, which includes making quality a key initiative in the strategic- and business-planning process as well as in the budgeting process. The budget must include financial resources necessary for training and rewarding employees.

Creation of an infrastructure, or framework, includes deciding whether there will be a quality council or a steering committee. Individuals on the quality council may vary from one organization to another. One recommended hierarchical structure for membership is as follows:

- Chief executive officer
- Chief operating officer
- Senior executives (line and staff)
- Medical staff liaison
- Quality coordinator or director
- Other members (may include representatives from the medical staff, board of trustees, department heads, and employees)

This type of QC is recommended to be installed for three to five years to assist with implementation and monitoring. Although the council will be important for implementing, monitoring, and nurturing CQI, it may wish to continue the reporting of CQI efforts through the organization's quality assessment committee established to review and monitor the organization's quality assessment activities.

The role of the quality council will evolve with the investigation and implementation of CQI. The initial role will be to create the vision, to develop the quality definition, and to develop the change strategy needed to create a continuous quality culture. This means creating the policies for reporting and monitoring quality initiatives, the plan for training and implementing continuous quality, and method(s) of continuous quality improvement to be adopted.

Once implementation of the CQI effort has begun, the council's role will change to include eliminating barriers, establishing guidelines for team activities, ensuring implementation of appropriate solutions, and supporting medical staff involvement. The QC also may recommend changes in the facility's management structure. The council is an important resource for training, reward and recognition, budgeting guidelines, communication of CQI activities, and ensuring that teams are given the time they need to fulfill their commitments.

As a monitoring body for assessment of CQI progress, the QC communicates plan updates to reflect changing directions based on improvements made. Although reporting may be accomplished through the organization's QA committee, the QC must perform monitoring activities that ensure organizationwide involvement. A sample reporting structure is shown in figure 4-4.

Figure 4-4. CQI Flowchart

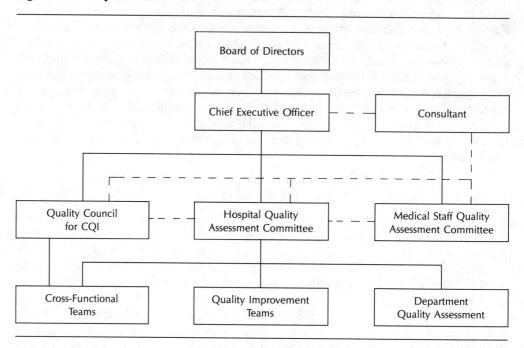

The board of directors reads the flowchart because, to meet JCAHO standards, the board must be informed of quality activities within the organization. Whether an organization is JCAHO certified or not, reporting would likely occur at the board level. The CEO (or his or her designate), the next reporting level, is informed of the implementation and training activities for CQI, of the consultants' progress or role, and of the quality assessment activities of both the medical staff and the hospital.

Although the chart becomes slightly more complicated below the CEO level, keep in mind that the structure is short term. Both the consultants and the quality council will cease to exist when the organization's culture has changed sufficiently to emphasize quality in all activities. Once this transition has been made, the medical staff quality assessment committee and the hospital quality assessment committee will continue to work together and interact with quality improvement teams. Existing hospital and medical staff committees can be utilized to process information or to act as quality teams for process improvement. Nonclinical departments should be included in the reporting process to allow full organizational participation in quality improvement.

The quality council may decide to create critical indicators for the organization to determine whether customer satisfaction is being met. This may include developing and administering—or contracting with an outside source to develop and administer—a customer satisfaction survey. The council must decide whether the survey will be used to assess internal performance only or to benchmark performance against other similar institutions. The QC also will interface with the human resource department to develop a performance management system that supports and encourages participation in quality initiatives by all individuals throughout the institution.

☐ Components of the Food Service CQI Plan

A continuous quality improvement plan for health care nutrition and food services has three components: quality control to ensure safe and wholesome products, customer service, and clinical quality assessment. The following sections describe each component.

Quality Control

Quality assessment measures the overall quality of care delivered to patients, whereas *quality control* as it relates to food service management measures systems for handling, preparing, and serving food. Customer satisfaction is gauged by addressing quality from the customer's point of view, for example, food temperature, appearance, palatability, and nutrition content. The handling, preparation, and service of food also are measured against standards for infection control, aesthetic appeal, and safety. Feedback tools in a quality control program may include the following:

- Sanitation reports (internal, external)
- Safety reports
- Temperatures of refrigerators, walk-in refrigeration units, and dish machines
- Downtime on the tray line
- Cart delivery time
- Trays per labor minute
- Portion control
- Food temperatures
- Patient questionnaires and/or surveys
- Verbal compliments and complaints
- Comment cards
- Observation of customer service as measured against preestablished guidelines
- Timeliness of cafeteria service and other meal service

The quality control program must be adhered to in every food and nutrition service department. If the program is carefully developed, monitored, and evaluated, and if it has built-in routine follow-up procedures, continuous quality improvement and customer satisfaction are enhanced.

A comprehensive quality control program includes written policies and procedures with established standards that help identify strengths and weaknesses in food and service quality. Once standards or guidelines are in place, appropriate training must be completed to convey responsibility and expectations to staff and supervisors. The standards are then utilized to measure compliance so as to ensure consistent and safe operations.

Quality Control of Food Products

The sampling of food products, measurement of food temperatures, and sensory appraisal of product characteristics allow comparison of observed quality with the standard established for each item. Inspection criteria for food production and service include food appearance, taste, texture, and safety and tray appearance. Through evaluation and analysis, food service directors can identify what went wrong, how often, and why. For example, evaluating a patient tray would include making sure that an attractive garnish is present, that the meat is adequately brown, that the vegetables complement the meal in color and are not overcooked, and that everything is at appropriate serving temperature. Then corrective action can eliminate or reduce quality deficiencies.

Success of a quality control program depends on the commitment of all employees to the provision of high-quality food. Quality control activities should be incorporated into regular job routines and duties for each position. For example, each position on the tray line can be responsible for checking temperatures and ensuring that each menu item is attractively served on the plate. Failure of staff members to follow established criteria for food product safety should be documented and addressed. The director should prepare a food service quality checklist as a routine evaluation tool. Figure 4-5 is an example of quality checklist inspection criteria.

Figure 4-5. Inspection Criteria for Food Production and Service

Food appearance

☐ Satisfactory and appropriate color and texture

☐ Pleasing and varied food color/texture combinations

☐ Attractive garnishes

☐ Variety in shape and size of food items

☐ Adequate portion size

Food taste

☐ Pleasant flavor combinations

☐ Taste integrity of each item

☐ Adequate seasoning

☐ No undesirable or odd flavors

☐ Pleasing aroma

☐ Proper temperature

Food texture

☐ No item overcooked or undercooked

☐ Variety of textures

☐ Suitable moisture content

☐ No toughness or stringiness

☐ Suitable for consumers being served

Food safety

☐ Proper hot serving temperatures: for liquids, 185°F (85°C); for cooked cereals, 175°F (79°C); for soups, 180°F (82°C); for meats, 150°F (65°C); for eggs, 145°F (63°C); for vegetables, 160°F (71°C)

☐ Proper cold serving temperatures: for liquids, 35°F (2°C); for solid foods, 45°F (7°C)

☐ Foods prepared and portioned using utensils or disposable gloves to avoid contamination by employees' hands

☐ Two clean spoons used for tasting food products

☐ Special care used in handling clean dishes and flatware to prevent contamination

☐ Unused raw ingredients or cooked leftover foods labeled, refrigerated promptly, and used within 24 to 48 hours, frozen immediately, or discarded

☐ No reuse of single-use utensils and containers

☐ Employees' clothing and personal hygiene at established standards

Tray appearance

☐ Adequate tray size, no overcrowding

☐ Specified setup used

☐ Each item placed on tray correctly and arranged for eating convenience

☐ Dishes and/or flatware in good condition

☐ Food neatly served

☐ Separate dishes for foods that contain liquid

☐ Neat overall appearance, no spills

Tray accuracy

☐ All food items specified on menu present on tray

☐ Food on tray allowed on patient diet

☐ No unnecessary utensils on tray

Customer Service and Satisfaction

Whether it is called guest relations, customer service, or customer relations, the concept is the same. It is estimated that more than 60 percent of the nation's hospitals have introduced some type of customer relations training for their employees. The purpose of these programs is to improve customer satisfaction in order to obtain repeat business and to increase market share through word-of-mouth referrals. Often customer satisfaction is based on the interaction between the customer and service personnel and occurs at the time service is delivered. In this respect, customer satisfaction depends on employee performance. Research conducted on the results of meeting customer needs has shown measurable benefits in profits, cost savings, and market share. Customers often do not complain when they have received less-than-satisfactory service; however, they do tell 9 or 10 other people about the problem. It is estimated that it costs an organization five to six times as much to gain a new customer as it does to keep a current one. To retain current customers while attracting new ones, health care food service managers must strive toward two goals. First, they must instill in employees the fact that customer orientation drives customer satisfaction. Next, they must design and launch a strategic quality service plan.

From Customer Orientation to Customer Satisfaction

To embrace the concept of customer relations, employees must first recognize that they have customers. Customers include patients, residents, their families and significant others, physicians, and other staff members. The thought of identifying a patient as a customer has been disconcerting for some health care professionals, but without viewing patients as end users of their services, providers do nothing more than develop systems and processes for their own convenience. Although these systems and processes may be based on the best medical practice and perceived need, they often are created at the expense of customer satisfaction. Referring to patients as customers recognizes their autonomy and capability of demanding high-quality care and information about the services they buy.

The nutrition and food service department can play a key role in developing a positive image for patients and their caregivers. Although much of what customer/patients come in contact with in the hospital setting is technical and beyond their general understanding, food is the one thing they *do* know. They know whether the food is prepared to their satisfaction, whether it is delivered when they are hungry, whether it is at the right temperature, and whether the person delivering the meal is polite and attentive to their needs. Therefore, it is vitally important for the food service manager to ensure that staff understand their role in customer satisfaction.

Although the customer/patient is certainly a key focus, this is not the only type of customer encountered by food service employees. Physicians, family members, and other hospital staff are served in the cafeteria, physician dining rooms, coffee shops, and so on. Service quality can be compromised not only because it may be difficult to persuade food service staff to accept other hospital employees as customers but also because satisfaction is based on customer expectations and perceptions. By comparing their expectations of service quality with actual service delivery, they judge whether satisfaction has been attained.

From Service Plan to Customer Satisfaction

In the book *Service America,* Karl Albrecht and Ron Zemke identify three features of outstanding service organization:

1. A defined, customer-focused service strategy
2. Customer-oriented frontline employees
3. Customer-friendly systems

It is impossible to expect employees to provide exemplary service if no quality service plan or strategy is in place. A service strategy is based on feedback from the customer and also on the organization's strategy and mission. The plan should include a written statement or mission that all employees can understand and support. A health care food service strategy may include the following elements:

- Greeting customers appropriately, making eye contact
- Extending extra effort to be helpful
- Providing timely and prompt service
- Listening to customers' needs and responding to them
- Maintaining appropriate appearance according to departmental policy
- Maintaining a safe and pleasant environment
- Providing what was promised

Once the departmental strategy is written, employees must be trained to deliver the service as outlined. Training may be done through modeling behavior, scripting phrases for greeting customers, or practical examples of ways to handle specific customer issues or requests. This strategy and training are useful in developing customer-oriented frontline employees.

Comment cards on patient trays or on cafeteria tables can be used to identify what customers want. Traditionally, institutional food service has been viewed as less than satisfactory by the general public, a perception confirmed by national surveys on hospital food service. This perception can be overcome by a commitment to ask customers consistently what they want and whether their expectations are being met. This can be done with written surveys or, for inpatients or residents, through one-on-one interviews during meal rounds. Cafeteria customers can be given a written survey or asked by frontline employees to participate in a focus group to gauge their acceptance of meal items and the quality of service provided.

Used consistently as monitoring and measuring devices for service performance, these feedback mechanisms keep managers up to date regarding customer perception of timeliness of meal service, temperature of food items, and staff courtesy. Once surveys are tabulated, they should be analyzed for potential problem areas so that action plans can be created and implemented for improvement. Ongoing surveys provide feedback to determine in turn whether the action plans were effective.

Customer-friendly systems are based on understanding what the customer wants, and in a quality-oriented and participative work environment, feedback is encouraged so as to get this information. Employees are best positioned to know which systems or processes are not customer friendly and in some instances can work around these systems to offer better service. Policies and procedures are developed to ensure safe, consistent service, but before being implemented they should be evaluated from both the customer and employee points of view so that management can evaluate how relevant these guidelines are to promoting customer satisfaction. Once a system or process is identified as not being customer friendly, the customers' input must be obtained to correct the situation.

Clinical Quality Assessment

The quality assessment (QA) program, according to the JCAHO, is an ongoing, planned, and systematic process to monitor and evaluate the quality and appropriateness of patient care. It is used to improve clinical patient care and to identify problems. The minimum requirements of the QA plan include:

- The use of relative indicators or performance measures
- Ongoing monitoring (that is, a process that tracks QA system components to determine the system's level of compliance to the indicators)
- Analysis of performance data against reference data bases (benchmarking)
- The use of multidisciplinary teams when processes and systems are being evaluated across departmental lines
- The use of individual peer review when the performance of an individual practitioner is being evaluated
- Annual review and revision of the plan to ensure effectiveness

Although the JCAHO appears to be moving away from thresholds, currently it requires ongoing monitoring against established thresholds. Continuous quality improvement, on the other hand, emphasizes changing the target as improvement occurs. However, ongoing monitoring is compatible with the quality control aspects of CQI. The JCAHO is looking for sustained improvement over time, and if the threshold is met consistently, monitoring can be deferred until a later date but must occur again to ensure sustained improvement or compliance.

The JCAHO still emphasizes the concept of individual competency, that good results occur when competent people work in effective systems. The JCAHO also recognizes that ineffective systems can hinder good performance and results. Thus, when individual weaknesses do occur, the organization is expected to identify them and provide guidance or training for improvement.

Peer review continues to be a part of the JCAHO's standards, indicating the persistent need for professional judgments in the review of process and of individual performance. The best judgments must be made based on the latest information available. Those best qualified to determine whether the best judgment was made are peers, in the JCAHO's view.

JCAHO's 10-Step Process for Developing a Department Plan

Figure 4-6 shows the JCAHO's 10-step process for continuous quality improvement. Although the JCAHO no longer requires this approach, the model does provide a starting point for developing a plan to blend CQI and traditional QA.

Step 1 assigns responsibility for quality activities. The new emphasis on CQI means that in addition to identifying departmental responsibility, the organization's leadership is responsible for the oversight and coordination of all quality-related efforts. This coordination allows the best utilization of resources and helps ensure that all parties to the process are included on the teams.

Step 2 identifies the department's scope of care, that is, those functions or activities having the greatest impact on the care patients receive. To incorporate CQI, this section should be expanded to include the scope of service for patients and other customers. This section takes into consideration the type of patients (including age) served. For food service departments this would include everyone who receives meal service along with where the service is provided.

Step 3 identifies the important aspects of care and service, using the scope of care and service delineated in step 2. Important aspects are high-priority key functions, processes, treatments, and activities to be monitored. Items should be selected based on their high-frequency, high-risk nature, or because they are problem-prone aspects of care. Clinical examples may include nutrition education or hyperalimentation. Service items may include patient meal temperature maintenance processes or late tray delivery.

Step 4 requires that indicators be established for each important aspect of care and service identified in step 3. Indicators are used to measure deviation from accepted standards or thresholds and help to identify potential quality problems. Although the indicator is the overall measurement of quality care, it may consist of several criteria that must be met and are the basis of monitoring and evaluation. Criteria, usually a series of questions that can be answered yes or no, must be objective, valid, preestablished, and measurable.

Step 5 requires that thresholds be established for each indicator identified. Thresholds continue to be stressed by the JCAHO but should not be the only method used to trigger further evaluation and investigation. When an issue is resolved to 100 percent satisfaction of the team or management, it should be revisited after an appropriate period to ensure sustained improvement. Another important point to remember when using thresholds is that customer expectations and needs change over time. Therefore, even if the threshold is met 100 percent of the time, the customer may not be satisfied with service. Customer service and quality are moving targets, assessable only by continued customer feedback.

Step 6, data collection and analysis, includes collecting feedback from ongoing monitoring as well as from customer satisfaction information, meal rounds, and patient contacts. Once

71

Figure 4-6. JCAHO 10-Step Process for Quality Assessment and Continuous Quality Improvement

Step 1: Assign Responsibility
Current: Each department/service is assigned responsibility for overseeing and carrying out monitoring and evaluation within the department.
For CQI: Organization leaders oversee the design of, and foster an approach to, CQI, which includes both intra- and interdepartmental activities.
Step 2: Delineate Scope of Care and Service
Current: Each department/service delineates its separate scope of care.
For CQI: Add scope of service (customers).
Step 3: Identify Important Aspects of Care/Standards
Current: Identify high-volume, high-risk, and problem-prone aspects of care.
For CQI: In addition, identify high-priority key functions, processes, treatments, and activities to be monitored for service.
Step 4: Identify Indicators/Standards
Current: Identify indicators to correspond to the important aspects of care.
For CQI: Action teams of inter- or intradepartmental experts identify indicators for service.
Step 5: Establish Thresholds for Evaluation
Current: Establish the level, pattern, or trend in data for each indicator that would trigger intensive evaluation.
For CQI: Statistical methods are emphasized; therefore, thresholds are not the only way evaluation is triggered.
Step 6: Collect and Organize Data
Current: Establish a data-collection methodology.
For CQI: Data collection includes feedback from sources other than ongoing monitoring for evaluation and improvement (for example, patient surveys).
Step 7: Initiate Evaluation
Current: Care is intensively evaluated only when the threshold for a given indicator is reached.
For CQI: Evaluation occurs when any opportunity for improvement presents itself. Teams are established to evaluate patient care and service according to customer feedback.
Step 8: Take Action to Improve Care or Service
Current: Those with authority take action, based on recommendations of those who evaluate care.
For CQI: Emphasis on process improvement, especially between departments. Action taken by employees as well as managers.
Step 9: Assess Effectiveness of Action for Improvement
Current: Continued monitoring determines if action was effective.
For CQI: Emphasis is placed on ensuring that improvement is sustained over time.
Step 10: Communicate Results to QA Committee and Others
Current: Results reported to hospital QA committee, which disseminates the findings as necessary.
For CQI: Findings of those performing monitoring and evaluation are forwarded to the QA committee and to involved individuals or teams. The QA committee also disseminates information as necessary.

data are gathered, *step 7*—evaluating the data for trends—follows. Trending identifies repetition or patterns of a specific problem. Once the trend (or trends) has been established, a focused analysis or evaluation should be written documenting the outcome of efforts expended to provide improved quality of care. This step also may include convening a team to further evaluate or provide action on the trend identified. This action represents *step 8* of the plan. If the trend is related to inadequate staff knowledge, for example, appropriate training and counseling efforts should be undertaken to prevent recurrence of the problem. Once an action plan has been identified and implemented, follow-up monitoring should be completed to assess whether the action was effective, which constitutes *step 9*.

Step 10 concerns the reporting of quality activities within the facility. Quality assessment reporting by JCAHO standards requires that information be processed through a hospitalwide committee for dissemination of findings as appropriate. The department's plan, policies, reports, and action plans should be documented and kept in the department. Reports should be completed at the end of each quarter for the hospital committee and should be shared with the department quality committee. Reports are the documented results of the monitoring and evaluation process. Although there is no JCAHO requirement for a department quality committee, results of the findings must be shared and discussed with staff members for their input.

If a department committee is established, membership should be representative of all levels of the department's clinical management and food service units. This committee may participate in establishing criteria and monitoring procedures as well as in analyzing and evaluating the results of action plans, making recommendations for change, performing follow-up activities, resolving problems, and identifying trends. Minutes of all committee meetings become a part of the overall program documentation.

In an environment of participative management with an organizationwide focus on quality, teams and managers will share information with individuals as necessary. If another department is involved in the process or issue under investigation, members of that department should be included on the team to establish the criteria used for monitoring. This prevents one department's performance from being monitored by another department.

☐ Methods and Tools for Assisting with CQI

Health care quality programs are following many paths to provide improved care at the lowest cost. Some programs strictly adhere to the TQM model established for industry, and others adapt some of the tools from TQM or other methods. Alternative methods in use include (but are not limited to) critical paths, comparative outcome measures, case management, and process reengineering. This section will first examine the role of consultants and their value to the CQI effort. Then a brief overview of each of the four cited tools and methods of achieving CQI will be presented.

The Role of Consultants

As more health care organizations implement a CQI process, more individuals will become proficient in its implementation and facilitation. When this occurs, consultants may not be the first choice for health care institutions, especially if the organizations have strong management teams capable of coaching, teaching, and facilitating. However, it may be necessary for an organization to contract consultants to begin the quality improvement process. If this is the case, care should be taken to ensure that dependence on their expertise is not created. As soon as possible, the organization should move to in-house trainer–facilitators to promote a sense of ownership and to reduce cost. Consultants should be selected based on the quality of their training materials and on their commitment to make the organization self-reliant. Future support from the consulting firm also must be considered. For example, if the company continues to revise and update training materials, what provision will be made for the health care facility to acquire those materials?

A consultant can be beneficial to a facility seeking to implement a CQI process. The consultant can serve many roles and offer an outside unbiased assessment of the organization. Roles might include:

- Providing expert advice and information on CQI processes as they relate to health care
- Providing information about what has and what has not worked based on their experiences with other health care institutions
- Using their expertise and objectivity to identify barriers and problems within the organization that may hamper the implementation of CQI
- Assisting with an audit or assessment of organizational culture and acting as an agent of change to move to a culture that supports CQI
- Assisting individual managers and departments that may have difficulty accepting or persuading employees to accept the CQI philosophy
- Providing initial training and assisting in-house trainer–facilitators with techniques for becoming self-sufficient
- Customizing quality processes and concepts to meet the needs of the facility
- Serving as continued outside support for training material, networking with other facilities, and promoting a positive image of the organization and its CQI efforts

Before hiring a consultant, management must evaluate the pros and cons of its decisions. On the positive side are those reasons cited above. In addition, an outside consultant may be seen as more knowledgeable and creditable than anyone inside the organization. To "groom" an internal expert will be both time-consuming and costly. Even after he or she is trained, an in-house expert may be confronted with organizational politics and/or resistance from managers who reject them as experts. Qualified outside consultants can speed the learning process, thus accelerating the CQI effort. Though sharing information from other industries is helpful, it is important that the consultant hired have experience in health care. If hired specifically for food service, the consultant should be knowledgable of health care food service operations. Finally, a consultant can help assess readiness of the management team and the organization to move toward a quality-focused culture.

Disadvantages to using a consultant also must be weighed before the decision is made. Using consultants can be expensive for the organization and, if not handled carefully, consultant dependency can occur. Because the consultant is there to answer all the questions that arise, internal knowledge may be slow to develop and employees may be slow to take ownership of the process. Ownership also may be hampered because employees view the approach as canned and not responsive to the organization's individual needs. This may lead them to believe that once the consultants are gone, the "program" will be over and gone. In addition, consultants unfamiliar with the priority of organizational commitments may fail to consider the time constraints on managers.

Total Quality Management

Total quality management provides the techniques, concepts, and tools to analyze data for application in continuous quality improvement. The tools of TQM help identify and analyze current processes either within or across departmental lines. Once data are collected and analyzed, steps can be taken to improve a complex process. Unnecessary or non-value-added steps can be eliminated and the process streamlined to provide better care or service.

TQM Tools

Statistics-based process control is the foundation of total quality management. Tools of TQM, such as flowcharts, pareto charts, and cause-and-effect diagrams, provide a common statistical language and visual aids when analyzing a process or problem. Not all TQM tools are required to evaluate any one process or problem, and only those that clearly will facilitate decision making should be selected for the issue in question. Quality improvement tools can be broken into two general categories: those used for *problem identification* and those used for *problem analysis*. However, some tools can be used for problem identification *and* analysis.

Tools used for problem identification include flowcharts and brainstorming. Recall from chapter 2 that brainstorming is a group session devoted to sharing ideas and information without judging their value. A top-down flowchart is explained in chapter 5. Another type of flowchart is a detailed flowchart, used to identify steps or tasks in a process. This flowchart may identify the current path or establish a new road map or direction. Flowcharts are usually drawn using squares, rectangles, diamonds, and circles, with circles specifying the beginning and final steps in the process. Squares or rectangles represent the in-between steps, and diamonds represent decision points and questions. Flowcharts are beneficial in that they disclose duplicate steps and steps that can be combined or performed in a different order to prevent unnecessary feedback loops. *Feedback loops* are steps or events that require a product or customer to return to a previous step in the process. An example of a flowchart for the late tray process is shown in figure 4-7.

Tools used for problem identification or analysis include pareto charts, cause-and-effect diagrams, and run charts. A *pareto chart* is simply a bar graph used to prioritize problems and determine which should be solved first. In constructing a pareto chart, categories must be designed and the unit of measure (for example, hour, error, dollar, or job category) selected. After data are gathered they must be broken down, or aggregated, by category; items should be ranked in descending order from left to right. Efforts can then focus on the categories with the greatest impact or frequency. An example of a pareto chart reflecting the problems associated with late tray delivery is provided in figure 4-8.

Cause-and-effect diagrams, also called *fishbone* or *Ishikawa* diagrams, are used to represent the relationship between an effect and all the possible causes contributing to it. Team brainstorming may be used to create a fishbone diagram. Causes are generally divided into four categories: materials, methods, equipment, and employees. An example of a cause-and-effect diagram related to late tray delivery is provided in figure 4-9.

A *run chart* can be used to identify trends or shifts over several observation periods. Run charts provide information regarding long-range averages to determine whether changes are occurring. This allows for investigation of increases and decreases in averages. For example, a run chart can disclose the number of patients over a 12-month period who waited longer than 15 minutes to receive a late tray. Figure 4-10 charts this scenario.

Another common tool used for problem analysis is the control chart. *Process control charts* are run charts that allow the use of probability and statistics to set upper and lower control limits for tasks in order to study those above or below the norm. The control chart assists in determining which variations are acceptable and to be expected versus those that are unacceptable. Unacceptable variations are usually unpredictable and are related to a special cause. Correction of the variation will require removal of the special cause. Acceptable or expected variations are usually caused by the process itself, and the only way to correct these variations is to change the process. Special causes must be eliminated before the control chart can be used as a monitoring tool because as a monitoring tool, chart measurements are expected to stay between the upper and lower limits established. For example, the start of a tray line may be within plus or minus 10 minutes of the preestablished time. If a time occurs outside this control, investigation should occur (see figure 4-11, p. 78).

Some food service employees may require training in proper use of improvement process tools of TQM. A manager or supervisor should work with these individuals to model the behavior of conducting a meeting, using the tools, and making decisions for improvement based on the results.

Figure 4-7. Flowchart for Patient Late Tray Process

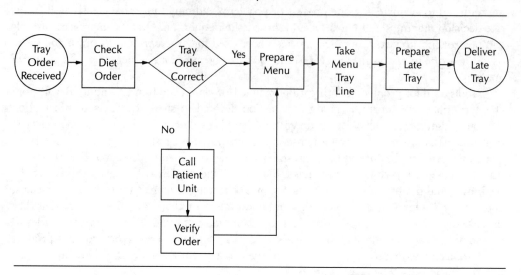

Figure 4-8. Pareto Chart – Problems Associated with Patient Late Trays

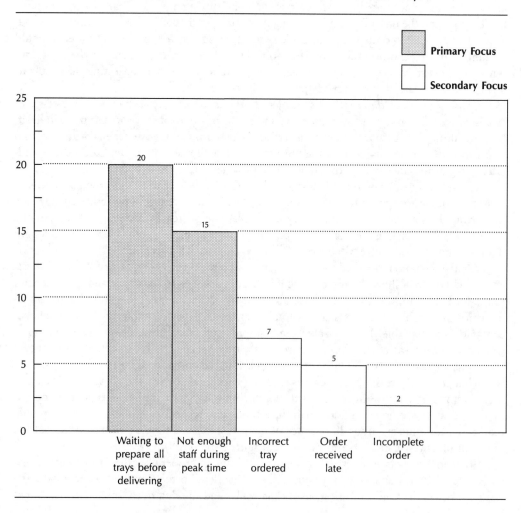

Figure 4-9. Cause-and-Effect Diagram for Patients Not Receiving Late Trays

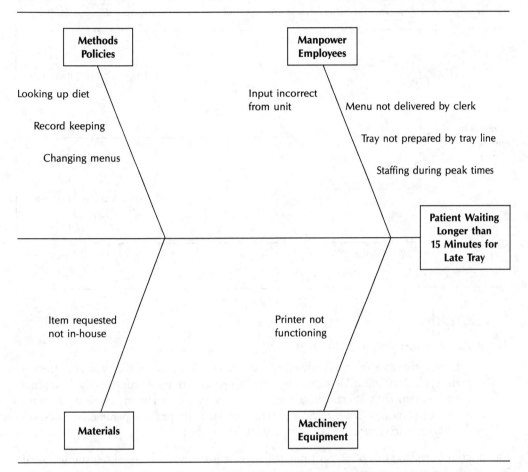

Figure 4-10. Run Chart for Late Trays Longer than 15 Minutes

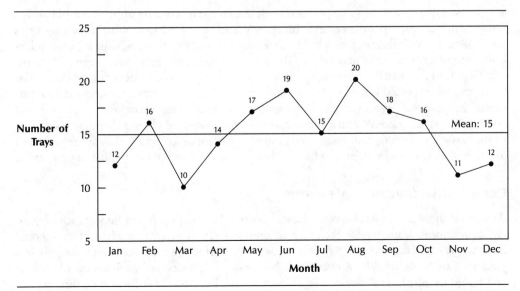

Figure 4-11. Control Chart of Tray Line Start Times

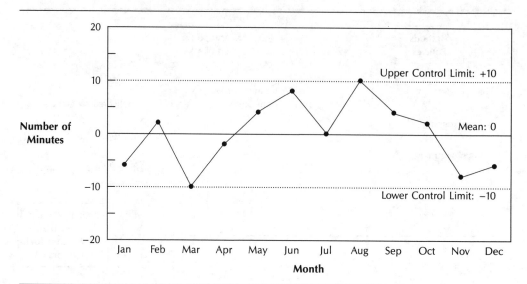

Critical Paths

The JCAHO defines *critical paths* as a

> Descriptive tool or standardized specification(s) for care of the typical patient in the typical situation; developed by a formal process that incorporates the best scientific evidence of effectiveness with expert opinion. Synonyms or near-synonyms include clinical policy, clinical standard, parameter (or practice parameter), protocol, algorithm, review criteria, and preferred practice pattern.

Interdisciplinary standards of care for particular patient types can be used to establish quality criteria for measurement. If data bases that include a large number of facilities are utilized, practice patterns can be developed and tracked for improved patient outcomes. Dietitians should be involved in developing critical paths to ensure that the appropriate nutritional intervention is included.

These types of protocols or practice guidelines provide a means of bringing physicians into continuous quality improvement. Independent of the TQM movement, for many years the American Medical Association has been a proponent of practice guidelines. These guidelines become critical paths and help to define when there are variations in care. Once the critical paths have been used for long periods of time, it is possible to identify expected variations versus unexpected variations in care and outcome. Critical paths are used to reduce variations in treatment from a clinical standpoint. However, these variations should not just concentrate on variations of practitioners but also on the hospital systems that may contribute to the variations. Health care institutions must pay attention to operational systems as well as to clinical systems in order to effect a true picture of continuous quality improvement.

Comparative Outcome Measures

As stressed throughout this chapter, information and data are of primary importance in quality improvement. Data provide the information necessary to determine where efforts should be concentrated. Severity-adjusted data bases have become more common over the past few years and are being used by a number of businesses to provide comparisons on physicians and hospitals during provider contract negotiations. Health care institutions, through cooperative partnerships, have established comparative data bases to assess variations in practice patterns that are used as indicators of quality. Through the use of these data bases, hospitals can determine which diagnosis-related groups should receive special emphasis and will have the greatest return in improving patient care and reducing associated costs.

Standards established by data bases with many contributing hospitals can provide information on length of stay, charge or cost of care, and mortality. This information can be used to focus quality initiatives within a facility. Morbidity can be indirectly assessed by length of stay. No outcome data currently in use can define absolute medical quality, but measurements of these aspects of quality can be useful for physicians and health care organizations to use their time and other resources more wisely and begin problem solving. Such comparisons must be adjusted for severity against an established norm. There is no consensus among health care practitioners regarding the use of severity-adjusted data bases because of fear that not every variation between facilities can be taken into consideration and boiled down for a simple comparison. However, these types of comparisons seem inevitable, and at least 12 states currently have established severity-adjusted data bases.

The federal government uses a similar data base, called MEDPAR, with Medicare patient information. Although proponents recognize that only practitioners with the patient and chart in front of them can truly define the quality of care, they think that some aspects of care are measurable.

Case Management

Closely related to critical paths is the concept of case management, which furthers continuous quality initiatives by allowing coordinated prospective review of patient care, that is, review *prior to* admission. A case manager participates in planning for a patient's admission, monitoring the concurrent stay using critical paths and retrospectively evaluating the stay after discharge. A nurse or other health care professional is responsible for coordinating all aspects of care during the patient's stay.

Case management is seen as a method to improve inpatient care, decrease length of stay, reduce rate of readmission and/or negative outcome, and provide cost-effective care. Discharge planning begins at the time of admission to ensure a smooth transition to home with no additional care, to home with home care services, or to a long-term care facility.

Process Reengineering

Total quality management stresses utilization of statistical tools to identify and modify work processes on a continuous basis. These modifications are generally incremental in nature and implemented over short time frames. Process reengineering, on the other hand, makes radical changes by creating new processes to replace inefficient ones. Accomplished through team effort in a concentrated time frame and generally taking longer than the time needed to make minor quality improvements, process reengineering is most useful when the scope of the project is cross-functional and complex. Reengineering may require a structural change as well as a cultural change in the organization. Rather than using statistical tools, a modeling process using computer technology is utilized.

Process reengineering is an analytical approach to quality improvement, with analysis occurring from the top down. For example, the late tray process diagrammed in figure 4-7 would begin with providing a patient with a late tray. From this point the various steps would be charted with second-level steps and possibly even substeps to the process. This breakdown allows for each activity to be subcategorized to the lowest level necessary to facilitate transformation or improvement. Process reengineering also provides information regarding the inputs to the process, outputs of the process, controls affecting the process, and mechanisms used to complete the process.

☐ Summary

In the past, health care institutions measured the quality of clinical care with an emphasis on quality assessment (QA). Quality assessment focused on reactive or retrospective monitoring of individual variance and performance. The recent emphasis on continuous quality improvement (CQI) views quality in terms of both process improvement and customer perspective.

Continuous quality improvement is influenced by regulatory agencies, but a quality-committed organization will practice it with or without outside influence. Benefits of CQI include customer satisfaction, employee morale through involvement and ownership, and a cost-effective business approach that offers better value to the customer. The best reason for an organization to adopt a CQI agenda is to compete at a higher level, improve quality, and reduce cost.

An organization can expect to generate from 20 to 30 percent in cost savings by implementing a CQI process. The costs of implementing a CQI process include the labor for training and conducting team meetings, training materials, and possibly the use of a consultant. These costs are more than offset by the savings generated when processes are improved to decrease non-value-added steps. It should be noted that occasionally the solution to a process or system problem will end up costing more in the short term to correct than to leave it as is. But when the cost of the solution is considered over the long term, with the customer in mind and in regard to total savings from process improvement, it may be determined to be the best solution.

☐ Bibliography

Albrecht, K., and Zemke, R. *Service America.* Homewood, IL: Dow Jones-Irwin, 1985.

Anderson, C. A., and Daigh, R. A. Quality mind-set overcomes barriers to success. *Healthcare Financial Management* 45(2):21–23, Feb. 1991.

Brown, B. J., and Lehmann, R. S. Case management: a product line. *Nursing Administration Quarterly* 15(2):16–20, Winter 1991.

Causey, W. B. Accreditation leading to evolution of alternate CQI model. *Quality Improvement through Total Quality Management* 2(9):136–38, Sept. 1992.

Causey, W. B. *An Executive's Pocket Guide to QI/TQM Terminology.* Atlanta: American Health Consultants, 1992.

Causey, W. B. Business coalitions pushing Deming-style "bonding" with hospitals. *Quality Improvement through Total Quality Management* 2(9):129–31, Sept. 1992.

Causey, W. B. Cascade training provides trained facilitators, improved morale among managers. *Quality Improvement through Total Quality Management* 2(7):101–03, July 1992.

Causey, W. B. Clinical guideline movement merging with, supporting TQM. *Quality Improvement through Total Quality Management* 2(12):179–80, Dec. 1992.

Causey, W. B. Converting patients to customers a hard struggle in health care. *Quality Improvement through Total Quality Management* 3(1):8–10, Jan. 1993.

Causey, W. B. CQI or QA? JCAHO having difficulty communicating its position. *Quality Improvement through Total Quality Management* 2(11):161–62, Nov. 1992.

Causey, W. B. Joint Commission says it has not shifted back to QA. *Quality Improvement through Total Quality Management* 2(12):182–83, Dec. 1992.

Causey, W. B. Joint Commission says some people are getting the wrong CQI message. *Quality Improvement through Total Quality Management* 2(7):99–101, July 1992.

Causey, W. B. Severity-adjusted databases gaining favor as TQM tools. *Quality Improvement through Total Quality Management* 2(9):131–33, Sept. 1992.

Causey, W. B. Small hospitals face unique challenges in implementing TQM. *Quality Improvement through Total Quality Management* 2(7):108–10, July 1992.

Causey, W. B. Tracing the cost of quality isn't hard, two hospitals show. *Quality Improvement through Total Quality Management* 2(11):163–65, Nov. 1992.

Causey, W. B. Tremendous strides made but there is still a long way to go, experts say. *Quality Improvement through Total Quality Management* 2(12):173–75, Dec. 1992.

Causey, W. B. Warning: TQM can fail—how to see it coming. *Quality Improvement through Total Quality Management* 2(11):165–66. Nov. 1992.

Causey, W. B. You can't separate administrative, clinical systems, TQM experts say. *Quality Improvement through Total Quality Management* 3(1):1–8, Jan. 1993.

Crosby, P. B. *Let's Talk Quality.* New York City: McGraw-Hill, 1989.

Deming, W. E. Improvement of quality and productivity through actions by management. *National Productivity Review* 2(1):12–22, 1982.

Dougherty, D. A. Joint Commission accreditation manual for hospitals. *Hospital Food & Nutrition Focus* 9(3):1–5, Nov. 1992.

Dougherty, D. A. Reorganization of JCAHO's standards manual slated for 1995 finalization. *Hospital Food & Nutrition Focus* 9(7):1–4, Mar. 1993.

Dougherty, D. A. The new JCAHO standards for information management. *Hospital Food & Nutrition Focus* 9(8):4–5, Apr. 1993.

Espinosa, J. Physician's notebook: developing protocols leads to effective quality indicators. *Quality Improvement through Total Quality Management* 2(9):142–44, Sept. 1992.

Garvin, D. A. *Managing Quality: The Strategic and Competitive Edge.* New York City: The Free Press, 1988.

Gaucher E., and Kratochwill, E. The progress in total quality of the original 21 participating organizations, National Demonstration Project on Industrial Quality Control and Health Care Quality. *Journal of Quality and Participation,* Jan.–Feb. 1991, pp. 32–34.

Hammer, M., and Champy, J. *Reengineering the Corporation.* New York City: Harper-Collins Publishers, 1993.

Hillman, A. L. Continuous quality improvement and total quality management. *Quality Health Care & Outcomes* 1:4–5, Oct. 1991.

Hogue, M. A. Guidelines to service quality control. *Hospital Food & Nutrition Focus* 6(7):1–4, Mar. 1990.

Joint Commission on Accreditation of Healthcare Organizations. *1993 Joint Commission Accreditation Manual for Hospitals.* Vol. II, *Scoring Guidelines.* Oak Brook Terrace, IL: JCAHO, 1992.

Joint Commission on Accreditation of Healthcare Organizations. *Proposed 1994 Joint Commission Accreditation Manual for Hospitals.* Vol. II, *Scoring Guidelines.* Oak Brook Terrace, IL: JCAHO, 1992.

Juran, J. M. *Quality Control Handbook.* New York City: McGraw-Hill, 1951.

Kazemak, E. A., and Charney, R. M. Quality enhancement means total organizational involvement. *Healthcare Financial Management* 45(2):15, Feb. 1991.

Koska, M. T. JCAHO introduces three new areas of survey concentration. *Hospitals* 66(19):62–66, Oct. 5, 1992.

Leebov, W., and Scott, G. *Service Quality Improvement: The Customer Satisfaction Strategy for Health Care.* Chicago: American Hospital Publishing, 1994.

Martin, C. A., and Dent, J. N. The impact of TQM implementation on JCAHO accreditation. *Total Quality Management* 18(4):357–63, Apr. 1993.

Rodriguez, S. Culture shock—the road to TQM. *Quality Management* 58(4):8–9, July–Aug. 1992.

Scholtes, P. R. *The Team Handbook: How to Use Teams to Improve Quality.* Madison, WI: Joiner Associates, 1988.

Sinnen, M. T., and Schifalacqua, M. M. Coordinated care in a community hospital. *Nursing Management* 22(3):38–42, Mar. 1991.

Walton, M. *The Deming Management Method.* New York City: Dodd, Mead & Company, 1986.

Chapter 5

Planning
and Decision Making

☐ Introduction

Planning has been identified as the first function or step in management and is applicable at all levels of management. Generally speaking, the higher the level of management, the more time is spent in formal planning activities. Formal planning is performed on a regular time cycle by a group of people working together. Formal planning involves the use of systematic procedures and comprehensive data and is recorded in writing. Upper management may spend as much as 50 percent of the time planning, compared to less than 10 percent by first-line managers. *Planning* can be defined as the process of identifying expected outcomes and determining possible courses of action utilizing appropriate resources to achieve the desired outcome.

Planning involves setting goals and objectives for the organization and/or its various units. A *goal* is a broad term used to describe what an organization hopes to accomplish over a relatively long period. *Objectives* are more concrete and specific statements of how an organization or a unit in the organization intends to accomplish a goal. In addition to setting goals and objectives, planning involves developing strategies. *Strategies* are precise action plans for achieving the organization's goals and objectives while making the best use of its resources.

Health care food service planning is designed to support organizational goals or mission, meet customers' needs, and provide for efficient and effective utilization of departmental resources. To accomplish this, planning must respond to the demands of the external and internal environmental trends and issues addressed in chapter 1. Knowledge of these trends allows the manager to be proactive in establishing future objectives and strategies or action plans that take advantage of projected shifts in the business environment. Planning sets the framework within which the other management functions—decision making, organizing, staffing, leading, and controlling—can be accomplished.

Planning applies to diverse activities in the food service department and varies in complexity from writing an annual business plan to preparing daily menus or work schedules. Food service managers may be required to plan or help plan any number of organizational agendas. Some of these are:

- Annual objectives as part of the institution's business plan
- Policies and procedures
- Projects or new business opportunities
- Human resource recruitment and retention

- New or remodeled facilities
- Departmental safety
- Continuous quality improvement and customer satisfaction activities
- Strategies for support of a new product line
- Patient-centered care strategies
- Employee performance planning

This chapter will discuss steps in the planning process, including key types of planning and how they apply to nutrition and food service department operations. A model and steps are provided for writing a department business plan based on the organization's strategic focus. An approach to writing up departmental policies and procedures is presented, as are tools for monitoring planning efforts and specific suggestions for writing effective objectives. Finally, the chapter will review the decision-making process, including group decision making, and planning for change.

☐ The Planning Process

The planning process in a participative organization is characterized by involvement from managers and employees at as many levels as is feasible. Chapter 2 identified three levels of employee empowerment (participation) as suggestion involvement, job involvement, and high involvement. The extent of involvement by various levels of management and employees will depend on the type of planning and the level of participation with which the organization or department is comfortable. In most organizations, top managers set the organization's overall goals, middle managers set their departments' objectives for meeting those goals, and first-line managers make everyday strategy decisions in fulfilling their departments' objectives.

Kinds of Planning

There are three basic kinds of organizational planning: strategic planning, operational planning, and individual performance planning. *Strategic planning* assists management in making nonrecurring, significant decisions that affect the culture and direction of the organization. It also assists the organization in adapting to the external business environment. Strategic planning is based on the values and purpose of the organization, in addition to the expectations of customers and the community at large.

Operational planning deals with the process by which the organization's larger mission and long-range goals are broken down into shorter-range objectives and activities. This type of planning is accomplished by members of the particular department or unit.

As they develop operational plans, managers prepare standing plans, periodic plans, or single-use plans. *Standing plans* guide activities that tend to be repeated frequently in the organization over long periods. Standing plans include policies and procedures, and standards of operation. *Periodic plans* identify a specific course of action for a designated period and are rewritten at the end of that period. Annual department business plans and budgets are examples of periodic plans. *Single-use plans* define a course of action that is not likely to be repeated, such as program or project plans (for example, remodeling the cafeteria). Standing plans, periodic plans, and single-use plans represent the major outcomes of operational planning.

The third kind of planning, *performance planning* with individuals within the department, is often overlooked by managers but is essential in setting goals for individual performance. Performance planning attempts to elicit maximum motivation and commitment from individual employees to contribute to departmental and organizational goal achievement. Individual performance planning as it relates to coaching is discussed in chapter 8. The remainder of this chapter will focus on strategic and operational planning.

Steps in the Planning Process

To plan effectively, it is important to know the organization's current status; what factors influence its future; and how the organization, department, or employees must be positioned to attain success in that future. Although the following six basic steps apply more directly to strategic planning than to operational planning, they have applicability in all levels of organizational planning:

1. *Collect data.* Gathering information to identify the organization's or department's current status and strategies and to predict future implications will yield details of internal strengths and weaknesses and external opportunities and threats.
2. *Analyze the data collected.* Analyzing the information assesses what impact it has on current organizational strategies and identifies alternative or new strategies.
3. *Develop goals and objectives.* Based on the information gathered and the strategic focus established, long-term and short-term desired outcomes can be identified. This step also includes assigning specific time lines for meeting objectives.
4. *Develop action plans.* These delineate specific assigned responsibilities and contingency plans, as well as time frames for task completion.
5. *Implement the action plans.* This step begins movement toward the established objectives.
6. *Evaluate plan effectiveness.* Was the action plan appropriate to the objectives set and to the degree of goal attainment accomplished? If not, the action plans and objectives should be reevaluated.

The six steps of the planning process can be examined by grouping similar activities into three phases: (1) data gathering and analysis, including current status, strengths and weaknesses, and opportunities and threats; (2) development of goals and objectives with appropriate strategies or action plans; and (3) implementation, evaluation, and modification of the goals and action plans.

Time and the Planning Process

The dimension of time is a major element in all planning activities. Time parameters serve to enforce operational controls, structure, a sense of focus, and direction for everyone charged with carrying out plan objectives. The terms *long-range planning* and *short-range planning* are sometimes used to describe strategic planning and operational planning, respectively. As mentioned, long-range planning involves the major activities or strategic changes an organization will undertake during the next two to five years, sometimes even as far as 10 or more years into the future. Long-range planning, such as deciding on the organization's mission and goals, rests in the hands of top-level managers and the board of trustees. Intermediate-range planning is a type of operational planning that covers shorter periods, perhaps one to three years. Responsibility for intermediate-range planning is shared by top- and middle-level managers. Finally, short-range planning covers operational activities that are to take place in the near future, for example, the next week or the next fiscal year. Such planning usually involves the participation of first-line managers and employees.

The time frame for long-range planning depends on the degree of uncertainty in forecasts and predictions. The further into the future planning efforts extend, the more they are based on speculation and guesswork and, therefore, the less valid the predictions and subsequent planning become. For this reason, careful research is conducted to validate forecasts and predictions before long-range planning is undertaken.

Planning time frames also are influenced by need. This is especially true for short-range planning. For example, in planning departmental involvement in implementation of a new organizationwide safety program, dates for implementation may be set by upper management based on immediacy of need for the program to control injuries. Department managers would then be required to develop and implement the necessary objectives and action plan within the established time frame. Time lines may be influenced by the item being planned, such as the development and implementation of a particular product line. The organization may wish to have the new product line available in six months to meet the demands of the market and customers. However, the influence of technology, need for infrastructure changes, or difficulty in attracting the appropriate human resources may prevent meeting the established time line. In this case, the nature and complexity of the planning event set the time frame.

☐ Strategic Planning

In health care organizations, the chief executive officer usually is responsible for strategic planning, together with the board of directors (also referred to as the board of trustees, the governing board, or the board of commissioners). Most of the time, the board has ultimate responsibility for how the institution is run, with the CEO representing the board in his or her management capacity.

Depending on the size of the organization and the complexity of its structure, there may be a planning committee or a department responsible for planning activities. Commonly, a planning department led by a vice-president or director is responsible for gathering and disseminating information for individuals at various levels who assist in planning activities. Often large organizations use outside consultants to conduct an internal analysis and make suggestions for areas that need attention. The following sections describe the three phases of strategic planning.

Phase 1: Data Gathering and Analysis

Collecting and analyzing data is the basis of long-term strategic planning for the organization. Organizations with planning departments have the capacity to gather and analyze data on an ongoing basis. Others may assign this responsibility to individuals in the organization or rely entirely on consultants. Either way, a number of activities must be carried out continuously to ensure availability of adequate information for long-range planning. These include:

- Conducting market research and analysis to identify current and potential customers; this includes collecting data on consumer markets
- Gathering information on customers' profile including average age, which services they use, their sources of payment for these services, how long they stay in the institution, why they choose to use the services, and what other services they may want
- Monitoring current market share and forecasting future market share activity; *market share* is defined as the percentage of patients using the institution compared to the total number of possible patients in a designated area
- Conducting an internal analysis of the services offered, number of admissions (inpatient and outpatient), emergency department visits, length of stay, patient days, surgical procedures, meals served, and other specific departmental activity and financial reports that may help guide strategy
- Gathering information on physician referral patterns to other hospitals and physicians; other physician-related information includes average physician age, specialties, number of admissions, and level of satisfaction with the services offered by the institution
- Studying the market for new business opportunities or product lines and making feasibility, pricing, and promotion recommendations
- Collecting information on the external environment (competition, business environment, political and economic trends); information about other health care organizations may include their past growth and performance, their current position and image in their service areas, and their current services and future plans
- Collecting information on new technology developments and their impact on the future of health care delivery
- Collecting and analyzing data on work force issues to predict labor requirements

- Monitoring and collecting information on the facility's financial operation; for example, data on expenditures for personnel, and equipment and supplies

Designing systems and methods for gathering the above information may fall to the planning department or committee or be handled by the institution's marketing department. The methods for acquiring this information are reviewed in detail in chapter 3.

Once the appropriate data have been gathered, the organization's current business position must be evaluated. This evaluation is conducted by the board, the CEO, top-level managers, and possibly a consultant. Analysis of the internal environment includes identifying the organization's current strengths and weaknesses as well as opportunities and threats posed by the external environment. The external environment is influenced by events and circumstances beyond the organization's control. In contrast, the internal environment, although based on external pressures, is within the organization's control. Analysis is taken a step further to predict what probable effect environmental pressures will have on the organization's operation in the foreseeable future. Based on the information collected, the strategic planning team will prepare strategies for responding to the projected environment influences. For example, the shift from inpatients to outpatients is an external factor that affects the organization's future plans for delivery of service.

As part of the strategic planning process, managers and the board may reconsider the institution's mission as represented in its mission statement. Typically, the *mission statement* is an inspirational description of the institution's purpose, intended to instill in all who work there a shared sense of purpose and to foster commitment to a shared ideal. A mission statement usually includes a set of goals that specify in broad terms how the mission is to be accomplished. For example, the statement may include a description of the hospital's primary functions, its philosophy and values, the levels of care and types of service it offers, the population or special groups it intends to serve, and its special relationship with other organizations. A mission is defined by what organizations stand for and how they perceive their function in the community and to their customer base.

In addition to a mission statement, an organization may write a vision statement. The *vision statement* is designed to denote where the organization would like to be positioned in the future. Without a vision of where the organization is going, it is impossible to devise a plan to get there.

The JCAHO guidelines proposed for 1994 identify setting a written organizational mission and vision as a measurement standard. This guideline is listed in the new leadership section and further states the organization's planning will provide "the strategic, operational, programmatic, and other plans and policies to achieve the mission and vision." (Programmatic planning would be included in the single-use planning described earlier in the chapter.) Proposed JCAHO guidelines also include standards for information management, including the gathering of data and extraction of meaningful information.

Phase 2: Establishing Goals, Objectives, and Strategies

Based on evaluation of the data, goals and strategies are set for the entire organization and are the basis of the departmental business plan and objectives. Strategic options are established and evaluated based on the organization's ability to meet the identified opportunities and threats. Once goals and strategies are written, they are evaluated to determine whether and how they best fit the organization and their potential for leading the organization to success. Selection of strategies should reflect the best balance between the organization's potential for taking advantage of the opportunities or overcoming threats and the values of its management and established mission.

In addition to forming the basis for department planning, identification of goals and strategies for the entire organization will require upper management to form and be responsible for specific action plans at their level. An example of an objective and action plan is development of the organization's long-term capital expenditure plan. This budget is based on the need for resources identified in both the long-range strategic planning and the departmental planning process. The long-term capital budget must be approved by the governing body or board. The capital budget is the organization's action plan for fiscal and other resource allocation.

Action plans focus on how the goal and objectives of the strategic planning process are to be accomplished. The department director can expect to become involved in this phase when the chosen strategic alternatives affect his or her department or are relevant to all managers throughout the organization. For example, the planning committee may decide that the institution must improve its management competence at all levels and, therefore, establishes a plan for organizationwide management training.

Action plans include designation of the person (or group) responsible for completing the activities, along with specific statements of the measurements used to identify when the objective has been met. Time lines are specified for each step in the action plan to ensure that objectives are met according to the established strategic plan.

Phase 3: Implementing, Evaluating, and Modifying Goals and Action Plans

Once an organization knows its mission and strategic direction, it has a strong foundation for implementation of operational planning and setting of objectives. However, an organization concerned with long-term success will not stop at implementation but will continue to gather information, evaluate its mission in light of that information, and adjust its strategic plan as necessary.

Strategic thinking moves with the environment; as the environment changes, the organization must respond and adapt accordingly. An example of change in external environment was experienced with the 1992 presidential election. Although health care had been an issue of national debate for many years, this election clearly established a major shift in the environment, forcing health care institutions to rethink their strategic direction and how well they were positioned to deal with these changes. Another example is a change in an organization's financial status, a real issue for many institutions across the country in the past decade. Even organizations that were once in financial trouble but managed to recover will have to modify their strategic focus for future advancement, not just recovery.

The Middle Manager's Role in Strategic Planning

Although information collection is important to strategic planning, much of it also is valuable to operational planning. Department managers must be aware of what is being monitored or surveyed in their organizations and use these data in operations planning. Upper management must communicate to department managers and staff the organization's future direction and provide regular updates on goal accomplishment. Providing communication on these issues is important to having a highly committed and motivated work force.

During the early phases of strategic planning, middle managers are often a source of data, reports, and knowledge for strategic planners. If appropriate for the alternatives being considered, department directors also may be asked to respond. For example, the food service director might be called on to find outreach contracts for the delivery of nutrition services in physicians' offices, wellness centers, and extended care facilities. A food service director might need to answer any number of questions about suggested alternatives. For example:

- How would the new strategy fit the established objectives of the department as well as the values and beliefs of its staff?
- Would the department be able to implement the new strategy with its current resources, or would new resources be needed?
- How much would it cost the department to implement the strategy, in terms of human resources, time, money, equipment, training for new methods, and other support systems?

- How would the department need to change its structure or its relationship with other departments to ensure that the strategy would be implemented most effectively?
- Would this strategy be relevant to the market the department currently serves?
- Would the strategy represent a risk that the department is ready to assume?

These questions would be addressed in the department's business plan, and objectives would be written to meet the challenges identified. The department director needs to have a considerable amount of information before responding to such questions and making recommendations to strategic planners. In addition to increased commitment, motivation, and involvement of others in the department, gathering this information and evaluating the suggested changes offer two other advantages for the director: having access to more comprehensive information and being equipped to inform and prepare department employees for major changes that might take place over the long term.

☐ Standing Operational Planning

Primary responsibility for operational planning rests with the manager or director of the food service department. Standing operational planning is the basis for daily recurring department functions and assists in establishing structure and accountability for all members of the department. The largest portion of this planning is policies and procedures, in addition to which are departmental reports that monitor financial success and provide information to others within the organization. These reports also form the foundation for information necessary for periodic planning, such as budgets or business plans. Examples of various reports include productivity reports; cash register reports; turnover, overtime, and other payroll reports; and meal equivalent information (that is, the number of meals served).

Policies and Procedures

Policies are general guidelines—usually written—for carrying out essential and frequently repeated activities. Policies give direction for action and therefore are helpful in reducing the need to make operating decisions each time an activity takes place. *Procedures* can be defined as prescribed ways to accomplish an objective. Procedures specify how to do something; who will do it using what skills, materials, equipment, and other resources; and what the time frame for accomplishing the task will be. In contrast to policies, procedures list in chronological order the steps required to achieve an objective or to carry out a policy.

Although the policies of the food service department must be relevant to its activities, the policies also must be consistent with policies of the institution and reflect the requirements of standard-setting organizations (for example, the Joint Commission on Accreditation of Healthcare Organizations, discussed further in chapters 4, 9, and 11). The JCAHO's standards for dietetic service mandate that policies as well as procedures be in written form for at least the following areas in nutrition and food services:

- The responsibilities and authority of the food service director and, when the director is not a dietitian, of the qualified dietitian
- Food purchasing, storage, inventory, and preparation and service systems
- Diet orders, which are recorded in the patient's medical record by an authorized individual before the diet is served to the patient
- Proper use of and adherence to standards for nutrition care, as specified in the diet manual
- Nutrition assessment, counseling, and diet education
- Menu planning
- The role, as appropriate, of the dietetic department/service in the preparation, storage, distribution, and administration of enteral tube feedings and total parenteral nutrition programs

- Alterations in diets or diet schedules, including the provision of food service to persons who do not receive the regular meal service
- Ancillary dietetic services, as appropriate, including food storage and kitchens on patient care units, formula supply, cafeterias, vending operations, and ice making
- An identification system designed to ensure that each patient receives the appropriate diet as ordered
- Personal hygiene and health of dietetic personnel
- Infection control
- Safety procedures, including control of electrical, flammable, mechanical, and, as appropriate, radiation hazards
- Compliance with applicable laws and regulations

This list represents the requirements in the 1994 standards. A review of the standards must be made annually to ensure departmental compliance.

Department Policies and Procedures Manual

Writing a policies and procedures manual is the final phase in a long process of planning departmental activities. A well-written manual depends on input from a number of sources:

- Managers and professionals in the department
- Information gathered from the department's records
- Requirements imposed by relevant standard-setting organizations and regulatory agencies
- Suggestions gleaned from manuals written for other departments
- The food service director's own experience

Although each department's manual is based on input from many sources and can be written by different individuals, the final editing and approval of each policy and procedure is completed by the food service director. Having only one editor will ensure that the writing style and format are consistent throughout the manual. Figure 5-1 illustrates the basic format for a policy and procedure statement. Figure 5-2 shows an example of a food service policy.

Once policies have been established, procedures can be developed for carrying them out. Like policies, procedures should be written for every area of the food service department's activities—purchasing, production, service, clinical care, sanitation, and personal hygiene, among others.

Procedures are usually specific, step-by-step descriptions of a particular technique (see figure 5-2) and often include illustrations that enhance the description. Each procedure should be described in a separate entry in the manual.

In addition to a written policies and procedures manual, the JCAHO also requires the food service department to review and update the manual annually. (State licensing agencies have similar requirements.) The department director is responsible for this process but may enlist the help of the food service staff. Policies and procedures no longer relevant or now obsolete must be revised. Once revisions have been approved by appropriate administrative and medical staff in accordance with the organization's policy, their signatures must appear on the relevant pages of the manual or on a cover page. Such changes include, for example, price increases in the cafeteria, changes in nutrition care policies, and changes in the services offered that would affect staffing levels and budgets. Finally, the director must communicate changes to department employees to ensure that everyone involved in implementing the changes knows how they are to be carried out.

In that the manual is a tool for routine decision making, new employee training, and veteran employee retraining, regular updating of the policies and procedures manual also is important to ensuring smooth department operations. Finally, the manual serves as documentation of the standards against which employee performance will be evaluated.

Figure 5-1. Policy and Procedure Format for the Food Service Department

Department of Food and
Nutrition Services,
Community Hospital

POLICY MANUAL

Policy Number: _____

Effective Date: _____

Subject: _____

Area of Responsibility: _____

Classification: _____

Approved by: _____

Primary Responsibility: _____

Distribution: _____

Review Date: _____

Revise Date: _____

Person Responsible: _____

Purpose:

Policy:

Procedure:

Special Instructions or Illustrations:

Figure 5-2.   Sample Policy and Procedure for the Food Service Department's Policies and Procedures Manual

Department of Food and Nutrition Services, Community Hospital	Policy Number: 1306

Department of Food and
Nutrition Services,
Community Hospital

Policy Number: 1306
Effective Date: March 1988

POLICY MANUAL

Page 1 of 2

Subject: Taste Panels

Area of Responsibility: General administration

Classification: Purchasing

Approved by: Director, Food and Nutrition Services

Primary Responsibility: Assistant Director,
             Procurement and Production, and
             Food Stores Manager

Distribution: Standard

Review Date:					
Revise Date:					
Person Responsible:					

Purpose: To determine the acceptability of a product before purchase and service.

Policy: Taste panels will be conducted at least monthly, more often if deemed necessary, to objectively evaluate products.

Procedure:

1. Taste panels will be regularly scheduled on the third Friday of each month at 1:30 P.M.

2. A group of no more than 10 and no fewer than 5 people will be selected prior to the date of the panel by the Food Stores Manager and as appointed by the Director.

3. The panel will include representatives from Purchasing, Nursing Services, Food and Nutrition Services, Administration, and other interested personnel.

4. Tabulation of the results of the panel will be completed by the Food Stores Manager and kept on file for future reference.

5. Results of the panel will be discussed with the Director, Assistant Director, Clinical Dietitians, and/or Production Manager.

6. The Clinical Dietitian, Production Manager, Assistant Directors, and Director may recommend products for testing. This should be done at least a month prior to scheduled panel.

7. Procedure outlined in policy for taste panels dated 10/04/87 is still applicable (attached).

Figure 5-2. *Continued*

Department of Food and Nutrition Services, Community Hospital	Policy Number: 1306 Effective Date: March 1988
POLICY MANUAL	Page 2 of 2

Before a new product is to be utilized on the menu, it will be tested for acceptance.

Procedure:

1. Except on approved occasions, the taste panel will be conducted on the third Friday of each month at 1:30 P.M.

2. The Assistant Director for Production and Service will have the *overall* responsibility of the panel.

3. Assistance will be given by the Food Stores Manager (that is, she will invite participants, tabulate forms, and so on).

4. Water, cups, plates, napkins, and utensils will be made available for each participant.

5. There will be no talking, except to ask questions, during the taste panel.

6. Each product is to be individually evaluated by each participant.

7. Each individual is to independently score the results.

8. There will be no joking, horseplay, and so forth, allowed during the meeting.

9. Answering pages and telephone calls will be kept to a minimum.

10. There will be no more than 12 people at each panel (including the Production Manager and the Assistant Director, Procurement and Production).

11. No food is to be taken out of the conference room by the participants.

12. The panel will be made up of:

    Director
    Assistant Director, Procurement and Production
    Assistant Director, Nutrition Services or Clinical Dietitian
    Food Stores Manager
    Production Manager
    Other food service personnel as invited
    Nursing Services representative
    Purchasing representative
    Administration representative

The Assistant Director, Procurement and Production, will invite persons from the preceding list to participate. Invitations will be issued a week in advance. Those unable to attend should notify the Assistant Director as soon as possible. After participants have tasted products and finished the evaluation phase, they are to return to their work area.

Everyone should be honest and objective in the evaluation.

Periodic Operational Planning

Periodic operational planning is conducted for specific purposes and within designated time frames. Examples of this type of planning include development of the department budgets (including operating budget, capital budget, and cash budget, for example) and the annual department business plan. Annual department business planning is similar to strategic planning in that the same six steps are applied in the three phases previously identified. Information affecting the department must be gathered and analyzed, objectives and action plans must be developed and implemented, and evaluation and modification of goals and action plans must occur as deemed necessary.

Department Budget

The budget, a relatively simple and familiar planning tool, is a good means of forecasting long-range expenditures for personnel, equipment, supplies, and other resources. Therefore, it is important for managers to learn to use department budgets to ensure that necessary resources are available to meet department objectives.

The department budget actually is a composite of different types of budgets. The *operating budget,* for example, projects the number, types, and levels of service to be offered over the defined period and the resources needed to support service delivery. The *capital budget* forecasts major purchases in plant and equipment, new construction and/or facilities renovation, and furnishings. The *cash budget* estimates cash income and expenditures over the budget period so as to ensure sufficient cash availability to meet the department's and organization's financial obligations. The operating and capital budgets are primary components of the department's financial plan and become part of its business plan.

Because the overall department budget also is a tool for controlling departmental performance, each of these components will be discussed at greater length in chapter 11.

Department Business Plan

A department business plan is a tool or process that can be used to organize department-specific operational planning. As mentioned earlier, the strategic direction is set by upper management and the board of directors and is the foundation for department operational planning. During the strategic planning process, specific areas are targeted for development or concentration of effort. Based on the direction set and the specific goals the organization wishes to accomplish, the department must assess how its role fits in the larger picture and plan accordingly. Once the strategic focus has been determined, the food service director must evaluate his or her current ability to assist in accomplishing the organizational goals and then set the necessary objectives to assist in goal attainment.

Depending on an organization's size, structure, and level of service offered, departmental business planning may or may not be part of the organization's process and may or may not be required of managers. However, a number of benefits are to be gained by developing a business plan. One benefit is improved performance by clearly identifying and understanding the strengths and weaknesses of the department, which allows management to plan proactively for potential problems instead of becoming embroiled in crisis management. Clarity of objectives as delineated in a business plan in turn sets clear performance, priority, and accountability expectations by providing standards against which to measure. The instrument coordinates the planning effort throughout the department and provides a framework for making key decisions. As an educational tool, the business plan can present an opportunity to promote staff involvement and ownership in the department's future.

The department business plan can be utilized externally. For example, in a business expansion effort to provide meal service to a smaller organization, a well-written business plan could help "sell" the idea to the potential client. The complexity of the business plan is directly related to the size and makeup of the organization and department.

Lessons from Other Industries

To better understand business plans, it is helpful to look at their use in other industries. Generally, business plans are composed of five components:

1. Market strategy
2. Production or service strategy
3. Research and development strategy
4. Organization and management strategy
5. Financial strategy

Each of these areas can be applied to health care food service and included in the planning process. The market strategy (or plan) identifies who customers are; what products or services will be sold to them; and the policies regarding pricing, promotions, and distribution as explained in chapter 3. Marketing strategy information will apply to both the data gathering and analysis phase and the objective and action plan phase.

As in other planning activities, production strategy begins with gathering and analyzing data to identify current capabilities of meal production and service and to predict future needs based on the objectives. The food service director must learn whether changes are needed in the department's infrastructure, whether additional capital equipment or technology is needed, or whether changes in the marketing mix are needed. For example, if a department was using a hot pellet system for meal delivery and determined there was a need to change to cook–chill, changes would be necessary in the production strategy so as to modify preparation, storage, tray assembly, and service.

The third strategy in the general industry model is research and development. This applies to food service departments that wish to develop new programs for clinical services or new revenue-producing ventures. New development may include expanding catering to the outside, implementing a vending program, opening a coffee shop, or opening a branded chain operation within the facility. The research and development portion of the business plan is based on market analysis of who customers are and what they want. Often this portion of the business plan is completed by managers as a single-use program plan. However, in order to monitor its effectiveness, it must be an ongoing element of the overall business plan.

The organization and management strategy of the business plan includes an explanation of the functions that must be performed and who is to perform them. This portion includes staffing needs, training and skill development needs, procedures and control measures necessary to support the department or new programs, and the level of employee involvement. The organization and management strategy may include an explanation of how things currently are done in the department and what procedural changes will be necessary to support new objectives. This portion of the business plan may include training programs that will be needed or will assist in translating customer needs into continuous quality.

The last strategy of the model used by business and industry is the financial strategy. As mentioned above, both the operating and capital budgets become a part of the annual business plan. Furthermore, when new programs or products are proposed, the financial plan must address revenues and cost of the investment. It may be necessary to establish a pro forma, or projected profit and loss statement. The pro forma is usually based on one budget year and on the projections made from the marketing, production, research and development, and organization and management strategies.

Business Planning Phases

Although the five components mentioned above should be addressed in the department business plan, the three phases utilized for strategic planning earlier in this chapter should be used to develop the business plan. Figure 5-3 illustrates a top-down flowchart of the business planning process for the department. A top-down flowchart is another tool that can be used by the manager, especially for project planning.

Figure 5-3. Top-Down Flowchart for the Major Steps in a Business Planning Process

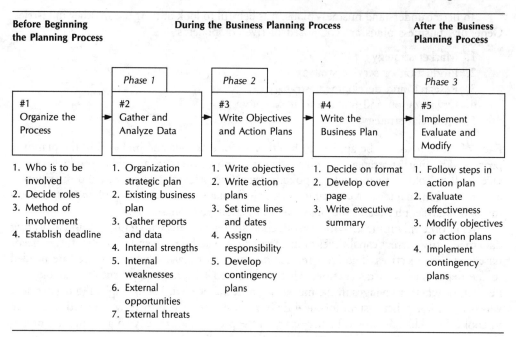

Before Beginning the Planning Process	During the Business Planning Process			After the Business Planning Process
	Phase 1	*Phase 2*		*Phase 3*
#1 Organize the Process	**#2** Gather and Analyze Data	**#3** Write Objectives and Action Plans	**#4** Write the Business Plan	**#5** Implement Evaluate and Modify
1. Who is to be involved 2. Decide roles 3. Method of involvement 4. Establish deadline	1. Organization strategic plan 2. Existing business plan 3. Gather reports and data 4. Internal strengths 5. Internal weaknesses 6. External opportunities 7. External threats	1. Write objectives 2. Write action plans 3. Set time lines and dates 4. Assign responsibility 5. Develop contingency plans	1. Decide on format 2. Develop cover page 3. Write executive summary	1. Follow steps in action plan 2. Evaluate effectiveness 3. Modify objectives or action plans 4. Implement contingency plans

Before the process can begin, deadlines must be set and the manager must determine who is to be involved, when, and in what capacity. Involvement from staff may take place in small group meetings, employee meetings, management meetings, or one-on-one sessions with the director. The director in a high-involvement department may ask employees to participate in the data-gathering and analysis phase or wait and include input on objective and action plan writing.

Either way, providing opportunity for involvement will ensure commitment from the staff who will have to assist in carrying out the action plan. Once the method and time for employee involvement have been established, the director will need to provide the necessary information regarding the organization's strategic plan, without which managers and employees will be unable to contribute informed suggestions.

Once deadlines are set and staff involvement has been identified, *phase 1* of the planning process begins. A situational diagnosis is conducted to determine internal strengths and weaknesses and external opportunities and threats. This portion of the situational (SWOT) analysis might be conducted through staff brainstorming. A list of strengths, weaknesses, opportunities, and threats may look like the one in figure 5-4. This portion of the analysis and the next portion, defining the current business definition, form the foundation of objectives needed for the coming year for improvement and those needed to support the organizational strategy.

The internal analysis will include the business definition—what is being done now—and the number of meals served, customer groups served, where services are being provided, and the clinical services provided. Analysis also will include the number of employees, hours of operation, and service. Internal environment will include the strategic plans made by the organization. An example of a strategic goal for the organization that affects departmental planning is focusing on the customer while implementing continuous quality improvement. The department is then responsible for making its contribution and setting specific objectives for how its members will contribute. Questions to be asked may include:

- What does the strategic direction mean in relation to what is going on in the department now and the forces in the external environment?
- What objectives must be set to assist in organizational goal accomplishment?

Figure 5-4. Food Service Department SWOT Analysis

Strengths

- Highly qualified and concerned staff
- Low employee turnover
- High employee morale
- Positive internal image, especially in catering and cafeteria
- Ability to function within operating budget
- Strong inventory control and purchasing procedures
- High department productivity

Weaknesses

- Timeliness of patient late trays
- Timeliness of food production
- Constraints of the physical plant in relationship to meal delivery
- Aging equipment
- Limited computer access

Opportunities

- Train employees for enhanced quality of service
- Replace current patient tray line
- Improve patient satisfaction with a new patient tray delivery system
- Convert production to a cook–chill system

Threats

- Shortage of qualified service employees due to changes in the work force
- Difficulty of serving patient meals if tray assembly and delivery systems are not updated

Another example of building on strategic plans is the organization's decision to undertake a major building project. The department director would have to assess whether adequate facilities and staff are available to provide the needed meal service. If not, necessary data would be gathered and analyzed to determine needs. Objectives for the department would be based on the information gathered.

In *phase 2,* specific departmental objectives are written to assist in organizational goal accomplishment. The objectives must be measurable and include time frames for accomplishment as well as specific action plans. Action plans are then developed to support the objectives. The action plan must be specific in terms of time frame for accomplishment, specify who is responsible, and state how success will be measured. Also included will be contingency plans in the event the initial plan was either ineffective or the objective needed to be modified. If the objective involves capital expenditures, the appropriate financial information is included in the action plan. Details for writing appropriate, measurable objectives will be covered later in this chapter.

Phase 3 of the business plan, like the strategic organizational plan, requires the manager to provide leadership for implementing the agreed-on action plans. The steps of the implementation process are delegated by the manager. The food service director's responsibility does not end with implementation of the action plan, the effectiveness of which in meeting established objectives must be monitored and changes made as necessary. As mentioned, the validity of the objectives must be continuously evaluated in relationship to the changing environment. For example, if the food service department based one of its objectives on providing meal service to a long-term care facility to be acquired by the institution, but upper management decided to forgo the purchase, the objective and action plan would need modification.

Business Plan Format

A written plan should be made even if only for inside use. This will help solidify the importance of the planning process and provide documentation for coordination of efforts. The format for the business plan may vary by organization, but the fundamentals are similar across organizations. The first thing the manager needs to do is determine whether the organization has adopted a format. If not, guidelines built on the five components mentioned previously—market plan, production plan, research and development plan, organization and management plan, and financial plan—may be used. Another approach, used by Rotanz Associates and specific to health care, is represented in figure 5-5. Not utilized in the Rotanz model but added by the author is a table of contents and an executive summary briefly highlighting each major section.

Figure 5-5. Sample Business Plan Outline for the Food Service Department

I. Title page

   A. Name of the institution
   B. Name of department or functional areas
   C. Date of preparation and time period covered by the plan
   D. Name(s) of person(s) preparing the report

II. Table of contents

   A. Major headings with page numbers
   B. Appendix of figures, charts, graphs, tables, or other supporting documentation

III. Executive summary

   A. Brief description of the department (business definition)
   B. Current position or changes, or how plan is consistent with current status
   C. Significant strengths, weaknesses, opportunities, and threats that directly affect goals
   D. Financial and other resource requirements
   E. Main objectives, strategies, or plans

IV. Development process

   A. Details how the information was gathered
   B. Identifies sources used to develop the plan

V. Business definition

   A. Overview of current department status
   B. Resources

      1. Technologies that affect services
      2. Facilities that affect services
      3. Human resources
         a. Department-based employees
         b. Common interfaces with other departments
      4. Current budget
         a. Capital
         b. Operating

   C. Principal customers

      1. Identify various groups (patients, physicians, employees, and so on)
      2. Identify characteristics (age, needs, changing environment, and so on)

   D. Sustainable competitive advantage

      1. Strengths that have long-term effects

VI. Strategic focus of the department

   A. Brief statement of major emphasis for department

VII. Key results areas (identify those areas important to department—may come from strategic plan or department environmental analysis). Examples:

   A. Human resources (attraction, retention, or training)
   B. New products or business opportunities
   C. Financial performance
   D. Facilities development
   E. Quality and customer satisfaction

VIII. Environmental assessment

   A Business/health care environment
   B. Market segmentation

      1. Specific breakdown of groups served
      2. Brief details that identify differences

   C. Market needs assessment

      1. How were needs of the specific markets determined?
      2. Do these needs vary?

   D. Customer concentration

      1. Location of customer groups
      2. Demographics
      3. Common disease entity
      4. Age category
      5. Professional category

   E. Competitive (SWOT) analysis

      1. Strengths
      2. Weaknesses
      3. Opportunities
      4. Threats

IX. Business objectives

   A. Action steps
   B. Person(s) responsible
   D. Completion dates
   E. Measurement of success

X. Appendix

Source: Adapted from Rotanz, R. J. *Seminar on Business Planning.* Berkeley Heights, NJ: Rotanz Associates, 1990.

Scheduling Techniques

Managers often find that a visual representation of work over time is helpful in scheduling routine activities. The Gantt chart is one such device that can help a manager plan a variety of related tasks or schedule the work of a group of employees who perform the same task. The chart in figure 5-6 is an example of a schedule for a catering service. The Gantt technique is useful for relatively simple planning tasks. More sophisticated methods must be applied as a project grows more complex.

A planning technique used for short-term projects is the planning grid, shown in figure 5-7, which provides the planning team with an organized format for reaching a goal. The first step in completing the planning grid is to identify the objective or outcome of the planning effort. Achievement of outcome with the final action step is the measurement that determines when the planning is complete. The first action step might simply be to schedule the first planning session with the relevant team. The remainder of the planning grid is completed by the team using various techniques of teamwork participation (see chapters 4 and 6).

Another tool, the *program evaluation and review technique* (PERT), can be used for planning as well as for controlling more complex departmental activities. Much more quantitative than the Gantt chart, PERT is best used by managers who are skilled in using mathematical methods for planning complex projects. Briefly, PERT helps to define a network of relationships among activities and events that occur in the course of a project and then to calculate the time needed for each event and the time lapse between one event and another. The PERT technique is often used to reduce the total time needed to complete a project and to keep the project on schedule by making adjustments in the network of relationships. A similar quantitative planning tool for sophisticated, nonrepetitive technical projects is the *critical path method* (CPM). Both CPM and PERT are used by industrial and management engineers to plan and schedule activities for a one-time project (such as a major renovation of a department) and can, therefore, be considered methods for single-use planning.

Figure 5-6. Sample Gantt Chart for Planning a Catered Dinner

	Week 1	Week 2	Week 3	Week 4	Week 5	Week 6
Activity A	XXXXXX					
Activity B		XXXXXX				
Activity C			XXXXXX			
Activity D				XXXXXX		
Activity E					XXXXXX	
Activity F						XXXXXX

Activity A: Plan menu.

Activity B: Order supplies (including tables, linens, chairs, and flowers).

Activity C: Order food (after checking recipes).

Activity D: Make arrangements for security (including parking facilities and coatroom).

Activity E: Hire and train additional workers.

Activity F: Set tables and make general arrangements.

Figure 5-7. Sample Planning Grid Format for Short-Term or Project Planning

Objective or Outcome:								
Team Members:								
Item #	Action Step	Product Outcome	Responsibility	Due Date	Whom to Involve/Contact	Budget or Cost	Other Resources	Other Categories
1								
	Final Step	Objective Achieved						

Objectives

Although the use of a business plan can assist the department manager in determining which areas need attention and what specific objectives should be, a business plan is not necessary to establish operational objectives. Operational objectives are the foundation for directing performance expectations. Writing and executing clear objectives avoids crisis management and allows managers time to further develop employees. Objectives also assist in bringing the department together, with everyone moving in the same direction.

Characteristics of a Well-Written Objective

Objectives must be specific statements that explain how the broader goals of the organization are to be accomplished. The more specific an objective is, the more efficiently it can be reached. In addition, specific objectives are essential as tools for adequately evaluating and controlling the performance of the organization as a whole, of specific departments, and of individual employees. A well-written objective has the following characteristics:

- *Specificity:* The objective identifies the specific outcome of an activity. The results of quantitative objectives (that is, those whose results can be measured mathematically) are easier to determine than the results of qualitative objectives. For example, the objective of increasing the productivity of the tray preparation line by 2 percent is a quantitative objective. The objective of improving employee morale is qualitative and is, therefore, somewhat harder to measure. However, a manager should not be discouraged from setting qualitative objectives because other factors can be measured that are good evidence of employee morale, such as the number of employee grievances filed or the rate of absenteeism.
- *Conciseness:* The objective is succinct, uncluttered by identification of the method for accomplishing a task, for example; that is, it contains no extra information.
- *Time dimension:* The objective is time related in that everyone involved understands by what point a task must be accomplished.
- *Reality:* The objective is achievable and within the work group's capabilities and available resources. On the other hand, an objective should not be so easily achieved that the work group does not feel challenged to give its best performance.
- *Method:* Each objective is accompanied by an action plan that outlines the steps for achieving the objective.
- *Value dimension:* Objectives should have value to the department and to those responsible for carrying them out.

In the following example, a food service department objective reflects one of the hospital's overall goals: to provide service in a cost-effective manner. The department implements this goal by stating its own objective:

> To reduce the overall cost of each patient meal by 1 percent by the end of the current fiscal year.

This objective is specific and its achievement can be measured (quantified) against the financial information from department records. The objective is stated concisely, clearly, and within a designated time frame. To decide whether the objective is realistic, the food service director would need to assess the costs involved in current meal preparation and delivery and decide whether a 1 percent reduction is feasible and if so, through what means—reductions in staff, changes in methods of preparation, or some other adjustment. Devising or amending production methods involves creation of action plans. It also incorporates a value element in that doing so must be worthwhile to those who must perform the tasks that lead to attainment of the objective.

To implement department objectives effectively, each one must be prioritized in relation to the others. In addition, each objective must be broken down into its component tasks in an action plan. The resources available for accomplishing each task should be assigned according to the objective's relative priority.

Steps for Writing Objectives

A manager who uses a department business plan will have a clear idea of what areas would benefit from having objectives established. Otherwise, the first step is to determine which areas need objectives. Experts estimate that approximately 20 percent of the activities in any business necessitate having specific objectives in place. Setting objectives for everything in the department is extremely time-consuming and can frustrate the monitoring process. Once the determination is made as to which areas need objectives, five steps can be used to establish clear ones:

1. State the problem or opportunity clearly.
2. Decide what the expected outcome is to be.
3. State the end product—what will be achieved by the outcome.
4. Establish possible action steps, including the measurement to be used.
5. Refine the possible action steps into a concrete plan.

After the target areas for objectives have been identified, the next step is to identify the challenge or opportunity at issue. A general statement is then written to identify what the desired outcome or change would look like. The next activity is to refine the general statement, keeping in mind to determine how the outcome will be tracked and measured. Once the objective is clearly written, all possible actions are listed. From this list an organized sequential list is formed. The action steps to be followed to accomplish each task should be described in specific procedures (discussed previously in this chapter). A time frame for completing each task also must be established. Scheduling becomes a more complex process as tasks require more steps and more people to perform them. Action plans that lead to attaining objectives identify who is responsible for each step and provide time lines for completion.

Assigning responsibility for fulfilling each objective and completing its component tasks is the food service director's role. One person may be involved in a task, or the whole department may work to fulfill the overall objective. It is vital that the person assigned primary responsibility for completing the task be given sufficient authority and resources. As mentioned earlier in this chapter, once the action steps have been outlined with responsibilities and time lines, monitoring must occur to ensure success. Progress reports should also be kept as records of the department's objective-setting and fulfillment process so as to document for top-level managers the department's progress in fulfilling institutional goals. The reports can also be used as part of the institution's evaluation and control system. The objective and action plan should be put in writing and shared with everyone who will be affected either directly or indirectly.

Management by Objectives

Peter Drucker is usually credited with developing the systematic technique of goal setting and implementation called *management by objectives* (MBO). This tool is best applied by a department director as part of an organizationwide program for meeting the organization's goals. Briefly, MBO is a method by which a manager and a subordinate (a person directly supervised by that manager) cooperate in setting objectives that the subordinate intends to accomplish in his or her position. Usually, both agree to document in the subordinate's personnel file the objectives to be reached by a certain date, at which time the manager evaluates the subordinate's success in achieving the objectives. If performance has been satisfactory, the manager can reward the subordinate according to the personnel policies established by the organization for salary increases, benefits, promotions, and so forth. If performance has not been successful, both must reach agreement about the problem and identify ways to solve it. That is, they must define a new set of objectives.

The MBO tool has several advantages when used carefully and cooperatively. First, it is a powerful morale booster and motivator of employee productivity. By involving employees in defining objectives, MBO fosters a greater commitment to the organization by demonstrating how the employees' objectives are intertwined with the organization's goals and strategies. Furthermore, MBO makes a clear connection between performance and reward, thus ensuring for both employee and manager that evaluation is an objective and fair process rather than a subjective one. Finally, MBO provides a systematic tool for planning employee activities as well as for controlling them and keeping them on the same course as the department and the organization.

☐ Decision Making

Decision making can be defined as the process of assessing a situation or objective, considering options or alternatives, and selecting the one most likely to provide the best possible outcome for those involved. As discussed in chapter 2, decision making is a key managerial activity and a significant part of the four basic management functions of planning, organizing, leading, and controlling. The purpose of decision making in health care food service is to coordinate objectives and activities of the department so that its members deliver optimal nutrition care and meal service to designated customers.

Managers are required to make decisions for problem or conflict resolution and for identifying objectives. Throughout the planning process, managers make decisions when determining which objectives the department should pursue in the future. They also make decisions during implementation of the objectives. Additional decisions will be made regarding effectiveness of the objectives, appropriateness of the action plans, and alternatives in the event neither is determined to be appropriate.

Planning drives much of the daily work in health care food service by establishing appropriate written policies and procedures. However, problems may occur that require decisions and changes in these policies and procedures. Even with problem resolution, decision making is more effective when based on information-gathering procedures that contribute to developing appropriate actions.

Three Elements Essential to Effective Decision Making

Three elements are critical to making decisions effectively and in a timely manner. These are:

1. Authority or freedom to take action
2. Knowledge of the situation or issue under consideration
3. Motivation to make the decision

Having authority to act is especially important if employees are to participate in the decision-making process. For instance, unless authorized to do so as part of his or her job description or as defined under a specific policy or procedure, a tray line worker cannot make menu substitutions for patients receiving a diabetic diet. Even if so authorized, the employee cannot do so without knowledge and expertise in diabetic diets and in the nutritive value of foods and food equivalents. Even if authorized and properly trained, without sufficient motivation—for example, a line employee being evaluated for promotion to a supervisory position requiring more of a decision-making role—there is little or no will to make the decision.

Obstacles to Effective Decision Making

Unfortunately, more obstacles can preclude good decision making than there are factors that promote it. This section identifies six such roadblocks.

One obstacle is individual bias that locks a decision maker into a perspective that can sabotage the best choice for a given situation or even eliminate other alternatives from consideration. Another, obvious from the preceding section, is lack of knowledge or ability. Third, the lack of clear objectives can inhibit the decision-making process. Fourth, without availability of crucial resources (for example, finances, time, or staff), less-than-satisfactory decisions can result. One barrier that should be avoided, especially by new managers or new line employees, is fear of taking risks or making mistakes. Finally, resistance to change can bottleneck even the simplest decisions. (Planning and managing for change will be covered later in this chapter.)

Influences on Decision Making

When making decisions that will affect the entire organization, the manager must be able to identify elements that may influence the decision-making process and understand how their influence plays a part. For example, decisions are often made based on past experiences of the decision maker; a manager who tried an approach that proved to be ineffective may be reluctant to make that choice again (even if the situation is different). Although learning from the past is desirable, it is also important to ensure that logical choices are not precluded because of limited failures. The same is true for experimentation: A manager who tries a decision in a limited setting and finds it to prove effective may fear applying it in a larger context. Each person brings to the decision-making process his or her own personal and social views and values that will have an effect on the outcome. In addition, decisions are influenced by the departmental or organizational values. The final influence on the decision-making process comes from other managers or people whose judgment the decision maker trusts.

The Decision-Making Process

The decision-making process follows the same steps whether a first-line manager is solving a minor production problem or a top-level manager is deciding what the objectives are to be for the coming year. There are five steps to any decision-making process that should be followed to provide for optimal outcome. These steps are:

1. Establish objectives or define the problem.
2. Identify alternative solutions or outcomes.
3. Evaluate relative values of alternatives.
4. Activate action plan to implement best choice.
5. Follow up and evaluate the decision.

Establish Objectives or Define the Problem

Decisions are made based on a clearly defined expectation of the outcome. This is true whether the decisions are being made in connection with solving a problem, resolving a conflict, or allocating resources. To make the best possible decision, it is necessary to establish clear objectives that will lead to the optimal outcome or resolution. Defining the problem allows the manager to understand the full implication of his or her decisions. What may appear to be a small, simple problem can turn out to be much larger and involve multiple processes or systems. For example, upon noticing a rise in employee complaints about work conditions, higher-than-average absenteeism, an increase in number of kitchen accidents, or a falling off of employee dependability in timely task completion, a manager might easily jump to the conclusion that "today's employees are unreliable and careless." In fact, such symptoms may signal an operational crisis on the horizon.

An alert manager thoroughly explores a problem to find its possible causes. For instance, rumors of layoffs, a wage freeze, or employee perception of supervisor apathy could explain any one of the observations cited above. Whatever the cause of disruptions or negative changes in the department's operations, investigating beyond the first impression probably is worth the time and effort. This way the manager avoids wasting time on treatment of symptoms while the real problem remains undetected. It also avoids time spent in crisis management once the problem erupts. Clarity in defining the problem simplifies the rest of the decision-making process and, indeed, may make the rest of the process unnecessary.

Identify Alternative Solutions or Outcomes

With the problem clearly defined, the manager can move on to the second step in the decision-making process, developing alternative courses of action to deal with the problem. In some situations, alternatives may already have been defined by the organization's policies and procedures, and the manager must simply carry them out. For example, if an employee repeatedly ignored a work schedule by arriving late and had received first an unofficial reprimand and later a written warning about the consequences of repeated tardiness, the manager usually would have only one choice in dealing with the problem, according to the organization's personnel policies.

In other settings, however, the manager will have to collect information to arrive at relevant and valid alternatives. Depending on how quickly the decision must be made, the manager may involve employees or other managers to brainstorm ideas and possible alternatives. Decisions made for nonroutine problems or conflicts must consider all possible outcomes of the alternatives outlined to ensure a winning situation.

Evaluate Relative Values of Alternatives

Each alternative must be carefully examined for its strong and weak points. To do this, the manager must gather all information pertinent to each alternative and then answer these questions:

- Is the alternative feasible? For example, does it violate any departmental policy or procedure? Does it conform to legal, regulatory, or code restrictions? Does the alternative risk overstepping firmly established bounds of authority?
- Is the alternative satisfactory? Even when an option is feasible—that is, even if no strict organizational barriers are in its way—the option may not suit the unofficial social norms of the work group. Implementing changes that are socially unacceptable to the staff would meet with stiff resistance.
- If the alternative is both feasible and satisfactory, will its consequences be acceptable to the manager? the department? the organization?

Information gathering for each option may require review of policies and procedures, examination of previous memos or other documentation on the same or a similar problem, or analysis of job descriptions. Additional information may be gained from personal experience and observation and from discussions with other managers in the organization.

Activate Action Plan to Implement Best Choice

Answering the above questions will help eliminate all but a few options. The best of these probably will be the one that allows the most positive answers to the questions of feasibility, satisfaction, and potential consequences. However, not all options are mutually exclusive. If two seem to be equally good solutions to a problem, perhaps they can be used in tandem or sequentially. For example, offering a new special diet menu to patients might require them to make choices that are somewhat more complicated than what they are accustomed to. Should the nutrition staff show the staff nurses how to help patients fill out their menus, or should the nutrition staff urge patients to call the food service department with questions or problems? The staff may be able to implement both alternatives and, in doing so, provide two options that will ensure that patient menus are filled out properly.

Implementing the most appropriate solution may in turn require another set of decisions. The manager may need to choose the most efficient and effective method for carrying out the solution from several possible alternatives. Upon learning that standing plans have already been developed that would be workable for the proposed activity, the manager may need to prepare a single-use plan for a brand-new effort. For example, the existing policy on the delivery of meal carts would need revision if the number of personnel assigned to cart delivery was reduced because of a low patient census.

Follow Up and Evaluate the Decision

The final step in the decision-making process is to evaluate the option(s) chosen. Do the chosen actions have the desired effect? If not, why? At this point, the decision-making process may have to begin again from step 1, and the problem may need to be reanalyzed in light of the failed attempt to solve it. If the chosen actions fail to meet expectations, the manager should not assume that the problem was incorrectly identified. Indeed, the action may have been well chosen and well planned but may have lacked good implementation. In any case, timely follow-up is essential to the decision-making process because it keeps poor decisions from wasting department resources and derailing its efforts.

☐ Team Decision Making

All steps in the decision-making process can be taken by an individual manager or by a team. For the sake of time and efficiency, a manager can and should make certain decisions independently. However, research studies and management experience have shown that the manager who involves subordinates significantly in the decision-making process has a more satisfied, committed, and productive staff. Research has further demonstrated that team efforts make for more sound decisions than does an individual effort to resolve the same problem.

Team decision making can offer other advantages as well. For one thing, individuals working together bring their *accumulative* knowledge and experience to the decision-making process. Therefore, a group is likely to generate not only more but better alternatives and be better able to evaluate them. Once a decision is made, group members are likely more motivated to implement it because of their ownership in formulating it. Also, routinely sharing decision making makes a stronger working team.

Team decision making has its limitations, however. A significant drawback is that it can be time-consuming and therefore not the best approach if a decision must be made quickly. Other problems arise if the decision-making process is not carefully carried out. For example, if decision makers fail to assign responsibility for specific tasks in the action plan, no one assumes responsibility, even though the manager's superiors will hold the manager responsible. Furthermore, fear of suggesting what may be workable but radical alternatives could discourage creativity in suggesting options. Therefore, the team may generate a decision that appears to be endorsed by a majority of members but is really a less-than-satisfactory compromise. Often this is a problem when a manager or other group member resistant to suggestions tries to dominate the decision-making process.

As a decision-making technique, brainstorming (discussed earlier) is applied most often to solving problems that are unusual and especially challenging. To generate the most creative alternatives for the group to consider, brainstorming encourages participants to suggest novel—even radical—ideas. Everyone in the group must agree in advance to conform to an important ground rule of brainstorming: Criticizing the ideas of other participants is not permitted. Instead, participants must try to build on the ideas advanced until a solution is found that is feasible, satisfactory, and has the fewest negative consequences.

Another technique that engages a work group in participative decision making is *quality circles*. Professor Powell Miland describes the quality circle as "a group of workers and their supervisors who organize themselves for the purpose of working on a specific quality control problem related to the work of their section of the plant." In a wider sense, however, a quality circle is an environment in which a team decision-making process takes place. Various decision-making techniques, including brainstorming, can be used by a quality circle to arrive at decisions, depending on what kind of problem the group is attempting to solve.

Whatever techniques are used, effective team decision making is characterized by the following, according to Megginson and others:

- It is fair to all members of the group.
- It provides an opportunity to gather together people with different attitudes.
- It permits members of the group to explain what they think should be done to solve the problem.
- It fosters group discipline through social pressure and persuasion.
- It permits the cooperative solution of problems.

In contrast, team decision making is ineffective when any of the following conditions result:

- It tries to give each member what he or she wants.
- The manager or some other group member tries to manipulate participants to reach his or her "right" decision.
- The manager considers the team decision-making process as only a forum to sell his or her idea to the group and does not listen to alternative ideas.
- Discipline is ignored in the process of exchanging ideas.
- The manager only appears to seek the advice of the group, without actually planning to implement it.

☐ Planning, Decision Making, and Resistance to Change

Most decisions, whether made by top-level managers, department heads, or groups within departments, require some change in the way things work. As in other aspects of everyday life, change is a constant in the work setting. Therefore, resistance to change, no matter how insignificant it is, might seem a curious phenomenon. Managers must contend with this resistance, both in employees and in themselves. A positive attitude toward change is critical to an effective management and leadership style. Change in products, equipment, methods, and clientele is a fact of life and a necessity for survival in health care institutions. The effective manager not only accepts change, but strives to be instrumental in bringing it about by constantly searching for ways to improve his or her department.

Managing change begins with a self-examination of the manager's own attitudes toward impending change and his or her sensitivity to the reasons why employees resist change. These reasons include a fear of losing status or economic well-being and a general fear of the unknown. Many times, employee concerns are unwarranted and are the result of the manager's failure to explain the changes adequately. Fear of change is further exacerbated if employees are not allowed to participate in making decisions that affect them. For this reason, group decision making is becoming an important element of effective management.

Attempts to change the way a group works often imply criticism of the status quo. Suggested changes in procedures or products may cause employees to feel that their past performance has been less than satisfactory and that their work is being criticized. Unfortunately, many employees have prior experience with poorly implemented procedural changes and tend to be suspicious, even angry, when new methods are proposed. An alert manager anticipates this problem and makes every effort to prepare employees for changes in procedures, products, or services. Extra effort should be made to assure employees that suggested changes are not a criticism of their past performance but merely represent more efficient procedures.

Because change almost always causes some negative reaction among employees, managing change well also means managing employee emotions, so that sensitivity to the emotional connotations of change helps a manager effect change smoothly. Setting the stage by creating a positive work environment within the food service department is the first step in the right direction.

The next step is for managers to cultivate employee awareness of, and interest in, the change process. This will make the trial and adoption stages easier for everyone involved.

Apprising employees of possible changes can help lessen their anxiety and distrust. Generating employee interest and their suggestions for ways to try out new plans can result in a more cohesive work group and in helping employees develop their own management skills.

Employees must feel that the change will be good for them. Therefore, changes that are well planned and well executed enhance growth and positive development toward the goals and objectives of the organization. In contrast, hasty or poorly planned changes may lead to problems and lack of productivity. A manager's effectiveness can be measured in part by his or her skill in initiating and leading constructive planning for change.

☐ Summary

Effective business plans rely on upper management's commitment and involvement. Objectives and action plans should address all significant factors that affect the department's short- and long-term performance. The business plan must be forward-looking and based on realistic analysis of the situation. Key management and staff members charged with implementing plans should be involved in plan development. Plans should foresee contingencies and outline courses of action in the event that organizational plans or direction change. For example, if you decide to remodel an existing part of the department and then the decision is made to build a new kitchen, contingency plans would be needed.

☐ Bibliography

Ashkenas, R. N., and Schaffer, R. H. Managers can avoid wasting time. *Harvard Business Review* 60(3):98–104, May–June 1982.

Baud, J. Quality circles may substantially improve hospital employee morale. *Modern Healthcare* 11(10):70–72, Sept. 1981.

Bolten, L., Aydin, C., Popolow, G., and Ramseyer, J. Ten steps for managing organizational change. *Journal of Nursing Administration* 22(6):14–20, June 1992.

Burack, E. H., and Mathys, N. J. *Introduction to Management: A Career Perspective.* New York City: John Wiley and Sons, 1983.

Capoor, R. Strategic planning: parts 1, 2, and 3. *Restaurant Business* 80(10, 12, 13), May 1, 1981; June 1, 1981; July 1, 1981.

Cohen, A. R., Fink, S. L., Gadon, H., Willits, R. D., and Josefowitz, N. *Effective Behavior in Organizations.* 4th ed. Homewood, IL: Irwin, 1988.

Cohen, M. W. Arguments for and against MBO. *Hospital and Health Service Administration*, Special issue, Jan. 1980.

Dougherty, D. A. Reorganization of JCAHO's standards manual slated for 1995 finalization. *Hospital Food & Nutrition Focus* 9(7):1–8, Mar. 1993.

Drucker, P. *The Practice of Management.* New York City: Harper and Row, 1954.

Fannin, W. R. Making MBO work: matching management style to MBO program. *Supervisory Management* 26:20–27, Sept. 1981.

Flippo, E. B., and Munsinger, G. M. *Management*. 5th ed. Boston: Allyn and Bacon, 1982.

Gibson, J. L., Ivancevich, J. M., and Donnelly, J. H., Jr. *Organizations' Behavior Structure Processes*. 7th ed. Homewood, IL: Irwin, 1991.

Griffin, R. W. *Management*. 2nd ed. Boston: Houghton Mifflin, 1987.

Gryna, F. M. *Quality Circles: A Team Approach to Problem Solving*. New York City: AMACOM, 1981.

Haimann, T., Scott, W. G., and Connor, P. E. *Management*. 4th ed. Boston: Houghton Mifflin, 1982.

Ingle, S., and Ingle, N. *Quality Circles in Service Industries*. Englewood Cliffs, NJ: Prentice-Hall, 1983.

Joint Commission on Accreditation of Healthcare Organizations. *1993 Joint Commission Accreditation Manual for Hospitals*. Vol. II, *Scoring Guidelines*. Oakbrook Terrace, IL: JCAHO, 1992.

Kerrigan, K. Decision making in today's complex environment. *Nursing Administration Quarterly* 15(4):1–5, Summer 1991.

Koontz, H., O'Donnell, C., and Weihrich, H. *Management*. 7th ed. New York City: McGraw-Hill, 1980.

Lakein, A. *How to Get Control of Your Time and Your Life*. New York City: Signet, 1974.

Lane, B. *Managing People*. Sunnyvale, CA: Oasis Press, 1989.

Longnecker, J., and Pringle, C. *Management*. 5th ed. Columbus, OH: Charles E. Merrill, 1981.

McCoy, J. T. *The Management of Time*. Englewood Cliffs, NJ: Prentice-Hall, 1982.

Megginson, L., Mosley, D., and Pietri, P., Jr. *Management: Concepts and Applications*. New York City: Harper and Row, 1986.

Mosley, D., Megginson, L., and Pietri, P., Jr. *Supervisory Management: The Art of Working with and through People*. Cincinnati: South-Western, 1985.

Munn, E. M., and Saulsbery, P. A. Facility planning. *Journal of Nursing Administration* 22(1):13–17, Jan. 1992.

Odiorne, G. S. *The Practice of Management by Objectives in the Eighties*. Westerfield, MA: MBO, 1981.

Peters, J. P. *A Strategic Planning Process for Hospitals*. Chicago: American Hospital Publishing, 1985. [Out of print.]

Pritchett, P., and Pound, R. *The Employee Handbook for Organizational Change*. Dallas: Pritchett Publishing Company, 1990.

Puckett, R. P. MBO. Presentation for consultant dietitians, ADA-HEW Workshop 12, 1980.

Puckett, R. P. Optimizing employee productivity through motivation. *Journal of Foodservice Systems* 1(3):205–20, Spring 1981.

Quality control circles. Part 2: a step by step approach to implementation. *Small Business Report*, Feb. 1982.

Rose, J. C. How to write a business plan: part 1. *Hospital Food & Nutrition Focus* 4(9):3–7, May 1988.

Rose, J. C. How to write a business plan: part 2. *Hospital Food & Nutrition Focus* 4(10):1–4, June 1988.

Rose, J. C. How to write a business plan: part 3. *Hospital Food & Nutrition Focus* 4(11):1–4, July 1988.

Rose, J. C. How to write a business plan: part 4. *Hospital Food & Nutrition Focus* 4(12):1–5, Aug. 1988.

Rose, J. C. How to write a business plan: part 5. *Hospital Food & Nutrition Focus* 5(1):1–6, Sept. 1988.

Rose, J. C. How to write a business plan: part 6. *Hospital Food & Nutrition Focus* 5(2):1–7, Oct. 1988.

Rotanz R. J. *Seminar on Business Planning*. Berkeley Heights, NJ: Rotanz Associates, 1990.

Scanlon, B., and Keyes, B. *Management and Organization Behavior*. 2nd ed. New York City: John Wiley and Sons, 1983.

Scholtes, P. R. *The Team Handbook: How to Use Teams to Improve Quality*. Madison, WI: Joiner Associates, 1988.

Thiagarajan, S. Take five for better brainstorming. *Training & Development Journal* 45(2):37–42, Feb. 1991.

Wheelright, S. C. Japan—where operations really are strategic. *Harvard Business Review* 59(4):67–74, July–Aug. 1981.

Chapter 6

Organization and Time Management

☐ Introduction

Organizing is the process of dividing the work done in an organization (or a unit within the organization) into smaller parts and assigning responsibility for those parts to specific positions. Historically, organizations believed work was accomplished most efficiently when divided into specialized tasks and given to specialists of those tasks. More recently, the idea of specialization is being questioned in light of job diversity that creates multiskilled workers, a more desirable approach. The change from a specialized skills approach to a multiple skills approach is attributed to a number of trends. These include demands for a customer orientation and patient-centered care, the movement toward continuous quality improvement, changes in work force demographics, and the demand for participative management.

To answer the question of how health care facilities should be organized to meet their goals efficiently and effectively, this chapter will explore various organizational structures. Each structure will be reviewed in terms of the extent and type of departmentalization within an institution, the degree to which decentralization of tasks and decision making is a prominent feature of an institution, and job design factors in a specific corporate climate. Organizational structure will be applied to how the role of a food service department is defined in the larger organization (for example, through teams). In addition, food service department organization will be addressed, including proper exercise of authority, staffing, and scheduling. Time management is discussed from the point of view of time as a resource whose function is to maximize productivity.

☐ Determining Organizational Structure

The system a facility chooses as most appropriate for conducting its work is called the *organizational structure*. Health care facilities are exploring various organizational structures to determine the one best suited to meet quality demands within limitations imposed by cost constraints. It is important that decisions be made quickly, that employees participate in decision making, and that customer demands (especially those of the patient) be met to ensure a health care institution's long-term viability. With these considerations in mind, the following sections discuss three common entities in health care organizational structure: departments, committees, teams.

Departments

The formation of departments, or *departmentalization,* can fall into any of several categories: functional, product, geographic, customer, process or equipment, and time. In the past, only functional and time departmentalization were relevant to food service departments in health care institutions. However, changes in health care focus have made product, customer, and process departmentalization pertinent components of a facility's structure. For departmentalization to be effective, the concept of separation and reintegration must be taken into account when deciding how to form an organization. *Separation* represents division of labor by pulling the organization apart, making it more complex. The value of separation becomes evident when groups are reintegrated, forming the support structure for operations. *Reintegration* refers to the degree of coordination, cooperation, and communication that flow among units in the organization.

Usually, it is up to top-level managers to determine which department structure is appropriate for their institutions. Most likely, a combination of categories will be the best choice. Six departmentalization types are briefly described here.

Functional Departmentalization

Functional departmentalization groups jobs into departments or units in which employees perform the same or similar activities. Most units within hospital food service departments are organized according to function, such as nutrition services, food production, purchasing and storage, and nonpatient services. (See figure 6-1.) A manager or supervisor is usually in charge of each unit's activities. Functional departmentalization makes sense from the standpoint of having like functions centralized. For example, although decentralizing meal service may be desirable, it does not make sense to decentralize food preparation.

Functional departmentalization can cause conflicts between departments in meeting customer demands. Those closest to the patient (for example, nurses) have a unique perspective of patient requirements and may fault another department, such as food service, whenever patient needs go unmet. Because food service staff are removed from the customer, they may not comprehend the urgency of nurse requests. For example, interrupting a work activity to get an item requested by a nurse interferes with getting items ready for the tray line. This type of functional cross-purpose does not allow employees to engage in the full cycle of their work. In this example there is a conflict between nursing and food service. However, if the food service employee were involved in the full cycle of fulfilling a patient's dietary needs, he or she would understand that both tasks are of equal importance. The employee could then understand that the choice is not between completing a department task versus a nursing request but a choice of meeting an immediate patient need and scheduling or postponing a task for a future need. With the patient in clear focus, the food service staff could see that the positive consequences of meeting the patient need would outweigh the negative consequences of not having all items ready for the tray line to start.

Product Departmentalization

Product departmentalization creates work units based on the product or service the unit delivers. This form of departmentalization is used most often in large manufacturing companies and financial institutions. In recent years, health care institutions have experimented with product line departmentalization, defined by body system units or by the traditional nursing care units. Therefore, product lines may include cardiac care, obstetrics, oncology, or orthopedics among others.

The idea of product line departmentalization is to coordinate the efforts of all health professionals involved in caring for a particular patient type. This coordination enhances the quality of care and improves costs associated with that care. Product line management is further enhanced by critical paths that standardize the intervention at various stages of the patient's stay. (Critical paths are covered in detail in chapter 4 on quality management.) Dietitians

Figure 6-1. Functional Organization of a Food Service Department

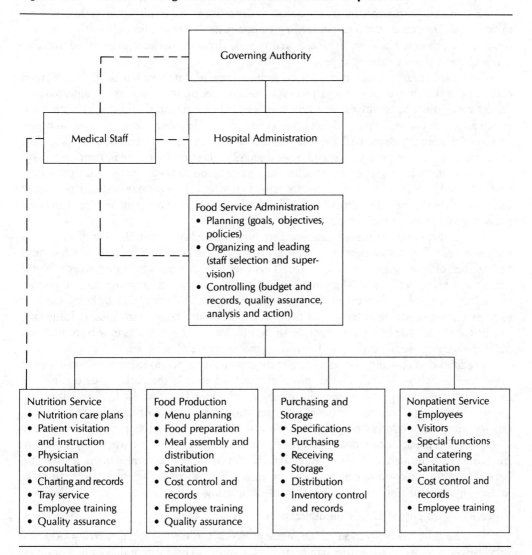

are among the practitioners who will have a role in product line management. Although most product lines will likely be managed by a nurse, other professionals may lead. An example of this type of product line is an orthopedic or rehabilitation unit, where a physical therapist may be the manager. Product line departmentalization may or may not require that dietitians and others from food service report to the manager of the product line. If, for example, 100 percent of a dietitian's time were devoted to a particular unit, he or she could conceivably report to the product line manager.

Geographic Departmentalization

Geographic departmentalization groups an organization's activities according to the places in which the activities are carried out. This type of departmentalization is used in fast-food operations, contract feeding services, and large school districts. For example, food may be purchased, delivered, and stored in a central warehouse. Preparation of the food may take place at a single second location or be disseminated to individual sites for preparation and service. Geographic departmentalization allows concentrated effort around fewer tasks.

Customer Departmentalization

Customer departmentalization focuses each department's or unit's work on the customer to be served. For example, a contract feeding company might service hotels, health care institutions, and schools. Therefore, it would structure its departments according to the different needs of these three customer types.

Customer departmentalization can be seen in large hospitals in which patient-focused care or patient-centered care groups professionals and nonprofessionals as a team around a patient care unit. The traditional term *nursing unit* is being replaced with *patient care unit*, which attests to the influence patients have on how care is delivered. During a typical hospital stay, the average patient will come in contact with more than 25 individuals a day. It is estimated that nursing personnel spend more than 52 percent of their time in nonprofessional tasks including ordering supplies, handling communication, housekeeping, and performing personal service duties. Services related to patient support take approximately 22 percent of their time, leaving only 26 percent available for direct patient care. This revelation has led many organizations to patient-focused care units.

Patient-focused care units are designed to rely on a highly cross-trained staff that functions as a team. Patients are treated by the same team members during their stay, which reduces the number of caregivers they have to see. This care allows a high level of comfort for the patient and his or her family. Many organizations have dissolved the nursing station, providing bedside terminals and decentralized supplies, allowing staff to "float," thereby being available to meet patient needs. With customer departmentalization, patient admission is frequently handled at the bedside by a clerical person in the unit. Support generalists may be responsible for housekeeping, food service, and stocking and ordering of supplies.

In addition to providing better care, patient-centered care acts to improve the staff's work environment. Everyone has an equal place on the team and in the patient's care. This can be especially rewarding to food service employees who have traditionally felt left out of caring for the patient. Rewards are based on team effort and quality of care. To ensure high-quality care, measurements must include clinical outcomes as well as patient satisfaction.

What this means for food service departments is that some of their work may be decentralized to these units, which also means that the staff may be decentralized. As team members, they will be allowed to contribute to the care of the patient while increasing their skills and the number of tasks they are capable of completing.

Process or Equipment Departmentalization

Process departmentalization divides work groups according to their different production processes or the specialized equipment their work requires. This form of departmentalization also is being explored by health care and food service departments. Employee involvement and teamwork has placed new emphasis on process departmentalization, and employees are grouped together to manage a process from beginning to end, rather than seeing only one specialized piece of the process. For example, a process team established for patient feeding would include not only servers on the tray line, but also cooks, dietitians, hostesses, purchasing personnel, and a supervisor or manager. This departmentalization requires the manager of the process to have a broad knowledge base and understanding of the interactions of various parts of the process. Process focus has been shown to improve not only the quality of work produced but also employee commitment to work. Teams and self-managed teams will be discussed later in this chapter.

Process departmentalization allows employees to cross-train and gain information about all steps of the process. This way, they no longer place blame on one step in the process; instead, they see how everyone working together can improve the overall process to improve outcome. This type of work unit division can go further than food service department units and can include nurses or other professionals on the patient unit. If the organization is using customer departmentalization and patient care units, the person on this work team may be the service generalist from the patient unit.

Time Departmentalization

Time departmentalization is often used along with another form of departmentalization when the work to be done fills more than a standard eight-hour workday. Hospitals use time departmentalization in grouping work according to shifts. In most food service departments, two shifts are needed to cover the 12- to 14-hour period of meal service for patients and nonpatients.

Committees

Although most work in health care organizations will continue to be accomplished in departments and intradepartmental units, some activities require that individuals from different departments (or from different units within a department) work together on a common task. In this case, a work team such as a committee, task force, or project team is formed. Historically, team members come from approximately the same level in the organization. However, with participative management and continuous quality improvement, this no longer may be the case. For example, a task force whose assignment is to explore a new process for preparing department budgets might consist of persons from the same level. Members of the work team would include all department directors and a representative from the finance department. A different type of work team might review the patient admission process for improvement. This team would include clerks who actually complete the process as well as managers, directors, and perhaps administrators.

Work teams can take several forms, some of which are listed below:

- *Ad hoc committees* are created for a short period of time to perform a specific task (for example, evaluating new computer training packages).
- *Standing committees* work together for a longer period than do ad hoc committees to deal with an ongoing subject of relevance to all committee members. For example, several departments might send representatives to a multidisciplinary patient education committee whose task is to develop materials and programs to teach patients about topics that draw from the department's knowledge. For example, a program on diabetic patient education might require help from the medical staff, nursing staff, pharmacy, laboratory, and a dietitian.
- *Task forces* are similar to ad hoc committees in that they are short term and have a narrow purpose. Usually, however, task forces are formal teams charged with solving or reporting on specific problems. Another difference is that a task force always has representatives from a variety of departments, whereas committee members may be from the same department. The purpose of a task force is to integrate the work of discrete departments that on a daily basis work independently. Another difference is that the task force membership may change as the team works through a project. For example, a task force whose purpose is to evaluate a hospital's eating disorders program might be composed of nutritionists, psychologists, and physicians initially, with marketing specialists brought in later to suggest ways the program could improve so as to better fulfill the community's needs.
- *Project teams* are similar to task forces and ad hoc committees in that their purpose and duration are limited. However, the task that the project team is to accomplish may take as much as a third or a half of members' work time. For example, development of an eating disorders program might be assigned to a project team so that the program can get under way as quickly as possible. A project team manager coordinates the work of the different specialists. These specialists must report to the project manager as well as to their regular department or unit directors until their work on the project is completed.

Work teams are useful in carrying out essential activities in organizations. Food service directors can benefit from both participating in such teams and using them to accomplish the work of the food service department. Such teams offer several advantages:

- They foster effective communication among departments that share common goals and objectives.
- They permit integration of departments with similar goals and objectives.
- They offer a medium for coordinating the opinions and experience of specialists from several different functional areas.
- They provide a forum for team decision making.
- They create broad-based support for projects that demand the involvement of several different departments or units within departments.

Generally speaking, the food service director is required to serve on various hospital committees, among them the disaster-planning committee, quality assessment committee, safety committee, or infection control committee. (The advantages of team decision making are discussed in chapter 5.)

Teams

The importance of teamwork in a participative management structure is emphasized throughout this segment of the manual. Teamwork is important at the job-involvement level of empowerment to help employees make decisions that affect their work group. Teamwork is valuable in health care food service because of department complexity and job interrelationships; the more complex the organization or department, the greater will be the return on an investment in teamwork. For example, because many individuals are involved in providing a patient with a meal tray, collaborating on the task provides a clear goal to be accomplished. In a complex department like health care food service, the various sections of the department have a variety of goals. For instance, those purchasing food see their goal as obtaining and providing raw materials to the cooks. The cooks see their goal as preparing food for the tray line to serve. The tray line server's goal is to complete the tray for a hostess to deliver. When all of these members act as a team, the goal becomes serving the patient. In addition, an organization with a focus on customers and continuous quality improvement can benefit from the ideas and accomplishments created by teams. Risk taking also is a positive outcome of teamwork, and research has shown that team workers are more likely to take risks than are individuals. These statements, while supported by the author, are based on the information presented by various leaders in business and specifically in health care and food service. (See the bibliography for specific references to teamwork.)

Characteristics of High-Performance Teams

A great deal of time and research has been devoted to singling out competencies or characteristics of high-performance teams. Stellar teams exhibit the following characteristics:

- *Clear definition of roles and purposes:* The team has clear goals and strategies for goal accomplishment.
- *Interpersonal relationships:* Interactions among team members and with key people outside the team are ruled by trust, collaboration, responsiveness, and support.
- *Member empowerment:* Team workers have access to necessary skills and resources. Policies and practices support team objectives.
- *Open and honest communication:* Members express understanding and acceptance of others, practice active listening, and value different opinions and perspectives.
- *Member participation:* Members perform roles and functions as needed, share responsibility for leadership and team development, are adaptable, and explore various ideas and approaches.
- *High performance:* High output, excellent quality, effective decisions, and an efficient problem-solving process are apparent.
- *Exemplary individual contributions:* Workers' efforts are recognized by everyone. Team accomplishments are recognized, and members feel respected and recognized by the organization.

- *Individual motivation:* Workers feel good about their membership, are confident and motivated, have a sense of pride and satisfaction, and have a strong sense of cohesion and team spirit.

Leader/Manager Responsibility to Teams

Creating an environment that fosters teamwork is accomplished through participative management and employee empowerment. The manager is responsible for communicating a clear vision or purpose for the team. (Communication related to teams is detailed in chapter 7.) The working environment culture must support team members and efforts for goal accomplishment. Many of the necessities for a participative work environment also are critical to effective teamwork. These include providing flexibility by eliminating unnecessary procedures and allowing employee freedom to develop new ideas, permitting people to take risks and make mistakes, setting challenging goals with clear standards for accomplishment, providing recognition and praise, clearly communicating expectations and plans, and being committed to provide whatever is necessary for goal accomplishment.

The manager is responsible for providing employee training so that employees have the skills needed for problem solving and team interaction. Education and reeducation are based on the demands and needs of the team members and individual levels of competency. It is the manager's responsibility to assess level of competency and, if needed, to provide individual coaching for employees. The manager must ensure that everyone is given ample opportunity to participate and that outspoken members do not make all decisions and dominate the group. Before asking employees to work in a team, they must be trained in how to conduct team meetings, how to participate, how to make decisions, and how to follow the ground rules for team meetings. (See chapter 7.) Once everyone is provided with the training, individual abilities can be addressed. The competency of team members can be assessed through observation by a manager and can frequently be measured by the output or lack of output by the team.

The manager may have to assist with resolving conflict and with providing problem-solving tools. Statistical tools used to measure and analyze problems (reviewed in chapter 4) and situational leadership (see chapter 2) should be kept in mind with teams.

Group Development or Team Stages

Blanchard and associates identify four distinct stages of team or group development: orientation, dissatisfaction, resolution, and production. (Other writers refer to these four stages as forming, storming, norming, and performing.) *Orientation,* or stage 1, characterizes a newly formed group whose members have high expectations and some enthusiasm but may experience anxiety about their role and feel a need to find their place. They test the leader but at the same time are dependent on authority and the hierarchy to provide guidance. During this stage, the group will have a low productivity level but a high commitment level. The leader will have to provide very specific directions and a clear vision with desired outcomes to decrease anxiety and allow members to understand what is expected.

At stage 2, *dissatisfaction,* teams are somewhat disillusioned about team accomplishment. They may feel dissatisfaction with authority; be frustrated with goals, tasks, or action plans; feel confused and incompetent; compete for power and/or attention; and experience dependence and counterdependence. Although their morale and commitment may be waning, their level of productivity is on the upswing. The manager or leader will have to create a supportive environment that allows members to explore their feelings of discontent while providing enough coaching to move the group forward. Understanding that this stage of team growth is normal will allow members to stay focused and committed.

At stage 3, teams have moved toward some *resolution* of what dissatisfied them at stage 2. Members begin to develop harmony, trust, support, and respect for one another. Self-esteem and confidence are strong, leading to more open communication and feedback. Responsibility and control are shared by group members and a team language begins to develop. The manager/leader must continue to provide support but from somewhat of a distance as team members begin to take active roles and become responsible for the outcome of the group.

The final stage, *production,* is represented by a high level of productivity and morale. Members feel excited about their team and collaborate and work interdependently as a whole and within subgroups. There is a feeling of team strength, leadership is shared, tasks are being accomplished, and the team members have a high level of confidence. The team leader will have to further remove him- or herself from the leadership role and move toward delegation, allowing team members to accomplish desired outcomes.

Team Building

Team building is important to producing a desired outcome or high performance. Otherwise, both loyalty and performance will be jeopardized. Trust is developed through team building, which allows open discussion and feedback among members. The first step to building high-performance teams is to nurture the collaborative relationship between managers and team members. Managers must share their power and authority in an effort to reinforce the responsibility given teams. A commitment from the manager means giving the time necessary for team development and always attending scheduled meetings.

To form a high-performance team, members must understand and believe in the purpose of the team and in their ability to influence work. Team building allows for personal growth of members and should provide enjoyment. To begin functioning in teams, the manager will have to ensure commitment from department members to join in. For the best results, participation in teamwork should be voluntary, because some individuals feel uncomfortable functioning in teams just as they feel uncomfortable giving opinions. These employees should be given other individual tasks to complete. It is also possible that individuals who are reluctant to join teams will come around after they see there is nothing to fear and after team members provide positive feedback.

Team-building efforts must focus on the task or content of the meeting and the process of how things are done. Usually, if team members are selected on the basis of their knowledge, the task portion of teamwork is effective. It is the process portion—or how members relate, go about the task, and communicate—that must be addressed in team building. The team process can affect the outcome. Team building should concentrate on how things are going, encourage full participation, and emphasize listening and building consensus rather than majority rule. Two ways to increase awareness of process have been suggested by author Byron Lane:

1. When process problems develop where people are dropping out, forming subgroups, or not listening, stop the meeting. Ask members to discuss how they feel about what is happening. They may be apprehensive at first, but as teams develop they will be more willing to share their concerns.
2. At the end of each meeting allow 10 to 15 minutes to discuss process. Ask the team members "How did we do today?" Once they realize process is important enough to discuss, they will pay closer attention.

Team building should be fun. If possible, off-site training and development sessions should be held with team members. If this is not possible, time should be set aside for the department to celebrate and reward team participation. Effective team building requires as much interaction time as possible for team members. Early meetings should focus on how they can work together, what they think they can accomplish, and what issues are important to them in terms of decision making. (Team decision making is discussed in chapter 5.)

Self-Managed Teams

The highest level of employee involvement or empowerment is self-managed or self-directed work teams. Historically, teams required employees to work within traditional job descriptions with traditional supervisor–employee reporting relationships. Self-directed work teams allow employees to control their own work schedules, and team members deal with employees at all levels of the organization. The team manages a budget and takes responsibility for productivity, cost, and quality. Members are empowered to make major changes in their work processes without going through management.

Self-directed work teams benefit the organization because people are taking more responsibility. Downsizing in organizations has caused a decrease in the number of middle managers, making self-directed teams more important.

Self-directed teams may work in some areas of the food service department. For example, dietitians, technicians, and clerical support personnel can be made responsible for making decisions that relate to the tasks they perform for patient care and supporting meal service to this customer.

☐ Organizing the Food Service Department

The division of work and its efficient coordination is important in every health care institution, and the JCAHO recognizes this importance in its standards. The JCAHO standards require that all departments/services be organized, directed and staffed, and integrated with other units and departments/services of the organization. For food service, the standards stress organization in a manner designed to ensure provision of optimal nutrition care and high-quality food services.

All health care employees must be aware of their place in the organization—who their supervisor is and who their peers are. This information must be posted in the food service department in the form of an organizational chart. An *organizational chart* is a visual representation of the division and coordination of work within an organization or department within an organization. The food service department's organizational chart should be reviewed and revised at least once a year or whenever changes are made in the department's structure.

An organizational chart is a useful tool because it shows the characteristics of the larger organization and its units. For example, the organizational chart in figure 6-2 shows how the various positions in one type of food service department relate to each other and to the administration of the hospital. However, no chart can show the dynamic interconnections and interactions among members of the organization. The items that the organization chart depicts are:

- *Chain of command:* The solid lines in figure 6-2 demonstrate that the upper levels of the organization are linked to each of the lower levels through a defined set of relationships.
- *Unity of command:* Each employee is linked by a vertical line to only one supervisor. This ensures that each employee reports to, and is accountable only to, his or her immediate superior.
- *Departmentalization:* The organizational chart also shows how jobs are grouped into logically related units. For example, figure 6-2 shows that the food service department is split into three units: nutrition care services, food procurement and production, and nonpatient operations. Each unit is further divided into areas of specialization.
- *Lines of communication:* In addition to showing the chain of command, organizational charts show how information should flow through the organization. Solid lines in all the flowcharts shown (see figures 6-1 through 6-8) indicate both the flow of authority and the flow of formal communication among different positions in the chart.
   Broken lines show that information must also flow outside the chain of command. For example, in figure 6-2, although the assistant directors of nutrition care services, food procurement and production, and nonpatient operations do not supervise each other, they must communicate and coordinate their efforts to ensure efficient operation of the whole department. In addition, the broken line in figure 6-2 between the medical staff and the food service director indicates that the medical staff advises the food service department on the most appropriate service for particular patients but does not have direct authority over the department.

Figure 6-2. Organization of a Food Service Department with a Food Service Director in a Large Hospital

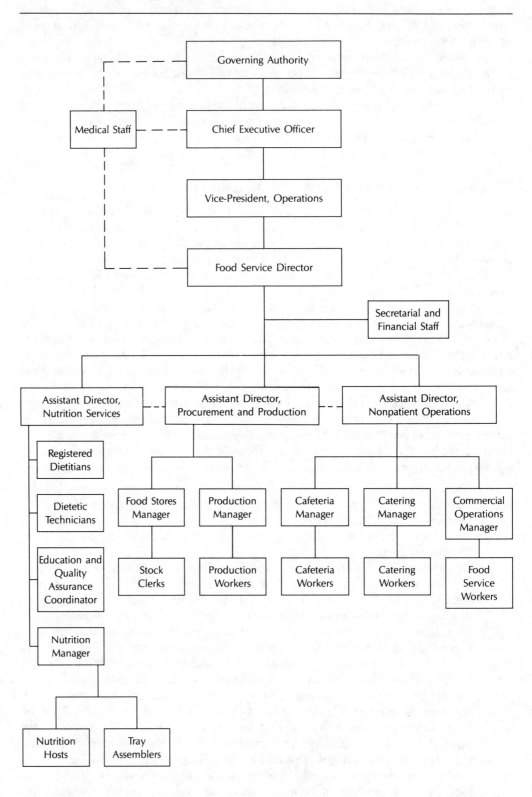

- *Span of control:* Span of control refers to the number of employees each manager must supervise directly. In a large organizational structure (see figure 6-2), each manager tends to have a narrow span of control, whereas in a less complex structure (see figure 6-4), each manager's span of control is wider.

Functional–Hierarchical Structure

Most health care organizations and food service departments continue to use the functional–hierarchical structure. The functional–hierarchical structure is present in organizations that group similar tasks (functions) together (for example, food production) with the chain of command and span of control increasing as one moves to the top of the pyramid (hierarchy). The more management levels there are in an organization, the more complex the organization is. For example, figure 6-2 represents five management levels: chief executive officer, vice-president of operations, food service director, food service assistant directors, and managers. A large organization such as this one has what is called a *tall* organizational chart. Smaller organizations tend to have what is called a *flat structure* because they have fewer levels of management.

Figure 6-3 is an example of an organizational chart for a small health care institution. Small hospitals and extended care facilities, particularly those in small communities or rural settings, frequently do not have the services of a full-time registered dietitian. Therefore, to meet the JCAHO's requirement for supervision of patient nutrition care, such institutions hire a dietetic consultant or part-time registered dietitian. A dietary manager has responsibility for the day-to-day supervision of the food service department in such institutions. (The dietary manager usually has completed a 90-hour food service management program approved by the Dietary Managers Association.) The organizational chart for a small food service department is shown in figure 6-4. Figure 6-5 illustrates two levels of management within a much larger food service department.

Figure 6-3. Organization of a Small Institution's Top-Level Management

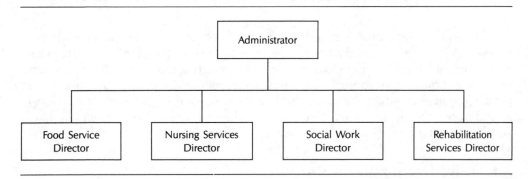

Figure 6-4. One Management Level in a Small Food Service Department

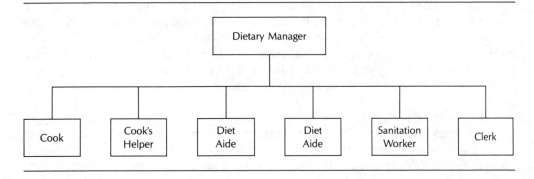

Figure 6-5. Two Management Levels in a Large Food Service Department

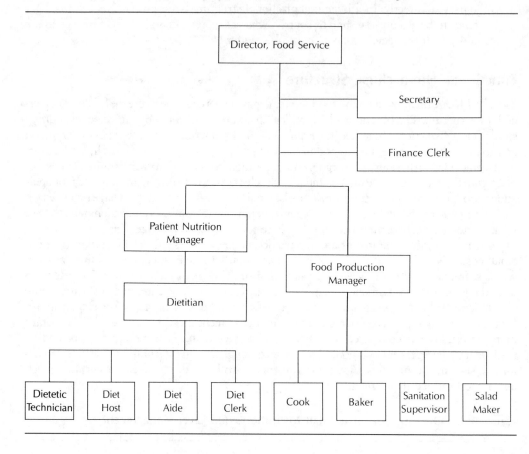

Although the functional–hierarchical structure has been credited with contributing to the large economic growth of the U.S. economy during the past 100 years, it appears to have outlived its usefulness. Its limitations include: turf orientation around departments or functions; limited information to employees, rendering them incapable of contributing to the big picture; communication difficulties due to the number of layers employees must go through; limited career growth; and rewards based on competitive individual or departmental progress, which limit contributions to the organization as a whole.

Alternative Organizational Structures

Changes in health care have required organizations to revisit the traditional functional–hierarchical structure to look for alternative structures. Options considered by some organizations have included removing a level of management by phasing out middle managers or reducing the number of managers at all levels, supposedly to improve communication with less vertical and horizontal boundaries. Still other attempts have been to invert the pyramid, putting employees at the top and the chief executive officer (CEO) at the bottom. However, this latter attempt did nothing with the direction of the power and authority. For managers to empower employees, a new structure must be developed, one that is not designed to direct and control.

One possibility, the *matrix model,* has been suggested to meet the needs of the participative organization more closely. This type of organizational chart allows for the continuation of the functional–hierarchical structure with the addition of project leaders. Top levels of the organization are still preeminent in regard to chain of command and span of control in these two models. These two models differ in that the matrix structure in figure 6-6 shows individuals or teams reporting to two different supervisors. Many of the relationships depicted in the matrix model occur in the traditional hierarchical structure without being "legitimized" on the organizational chart.

This type of structure is felt to be effective at cutting the time for decision making and is flexible enough to accommodate temporary teams such as committees, task forces, and project teams. It allows for changes in the informal structure without creating problems for the fixed hierarchical structure. It also allows a clear picture of product lines and customer or service units. Although the matrix model is more accommodating to organizational teams, there are problems associated with it. One such problem is ambiguity regarding the reporting structure. For this reason, the appropriateness of such a structure for frontline employees is questionable. The matrix model may prove more beneficial at the supervisory or professional staff level, where ambiguity regarding reporting structure is more comfortable. Good interpersonal skills and conflict management skills are essential for managers and employees if a matrix structure is used. These skills are helpful in improving communication and building relationships that facilitate dealing with ambiguity. For example, a dietitian may be asked to join a project team for developing a skilled nursing unit in the hospital. Conflict may arise if the team decides that meals should be delivered at a specific time. Good interpersonal skills will allow the dietitian to communicate the needs of the unit and the limitations of the department in meeting these needs.

Functioning in teams requires an organizational structure that is designed to depict cross-functional processes rather than functional departmentalization. It is difficult to assign a specific chain of command because process management functions tend to intersect. The organizational chart in figure 6-7 shows a *bubble diagram* for a nutrition and food service department. This structure represents different teams focused on the major core process of delivering patient care and food services. Comparing this diagram with the functional–hierarchical

Figure 6-6. Matrix Structure for a Health Care Institution, Showing Project Management

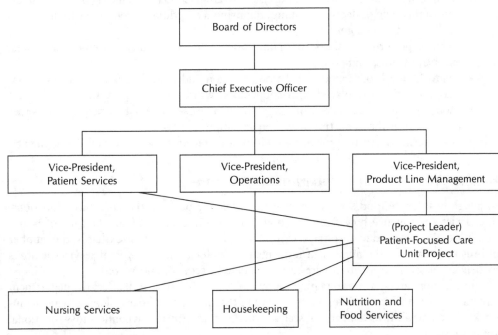

Figure 6-7. Bubble Diagram of Nutrition and Food Services Process Structure

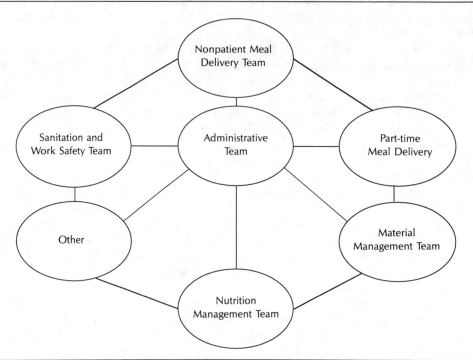

Note: The lines in this figure represent communication that may occur between any of the teams.

diagrams in figures 6-2 through 6-5 uncovers the following innovations afforded by a bubble structure:

- Management layers have been replaced with team leaders and facilitators who coach and facilitate rather than control.
- Team members are responsible for decision making. Consensus building becomes important in this type of decision making, requiring a coordinated communication process as discussed in chapter 7.
- Team empowerment allows communication with other teams, customers, suppliers, executive teams, and so on.
- Teams have a broader view of the organization and their contribution to its vision.
- Turf protection is replaced with cooperation within and across teams.
- Mobility of team members is increased through cross-functional participation on other teams within the department and organization.
- Team rewards can be provided in addition to rewards for individual development.

Factors That Influence Department Structure

Although health care food service departments typically perform the same basic functions, several factors influence how these functions are organized and staffed: the type of health care institution (acute care hospital, nursing home, for example); its size (that is, the number of beds it contains or the number of residents it cares for); and the type of services it offers (patient meal service, nutrition care service, cafeteria service, and so on).

In addition, an organization's philosophy and leadership style will affect the department structure selected. For example, an organization that promotes process development, teamwork, and employee involvement will seek a structure that depicts a dynamic, cross-functional approach.

Department Members and Responsibilities

As the sample organizational charts for food service departments demonstrate, the managers, staff members, and food service workers in various organizations have different titles. In addition, directors and managers have various levels of skill and responsibility and different levels of formal training and education. The food service director in figure 6-2 heads a large and complex department in a large acute care hospital. Two levels of management below the level of director manage numerous department services and employees. In contrast, a consultant (a part-time registered dietitian) advises the manager of a food service department in a small hospital or extended care facility like the one shown in figure 6-8. The consultant might work only 8 to 40 hours per month in such a facility.

The titles, responsibilities, and educational backgrounds of food service managers in various health care institutions can be described as follows:

- *Food service director:* In most large health care institutions and in many medium and small ones, the food service director is responsible for overall operation of the nutrition and food service department. The director usually holds a bachelor of science degree. In large organizations, advanced education in business management, health science education, institution administration, or other related field may be required. The food service director may or may not be a registered dietitian (RD). The director

Figure 6-8. Organization of a Food Service Department with a Dietary Consultant in a Small Hospital or Extended Care Facility

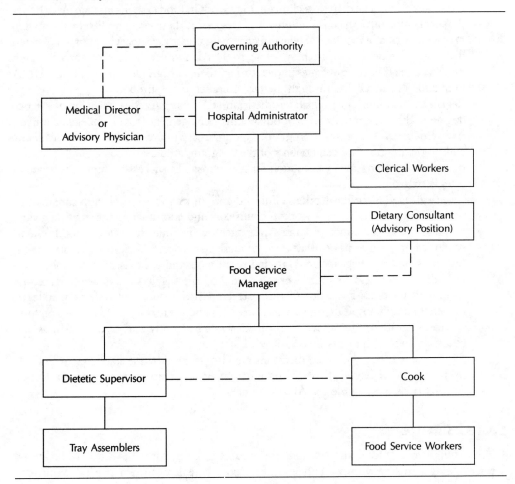

usually belongs to the American Society of Hospital Food Service Administrators, a subgroup of the American Hospital Association. Other titles that correspond to this position include director of dietetics, director of nutrition and food service, and food service administrator.

- *Certified dietary manager:* The certified dietary manager (CDM) has satisfactorily completed a course of study approved by the Dietary Managers Association (DMA). The approved course usually requires 90 classroom hours and 150 hours of on-the-job training. The dietary manager (DM) is certified by passing a national credentialing examination and earning 45 continuing education clock hours in each of the three years during the certification period. According to the DMA, a certified dietary manager "is a skilled and experienced generalist capable of assuming the responsibility of all aspects of food service operations other than the clinical and business aspects. In regard to the clinical or nutritional science areas, the DM would be required to utilize a dietetic consultant, with a recognition that this is a consultative service rather than occasional or visiting supervision. It is also assumed that the business aspects are the main responsibility of an organization administrator." Certified dietary managers belong to the Dietary Managers Association. Other titles that correspond to this position include food service supervisor, dietetic assistant, and lead cook.

- *Dietetic technician:* The dietetic technician has successfully completed an associate's degree program that meets the educational standards established by The American Dietetic Association (ADA) and has 450 hours of supervised field experience. The dietetic technician may become registered (DTR) by successfully passing a national certifying examination and maintaining 50 clock hours of ADA-approved continuing education over a five-year period. The dietetic technician may work in food systems management under the supervision of, or in consultation with, a registered dietitian. The dietetic technician may also work as a member of a health care team under the supervision of a registered dietitian. Dietetic technicians may belong to the ADA under the category of technician members. In addition, graduates of dietetic technician programs approved by the DMA may also become CDMs through the DMA credentialing process.

- *Registered dietitian:* The registered dietitian (RD) has earned a bachelor of science degree in dietetics, nutrition, or food systems management from a college or university with an ADA-approved program. Upon successful completion of the academic and on-the-job training components of the program, students become eligible to take the national registration examination for dietitians. The successful applicant becomes a registered dietitian.

  Registered dietitians work as clinical dietitians in a variety of health care institutions. Community dietitians work as counselors and coordinators of nutrition awareness and disease prevention programs. Management dietitians specialize in food systems or clinical management or other areas of management and work in health care institutions, schools, colleges, cafeterias, and restaurants and as advisers to the food service industry. Business dietitians work in related business areas such as sales, marketing, and public relations. Education dietitians teach nutrition and food systems in colleges, universities, and hospitals, and conduct research and write books and articles on food service. Consultant dietitians, who practice independently and advise business and industry, counsel patients in a variety of settings.

  In some states, registered dietitians are also licensed by the state and are entitled to use the LD (licensed dietitian) designation or other titles following their names. All dietitians are eligible for ADA membership.

Shared Services

Given the high cost of food and substantial increases in labor cost, it is difficult for a food service manager to stay within a budget and to forecast realistically for the following year.

The pressure to contain costs and at the same time improve the quality of food service is unrelenting. As a result, more and more food service managers are looking at shared food service systems as a means of providing high-quality food for patients and staff at a reasonable cost.

Shared service systems can be categorized according to the degree of control and responsibility exercised by the participating institutions. Thus, a shared service can be classified as a referred service, a purchased service, a multiple-sponsor service, or a regional service. Usually, shared food service systems are either a purchased service or a multiple-sponsor service. A purchased service is paid for directly by the institution. The purchasing institution acts as an intermediary between the patient and the provider and therefore assumes some responsibility for quality of service. In a multiple-sponsor service, several institutions jointly control and operate the service. Control can be established through an agreement among the institutions or through a separate corporation or cooperative. Although the nature and extent of shared food services vary, the major types of sharing are in professional and managerial expertise, food purchasing, and food production systems.

Shared Professional and Management Expertise

The sharing of professional and managerial expertise is of major importance to small and rural hospitals and extended care facilities. Opportunity to use the services of highly trained personnel on a part-time basis allows the health care institution to provide patient services that it otherwise could not afford to offer. Although large hospitals seldom share dietetic and other professional food service personnel among themselves, these institutions sometimes do so with small institutions. Usually, fees for this service are paid directly to the large hospital, which pays the shared personnel their salary, with additional compensation for travel when necessary. The shared personnel usually are required to submit reports to the administrators of both institutions, to meet accreditation requirements, and to evaluate the shared program.

Shared management services are similar to shared professional personnel services. Management services that can be shared include menu planning, financial record keeping, data processing for food service functions, payroll operations, in-service training and education, and policies and procedures planning.

Shared Food Purchasing and Production

Shared food purchasing systems are the most common of the shared services. Standardized and least perishable items are most often purchased through shared systems; but dairy products, frozen meat, poultry, fish, frozen entrees, and nonfood supplies are also frequently available. Agreement on product specifications among participating institutions is essential in attaining the greatest cost savings in shared purchasing arrangements. Shared food purchasing also implies sharing ideas about food quality, processing techniques, consumer acceptance data, and reliable information on new products. Management time is saved in shared purchasing arrangements because the buyer in the participating institution does not have to negotiate prices or see as many vendors, a benefit discussed further in chapter 17.

Shared food production systems are feasible, provided a comprehensive planning and evaluation procedure is used in the developmental stages. Food service managers and CEOs of the institutions involved must agree on long-range goals in level of service, quality, nutrition counseling, bacteriological control, menu variety, and flexibility of the system in the face of changing circumstances.

The decision whether to enter a shared production system or to maintain independent status should be documented. One method of documentation is to survey patients, medical staff, employees, and outpatients about availability, quality, and level of service currently being provided or desired. Opportunities for sharing often involve a shift to different food production and service systems. Careful consideration of the food service systems will help identify the strengths and weaknesses of the present or proposed system. Data to be collected include capital investment requirements, operating costs, quality and comprehensiveness of services, acceptability of services to client groups, and legal considerations such as taxes and contracts.

Multidepartments and Multifacilities

In an effort to flatten organizations, a facility may opt for multidepartment management, which has food service directors responsible for the management of more than one department within an organization. Another possibility is that food service directors may be required to provide management services to more than one facility within a corporation. For example, separate departments for wellness, weight management, or community education could be incorporated into the food service director's responsibilities in a large facility. A multifacility corporation that has a number of hospitals or extended care institutions may require the food service director to oversee more than one of the corporation's units. These services may include the shared management services mentioned earlier.

☐ Distributing Authority

Authority, the legitimate power an organization grants to some of its members, is used to direct and manage the actions of employees of the organization in achieving its goals. (Authority and leadership are discussed in chapter 2.) Just as there are patterns for grouping work in organizations, there are also patterns for the way authority is shared among managers at various levels depending on the structure selected.

Two terms are commonly used to describe the degree to which power is distributed in an organization: centralization and decentralization. *Centralization* refers to the concentration of authority at the top levels of management, where a high proportion of power to make important decisions lies. In contrast, *decentralization* refers to a more widespread sharing of decision-making power throughout the various management levels. Decentralization of authority is evident in organizations that promote teamwork, employee empowerment, and creative decision making and is effective for complex organizations that experience constant change (such as health care facilities). The process by which managers allocate authority to workers who report to them is called *delegation*.

Delegation

By allowing another person (for example, a line employee) to act for him or her in the workings of an organization, a manager is sharing authority and responsibility. A manager can share power through delegation but does not give power away. Delegation enables managers to accomplish more than they could if they attempted to do every task themselves. By delegating tasks, managers can spend time on the functions of planning and staff development. Delegation of responsibility and authority is especially important during a manager's absence, when an assistant (or understudy) can assume interim responsibility for the unit's performance and has the authority to carry out the responsibility. In large departments, a manager may need to train more than one assistant to assume certain portions of the manager's work.

Another advantage of delegation is that it permits the manager to share responsibility for a task with an employee who has more skill or training to perform that task. Delegation is important as a training device, providing employees with additional skills and knowledge.

If poorly managed, however, the process of delegation can have some negative side effects. The most obvious problem is that some essential task may not be accomplished, or it may be performed badly or late.

To work well, the process of delegation should follow these steps:

1. The manager must assign a clear objective or a well-defined task to the employee.
2. The manager must grant the employee the necessary authority to accomplish the task and must ensure that everyone involved in the activity understands that the employee has been given this authority.

3. The employee in turn must understand the objective and accept the authority and responsibility for accomplishing it. This acceptance creates an obligation on the part of the employee to accomplish the task.
4. The manager must hold the employee accountable for accomplishing the task satisfactorily.

In addition to these basic elements of delegation, managers should consider several other factors when deciding to share their responsibility. For example:

- Managers must select employees skilled to accomplish the task or willing to learn the required skills.
- Although managers should allow employees to assume responsibility for the whole task, they should monitor the employees' progress (especially if the employee is new to the assignment) to ensure success.
- Managers should anticipate some mistakes and be prepared to guide employees in correcting them.
- Managers should be certain that the lines of communication with employees are always open and that employees can rely on the manager's advice and support when needed and on praise when it is deserved.

Delegation becomes increasingly important as a manager rises to higher levels of management in the organization. How well the manager can accomplish the work of the organization is reflected by how well the manager leads the work of employees who report to him or her. Some management duties do not lend themselves to delegation and are better shared or left to the manager. They include:

- Establishing missions, goals, and objectives for the entire unit under the manager's responsibility
- Making policy decisions
- Defining standards of performance for the entire unit
- Monitoring the unit's achievement of these standards
- Taking corrective action when the standards are not met

Line and Staff Responsibilities

When managers delegate authority, they must consider the difference between employees in line positions and employees in staff positions. A line employee is part of the direct chain of command that has been established to accomplish the primary work of the organization. Staff support the line positions with their advice and special knowledge. In health care institutions, staff positions are found in departments of finance, human resources, marketing, legal affairs, planning, infection control, safety, management engineering, and data processing, among others. Staff positions usually do not have authority over line positions except when application of staff advice is crucial to the effective performance of line responsibilities. For example, the human resource director usually has no direct authority over tray line workers. However, because he or she has special knowledge about Occupational Safety and Health Administration (OSHA) safety standards, the human resource director knows that a worker without proper hair covering poses a risk and so apprises the food service director, who has authority in this case.

☐ Staffing the Food Service Department

Organizing the work of a department presumes that a competent staff is in place to accomplish the tasks that have been assigned. Building an effective staff involves making decisions about the tasks that need to be performed, the skills required to perform those tasks, the time needed to complete performance, and the number of employees needed to perform the work of the department.

Determination of Work Load

In a health care institution, several variables affect the type and number of job tasks to be performed by the food service department. In determining department work load, managers should ask the following questions:

- What types of service does the department offer? Is the department responsible for an employee cafeteria, a coffee shop, or a patient dining room in addition to patient tray service?
- What type of meal plan is required for the institution's patient population? Are patients offered three, four, or five meals per day?
- How varied are the menu items (for example, limited, moderate, or extensive variation)? How complex are the recipes (simple, average, involved)?
- In what form are foods purchased? Do prepared foods require less processing than do fresh or whole ingredients?
- How many and what types of modified diets will the department need to accommodate?
- Which type of service system is used, centralized or decentralized?
- How much time is available for meal preparation and service?
- How efficient are the department's physical facilities and equipment?
- What type of washing system is used for serviceware and dishware?
- To what extent are the department's information systems automated? What are the computer links with hospital information systems?

Determining work load, type and number of meals, service location, and so on provides information used to determine staff numbers. For example, a department that provided meal service to patients only will need less staff than the department that must staff a cafeteria. An organization using convenience food items would need fewer skilled cooks than one choosing to cook everything from scratch. All of the preceding questions assist in determining the number and skill level of employees needed by the department.

Job Analysis

Once work load has been identified, managers must perform a job analysis for each position. *Job analyses* define the positions in the department and determine the skills required for performing various job tasks. Each food service task must be evaluated according to the mental and physical effort it requires, the equipment it uses, and the time and work conditions it demands. A manager can gather this information by observing food service workers as they perform each task and by discussing their work with them. The manager should ask all relevant questions about the job:

- Who is responsible for performing the task?
- What supplies are needed, and what equipment is required?
- Why is the task performed, and why is it performed this way?
- When must the task be started, and when must it be completed?
- Where is the task performed?
- How exactly is the task performed?

Job analysis and recording of the information gathered during the analysis often benefit from the use of a questionnaire. (See figure 6-9.) Organizing the information in this way helps ensure that all tasks are analyzed on the basis of comparable observations.

Figure 6-9. Position Information Questionnaire

Purpose and Instructions

This form is designed to gather facts about the duties and responsibilities of your position. Your answers, the responses from other employees in the same position, and your supervisor's comments will be used as input into the evaluation of the positions at All Saints Health Care, Inc. This form will also help to update current position descriptions.

Keep in mind that this information will be used to help better understand the duties and responsibilities of your position within the organization. The form is not an evaluation of your performance.

Please be thorough and accurate. Try not to understate or inflate your answers. Base your responses on the duties and responsibilities that are most typical of your position under normal conditions, not special projects or temporary assignments. It might be helpful to imagine that you are explaining the requirements of your position to someone just hired.

Only your supervisor and certain members of the Human Resources Department will have access to these forms. If you have any questions about this form, please speak with your supervisor.

General Background Information

Please Print

Name: _____ Employee Number: _____

Position Title: _____ Date: _____ /_____ /_____

Cost Center: _____ Form Completed: _____

Your immediate supervisor's name and position title:

Name: _____

Title: _____

Your current shift [✓]:

[ ] days

[ ] evenings

[ ] nights

[ ] rotating

[ ] on call (PRN) or temporary

[ ] weekend

Your current employment status [✓]:

[ ] full-time

[ ] part-time (scheduled to work less than 32 hours per week in recent months)

[ ] other (specify)

Position Summary

Briefly describe the basic summary of your position (it may be helpful to complete this section last).

Your Basic Job Duties

List the most significant duties that you currently perform on a regular basis. Start each statement with an action verb; for example, draw, build, distribute, write, plan, process, administer, et cetera. Indicate whether that duty is *essential* or *marginal*. A job function may be considered essential because of the limited number of employees available to do that function or the function may be essential because the reason your position exists is to perform that function. Indicate the frequency of each duty by circling the appropriate number.

Use the guide below for frequency:

FREQUENCY

Once a Month	2 to 3 Times a Month	2 to 3 Times a Day	Once a Day	Many Times Day
1	2	3	4	5

129

continued on next page

Figure 6-9. *Continued*

Please rank your job duties from the most important to the least important job function. The number 1 would be assigned to your most essential job duty, 2 is the second most important, and so on until you have ranked each duty.

Duties	**Frequency**
	1 2 3 4 5
	E ____ M ____
1. _____	
	1 2 3 4 5
	E ____ M ____
2. _____	
	1 2 3 4 5
	E ____ M ____
3. _____	
	1 2 3 4 5
	E ____ M ____
4. _____	
	1 2 3 4 5
	E ____ M ____
5. _____	
	1 2 3 4 5
	E ____ M ____
6. _____	
	1 2 3 4 5
	E ____ M ____
7. _____	
	1 2 3 4 5
	E ____ M ____
8. _____	
	1 2 3 4 5
	E ____ M ____
9. _____	
	1 2 3 4 5
	E ____ M ____
10. _____	

Education and Training Demands

What is the minimum level of formal education required for your position? This is the minimum necessary educational level that would be required of a new person, not necessarily your own educational level. Please check one level.

Level	Definition	Examples
1 ( )	Some training, but less than a high school diploma	
2 ( )	High school diploma or equivalent	GED
3 ( )	Job-related course work after high school, up to 12 months	Word processing, data processing
4 ( )	Specialized training up to 24 months	ART, Surgical assistant
5 ( )	Associated degree of specialized training	RN, MLT, X-ray technician
6 ( )	Bachelor's degree obtained through formal four-year program	BSN, BSW, BA, BS
7 ( )	Specialized training beyond bachelor's degree	CPA, RDA
8 ( )	Master's degree; at least a two-year graduate program	MSW, MBA
9 ( )	Doctoral degree or equivalent	MD, PhD, JD

Figure 6-9. *Continued*

Indicate any specific certifications, licenses, registrations, or specialized skills (for example, 55 wpm typing) required of your position.

_____

Can previous experience be substituted for education/training requirements?

(Check one) _____ Yes _____ No

If yes, how much previous experience can be substituted? _____

Does this job involved reading ability in English?

(Check one) _____ Yes _____ No

(Check one) _____ Essential _____ Marginal

Describe the materials to be read:

_____

Does this job involve mathematical ability?

(Check one) _____ Yes _____ No

(Check one) _____ Essential _____ Marginal

Describe the mathematical functions to be performed.

_____

Does this job involve written language ability in English?

(Check one) _____ Yes _____ No

(Check one) _____ Essential _____ Marginal

Describe the writing assignments to be performed.

_____

Decision Making

Check the one statement that best describes the impact of the decisions and commitments you make.

Level   Definition

( )   Generally I follow specific instructions and make few decisions.

( )   I basically follow instructions, sometimes choosing which approach to use.

( )   I make decisions or recommendations within the limits of general instructions that have been provided to me.

( )   I make decisions or recommendations that require some interpretation of rules, policies, and procedures.

( )   Decisions and recommendations are of a broad nature and are made in accordance with general policies/procedures. My decision may affect the work of an entire department.

( )   I consult with others on very difficult decisions but have the responsibility for final decisions and recommendations; frequently I am required to provide input on policy decisions or a major impact. My decision can affect several departments or functional areas.

( )   I provide leadership to others and have ultimate responsibility for making final decisions.

Work Environment

Work environment includes things like lighting, noise, heat or cold, and exposure to harmful substances. In responding to this question, it is assumed that you do not take *unnecessary* risks and that all safety and protective procedures are followed.

continued on next page

Figure 6-9. *Continued*

For each type of exposure, circle the number that describes the frequency of exposure required to complete your position duties. (Please note that the frequency of exposure means how often you come in contact with the exposure compared to employees in other departments. For example, Radiology Techs would have frequent radiation exposure in comparison to most other employees.) Provide specific examples of the work exposures encountered in the course of completing your typical position duties.

Type of Work Exposure	Frequency of Exposure			Example
	Seldom	Normal	Often	
Cold	1 2 3 4 5 6 7			_____
Heat	1 2 3 4 5 6 7			_____
Heights	1 2 3 4 5 6 7			_____
Skin irritants	1 2 3 4 5 6 7			_____
Lung irritants	1 2 3 4 5 6 7			_____
Infectious diseases	1 2 3 5 5 6 7			_____
Electrical equipment	1 2 3 4 5 6 7			_____
Radiation	1 2 3 4 5 6 7			_____
Sharp instruments	1 2 3 4 5 6 7			_____
Loud noises	1 2 3 4 5 6 7			_____
Toxic materials	1 2 3 4 5 6 7			_____
Hazardous waste	1 2 3 4 5 6 7			_____
Solar radiation	1 2 3 4 5 6 7			_____
Laser radiation	1 2 3 4 5 6 7			_____
Rotating shifts	1 2 3 4 5 6 7			_____
Rotating weekends	1 2 3 4 5 6 7			_____
Permanent evening shift	1 2 3 4 5 6 7			_____
Permanent night shift	1 2 3 4 5 6 7			_____

Physical Demands

These physical demands deal with the type of physical activity required to perform the duties of your position. This may include for some positions an unusual requirement for visual focus or observations.

Please check whether the following physical demands are essential or marginal for your position duties. If the demand is essential please circle the importance of each demand.

Type of Physical Demand			If Essential Please Circle Importance						
			Minor		Important			Highly Important	
Seeing	_____ Essential	_____ Marginal	1	2	3	4	5	6	7
Hearing	_____ Essential	_____ Marginal	1	2	3	4	5	6	7
Touching	_____ Essential	_____ Marginal	1	2	3	4	5	6	7
Tasting	_____ Essential	_____ Marginal	1	2	3	4	5	6	7
Smelling	_____ Essential	_____ Marginal	1	2	3	4	5	6	7
Climbing	_____ Essential	_____ Marginal	1	2	3	4	5	6	7
Balance	_____ Essential	_____ Marginal	1	2	3	4	5	6	7
Color discrimination	_____ Essential	_____ Marginal	1	2	3	4	5	6	7
Finger dexterity	_____ Essential	_____ Marginal	1	2	3	4	5	6	7
Eye/hand/foot coordination	_____ Essential	_____ Marginal	1	2	3	4	5	6	7

Figure 6-9. *Continued*

Never	Occasionally 1–33% of shift	Frequently 33–66% of shift

During a typical work shift, does the job involve sitting?

(Check one) _____ Yes _____ No   (Check one) _____ Essential _____ Marginal

(Check one) (_____ Frequently; _____ Occasionally; _____ Never)

During a typical work shift, does the job involve standing?

(Check one) _____ Yes _____ No   (Check one) _____ Essential _____ Marginal

(Check one) (_____ Frequently; _____ Occasionally; _____ Never)

During a typical work shift, does the job involve walking?

(Check one) _____ Yes _____ No   (Check one) _____ Essential _____ Marginal

(Check one) (_____ Frequently; _____ Occasionally; _____ Never)

During a typical work shift, does the job involve kneeling?

(Check one) _____ Yes _____ No   (Check one) _____ Essential _____ Marginal

(Check one) (_____ Frequently; _____ Occasionally; _____ Never)

During a typical work shift, does the job involve crouching or stooping?

(Check one) _____ Yes _____ No   (Check one) _____ Essential _____ Marginal

(Check one) (_____ Frequently; _____ Occasionally; _____ Never)

During a typical work shift, does the job involve squatting?

(Check one) _____ Yes _____ No   (Check one) _____ Essential _____ Marginal

(Check one) (_____ Frequently; _____ Occasionally; _____ Never)

During a typical work shift, does the job involve twisting upper body or neck?

(Check one) _____ Yes _____ No   (Check one) _____ Essential _____ Marginal

(Check one) (_____ Frequently; _____ Occasionally; _____ Never)

Lifting

Assuming an average 8-hour shift with two 15-minute breaks and a 30-minute meal break, would your position perform the following activities:

1. Lift (Please state common item lifted) _____

	Never	Rarely 1–10%	Occasionally 11–33% of shift	Frequently 33–66% of shift	Continuously 67–100% of shift
Up to 10#					
11 to 24#					
25 to 34#					
35 to 50#					
51 to 74#					
75 to 100#					
100# +					

2. Carry (Please estimate distance in feet and state common item lifted) _____

Up to 10#					
11 to 24#					
25 to 34#					
35 to 50#					
51 to 74#					
75 to 100#					
100# +					

continued on next page

Figure 6-9. *Continued*

3. Push (State item being pushed and weight of item) _____

	Never	Occasionally 1–33% of shift	Frequently 33–66% of shift	Continuously 67–100% of shift
Sitting	_____	_____	_____	_____
Standing	_____	_____	_____	_____

4. Pull (State item being pulled and weight of item) _____

Sitting	_____	_____	_____	_____
Standing	_____	_____	_____	_____

5. Elevated work requiring reach above shoulder level, neck/back in extension position

(State task being performed) _____

Sitting	_____	_____	_____	_____
Standing	_____	_____	_____	_____

During a typical work shift does the job involve other plysical demands not mentioned? If so, what are the demands?

_____

Are these demands: _____ Essential _____ Marginal

Specific Equipment Used:

During a typical work shift, does the job involve operating or using any machinery or equipment (nonvehicle)? If so please list.

Is a license or certificate required to operate any identified machinery?

Is training provided by All Saints?

During a typical work shift, does the job involve operating or using a vehicle?

Other Position Characteristics:

Does this job supervise any other positions? If so how many FTE's. _____

During a typical work shift, the level of supervision over this position can be characterized as being: (Check one)

_____ Extensive (Much direct supervision; work with supervisor)

_____ Moderate (Access to supervisor and/or lead coworkers, when needed)

_____ Limited (Worker must be highly autonomous, show much independence)

Source: Used with permission of All Saints Health System, Fort Worth, TX.

Job Descriptions and Specifications

The results of job analyses are documented in the form of job descriptions and job specifications for all positions in the organization. A *job description* is a written record of the set of tasks to be performed by the employee and the conditions under which the tasks are to be accomplished. A *job specification* describes the qualifications required of the person responsible for performing those tasks. In most organizations, the job description and job specification are combined on one standard form.

An up-to-date job description and specification form must be kept for every job in the food service department. The form must be closely followed when a new employee is hired for a position, when a current employee and his or her supervisor develop objectives for the employee's performance, and when the employee's performance is evaluated by the supervisor. Figure 6-10 is an example of a combined job description and job specification for a position in the food service department.

Figure 6-10. Sample Job Description and Job Specification

Job Title: Tray Line Server   *Job Code:*
Department: Nutrition/Food Services
Reports to: Food Service Supervisor
Shift:

Position Summary: Responsible for food service to patients and other related duties including sanitation. Has a working knowledge of food service procedures and delivery. There are seven tray line positions, which are rotated either monthly or bimonthly.

Minimum Qualifications: Ability to read and write English in order to communicate with staff, patients, and other customers; a basic understanding of weights and measures. Experience is not required, but one year's experience in quantity food service is preferred.

Licenses, Certificates, or Similar Qualifications: None required

Essential Functions:

1. Checks daily assignment sheet for shift duties.
2. Prepares station for serving food. Physical requirements include:
   - Transporting 22.5-inch-by-16-inch trays of food weighing up to 25 pounds. Trays are stored at heights between 5 and 62 inches.
   - Stocking food steam tables. Requires lifting food pans weighing up to 20 pounds from heights of 11 to 62 inches and loading them onto a food bar 35 inches in height.
   - Stocking beverage/ice-cream cooling units. Requires reaching over edge of cooling unit 35 inches in height with a forward reach up to 28 inches.
   - Starter position responsible for placing hot pellets on the tray with the assistance of a delifter.
3. Checks quality, temperature, and appearance of food, relaying any problems to supervisor. Physical requirements include corrected visual acuity of 20–20 and good sense of smell.
4. Serves food from station on tray line. Requires using appropriate utensils, such as large spoons and knives, for proper portion control. Beverages are served from dispensers, pitchers, or taken from cooling units. All food and beverage items are placed on a tray on the conveyor belt. Full plates of food may weigh up to 2 pounds and are placed on a conveyor belt 33 inches in height.
5. Loads completed trays, weighing up to 10 pounds, into transport carts. Shelf heights are 8 to 50 inches from the floor.
6. Cleaning tech position or tray line server transports food carts weighing up to 730 pounds to patient floors for distances up to feet. Also returns carts with empty trays to the dish room. Porter duties include dish room duties and emptying 50-gallon trash cans in an outside dumpster. Trash can lift is 48 inches from ground.
7. Performs floor stocking duties. Requires reaching overhead to a 73-inch height and a forward reach of 13 inches. Boxes lifted may weigh up to 11.25 pounds.
8. Checks assigned stations hourly for cleanliness and operates equipment as required.
9. Performs dish room duties as assigned, including unloading and loading dishes between carts and various workstations. Maximum weight lifted is 50 pounds occasionally to move loaded bins to different shelves on cart (11 to 34 inches). Duties require a forward reach up to 40 inches and lifting ranges from 11 to 75 inches from the floor. Inspects dishes for cleanliness prior to taking to the serving line and prior to use.

continued on next page

Figure 6-10. *Continued*

10. Washes, drains, and dries empty food carts. Includes using spray hose and tilting 289-pound cart to drain water.
11. Cleans and sanitizes station before leaving area with approved cleaning solution.
12. Completes all line server shift assignments by end of shift. Responds to changes in the work load as assigned by the supervisor or manager. No eating or drinking in work area.
13. Uses disposable gloves and hair coverings. Facial hair and sculptured nails are not permitted in food service areas. Observes all sanitation, safety, and infection control procedures.
14. Complies with policies and procedures in departmental manual and ASH employee handbook.

Job-Related Equipment: Carts, trays, delifter, beverage dispensers, reach-in and walk-in refrigerated and freezer units, hot food storage units, steam tables, cartlift, dumbwaiter, microwave, dishmachine, pulper, conveyor belt, serving utensils, blender, knives, disposable gloves, hair coverings, and safety belts.

Work Environment: Working in hospital nutrition and food service increases the risk of exposure to sharp instruments and noise. Temperature varies in the area due to refrigerating and heating equipment. Cleaning duties include using various solutions to clean, disinfect, and polish surfaces. Tray line servers may be required to work different shifts including evenings and weekends. Standing and walking required for approximately seven hours out of an eight-hour day.

Safety Responsibility: All nutrition and food service employees must use good body mechanics and follow safe working procedures including infection control and OSHA guidelines. The employee must report any unsafe condition to a supervisor and demonstrate no on-the-job injuries due to a lack of good safety practices. On-the-job injuries must be reported immediately to the supervisor and an occurrence report completed.

Career Ladder: Through on-the-job training, advancement is possible to other positions including, but not limited to: hostess, cashier, vending, catering, cook, or clerk.

This job description reflects the general duties and principal functions of line server. It is not a detailed description of all the work requirements that may be inherent in the position.

Every job description and job specification form must include the following elements:

- Job title and its classification or code (usually established with help of the human resource department and used in defining salary levels and routes for promotion)
- Summary of major responsibilities of the position
- Clear statement of the minimum standards of performance for each essential function
- Description of the work environment—equipment used, possible health hazards involved, responsibility to safety, and other such essential information
- Outline of opportunities for promotion that are relevant to the position
- Minimum qualifications for eligibility to hold the job—education, training, experience, and any other special considerations

A job description and specification for every position in the food service department should be on file in the department director's office. In addition, employees should be given copies of their job descriptions and specifications on their first day of work and whenever the materials are revised. Using this document can lead to improved efficiency in the food service department by increasing the current employees' understanding of their responsibilities and by providing guidelines for training new employees.

As managers reevaluate current job descriptions and specifications or develop new ones, they must avoid establishing requirements that do not match the actual demands of the job. To cite an extreme example, managers cannot require that a patient nutrition aide have a college education or be a certified dietitian. Setting too high a standard for a position may violate certain of the regulations of the Equal Employment Opportunity Commission (EEOC). Job descriptions should clearly identify physical requirements for the position as a reference in screening job applicants with disabilities. The Americans with Disabilities Act (ADA) requires that Americans with disabilities be employed when they can perform essential functions and that reasonable accommodations be made to assist them in performing essential job functions. To ensure that job descriptions and specifications are in compliance with all federal and state laws, the food service director should work closely with the human resource department.

Work Division and Job Enrichment

The writing of job descriptions and specifications provides the manager with the opportunity to consider how the work can be divided in such a way that employee productivity and satisfaction are maximized. At one time, the traditional method of assigning work in the food service department was to have employees perform specific jobs that they followed through on from start to finish. Therefore, a cook was responsible for preparation, portioning, and service of specific menu items as well as for cleanup of the equipment and work space. In recent years, this method of assigning work has been replaced in many institutions by a greater division of labor that makes more efficient use of skilled employees. In this system, skilled employees are assigned work according to the degree of skill needed to complete each task. This division-of-labor method allows highly skilled employees to perform fewer unskilled tasks, such as preliminary preparation of recipe ingredients and cleanup. Instead, skilled employees are responsible for tasks that use their skills to greater advantage.

Both the traditional approach and the division-of-labor approach have inherent advantages and disadvantages. In the traditional approach, the employee who can do a task from start to finish feels more personal commitment to the job and may be more highly motivated and accountable for the quality of the work. However, skilled employees must spend a considerable amount of work time on portions of the whole job that do not require all of their expertise. From the manager's perspective, a greater division of labor is a more efficient use of the department's resources because preparation and cleanup tasks can be assigned to unskilled employees who are paid less than skilled employees.

The traditional approach is once again finding favor in food service departments. However, a combination of both approaches may be the most beneficial arrangement for managers and workers. In the food service department, for example, the measuring, weighing, and preparing of ingredients in a centralized ingredient area permits greater control of inventory and quality and modifies the division of labor so that all employees have more than one narrow set of tasks to perform. The repetitive tasks of measuring, weighing, and preparing the ingredients used in all recipes are transferred from skilled to less-skilled employees. Cleanup and maintenance responsibilities are also reassigned to those who are less skilled. To make the work of less-skilled employees more varied, their work assignments are typically enlarged to include a wider set of tasks. This process is called *job enrichment* or *job enlargement*. For example, a tray line employee may be assigned to patient service for part of the workday, or he or she may work in the ingredient area for some portion of the workweek.

Research on work in different kinds of organizations has demonstrated the feasibility and benefit of job enrichment to provide greater employee satisfaction and to increase productivity. Both benefits can help an organization better meet the pressures of rising labor costs and diminishing availability of skilled employees. Most employees are happier when work incorporates a challenge to them and permits reasonable flexibility in determining how an assigned task is to be performed. Worker satisfaction tends to reduce turnover and the costs associated with recruiting and training new employees.

To implement job enrichment effectively, managers must be aware of the work to be accomplished, the most efficient methods for accomplishing that work, the skills each task requires, and the best means for motivating employees. The processes of job analysis and work division must be an ongoing part of the manager's responsibility. They are also the bases for making decisions about staff size, schedules, and performance standards to be met. (Chapter 11 discusses performance standards in the context of financial management and control for the food service department.)

Determination of Staff Size

Once the type and number of food service tasks have been determined, job analyses have been performed, and job descriptions and specifications have been written, managers can begin to estimate the number of employees they need in each type of job. The variables that specifically affect how much labor time the food service department requires can be identified by answering the following questions:

- How much time is allocated for meal preparation and service? Is additional staff needed at certain times of the day?
- Is the service system centralized or decentralized? (Decentralized systems usually require more personnel owing to the staffing needed in areas outside the food service department.)
- How efficient is the department's physical layout and equipment?
- What type of washing system is to be used for serviceware and dishware? (When disposable serviceware is used, the time required for washing is greatly reduced.)
- What quality of work is expected from the employees?

Careful consideration of these variables will help ensure that the food service department has sufficient staff. The manager must next calculate productivity, full-time equivalent (FTE), and overtime needs based on the number of staff projected.

Estimating Productivity Levels

Staffing requirements must be based on the department's output. *Output* is defined as the end result of a work process, or the transformation of inputs. Output in the nutrition and food service department includes a variety of meal types and nutritional units of service. *Input* includes food and other resources, including labor. Transformation refers to the processes that convert input to output. The ratio of input to output is defined as *productivity*.

The use of a preestablished productivity factor allows the food service manager to determine the staffing required to produce the number of meals provided. The first step in determining a productivity level is to establish guidelines for calculating a single unit of service or a meal. Output can be determined as actual meals, which is usually the case for patient meals and late trays. However, for areas such as the cafeteria a meal equivalent is used. Meal equivalents are determined by first calculating a meal equivalent factor.

One accepted method of determining a meal equivalent factor for the cafeteria is using an average meal ticket. The average meal ticket is determined by dividing total sales by the number of customers over a predetermined length of time (average meal ticket = total sales ÷ number of customers). This figure represents the average ticket for meal service and can be used to establish meal equivalents. For example, if total sales for the cafeteria equal $550 for lunch and 200 customers were served over a defined period of time, the meal equivalent would be $2.75 ($550 ÷ 200 = $2.75). The average meal ticket meal equivalent should be established after gathering at least one week of ticket averages for lunch. The meal equivalent should be verified on a quarterly basis. Another method of determining an equivalent meal factor is to use the sum of the selling price for an entree, starch, vegetable, salad, dessert, bread, butter, and beverage at the noon meal.

Once the meal equivalent factor is determined, the number of meals produced can be calculated. Equivalent meals is calculated by dividing cafeteria sales for the period by the meal equivalent factor (equivalent meals = sales ÷ equivalent meal factor). Using the $2.75 meal equivalent factor calculated above and a sales figure of $45,000 for the month, equivalent meals can be calculated as follows:

$$\text{Equivalent meals} = \$45,000 \div \$2.75 = 16,364 \text{ meals}$$

The number of equivalent meals is used to calculate productivity. Productivity in food service is usually expressed as meals produced per labor hour or labor hours per meal produced:

$$\text{Meals per labor hour} = \frac{\text{Number of meals produced}}{\text{Number of labor hours}}$$

For the 16,364 equivalent meals produced in the cafeteria in the preceding example, a total of 2,975 hours were worked. Using the meals per labor hour calculation:

Meals per labor hour = 16,364 meals ÷ 2,975 labor hours = 5.5 meals per labor hour

Expressing this same productivity as labor hours per meal:

$$\text{Labor hours per meal} = \frac{\text{Number of labor hours}}{\text{Number of meals}}$$

Using the same numbers as in the preceding example:

Labor hours per meal = 2,975 labor hours ÷ 16,364 meals = .19 labor hours per meal

The following represent industry averages (from Sneed and Dresse, 1989) for various types of food service operations:

Facility Type	Meals per Labor Hour	Labor Hours per Meal
Cafeteria	5.5 meals	.19 hours
Acute care facility	3.5 meals	.29 hours
Extended care facility	5.0 meals	.20 hours

Calculating Full-Time Equivalent Needs

A *full-time equivalent* refers to an employee who works on a full-time basis for a specific period of time. The following hours and specific time periods are used in reference to FTEs:

- 8 hours per day
- 40 hours per week
- 173.33 hours per month
- 2,080 hours per year

Staffing needs are usually expressed as the number of FTEs needed for the department. Full-time equivalent needs are calculated using the productivity factor in the preceding section. First, the total number of labor hours must be calculated for the time period in question. Second, the number of labor hours is converted to FTEs needed. For example, if the cafeteria produced 16,364 meal equivalents in a month and the productivity standard being used is equal to 5.5 meals per labor hour, FTE needs are calculated as follows:

$$\text{Labor hours} = \frac{16{,}364 \text{ meals per month}}{5.5 \text{ meals per labor hour}} = 2{,}975 \text{ labor hours per month}$$

$$\text{Number of FTEs} = \frac{2{,}975 \text{ labor hours per month}}{173.33 \text{ hours per FTE per month}} = 17.2 \text{ FTEs}$$

The number of FTEs can be calculated for the day, week, month, or year by determining the number of labor hours needed in the period and dividing by the FTE equivalent factor identified earlier. For example, if department responsibilities require 40 hours of work per week, 40 hours ÷ 8 hours per FTE per day = 5 FTEs. For a department that needs 300 hours per week, 300 hours ÷ 40 hours per FTE per week = 7.5 FTEs.

Full-time equivalents required for the department are not necessarily reflective of the number of staff members employed by the department. For example, if the department needed 10.5 FTEs on an annual basis to run the department, it may have a total of 13 employees. Seven of the employees may be full-time employees working a total of 40 hours a week, and three of the employees may be .5 full-time equivalents, or work 20 hours per week.

$$
\begin{array}{rcl}
9 \times 40 & = & 360 \text{ hours per week} \\
3 \times 20 & = & \underline{60 \text{ hours per week}} \\
& & 420 \text{ hours per week}
\end{array}
$$

420 hours per week ÷ 40 hours per FTE per week = 10.5 FTEs

Anticipating Overtime Needs

The preceding examples calculated the number of FTEs required as regular productive hours. This figure represents core staffing based on the number of meals served. To determine complete staffing, the manager must consider the number of overtime, benefit, and nonproductive hours to be paid. (Budgeting is covered in detail in chapter 11.)

The amount of overtime used in the food service department depends on a number of factors, including fluctuations in demand, inefficient work processes or equipment, employee injuries, availability of workers, and department size. Some industry experts consider overtime above 2 percent of productive hours paid to be excessive and in need of attention. Most organizations establish an overtime percentage based on historical data and environmental information prior to completion of the annual operating budget. In an effort to lower the amount of overtime, the number of part-time or occasional (on-call) employees can be increased. To determine the number of FTEs required to cover overtime, the following formula is used:

$$\text{Total FTEs} \times \text{overtime percent} = \text{number of FTEs for overtime}$$

For example,

$$10.5 \text{ FTEs} \times 1 \text{ percent overtime} = .11 \text{ FTE}$$

Preparation for Outside Consultants

Effective control of labor costs requires a productivity measurement system to facilitate decision making. Many health care organizations have found themselves faced with outside consultants who have attempted to generate productivity standards for the food service department. To prepare for outside consultants, it is incumbent on food service directors to identify and establish productivity parameters for their departments. Having departmental statistics available for outside consultants allows the food service manager to be in control of productivity demands. Figure 6-11 represents a productivity form that can be used to track internal productivity. This type of internal monitoring provides the food service manager with information for consultants or for providing information as support documentation for staff or service changes.

☐ Scheduling Work in the Food Service Department

Because health care institutions require round-the-clock staffing, the food service director must make sure that the jobs in his or her department are filled at the appropriate times in each 24-hour period. Therefore, scheduling the workweek and specific hours each employee must be on duty is a key step in achieving efficiency in the use of labor dollars while meeting the institution's service objectives.

The 40-hour workweek is common for full-time employees in most of the nation's businesses. Actually, this period includes only 35 working hours because each hourly employee has a 15-minute paid rest period every 4 hours and a 30-minute unpaid meal period each day. Although the workweek has commonly been divided into 5 equal workdays, some innovative food service directors have developed schedules in which employees work 10½ hours per day and 4 days per week. Such schedules have produced notable improvements in employee productivity and job satisfaction. Another type of schedule calls for employees to work 4 days, take 3 days off, work 5 days, take 2 days off, and then begin the cycle again without working more than 8 days in any 2-week pay period.

Flexible Schedules

Overlapping schedules among employees can be avoided by retraining them to perform a broader range of duties as part of their job enlargement plan. For example, tray line workers could learn to perform production tasks and some sanitation duties, and sanitation workers

Figure 6-11. Sample Productivity Form

ABC Hospital
Food Service Department Productivity Report
for the Year:

Parameters	Jan	Feb	Mar	Apr	May	Jun	Jul	Aug	Sep	Oct	Nov	Dec	Annual Average
Worked hours													
Paid hours													
Inpatient meals													
Outpatient meals													
Other meals													
Cafeteria meals													
Cafeteria sales													
Meal equivalent													
Total meals													
Payroll costs													
Food costs													
Supply costs													
Other costs													
Total direct costs													
Adjusted patient days													
Internal Trends													
Worked hours/meal													
Meals/man-hour													
Paid time off (%)													
Total salary/meal													
Food cost/meal													
Supply cost/meal													
Total cost/meal													
Other meals (%)													
% labor/total cost													
Labor cost/adjusted patient day													
Total cost/adjusted patient day													
Total meals/adjusted patient day													
Worked FTEs													
Paid FTEs													

could learn to perform some food production and tray line duties. This flexibility in scheduling significantly reduces the total number of employees needed to meet labor needs. It also may result in less absenteeism and turnover because of improved employee morale and job satisfaction. The new schedule provides each employee with the opportunity for a wider set of duties and is an important element in any job enrichment effort.

Professional employees in the department also may wish to take advantage of flexible scheduling. For example, a registered dietitian might choose to work during the institution's most active period between 6:30 a.m. and 3:00 p.m. Two part-time professional employees might arrange their schedules so that together they meet the requirements of a full-time equivalent position; that is, one might work three 8-hour days, and the other two 8-hour days. This arrangement is called *job sharing* or *job splitting*. A nutrition host might choose to work four 10-hour days instead of five 8-hour days so that he or she could cover all three meals served on the days worked. Others might choose to work 9 hours for 4 days and then take half a day off on the day of the week when there are fewer rounds and admissions.

Master Schedules

No matter which system of scheduling is best suited for a particular institution, the work schedule should be charted and posted so that it is readily accessible to all employees. The schedule should indicate the days on duty for each employee, daily scheduled hours (when they vary from one day to the next), days off, vacation days, and so forth. A rotating master schedule should be developed to reduce the amount of time the director spends in scheduling employees each week. Rotating master schedules are used to regularly schedule employee days off. A rotating master schedule may complete the scheduling cycle every three, five, six, or seven weeks. It also helps ensure that employees share responsibility for working weekends so that the same people are not scheduled to work every weekend.

Master schedules are usually designed to correspond to the length of the pay period so that each employee is assured of working an equal number of hours during each period. In addition, the number of overtime hours can be minimized when the schedule is designed to coincide with pay periods.

The food service director should examine the schedule of every employee. The daily hours to be worked and the scheduled days off should be assigned fairly, without favoritism. Also, situations in which an employee has the late shift on one day and an early shift the following day should be avoided, as should split shifts because most employees prefer a continuous workday. Rotating shifts (in which an employee is scheduled for varying work periods from one week or pay period to the next) are frequently used to provide more flexibility for management and employees. Once the master schedule has been set, frequent major revisions should be avoided. Although rigidity is not the goal here, a relatively consistent work schedule that repeats with every pay period helps establish smooth work patterns for individual employees. Furthermore, within certain work groups, employees must depend on being familiar with one another's pace of work, to both ensure an adequate level of productivity and minimize the risk of accidents and injuries. Finally, consistent schedules permit employees to plan their personal time better, thus reducing the likelihood of absenteeism and employee turnover.

Other Schedule Types

In addition to scheduling employee workweeks, the food service director and his or her managers need to construct several types of schedules to ensure that all department work flows smoothly during a given day. The staggered daily schedule pattern illustrated in figure 6-12 indicates the different food service positions that need to be filled within the department and the daily hours during which the functions of those positions usually must be accomplished.

Figure 6-12. Example of a Daily Schedule Pattern

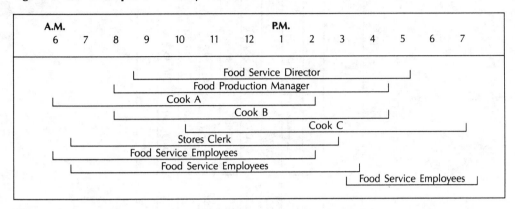

Figure 6-13 shows an example of a shift schedule for eight cooks working in a department that serves three meals per day, seven days per week. Cooks A, B, and C together cover the morning shift from 6:00 a.m. to 2:30 p.m. during which two cooks are usually needed. On the one day per week that all three are scheduled to work—Thursday on this schedule—they may perform extra cleaning duties or prepare special foods. The cooks on the afternoon shift, 10:00 a.m. to 7:30 p.m., are scheduled in the same way. Cooks D and E relieve each other so that four days per week only one of the two cooks is on duty. Cooks D and E prepare foods for modified diets and/or special salads and desserts.

Written daily work schedules guide each employee's activities during the workday, listing the duties to be performed during specified time periods and the routine cleaning tasks that must be completed. An example of an individual employee work schedule is shown in figure 6-14. Providing this type of breakdown for employees has several advantages:

- The employee has written instructions on hand for each task and does not need to rely on verbal orders, which are more easily misunderstood or forgotten.
- Deadlines help an employee set objectives for each portion of the workday.
- Work can proceed more smoothly, with less time spent waiting for a new set of instructions or explanations.
- The manager can use the individual schedule to maintain work-load balance among employees.

Some organizations set up separate cleaning schedules and rotate cleaning duties among employees. Rotating unpleasant jobs is usually desirable, but most of the daily and weekly cleaning tasks should be incorporated into individual schedules.

Computerized Scheduling

Scheduling for the food service department is a complex task requiring a large amount of information. Due to the complexity and time involved in scheduling, some departments have turned to computer software for this activity. Scheduling software can track the number of full- and part-time employees, the number of hours worked, vacation or other days off, specific times requested off by employees, and when an employee goes into overtime. Computerized scheduling also consistently provides management with timely reports of hours worked, which is necessary to track department productivity. In addition, work load and peak times can be predicted, allowing flexible staffing; management time is freed for other duties; and computer objectivity ensures scheduling equity among employees. Unlike manual schedules, computer scheduling can accommodate last-minute changes with little effort and time.

Figure 6-13. Example of a Shift Schedule

Week Ending: _____

Name/Classification	Sun.	Mon.	Tues.	Wed.	Thurs.	Fri.	Sat.
J. Lloyd—Cook A	6:00-2:30	6:00-2:30	D/O	D/O	6:00-2:30	6:00-2:30	6:00-2:30
T. Walker—Cook B	6:00-2:30	6:00-2:30	6:00-2:30	6:00-2:30	6:00-2:30	D/O	D/O
J. Foot—Cook C	D/O	D/O	6:00-2:30	6:00-2:30	6:00-2:30	6:30-2:00	6:30-2:00
I. Shenk—Cook D	9:30-6:00	9:30-6:00	9:30-6:00	D/O	D/O	9:30-6:00	9:30-6:00
M. Smith—Cook E	8:30-5:00	D/O	D/O	9:30-6:00	9:30-6:00	8:30-5:00	8:30-5:00
A. Frank—Cook F	10:00-7:30	10:00-7:30	10:00-7:30	D/O	D/O	10:00-7:30	10:00-7:30
B. Tyler—Cook G	10:00-7:30	D/O	D/O	10:00-7:30	10:00-7:30	10:00-7:30	10:00-7:30
B. James—Cook H	10:00-7:30	10:00-7:30	10:00-7:30	10:00-7:30	10:00-7:30	D/O	D/O

Figure 6-14. Example of a Work Schedule for an Individual Employee

---

WORK SCHEDULE FOR CAFETERIA COUNTER EMPLOYEE

Name: _____   Hours: 5:30 A.M. to 2:00 P.M.
                                                          30 minutes for breakfast
                                                          15 minutes for coffee break

Position: Cafeteria Counter Employee No. 1   Supervised by: _____

Days Off: _____   Relieved by: _____

5:30 to 7:15 A.M.	1. Read breakfast menu
	2. Ready equipment for breakfast meal
	a. Turn on heat in cafeteria counter units for hot foods, grill, and dish warmers at 6 A.M.
	b. Prepare counter units for cold food at 6 A.M.
	c. Obtain required serving utensils and put in position for use
	d. Place dishes where needed, those required for hot food in dish warmer
	3. Make coffee (consult supervisor for instructions and amount to be made)
	4. Fill milk dispenser
	5. Obtain food items to be served cold: fruit, fruit juice, dry cereals, butter, cream, etc. Place in proper location on cafeteria counter.
	6. Obtain hot food and put in hot section of counter
	7. Check with supervisor for correct portion sizes if this has not been decided previously
6:30 to 8:00 A.M.	1. Open cafeteria doors for breakfast service
	2. Replenish cold food items, dishes, and tableware
	3. Notify cook before hot items are depleted
	4. Make additional coffee as needed
	5. Keep counters clean; wipe up spilled food
8:00 to 8:30 A.M.	Eat breakfast
8:30 to 10:30 A.M.	1. Break down serving line and return leftover foods to refrigerators and cook's area as directed by supervisor
	2. Clean equipment, serving counters, and tables in dining area
	3. Prepare serving counters for coffee break
	a. Get a supply of cups, saucers, and tableware
	b. Make coffee
	c. Fill cream dispensers
	d. Keep counter supplied during coffee break period (9:30-10:30)
	4. Fill salad dressing, relish, and condiment containers for noon meal
10:00 to 11:30 A.M.	1. Confer with supervisor regarding menu items and portion sizes for noon meal
	2. Clean equipment, counters, and tables in dining area
	3. Prepare counters for lunch
	a. Turn on heat in hot counter and dish warmers at 11 A.M.
	b. Set up beverage area
	c. Place service utensils and dishes in position for use
	4. Make coffee
	5. Set portioned cold foods on cold counter
11:00 to 11:15 A.M.	Coffee break
11:30 A.M. to 1:30 P.M.	1. Open cafeteria doors for noon meal service
	2. Replenish cold food items, dishes, and tableware as needed
	3. Keep counters clean; wipe up spilled food
	4. Make additional coffee as needed
1:30 to 2:00 P.M.	1. Turn off heating and cooling elements in serving counters
	2. Help break down serving line
	3. Return leftover foods to proper places
	4. Clean equipment and serving counter as directed by supervisor
2:00 P.M.	Off duty

Scheduling software usually includes information about the job requirements for each position and information regarding employee capabilities. Based on this information, the manager can set parameters that allow the software to make the match of employees to days, times, and tasks to be performed. Scheduling software can offer many benefits to the department, as long as program users are adequately trained.

☐ Managing Time Effectively

Although managers assume responsibility for developing work schedules for their employees, they often fail to schedule their own time to best advantage. One step toward effective time management is for managers to analyze the way they currently use their time. A detailed log of daily activities, such as the one shown in figure 6-15, helps managers keep track of what they do, the amount of time spent on each activity, others involved in the activities, and how important each act is to the day's objectives. Analysis of these logs helps managers determine how effectively they spent their time and some of the reasons they do not reach their objectives during a particular week. For example, unnecessary phone calls, avoidable interruptions, or lack of a good work plan (see figure 6-16) all contribute to inefficient use of time.

Prioritizing Work

Once managers have monitored their daily activities, they are in a better position to list the essential tasks of the coming week and assign each a priority: *A* for tasks that are critical, *B* for tasks that are important but not critical, and *C* for tasks that might be delegated (see figure 6-17, p. 148). Priorities should be set for the tasks that are to be accomplished daily as well as for longer-term projects, such as recruiting a new staff member, developing a budget, or gathering information to plan a new program. Large projects are more easily handled and prioritized when they are broken down into their component parts and tackled one step at a time.

Another method of prioritizing work has been suggested by Stephen Covey in his book *7 Habits of Highly Effective People*. The focus of Covey's priority system is to manage "self" rather than time, using four quadrants for time management:

1. *Urgent and important:* This quadrant encompasses crisis situations or problems. Being problem oriented and driven by deadlines prevents managers from focusing on more important tasks.
2. *Not urgent and important:* This quadrant has to do with effective personal management as represented by planning functions. Functioning in quadrant 2 requires the manager to seek balance in work and personal activities and to undertake important activities that are not urgent.
3. *Urgent and not important:* Like quadrant 1, the driving force for quadrant 3 is urgency. Unlike quadrant 1, however, task urgency here is determined by others. That is, these tasks may be urgent to someone else but not for the manager's goals and focus.
4. *Not urgent and not important:* The activities in this quadrant are referred to as "comfort" activities, those tasks that require no great deal of thought and may be somewhat relaxing. The biggest problem with focusing on tasks in this area is that comfort tasks prevent managers from focusing on the tasks in quadrants 1 and 2.

With the self-management theory, time management is the responsibility of the manager and not determined by the tasks. Managers must choose the activities they will spend time on. To meet the challenges of a rapidly changing health care environment, managers should focus energy on the tasks of planning outlined in quadrant 2.

Figure 6-15. Example of a Manager's Daily Activity Log

Date: _____

Time of Day	Minutes	Activity	People	Important	Could Delay
8:00–8:10 a.m.	10	Talked on phone	Husband		X
8:10–8:30 a.m.	20	Took break with supervisor	Supervisor	X	
8:30–9:00 a.m.	30	Met with CEO	CEO	X	
9:00–9:20 a.m.	20	Returned three calls to food vendors	Sally, Bill Jim	1 call	2 calls
9:20–10:00 a.m.	40	Talked to assistant director about catering	Lloyd, Sam	X	

Total Minutes Wasted: _____

Figure 6-16. Example of a Manager's Daily Planner

Time of Day	Already Planned	Must Do	Comments/Carryovers
8:00	Staff meeting	1. Budget review	
:15		2. Write QA report	
:30		3. Procedure for	
:45		use of new	
9:00		dishwasher	
:15	Start budget review		
:30			
:45			
10:00			
:15			
:30			
:45			
11:00			
:15	Break		
:30			
:45			
12:00–1:00	Lunch		
1:15	Write QA report	Complete tomorrow	
:30			Complete QA report tomorrow
:45			See DB about figures
2:00	Complete budget review		Call engineer–dishmachine
:15			Infection Control Committee
:30			on Wednesday
:45			
3:00			
:15			
:30			
:45			
4:00			
:15			
:30			
:45			
5:00			

Figure 6-17. Example of a Food Service Director's Weekly Planner

Goals (Priorities)	Estimated Time	Day Completed	Comments
1. Complete budget (A)	6½ hours	Wednesday	Give budget to secretary to type by Wed. noon; review Thurs.; turn in by Fri., 3 P.M.
2. Discuss disciplinary action (A)	2½ hours	Thursday	Meet with Human Resource Department
3. Attend meetings (B)	3½ hours	Monday, Thursday	Be sure to go to staff meeting
4. Handle mail, meet with employees (B)			
5. Review magazines (C)	1 hour	Thursday	

	Monday	Tuesday	Wednesday	Thursday	Friday
9:00	Attend				Attend
9:30	nutrition	Complete	Complete		staff
10:00	support	budget	budget	Review	meeting
10:30	meeting			budget	
11:00					
11:30					
12:00					
12:30					
1:00		Complete	Discuss		
1:30		budget	disciplinary		
2:00			action		
2:30					
3:00					Turn in budget!
3:30				Review	
4:00				magazines	
4:30					
5:00					

Setting Limits

Managers should avoid the four biggest time wasters: excessive telephone calls, unnecessarily long meetings, unexpected visitors, and paperwork. To reduce the time spent on each, managers should set their own limits:

- If possible, schedule no more than one hour each day for returning telephone calls. Each conversation should be related to the work at hand.
- Although meetings can be useful, make sure that the meeting time is used productively by planning an agenda or proposing an outcome and by ending the meeting at a predetermined time.
- To better minimize unexpected visitors, avoid making them feel too welcome or too comfortable. When possible, a closed door and being screened by a secretary should do much to discourage unscheduled visitors. If that does not suit a manager's style or the institution's working climate, a manager might stand when an unscheduled visitor enters the room and remain standing until he or she leaves. Other options are to suggest a better time for a meeting, make an appointment to see the person in his or her own work area, and end the meeting as soon as the business is completed.
- Managers can reduce their share of paperwork by using several tactics. Have someone screen the paperwork and sort it according to its relative importance. Do not handle

any piece of paper more than once. Write responses directly on memos and return them to the sender. Whenever possible and appropriate, delegate responsibility for handling paperwork.

Time management, like any other management skill, can be learned with practice. Managers need to begin applying time management techniques to their own schedules to achieve the full range of their professional and personal objectives.

☐ Summary

The organizing function of management involves designing appropriate organizational structures, grouping work according to some common criterion such as function or product, and establishing relationships between the organization's activities and its job positions. In addition to divisions of authority and responsibility according to departments or units, managers often find that work groups such as committees, task forces, and project teams are useful in completing certain types of activities that require the expertise and cooperation of several departments. Food service departments benefit in many ways from participation in such work groups.

When coordinating work, managers also must organize the way authority is distributed throughout an organization. The sharing of authority by managers with their employees is called delegation and is instrumental in obtaining for managers the support, advice, and special knowledge of staff outside the direct chain of command.

The building of a competent staff to carry out the work of an organization involves assessment of the tasks to be performed and the employees needed for performing those tasks. Managers determine staffing needs by assessing work load, undertaking job analyses, and preparing job descriptions and specifications. The smooth flow of work throughout the organization is ensured through the careful scheduling of employees' time and by the managers' vigilance over the expenditures of their own time.

☐ Bibliography

Blanchard, K., Carew, D., and Parisi-Carew, E. *The One Minute Manager Builds High Performing Teams.* New York City: William Morrow and Company, 1990.

Burack, E. H., and Mathys, N. J. *Introduction to Management: A Career Perspective.* New York City: John Wiley and Sons, 1983.

Causey, W. B. Leading CQI hospitals now restructuring for latest innovation: patient-focused care. *QI/TQM* 3(2):17–28, Feb. 1993.

Coble, M. C. *A Guide to Nutrition and Food Service for Nursing Homes and Homes for the Aged.* Revised ed. Washington, DC: U.S. Department of Health, Education and Welfare, 1975.

Cohen, A. R., Fink, S. L., Gadon, H., Willits, R. D., and Josefowitz, N. *Effective Behavior in Organizations.* 4th ed. Homewood, IL: Irwin, 1988.

Covey, S. *7 Habits of Highly Effective People.* New York City: Simon and Schuster, 1989.

Dougherty, D. A. Organizational changes for the 21st century. *Hospital Food & Nutrition Focus* 9(6):1–3, Feb. 1993.

Dougherty, D. A. A new organizational structure for the 1990s. *Hospital Food & Nutrition Focus* 9(1):4–6, Sept. 1992.

Dougherty, D. A. Professionals, share positions! hospitals, share professionals! *Hospital Food & Nutrition Focus* 6(9):1–7, May 1990.

Dougherty, D. A. Time management—the fourth time around. *Hospital Food & Nutrition Focus* 9(11):1–4, July 1993.

Dubnicki, C., and Limburg, W. J. How do healthcare teams measure up? *Healthcare Forum Journal* 34(5):10–11, Sept.–Oct. 1991.

Flippo, E. B., and Munsinger, G. M. *Management.* 5th ed. Boston: Allyn and Bacon, 1982.

Haimann, T., Scott, W. G., and Connor, P. E. *Management.* 4th ed. Boston: Houghton Mifflin, 1982.

Hamilton, J. Inpatient unit adopts "patient-focused care." *Hospitals* 66(23):26, Dec. 1992.

Hamilton, J. Toppling the power of the pyramid. *Hospitals* 67(1):39–41, Jan. 1993.

Hammer, M., and Champy, J. *Reengineering the Corporation.* New York City: HarperCollins, 1993.

Hersey, P., and Blanchard, K. H. *Management of Organizational Behavior: Utilizing Human Resources.* 4th ed. Englewood Cliffs, NJ: Prentice-Hall, 1982.

Herzberg, F. *Work and the Nature of Man.* Cleveland: World, 1966.

Holpp, L. Making choices: self-directed teams or total quality management? *Training* 29(5):69–76, May 1992.

Kanter, R. M. Encouraging innovation and entrepreneurs in bureaucratic companies. In: R. L. Kuhn, editor. *Handbook for Creative and Innovative Managers.* New York City: McGraw-Hill, 1988.

Koontz, H., O'Donnell, C., and Weihrich, H. *Management.* 7th ed. New York City: McGraw-Hill, 1980.

Lane, B. *Managing People.* Sunnyvale, CA: Oasis Press, 1989.

Likert, R. *The Human Organization.* New York City: McGraw-Hill, 1967.

Moore, F. G. *The Management of Organizations.* New York City: John Wiley and Sons, 1982.

Mosley, D., Megginson, L., and Pietri, P., Jr. *Supervisory Management: The Art of Working with and through People.* Cincinnati: South-Western, 1985.

Oncken, W., Jr., and Wass, D. L. Management time: who's got the monkey? *Harvard Business Review* 75–80, Nov.–Dec., 1974.

Overman, S. Managing in the leaner organization. *H.R. Magazine* 37(11):39–43, Nov. 1992.

Puckett, R. P. *Dietary Manager's Independent Study Course.* Gainesville, FL: University of Florida Department of Independent Study by Correspondence, 1985.

Rapaport, R. To build a winning team. *Harvard Business Review* 71(1):111–20, Jan.–Feb., 1993.

Ritter, J., and Tonges, M. C. Work redesign in high-intensity environments. *Journal of Nursing Administration* 21(12):26–35, Dec. 1991.

Rose, J. C. Controlling overtime. *Health Care Supervisor* 2(1):54–66, Jan. 1984.

Scanlon, B., and Keyes, B. *Management and Organization Behavior.* 2nd ed. New York City: John Wiley and Sons, 1983.

Sneed, J., and Dresse, K. H. *Understanding Foodservice Financial Management.* Rockville, MD: Aspen Publishers, 1989.

Watson, P. M., Shortridge, D. L., Jones, D. T., Ress, R. T., and Stephens, J. T. Operational restructuring: a patient-focused approach. *Nursing Administration Quarterly* 16(1):45–52, Fall 1991.

Chapter 7

Communication

☐ Introduction

Communication can be defined as the process of conveying verbal or written information from one party to another. Communicating effectively is both a language process and a people process that requires interpersonal skills. Communication skills are vital to performing the basic functions of management: planning, organizing, controlling, and especially leading. In fact, managers spend most of their time in activities that involve some form of communication.

To run smoothly, organizations must have efficient information distribution systems that ensure that messages are received in the manner intended. The kinds of information disseminated throughout an organization include goals and objectives, change strategies, policies and procedures, behaviors and concerns, and problems and solutions. Communication is essential for obtaining information from customers because it allows managers to enhance service delivery. Furthermore, harmony, cooperation, and efficiency within a work team depend on effective communication as a means of ensuring that all members understand the team objectives and the tasks to be performed.

Communicating in health care organizations requires the manager to fulfill the following roles:

- Receptive listener in interactions with customers, superiors, peers, and employees
- Distributor of information, in both sending work plans and instructions to employees and reporting activities and results to peers and superiors
- Spokesperson for top-level managers in communicating with employees and spokesperson for employees in communicating with top-level managers

This chapter will examine the elements and process of communication, that is, factors that affect how messages are sent and how they are received and interpreted. Three barriers to effective communication—environmental, experiential, and behavioral—will be looked at. The two means of communication, the spoken word and the written word, will be discussed, as well as a third medium of nonverbal communication through body language. In discussing methods of communication, the chapter will give pointers on how to plan and conduct meetings, make oral presentations, and design effective written communications. The chapter will close with a brief description of the manager's role in mediating and resolving conflict.

☐ Communication Process

The communication process is complex, consisting of the formation, transmission, and translation of information. Five basic elements are involved in the communication process:

1. The message sender
2. The message (information)
3. The medium used to transmit the message
4. The message receiver
5. The feedback exchanged between receiver and sender (see figure 7-1)

Each element affects the creation, transmission, and translation of information in the communication process. Influences outside the communication process, called distractors or barriers, can affect each element of the process.

Both sender and receiver are influenced by their respective personal characteristics, shaped over a lifetime by language, education, religion, life experiences, culture, environment, work, and physical traits. Because lifetime experiences affect the perception of both sender and receiver, understanding the message sent means understanding the sender. Likewise, ensuring that the message is interpreted as intended implies understanding the receiver.

The medium selected often depends on the message to be conveyed. Sometimes—for example, when immediate feedback is desired—it is appropriate to convey a message verbally in person rather than via a written memo. Feedback is exchanged between sender and receiver to confirm whether the message received was the one the messenger intended. The feedback process is affected by the medium used and by the personal characteristics of sender and receiver. In other words, the five elements of the communication process are interrelated.

Communication Barriers

At any point the communication process could be interrupted or interfered with by distractors. These barriers are circumstances that draw the sender's or the receiver's attention away from, or that alter or otherwise compromise, the message. Barriers can cause miscommunication of even the simplest facts in the communication process, and as messages increase in complexity, the potential for miscommunication increases. Communication barriers can be categorized into three broad areas: environmental, experiential, and behavioral.

Barriers Due to the Environment

An obvious distractor in the communication process is an environmental interference that distorts or breaks the information flow between sender and receiver. There are two types of environmental barriers: physical (or mechanical) and operational.

Examples of *physical* or *mechanical* environmental barriers are broken connections or static on telephone lines, conversations interrupted by ringing phones or knocks on office doors, or loud laughter that disrupts a meeting. *Operational* barriers have to do with system breakdowns. Examples are letters lost in the mail, misplacement of a critical memo due to an inadequate filing system, or loss of data due to a programming error.

Figure 7-1. The Communication Process

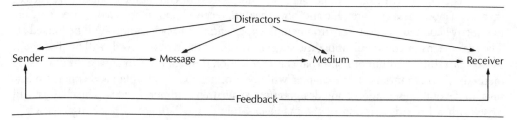

A food service manager whose office is near a cafeteria entrance can anticipate certain physical environmental barriers (such as noise). Therefore, the manager would schedule a one-on-one, manager–employee conference in a private conference room. Otherwise, it would be difficult for the sender (the manager) to communicate the message (the consequences of a specific inappropriate behavior and what must be done to change it) to the receiver (the employee) because the medium (the sender's voice) might be drowned out by the cafeteria's noise. Unless the message is conveyed and received accurately and without distraction, feedback would be virtually impossible.

Managers cannot anticipate *all* environmental distractors. In a situation where a patient with diabetes was given the wrong meal tray, the manager's responsibility is to recognize the probability of an operational environmental barrier. The manager should then investigate the food service department's information systems to discover the reason for the miscommunication of patient tray information.

Barriers Due to Experience or Personal Perception

Chapter 1 noted the increasing cultural diversity of the work force and the effect this will have on daily management functions and service operations. In the communication process, both sender and receiver are products not only of life experiences but also of accumulative cultural experiences. Collectively, these experiences define their personal perception in terms of who they are, how they feel about themselves, and how accepting they are of similarities and differences in customers, peers, coworkers, superiors, and subordinates.

Personal bias can create barriers to communication. For example, a cook asked to clean up a spill on the floor during lunch meal preparation to prevent someone from falling might interpret the request as a waste of time, even a form of punishment if the cook perceives the job of a cleaning technician to be less important than their own.

In the situation described above, the same message also might be received negatively if the cook is already busy preparing meatloaf. In addition to being influenced by personal outlook, messages and their interpretation can be affected by the circumstances of the moment. Pressures and stressors—those imposed by the work environment and those that are the result of personal perception—can affect all five elements of the communication process. Therefore, managers must be in touch not only with their own stress levels but also with those of others with whom they come in contact.

Savvy managers make every effort to suspend judgments that are based on differences in appearance or use of language, for example. Otherwise, they risk loss of opportunity that may be conveyed in information exchanges. A menu planner's suggestion to incorporate more ethnic entrees into patients' menus will be seen as a business opportunity because these managers are able to interpret the message with objectivity. Such managers demonstrate the valuable skill of separating the message from the messenger.

Barriers Due to Behavior

Personal perspectives and life experiences may precipitate certain behaviors that can block or distort the flow of information. Sometimes the behavior (the action) is the product of an emotion (a feeling). A tray assembler angry at being refused a promotion might deliberately miscommunicate patient menu orders. A cook denied approval to purchase precooked roast beef rather than preparing it might fail to take the meat out of the oven before it burns. In both cases, the flow of information is impeded because of what can be described as an *emotional behavior barrier to communication*. The emotions in the above examples are anger and disappointment, respectively.

An effective tool for removing the negative influence of emotional behavior is acknowledgment. Acknowledgment does not mean making judgments about the legitimacy of the feeling. If they tray assembler and the manager are "found out" and held accountable, their respective superiors should not judge the unacceptable behavior but simply state that the listener understands: "I understand that you are upset about _____; however, it is important to discuss how the situation can be handled."

Another method of handling emotional behavior is to continue the conversation while allowing—but not acknowledging—the behavior. For example, if an employee cries while the manager attempts to discuss a performance problem, the manager can simply continue the conversation. This is effective only if both manager and employee can continue to focus on the issue without allowing it to influence the outcome. If not, the conversation should be re-scheduled. In emotional situations, it is important to understand the other person's position before he or she can be expected to hear and understand your message.

Often behavior called *nonverbal communication* can communicate just as effectively as emotional displays. This behavior is conveyed through body language rather than spoken or written words. Facial expressions, gestures, and posture send "wordless transmissions" about attitudes, perceptions, and emotions. Smiling, shrugging, or sitting slumped in a chair are common expressions in the nonverbal vocabulary. Sometimes nonverbal communication can serve to support verbal communication, such as when a manager's words of encouragement to an employee are accompanied by smiles and nods.

However, nonverbal behavior also can contribute to creation of another behavioral barrier known as the *mixed message,* which results when a verbal message and a nonverbal message do not coincide. For example, while leaning back in a chair and shuffling papers without looking up, a manager might say to an employee, "I'm very interested in your suggestion." The employee leaves the office confused, having interpreted two contradictory messages: Although the manager's words convey interest, the manager's body language (absence of eye contact and preoccupation with desk papers) conveys apathy.

Workers throughout an organization rely daily on each others' nonverbal cues in gauging intent, acceptance, and comprehension of messages. All groups must remain alert to the information—verbal and nonverbal—they send.

☐ Methods of Communication

Direct communication can take two forms as determined by the medium used in the process. *Verbal communication* uses the medium of the spoken word, for example, in face-to-face conversations, telephone conversations, and meetings. *Written communication* includes letters, reports, proposals, justifications, and memos.

Verbal Communication

Verbal communication involves face-to-face contact between people in conversations or group discussions. Telephone calls are also common forms of verbal communication. The central avenue of communication for most managers, verbal communication is immediate in that it permits prompt feedback about the message, and it does not require the technical skills of typing or word processing. However, verbal communication is not always the best way to communicate messages in management situations. Aside from the environmental distractions of noise and static mentioned earlier, verbal exchanges provide no written record of conversations. Therefore, decisions and compromises reached verbally could be subject to debate later on. Verbal communication also may not give communicators time to reflect on their responses to questions raised and decisions discussed.

In organizations, verbal communication is used extensively when managers direct employee work activities, give instructions to employees, conduct meetings, lead work or process improvement teams, and make formal presentations. These formats are discussed in the following subsections.

Directing or Instructing Employees

Managers' verbal directions and instructions to employees should be thoughtfully prepared and carefully delivered to keep misunderstandings to a minimum. Every verbal direction given to an employee should be framed so that its meaning is clear, complete, and reasonable. The manager should always keep the employee's viewpoint in mind. New terms should be explained and simple words and sentences used. The manager should ask employees regularly whether they have any questions about the directions given.

When it is clear that the employees understand the directions, the manager should indicate when the task is to be completed and how the employees are to report back after it is completed. Complicated directions may require the manager to follow up and, if necessary, clarify the instructions to ensure that tasks are completed as directed. However, it is important that the manager show confidence in employees and allow them reasonable independence in performing their regular duties.

New or particularly complex tasks should be described in written detail in addition to being explained verbally. The manager should be careful to ensure that the written information matches the information given verbally. Conflicting sets of instructions for the same task can only cause misunderstanding and confusion.

Planning and Conducting Meetings

Managers spend a great deal of time attending meetings with superiors, peers, and employees in the organization. Many complain that most meetings are a waste of their time. However, meetings are the means by which organizations conduct a large part of their business. Planning is the key to conducting productive, informative, and cost-efficient meetings. For the purpose of this text, meetings will be categorized as business meetings and team meetings.

Business Meetings

The purpose of *business meetings* is to provide or share information and to delineate planning or development functions. For the most part, the department-level planning and development meetings that food service directors attend deal with menu planning, production planning, and nutrition care planning. The director or manager also attends informational meetings of the management staff and, depending on the size of the department, employee meetings. Meetings held for the sole purpose of providing information should be carefully evaluated. If the information easily could be shared in a memo, a meeting may not be necessary. However, many food service department employees appreciate and enjoy hearing information from the department manager. Also, this type of meeting allows for questions and discussion of the information presented to ensure understanding.

Each meeting requires a coordinated plan for conducting business and for decision making. The director or manager responsible for conducting such meetings should plan the meetings by routinely following a simple seven-step process:

1. *Clearly define the goal(s) of the meeting.* Be careful to avoid covering too much in any one session. It is better to thoroughly discuss and solve one problem than to discuss many subjects but reach no clear-cut conclusions.
2. *Determine how much time should be allotted for accomplishing the meeting's goals.* Most meetings should last no longer than 60 or—at most—90 minutes. When longer meetings are planned, a break should be provided after the first hour.
3. *Decide who should attend the meeting.* Factors to consider are the authority levels of the participants and the most cost-effective and efficient size for the group. Participants must have authority to make and act on any decisions that come out of the meeting. The number of attendants should be kept to a minimum to control the cost in terms of time expenditures. It should also be kept in mind that the larger the group, the *less likely* it is that the meeting's goals will be fulfilled.
4. *Determine the format that will best suit the goal of the meeting.* If the goal is to solve a problem, the meeting should be a free exchange of ideas and suggestions. If the goal is to distribute information, the meeting should be a preplanned discussion and explanation of data or other information. If the goal is to win the group's acceptance of a new proposal, the meeting should be a carefully constructed presentation of background materials and projections.

155

5. *Plan a strategy for accomplishing the goal of the meeting.* Anticipate potential resistance to change, conflict within the group, and other problems. Formulate methods for handling such problems and securing the support of other group members prior to the meeting.

6. *Write an agenda for the meeting.* An *agenda* is a written statement of the order of events in a meeting (see figure 7-2). If anyone other than the meeting planner is to be responsible for presenting topics, that person should be notified ahead of time. The final agenda should be distributed in advance to everyone who is to attend the meeting.

7. *Record meeting minutes.* If a written record of the meeting is required, appoint a group member to be the secretary prior to the meeting.

The person designated to conduct the meeting (referred to as the chairperson) is responsible for moving the meeting toward accomplishment of its goals. He or she should schedule the meeting room well ahead of time and make sure that it is large enough to accommodate the group and that the physical environment is comfortable. Any audiovisual equipment, displays, and handouts should be arranged for ahead of time. Equipment should be checked in advance to ensure that it is in good working order.

During the meeting, the leader should follow a few simple rules of courtesy:

- Arrive early so that he or she can greet people as they arrive.
- Start the meeting on time unless several people are late, in which case the leader should send out reminders and then proceed with the meeting.
- Direct discussions with open-ended questions that give everyone a chance to contribute.
- Stick to the agenda and make sure that other group members do so as well. If items or issues are raised that are not on the agenda, a "parking lot" can be created by writing on a board or flip chart a list of items that may need further discussion outside the meeting or may need to be added to the agenda in the future. This way, the meeting can move forward while providing a record of issues that require future attention.
- Limit the discussion to one point at a time to avoid conflict.
- Avoid unnecessary interruptions (such as telephone calls) and discourage distractions (such as shuffling of papers and whispering among attendees).
- Ask for input from attendees regarding how the meeting went, its structure, and whether they feel goals were met, topics were given appropriate time, and their participation was valued. Express sincere thanks to the group's members for their attendance and

Figure 7-2. Example of an Agenda Format

Agenda
Dietitian Meeting
August 20, 1994

Place: Conference Room   Time: 1:30 p.m.

1. Review and approval of minutes

2. Review and approval of agenda

3. Discussion items

   a. Nutritional supplement formulary

   b. Weight management classes

   c. Quality review

4. Old business

5. Other business

participation. Taking time to ask members to evaluate effectiveness can enhance future meetings of the group.

- End the meeting at the appointed time by reviewing key points, assigning follow-up tasks, and setting the date, time, and place for the next meeting.

After formal meetings, the minutes should be reviewed and then distributed to the participants to ensure accuracy. The names of those attending should also be recorded as part of the minutes, which should be signed by the chairperson and kept on file for future reference and follow-up.

At least once a year, the food service director should evaluate all formal meetings held in the department. Committees, task forces, and other formal groups should be dissolved if their goals have been met. The director should also review the cost of the department's meetings in terms of the supplies used, the salaries of the staff members who attended, the refreshments provided, and so forth. The director should ask two basic questions about the meetings to determine their effectiveness: Did too many people attend? Were the costs of the meeting justified by its results?

Team Meetings

Team meetings are conducted with employees in the department or as cross-functional teams with employees across the organization. Team meetings, which may or may not have a manager as the team leader, can be designed to discuss work methods, customer satisfaction, or process improvement. Their goal is to improve quality, that is, quality of work life, quality of customer satisfaction, or quality of work accomplishment. Before a quality improvement team can be initiated, several questions must be answered:

- What is the purpose or mission of the team? This question helps identify the process or issue under discussion, the background information surrounding the process or issue, and what information or data are available regarding the process or issue.
- What is the scope of the project? It is important to understand what is *not* being included in the activities. Once boundaries are identified, budget constraints must be explored. The decision-making authority of the team members and leader also must be clarified.
- Who should be on the improvement team? This question involves identifying who has ownership of the process, who knows what the issues and concerns are for the customer, and who is needed to offer a different perspective. This is the time to decide whether a facilitator is necessary.
- What are the expectations for improvement? Questioning the expectations identifies the outcome or goals, time lines for recommendations, the magnitude of improvement expected, and who is responsible for approval and implementation of the recommendations.
- What resources are available to the team? Resources may include consultants or internal experts, facilitators, coworkers who perform extra work so that team members can attend meetings, and support staff who can create presentation materials. Materials for data collection and analysis also are needed. They may include computers and software.

Answering these questions provides team members with a clear picture of their charter or mission. When the team meets for the first time, the information compiled from these questions is presented for review and discussion by the team leader. It also may be necessary to provide the answers in the form of a proposal to the quality council (QC) for its approval prior to the meeting, especially if the process requires a cross-functional team (see chapter 4). Once QC approval is obtained and the team members are clear of the team mission and purpose, ground rules for the meetings should be discussed. Ground rules may be a part of the training program provided for all employees involved in quality improvement but should be covered as a reminder in the first team meeting. Ground rules include:

1. *Attendance:* Time and place for meeting, how to notify team of absence, acceptable number of absences, designation of a replacement, and so on

2. *Time management:* Punctuality with regard to meeting start and end, timekeeper responsibilities, appointment of timekeeper, what must be accomplished during meeting, agenda for meetings
3. *Participation:* Being prepared for meetings, completing assignments, sharing responsibilities, and so on
4. *Communication:* Confidentiality, candor, orderly and focused discussion, one speaker at a time, active listening, respect for others' opinions
5. *Decision making:* How decisions are made (majority vote), open discussion permitted before voting, conflict acceptable and handled in the open, number of members who must be present for decision making
6. *Documentation:* Format for agenda, format used for minutes, distribution of agenda and minutes, storage of and access to documentation
7. *Miscellaneous:* Breaks, refreshments, room setup and cleanup, need for support services, how they will be coordinated

The same guidelines should be followed for conducting team meetings as those identified for business meetings. The leader (not necessarily the manager) is responsible for conducting the meeting, setting up the next meeting, and providing follow-up information or information needed prior to the next meeting. When conducting team meetings, the leader must keep individuals on target to reach established goals.

Making Presentations

Sometimes the food service manager may be asked to provide information in a formal presentation. Presentations may include training sessions for employees or students or delivery of information regarding the department business plan, budget, or special project to decision makers. Managers can give successful presentations by being prepared and by understanding how to deal positively with the anxiety or stress related to this activity.

A substantial body of literature is available to assist managers with gaining skills in business or technical presentations. The limited scope of this text prevents a detailed review of technique, but the following basic guidelines can serve to help the manager prepare to present information to a group.

1. *Plan the presentation by identifying objectives to be achieved.* Next, assess the needs and level of knowledge of the audience. For example, in speaking to students regarding the cook–chill process, a manager might relate the history or evolution of this food production method. On the other hand, in presenting a request to decision makers for conversion of the food production system to cook–chill, the focus might be on costs associated with the current system versus savings to be realized upon conversion.
2. *Organize the information to be presented.* Using the objectives for the presentation will help determine order of presentation. Organizing should include development of an outline, and main ideas should be developed with their subpoints. The presentation should have an introduction and a conclusion that summarize the main idea(s) from the body of the presentation. In other words, to use a well-known phrase: "Tell them what you're going to tell them—tell them—then tell them what you told them."
3. *Use handouts and visual aids to enhance the presentation.* Visual aids focus the audience's attention, reinforce the verbal message, stimulate interest in the topic, or illustrate hard-to-visualize factors. They should not be used if they do not improve the presentation's effectiveness. Nor should they be used to avoid interacting with the audience. If handouts are used, the manager must decide at what point to distribute them: If they are handed out in the beginning, the audience may spend time reviewing rather than listening; if they are handed out during the presentation, they should be distributed quickly to prevent distracting from the presentation. It also may be appropriate to distribute handouts at the end to provide written support of the verbal presentation.

4. *Gather in advance all handouts, visual aids, supplies, and equipment necessary.* Visit the meeting room ahead of time so as to be familiar with the room layout. If this is not possible, arrive early and organize notes, handouts, and visual aids. Practice the entire presentation beforehand to uncover possible difficulties with terminology or ambiguous points. Practice also gives a clue as to whether the predetermined time frame is realistic.

5. *Be natural and show enthusiasm for the topic.* Avoid standing stiffly or speaking in a monotone. Maintain eye contact with the audience and move naturally using hand movements and a conversational style of speech.

It is natural to have some anxiety about presenting to a group. However, effective speakers have learned to use this anxiety to their advantage. Following the steps listed above will help to decrease anxiety by being prepared for the presentation. In addition, use positive visualization and imagery, which have been shown by researchers to ensure success with accomplishing a task. Other techniques for decreasing anxiety include deep breathing and tightening and relaxing muscles.

Written Communication

Written communication has benefits for writer and reader alike. The writer has the satisfaction of immediacy, of communicating his or her message right away without waiting to see the receiver in person. The receiver benefits from having a written record, especially of complex information. Although written communication is unavoidable much of the time, it has some disadvantages. One key disadvantage is that written communication takes longer to reach its destination than does verbal communication. A second and related disadvantage is that feedback for written communication is delayed. However, when important details must be communicated, written messages provide a record of facts that can be referred to again and again, and they give the receiver time to study and absorb those facts before responding to the communication.

At its best, good written communication is clear and concisely worded, with short sentences and simple words. Jargon should be avoided except, of course, for use of appropriate technical language. The ultimate measure of a good exchange is that both sender and receiver understand the message.

Effective written communication anticipates and answers any questions the reader might have, not only to better communicate the whole message, but also to avoid delays in the receiver's response. The tone of the written message is also important, in the same way that it is important for a sender to consider the receiver's point of view. In the age of word processors and personal computers, managers should use all the technical support that such equipment provides to make sure that their written messages are not distorted by poor spelling and grammatical errors that might reflect poorly on their abilities to communicate with and influence others.

Types of Written Communication

The kinds of written communication used most often in the food service department, and in most business operations for that matter, include letters, internal memorandums, proposals, justifications, reports, policies and procedures, and materials for distribution to customers. Figure 7-3 illustrates a sample letter format for formal business correspondence. Figure 7-4 shows a sample format for an interoffice memorandum.

In writing *business letters,* the sender should clearly state the purpose of the letter in the first paragraph or sentence. The rest of the letter should be organized logically, and each paragraph should contain one main idea. Short paragraphs are usually better than long paragraphs. A letter should be no longer than it needs to be to make its point. Extra information or materials should be attached as addenda to the main letter.

Internal memorandums are an efficient way to communicate with department employees, with higher levels of management, as well as with peers in other departments. Note that everyday communications with employees for the purpose of giving directions and feedback should be more informal, and verbal communications are best on the supervisory level. A few basic guidelines for writing memorandums follow:

- There should be just one subject per memorandum.
- The memorandum should be direct, concise, and to the point.
- It should be typewritten or prepared on a word processor.
- It should be kept to one page in length if possible.
- It should ask for a response and feedback if required.
- It should close with a thank-you.
- A copy of the memorandum should be kept on file in the manager's office for future reference.

Figure 7-3. Sample Business Letter Format

ABC Hospital
300 Main Street
Any City, State 55555

August 20, 1994

Jane Smith, Sales Representative
XYZ Food Service Company
xxx Street
Any City, State 55555

Dear Ms. Smith:

I am writing to follow up on our telephone conversation on August 5, regarding. . . .

During our conversation you indicated that your company would be willing to supply the following items. . . .

Please contact me if any other information regarding. . . .

Sincerely,

Bob Jones, RD
Director, Nutrition and Food Services

Figure 7-4. Sample Memorandum Format

MEMORANDUM

To: All Department Managers

From: Julie Jones, RD, Director Nutrition and Food Services

Re: Ordering Food Supplies via the Fax Machine

Date: August 20, 1994

Attached are the new forms for obtaining food supplies for your department or unit. Use of the forms will begin effective September 1, 1994. Additional forms can be obtained by calling extension 0000. The completed form can be faxed to the department storeroom by _____ . Your order will be filled by _____ .

Thank you in advance for supporting this new order system designed to benefit the department in better meeting the needs of our customers. Please contact _____ at _____ if you have any questions or problems with the new process.

Written communication is often used to make a position known or to persuade someone of something, for example, written proposals and justifications. Skills for writing persuasive communications are increasingly important to the food service director whose purpose might be to inform and provide rationale for a decision that may require input from upper management. For example, a manager may wish to develop an outpatient nutrition education program in conjunction with the rehabilitation department or outside fitness center. To move forward with this decision, a *proposal* must be submitted to top managers to outline the need for such a program, the benefits of the program for the organization and community, the costs of the program, and the resources needed to implement the program.

A *justification* may be necessary to receive approval for capital equipment investments or for the addition of staff. With each of these types of justifications, the manager must present the facts used in making the decision for the request and answer questions that may be asked by administration. Anticipating questions will prompt the director to include information that can speed up the approval process. Justifications and proposals are designed to influence the decision maker based on the needs of the department. A sample justification for an additional cook's position is provided in figure 7-5 (p. 163). When writing justifications or proposals, the sender should be clear what action is expected from the receiver. For example, if it is necessary to have a signature on a requisition for an additional position, clearly state that the requisition is attached for signature. A statement inviting questions or requests for further information can be helpful, as would an offer to pick up the requisition upon being notified that it has been signed. This type of clarification allows the manager to know when the next step has been taken and when the issue has been closed.

Reports are another form of written communication frequently prepared by managers. Financial and departmental activity reports are generally completed on a monthly basis. (Financial reports are discussed in chapter 11.) Another type of report generated by the nutrition and food service department is the quarterly quality report. The format for this report is usually determined by the organization. (See chapter 4 for details.)

Written materials are often prepared and distributed to patients and other customers of the department. These materials include dietary instructions, menus, brochures of services offered, and, in some cases, department newsletters. Because these materials represent the department, it is important that the materials are professional in appearance. Although many large organizations have in-house print shops, most small organizations use outside sources. Regardless of where printing occurs, development should be the responsibility of individuals professionally trained to create high-quality materials. Large organizations generally have a marketing department to assist the manager. Small organizations can take advantage of preprinted materials or support from food vendors willing to supply materials, or they can work with outside printing companies.

Although most written communication is in paper form, it also can be in the form of output from personal computer networks. Electronic mail (e-mail) can communicate information to a single department or distribute information to every department. With the use of a modem (a telephone line that connects to the personal computer), facilities can link with other facilities and leave computer messages. Facsimile (fax) machines also have enhanced the capability to send information within and outside organizations. A memorandum may be typed as usual but distribution of the information is accomplished not through the mail system but through a facsimile machine. Hard-copy fax machines have enhanced this form of written communication, making permanent copies available. Regular fax paper will not hold the image transmitted, which necessitates copying the memorandum or using another form of communication if a long-term copy is needed.

□ Rules for Effective Communication

It is important to remember that communication depends on two dynamics. One has to do with how a message is sent, and the other has to do with how the message is received. As senders of messages, managers should consider the following guidelines:

- Plan the message by identifying the objective to be achieved through the communication. For example, if the objective is to seek information, formulate specific questions about the subject on which information is needed. If the objective is to change employee behavior or persuade decision makers, plan well-reasoned arguments in support of the change or decision.
- Determine the type of language appropriate to the communication. For example, if a manager is seeking to persuade hospital administrators to approve implementation of a cook–chill system, the language should be in layman's terms. But in a conversation between two technicians, technical language is entirely appropriate.
- Seek to maintain credibility by being honest and accurate, by gathering facts to support opinions, and by not pretending to be an expert on subjects on which the sender has limited knowledge. Managers who fail to follow this simple rule are likely to find their messages met with suspicion from employees, peers, and superiors.
- Be aware of the message behind the message; that is, the one conveyed by tone of voice and body language. Ensure that body language is congruent with the spoken message. Anticipate different ways the message might be interpreted and ask questions to ensure that it is received as intended. Avoid letting minor points of disagreement distract from the message.
- Be sensitive to the receiver's perspective, especially when the message deals with a sensitive issue, such as an employee denied a promotion. Avoid raising "heavy" issues when the receiver appears preoccupied or when time does not permit dealing with the issue adequately.
- Ensure that the setting is appropriate to the conversation. If it is too public and surrounded by distractions, relocate. For example, it would be inappropriate to discuss performance with a cafeteria tray line worker during a heavy-traffic period.
- Encourage feedback in communications. Invite receivers to ask questions, request clarification, or express opinions.

As receivers of messages, managers should fine-tune listening skills, try to remain open and receptive, and accommodate the sender. Here are some pointers:

- Listen carefully. Do not interrupt the sender unnecessarily. Show interest by eliminating distractions and asking appropriate questions. Most of all, listen without making premature judgments about the speaker or the message.
- Consider the sender's perspective to avoid distortion of how the message is received. This applies to communication between managers and their employees as well as exchanges between managers and their superiors.
- Create a supportive atmosphere for the sender. "Listen" for feeling as well as words. Be aware of body language—gestures, tone of voice, body position, eye movements, and breathing pattern—without underreacting or overreacting to it.
- Summarize and ask exploratory, open-ended questions to confirm the meaning of the message. "Is this what I heard?" or "What I hear you saying is . . . ?" This technique, called *mirroring*, validates the sender's effort to communicate by allowing him or her to confirm, correct, or clarify intent.

Both senders and receivers should remember to:

- Follow up on a message to make sure it was sent as intended and received as intended. In face-to-face communication, this is simply a matter of asking a question. In written communication, follow-up can be accomplished with a telephone call, a brief office (or hallway) conference, or written confirmation.
- Avoid the temptation to provide too much information in sending the communication or in giving feedback on it.

This last guideline suggests a common problem, especially in large organizations: the burden of handling too much paperwork and trying to process too much information. Simple written

Figure 7-5. Sample Justification Statement

Justification for an Additional Position
August 20, 1994

Need for an Additional Cook's Position

Based on departmental productivity and meal equivalents, I would like to add 1 FTE as a cook's position. Maintaining coverage for the production area for meal preparation and sanitation has become increasingly more difficult as the number of meals continue to increase.

Productivity for the department has met or exceeded the 100% goal set with man-hours per meal at .21. The man-hours per meal goal set for this year is .23. The total complement for paid FTEs is currently 70, which is well below the 73 to 77 shown as required on the productivity reports.

Validity of Productivity Figures

I have reviewed the validity of the paid FTE number with the changes made in the cafeteria renovations. It stands to reason that enough efficiencies have been gained with the renovation and number of meals served to make adjustments in the factor used to measure departmental productivity. The following steps have been taken or are in the process of being taken to ensure accuracy of our productivity numbers.

1. A two-week review of sales and counts in the cafeteria was conducted using figures from _____ through _____ . The attached chart shows the current average meal or meal equivalent to be $ _____ , slightly below the $ _____ now used to determine cafeteria meals. These numbers also indicate that roughly 2,000 more individual customers enter the cafeteria than is verified by the average ticket or meal.
2. The number of meals prepared for patient and all nonpatient areas have been charted and compared to the counts from a year ago. The attached table shows an increase in meals for all areas except vending. The total increase is 4.11% over last year. Patient meals show a significant increase and also are the most labor intensive.
3. In addition to the above two steps, observations will be made to determine the overall impact of changes made with the layout of the new cafeteria service area. If it is determined that these meals are now being served more efficiently, I will evaluate and modify the other meal factor used to determine departmental productivity.

Benefits and Rationale for Adding a Cook

The cook's position is being requested at this time based on the following:

1. Meal preparation for the physician's dining area is consistently being done by the production supervisor.
2. Either the production supervisor or the purchasing supervisor must fill a line slot when time off is granted to a cook, baker, or salad maker.
3. Cooks are voicing concern that they are unable to complete their meal preparation in a timely manner. They also state they are under excessive stress and feel overworked.
4. Although we have been able to decrease our injuries, last year's experience revealed that a high level of productivity directly impacts the number of injuries.
5. Efforts to increase sales and therefore the number of customers in the cafeteria will continue. These efforts have been shown to increase counts over the past three months.
6. Meal counts are higher in all areas other than vending. Patient meals are more labor intensive and are higher than budgeted due to an increased census.

Effect on Departmental Budget

The budget for this fiscal year will not be negatively impacted by the addition of a cook for the next six months. We are currently $32,000.00 under budget for the year. Adding a cook for the remainder of the year will cost $6,240.00.

Average cook salary = $6.00/hour × 1,040 hours = $6,240.00

Thank you for your consideration in filling this position. Please let me know if this position is approved or if additional justification is needed.

Julie Roberts, RD, Director
Nutrition and Food Services

messages probably do not require written responses, and it wastes everyone's time to ask for them. Not all telephone conversations require confirming letters. In addition, a manager should not expect to read from cover to cover every journal that crosses his or her desk. Some sensible decisions must be made about what kind of information exchange is essential, what kind must be committed to paper, what types of information employees need, and what might be left to casual conversation.

As noted earlier, managers should choose the medium that is best suited to a particular message. For example, a sudden and drastic change in an employee's work schedule might best be announced in a face-to-face conversation rather than in an impersonal memorandum. However, a request for funds to hire a consultant for a special project should be formally presented in writing, with solid supporting evidence for the request, rather than in a drop-in conversation. The choice of appropriate medium should always be made with the receiver's perspective in mind.

☐ Channels of Communication within Organizations

Because information exchange is essential to the operation of an organization, formal and informal channels of communication ensure that information moves from one point to another efficiently. Formal channels include a vertical track of communication and a horizontal track. The vertical track runs in two directions, upward and downward from the top of the organizational structure to the bottom. The horizontal track carries communications laterally across the organizational structure between departments and individuals on about the same levels. The most common informal channel of communication in organizations is the grapevine.

Upward Communication on the Vertical Track

Upward communication includes verbal and written messages (problems, perceptions, or suggestions) that subordinates send to superiors. Sometimes messages may seek clarification of instructions or advice. Top-level management depends on this vertical flow as a way to monitor each department's or unit's performance so as to make the best decisions possible in planning future activities of the organization.

Activity and performance reports are the most frequent form of upward communication. These provide information necessary for making decisions regarding capital purchases, FTE additions, or other such operational changes. Directors are responsible for adequately communicating to upper management the goals and objectives of the department and how these interface with other departments and with the broader vision of the organization.

Research has shown that the greater the difference in level between the employee and the superior to whom the message is being sent, the more likely it is that the message will be distorted or incomplete. Although department directors should communicate a sincere desire to listen to employees' suggestions and ideas, they must be conscious of employees' tendencies to provide incomplete or inaccurate information. The director should also avoid depending on lower-level employees for essential information.

Downward Communication on the Vertical Track

Downward communication occurs when information flows from superiors in the organizational hierarchy to employees. Top-level managers communicate the organization's goals and objectives and specify policies and procedures. They also explain the rationale for various operational decisions, give instructions about specific tasks, provide feedback to employees about their performance, and respond to messages from employees. Research suggests that most managers believe that they communicate information to their employees better than they actually do. Because information is often the lifeline of an operation and because accurate information is especially crucial in health care institutions, food service directors should examine their own patterns of downward communication for any possible shortcomings. For example, they should never assume that information supplied to higher-level managers will automatically be communicated to lower-level employees. Information that affects employees should be communicated to them deliberately and directly.

Horizontal Communication Track

Communication that follows the horizontal channel consists of a verbal and written information flow between organizational units that are at about the same level. This flow is particularly important in health care institutions, because service to the patient depends on efficient communication among several different departments. For example, the food service department cannot provide appropriate nutrition care services without information about the patient from the nursing staff. Such interdependence is apparent in daily activities such as meal service, but it also influences the department's long-term ability to plan major projects.

In addition, horizontal communication between units is more direct, thereby relieving some of the strain imposed on the vertical track. Interdepartmental communication minimizes the distortion and slowness of message relay that can hamper upward and downward communication. For example, the food service director and the nursing service director can communicate with one another directly and more immediately about a common project without necessarily exchanging information through their respective superiors.

The Grapevine

The grapevine is an important route for informal information flow in organizations. It is a natural result of the universal human need for social contact. Unlike formal communication channels, the grapevine operates without planning or documentation. Despite its haphazard nature, the grapevine is sometimes more informative than the messages sent through formal channels. In this sense, the grapevine can work either for or against the interests of management and the well-being of the organization.

Managers can use the grapevine to get a sense of the attitudes and perceptions among their subordinates and respond to them more quickly than if they waited for problems to surface through formal methods. To minimize the potentially negative effects of grapevine information, managers should share as much information as possible with subordinates about organization activities. If everyone in the organization has appropriate access to up-to-date and accurate information, the speculation that leads to rumor can be dispelled.

☐ Conflict Resolution

Occasionally, a manager must act as a mediator and resolve conflicts between employees or between an employee and a supervisor. (*Mediation* is the process of working with conflicting parties to suggest settlements and compromises.) Although full treatment of conflict resolution is beyond the scope of this book, this is an important management role. Mediation should be conducted so that, if possible, both parties can be winners. There are times when the manager will be required to end a conflict by making a decision that will be unpopular with one of the parties involved.

Generally, when conflict arises most people make a "fight-or-flight" decision. If they choose to fight, they expect to win. If they choose flight, they will ignore the person with whom they are in conflict and refuse to talk about the issues. For effective teamwork and management, the manager must have an empowered response to conflict resolution, and should understand that neither fight nor flight is appropriate for creating winning solutions to conflict.

Communication is the key to resolving conflicts. In meeting privately with opposing parties to mediate the issues, the manager should make it clear at the beginning that both parties will have an opportunity to state their point of view. He or she also must emphasize that it is unacceptable for one party to interrupt the other. The meeting should be held in an appropriate location, such as the manager's office or a conference room. Adequate time must be set aside to work out the conflict.

When the mediation session begins, the manager should express concern about the effects the conflict has on both individuals. The manager also should express optimism that a solution can be reached that is in the best interest of both individuals. The outcome should be a solution that both parties can agree to.

In a conflict situation, reactions can be displayed in an eruption of emotions and hurt feelings. Again, these feelings probably are tied to past experiences. The issue at conflict may remind the parties involved of previous situations or topics that although unrelated nevertheless are present in their subconscious. In dealing with conflict, it is important to get the individuals to understand why they are angry and what they would consider a suitable outcome.

☐ Summary

Communication is the process of sending verbal and written information from one person to another. Effective communication is achieved when the message received is in harmony with the message sent. The basic management functions all depend on the communication of information, especially the function of leading and directing employee activities.

Communication among people on all levels in the organization is vital to accomplishing the organization's work and achieving its goals. In their working relationships, successful managers tend to find and use the most appropriate and effective channels for communication within their organizations. They also develop and use effective interpersonal communication skills while remaining objective and nonjudgmental, always separating the message from the messenger.

☐ Bibliography

Babnew, D. What motivates people to work effectively? *Hospital and Health Service Administration* Special II:43–53, 1980.

Blake, R. R., and Mouton, J. S. *The New Management Grid.* Houston: Gulf, 1978.

Blanke, V. Political power and hospital dietitians. *Ross Dietetic Currents* 19(5):21, Sept.–Oct., 1982.

Boss, D., and Moore, D. The body speaks. *Food Management* 16:39, Apr. 1981.

Brill, L. *Business Writing Quick and Easy.* 2nd ed. New York City: American Management Association, 1989.

Bronstein, H. *How to Manage a Winning Team.* New York City: National Institute of Business Management, 1991.

Bureau of Business Practice. Communication: face-to-face is best. *Hospital Supervisor's Bulletin,* Issue 460, Apr. 30, 1983.

Burns, J. M. *Leadership.* New York City: Harper and Row, 1978.

Cassidy, R. How we're viewed by the men we boss. *Savvy,* July 1982.

Cornell, D. Say the words: communication techniques. *Nursing Management* 24(3):42–44, Mar. 1993.

Currall, M. B. Diplomacy in the office: how to get on with your boss. *New Woman,* Nov. 1984.

Currall, M. B. Privacy in the office. *Working Woman,* May 1982.

Curtin, L. L. "I know you think you heard. . . ." *Nursing Management* 24(3):7–8, Mar. 1993.

Dauw, D., and Fredian, A. J. *Creativity and Innovation in Organizations.* Dubuque, IA: Kendall/Hunt, 1976.

Davis, K. Cut those rumors down to size. *Supervisory Management* 20(6):2, June 1975.

Dougherty, D. A. Are you listening? *Hospital Food & Nutrition Focus* 8(9):1–5, May 1992.

Dumaine, D. *Write to the Top: Writing for Corporate Success.* New York City: Random House, 1989.

Employee motivation—"whatcha done for me lately?" *Institution* 92(3):16–17, Feb. 1, 1982.

Eubanks, P. Managing the participatory-style meeting. *Hospitals* 66(15):45, Aug. 5, 1992.

Fader, S. S. What your boss wishes you knew. *Working Woman,* May 1982.

Feinberg, M. R. Your communication quotient. *Restaurant Business* 84(1):84, Jan. 20, 1984.

Feinberg, M. R. The craft of communication. *Restaurant Business* 84(3):108–12, Feb. 10, 1984.

Feinberg, M. R. The exercise of power. *Restaurant Business* 80(15):120, Oct. 1, 1981.

Fink, C., and Willits, G. *Effective Behavior in Organizations.* 4th ed. Homewood, IL: Irwin, 1988.

Gabarro, J. J., and Kotter, J. P. Managing your boss. *Harvard Business Review* 58(1):92–100, Jan.–Feb. 1980.

Gellerman, S. W. *Management by Motivation.* New York City: American Management Association, 1968.

George, C. S. *Supervision in Action: The Art of Managing Others.* Reston, VA: Reston, 1981.

Gottlieb, L. Let's groom good communications. *Restaurant Business* 81(14):92–94, Sept. 15, 1982.

Grazian, F. Are you really listening? *Communication Briefings* 9(11):3, Sept. 1991.

Greene, C. Questions of causation in the path–goal theory of leadership. *Academy of Management Journal* 22(1):22–41, Mar. 1979.

Griffin, R. W. *Management.* 2nd ed. Boston: Houghton Mifflin, 1987.

Hayes, J. L., Jr. Mastering the effective memo. *Restaurant Business* 82(14):109, Sept. 15, 1982.

Hayes, R. H. Why Japanese factories work. *Harvard Business Review* 59(4):56–66, July–Aug. 1981.

Hersey, P., and Blanchard, K. *Management of Organization Behavior: Utilizing Human Resources.* 4th ed. Englewood Cliffs, NJ: Prentice-Hall, 1982.

Herzberg, F. One more time: how do you motivate employees? *Harvard Business Review,* Jan.–Feb. 1968.

Jay, A. How to run a meeting. *Harvard Business Review,* Mar.–Apr. 1976.

Kerr, S., and Jermier, J. M. Substitutes for leadership: their meaning and measurement. *Organizational Behavior and Human Performance* 22(3):375–403, Dec. 22, 1978.

Lane, B. *Managing People.* Sunnyvale, CA: Oasis Press, 1989.

Longnecker, J., and Pringle, C. *Management.* 5th ed. Columbus, OH: Charles E. Merrill, 1981.

McConnel, C. R. *Effective Communication.* Gaithersburg, MD: Aspen Publishers, 1993.

McGregor, D. *The Human Side of the Enterprise.* New York City: McGraw-Hill, 1960.

Mandel, S. *Technical Presentation Skills: A Practical Guide for Better Speaking.* Los Altos, CA: Crisp Publications, 1988.

Maslow, A. H. *Motivation and Personality.* 1st ed. New York City: Harper and Row, 1954.

Maslow, A. H. *Motivation and Personality.* 2nd ed. New York City: Harper and Row, 1970.

Megginson, L., Mosley, D., and Pietri, P., Jr. *Management: Concepts and Applications.* New York City: Harper and Row, 1986.

Moore, F. G. *The Management of Organizations.* New York City: John Wiley and Sons, 1982.

Mosley, D. C., Megginson, L. C., and Pietri, P., Jr. *Supervisory Management: The Art of Working with and through People.* Cincinnati: South-Western, 1985.

O'Brien, M. *The Skill of Communication.* 2nd ed. St. Louis: C. V. Mosby, 1978.

Odiorne, G. S. *How Managers Make Things Happen.* Englewood Cliffs, NJ: Prentice-Hall, 1961.

Odiorne, G. S. *Personal Effectiveness: A Strategy for Success.* Westerfield, MA: MBO, 1979.

Ouchi, W. *Theory Z: How American Business Can Meet the Japanese Challenge.* Reading, MA: Addison-Wesley, 1981.

Puckett, R. P. Are meetings necessary? *Contemporary Administrator* 6(6):18–20, June 1983.

Scanlon, B., and Keyes, B. *Management and Organization Behavior.* 2nd ed. New York City: John Wiley and Sons, 1983.

Shipper, A. Effective communications: a powerful tool for dietitians. *Ross Dietetic Currents* 13(4):17–20, 1986.

Siegel, D. *Are You Listening to Me?* Nursing Corps Publishing, Inc., and Nursing Horizons, Inc., Dec. 1992, pp. 16–27.

Skinner, B. F. *Beyond Freedom and Dignity.* New York City: Knopf, 1971.

Strauss, G., and Sayles, L. R. *Personnel: The Human Problems of Management.* Englewood Cliffs, NJ: Prentice-Hall, 1980.

Tairant, J. S. *Drucker: The Man Who Invented Corporate Society.* Boston: Cahners, 1976.

Vroom, V. H., and Yetton, P. W. *Leadership and Decision Making.* Pittsburgh: University of Pittsburgh Press, 1973.

Webber, A. M. What's so new about the new economy? *Harvard Business Review* 71(1):24–42, Jan.–Feb. 1993.

Human Resource Management

☐ Introduction

An organization's most valuable resources are the people who perform the work—its *human resources*—without whom no organization could function. Employers who recognize this fact understand the importance of involving employees in meaningful work to ensure their long-term retention. Consequently, human resource departments have become a mainstay in organizations of all kinds. The department advocates employee rights and serves as a source of counsel for managers on all levels.

The structure of a health care organization's human resource department varies with the size of the institution. Specific departmental activities also vary with type and size of the facility. In any case, a food service director must work closely with human resource specialists to make sure that the department's service delivery complies with labor laws and with the organization's personnel policies and procedures.

This chapter will discuss specific areas of concern in human resource management. These include:

- Laws that affect the employer–employee relationship
- Role of the human resource department
- The employment process (recruiting, screening, interviewing, hiring, orienting)
- Employee training and coaching
- Employee performance evaluation
- Maintenance of personnel records
- Development and application of personnel policies and procedures
- Compensation and benefits administration
- Labor relations

Although the food service director may not be directly responsible for performing all of these activities, he or she is involved in or affected by each one in some way. In small health care organizations, the food service department may be directly responsible for performing some of the activities usually performed by human resource departments in large organizations—for example, conducting its own training and orientation programs. In addition, food service supervisors may be charged with interviewing and hiring new employees they will supervise directly, evaluating employee work performance, and maintaining certain employee records.

☐ Laws That Affect the Employer–Employee Relationship

Federal, state, and local laws and regulations affect the way employers hire, pay, and manage their employees. In most health care organizations, the human resource department is primarily responsible for making sure the organization's personnel policies are fair and legal. However, anyone whose job is to supervise or manage other people also must be aware of workers' legal rights.

Most of the laws that affect human resource management fall into one of five areas. These are:

- Equal employment opportunity
- Compensation and benefits
- Labor relations
- Health and safety
- Immigration reform

The remainder of this section will describe briefly the major federal laws that affect human resource management.

Equal Employment Opportunity Legislation

Equal employment legislation forbids employers to discriminate against employees on the basis of race, color, religion, sex, disability, or national origin. The Equal Employment Opportunity Commission (EEOC) is the federal agency charged with making sure workers are not discriminated against unfairly. All areas of employment are regulated, including:

- Hiring
- Dismissals, work reductions, and layoffs
- Disciplinary actions
- Compensation policies
- Access to training and advancement

The EEOC's regulations are based primarily on Title VII of the Civil Rights Act of 1964. Several other laws have made other kinds of discrimination illegal as well.

Civil Rights Act of 1964

Title VII of the Civil Rights Act of 1964, and later laws that amended (or legally changed) the act, regulates the employment practices of most U.S. employers having 15 or more employees. (The Equal Employment Opportunity Act is one of the laws that amended Title VII.) Under Title VII, it is illegal for employers to practice the most obvious forms of discrimination based on race, color, religion, sex, or national origin.

Age Discrimination in Employment Act of 1967

The Age Discrimination in Employment Act (ADEA) prohibits employers with 20 or more workers from discriminating against employees age 40 to 70. Amendments to ADEA, effective January 1, 1987, eliminated the age 70 ceiling.

Rehabilitation Act of 1973

Section 503 of the Rehabilitation Act of 1973, as amended by the Rehabilitation Act Amendments of 1986, affects all companies that hold federal contracts for $2,500 or more. According to the amendments, such employers must take *affirmative action* to avoid breaking the law. That is, they must seek out, hire, and advance reasonably well-qualified individuals who belong to racial, sexual, or ethnic groups that because of discrimination have been underrepresented in the past. Also protected by the affirmative action mandate are individuals with physical and mental challenges.

Vietnam Era Veterans Readjustment Assistance Act of 1974

Section 402 of the Vietnam Era Veterans Readjustment Assistance Act prohibits discrimination against disabled veterans in general. It applies specifically to veterans of the Vietnam War.

Pregnancy Disability Act of 1978

The Pregnancy Disability Act represents an amendment to Title VII of the 1964 civil rights act. This law prohibits discrimination against workers on the basis of pregnancy, recent childbirth, or related medical conditions. It applies to employment practices and to qualification for employee benefits.

Civil Rights Act of 1980

Under Title VII of the Civil Rights Act of 1980, EEOC guidelines prohibit the sexual and ethnic harassment of employees. *Sexual harassment* in the workplace is defined as subjecting a person to unwelcome sexual advances, requests for sexual favors, and other verbal or physical conduct of a sexual nature. Sexual harassment is illegal under any one of the following conditions:

- When an employee is required to submit to such conduct as a condition of his or her continued employment
- When an employee's submission to such conduct is made the basis of a hiring decision
- When an employee's subjection to such conduct has the purpose or effect of unreasonably interfering with his or her work performance
- When such conduct creates an intimidating, hostile, or offensive working environment for employees

In 1990, EEOC policy guidelines on sexual harassment required employers to install a distinct policy against sexual harassment. To meet this requirement, the policy should demonstrate examples of exactly what is considered sexual harassment, an explanation of whom to talk to (other than a direct supervisor), the importance of confidentiality, and the fact that reprisal actions against a person claiming sexual harassment are not tolerated by the organization. The policy also should state that disciplinary action could include termination and that management is responsible for monitoring and preventing sexual harassment in the workplace.

Ethnic harassment is defined as subjecting an employee to negative comments or actions based on that person's physical, cultural, or linguistic characteristics. Racial jokes are one example of what might be construed as ethnic harassment.

Americans with Disabilities Act of 1990 (Title I)

Title I of the Americans with Disabilities Act (ADA) became effective on July 26, 1992, for employers with 25 or more employees and as of July 26, 1994, is in effect for employers with 15 to 24 employees. Title I of ADA prohibits employment discrimination against disabled workers who are qualified to perform the essential functions of a job. The law in this regard covers all aspects of employment including the application process and hiring, on-the-job training, advancement and wages, benefits, and employer-sponsored social activities. An employer must provide reasonable accommodations, unless it can be proven that such accommodations would impose undue hardship on the employer.

Disability under the ADA is defined as:

- Any physical or mental impairment that substantially limits one or more major life activities
- A record of such impairment
- An individual regarded as having such an impairment

In this definition, *major life activities* include—but are not limited to—seeing, hearing, speaking, walking, breathing, learning, working, performing manual tasks, and caring for oneself.

Employers are required to make reasonable accommodations or modifications that help impaired individuals in completing essential functions of a job. *Reasonable accommodations/modifications* are identified as adjustments to a job or the work environment that will allow a qualified, disabled person to perform essential job functions if these accommodations do not create undue hardship. With respect to the provision of an accommodation, *undue hardship* is defined as significant difficulty or expense incurred by a covered entity.

As related to nutrition and food service, department directors are required to consider carefully what are outlined in job descriptions as essential job functions and what could be reassigned so as to provide reasonable accommodations. During an interview, neither employers nor their representatives can ask whether an applicant has a disability, but they may ask whether the applicant can perform the job with or without accommodation.

Compensation and Benefits Legislation

Several important federal laws regulate how employers pay their employees and provide employee benefits. The following subsections briefly describe this body of legislation.

Social Security Act of 1935

The Social Security Act established a nationwide system for setting aside postretirement income for the majority of the nation's workers. According to the act, employers and employees make regular contributions to the Social Security fund. After retirement, individual workers qualify to receive monthly payments from the fund for the rest of their lives. The act also established a fund for unemployment compensation to protect wage earners and their families against loss of income due to unemployment.

Fair Labor Standards Act of 1938

The Fair Labor Standards Act (FLSA), also called the Wage and Hour Law, requires all organizations covered by the act to pay nonsalaried employees at least the *minimum wage,* an hourly wage that is fixed by the federal government and is considered to be the lowest wage on which an individual could live under current economic conditions. The federal minimum wage was $4.25 per hour in 1993. However, in August 1993, a bill introduced in Congress would raise the federal minimum wage to $4.50 and tie future increases to the rate of inflation.

Fair labor law also requires the employer to pay hourly employees at the overtime rate for the number of hours worked beyond 40 hours in one week. The usual overtime rate is time and a half. Most professional employees, however, are exempt from this requirement.

Equal Pay Act of 1963

The Equal Pay Act, an amendment to the FLSA, requires employers to pay equal wages to men and women for doing the same jobs. The jobs must require equal skill, effort, and responsibility, and they must be performed under similar working conditions.

Employee Retirement Income Security Act of 1974

The Employee Retirement Income Security Act (ERISA) sets standards for companies that provide private pension plans for employees. However, ERISA does *not* require companies to offer employee pension plans. As mandated by the act, employers must have a system for providing federal retirement insurance for cases in which employers' pension plans go bankrupt. The goal of ERISA is to ensure that employees who are covered by pension plans receive all of the benefits to which they are entitled.

Family and Medical Leave Act of 1993

The Family and Medical Leave Act (FMLA) requires employers with at least 50 employees to provide up to 12 weeks of unpaid, job-protected leave to eligible employees for certain family and medical reasons. Employees are eligible if they have worked for a covered employer for at least one year, and for 1,250 hours over the previous 12 months. Reasons for taking the leave include the employee's need to care for his or her newborn child or a child placed with the employee for adoption or foster care; to care for a spouse, son, daughter, or parent who has a serious health condition; or to attend to the employee's own serious health condition that makes the employee unable to perform his or her job.

Labor Relations Legislation

The federal government regulates how unions conduct their activities and how companies deal with unions. Managers should understand the requirements of the three main labor relations laws, as described below.

National Labor Relations Act of 1935

The primary purpose of the National Labor Relations Act (NLRA) is to prevent management from taking unfair actions against employees who wish to join unions. Unfair management practices are defined by the NLRA in an attempt to balance power between management and labor. Unfair management practices include firing employees who support unionization, threatening or bribing employees, and sending spies to union meetings.

Lawmakers gave the National Labor Relations Board (NLRB) the power to enforce the act. The NLRB can look into any labor dispute that affects interstate commerce (business dealings between companies in different states).

Labor–Management Relations Act of 1947

The NLRA was amended in 1947 by the Labor–Management Relations Act, better known as the Taft–Hartley Act. After a series of violent strikes in 1946, the act was passed the following year so as to limit the power of unions. Among other things, the law defines specific unfair labor practices by unions, bans union shops, and establishes procedures for secret ballot elections. In *secret ballot elections,* employees decide whether a union will represent them in collective-bargaining negotiations with management.

Labor–Management Reporting and Disclosure Act of 1959

The Labor–Management Reporting and Disclosure Act was passed to strengthen democracy within unions. The act protects the individual rights of union members and limits the economic and political power of unions. It also requires that unions report their financial status to the government. Regulations based on the law affect secondary boycotts, informational picketing, and recognitional and jurisdictional strikes. (A discussion of these regulations is beyond the scope of this book. D. D. Pointer and N. Metzger have discussed this subject in detail in their book *The National Labor Relations Act: A Guidebook for Health Care Facility Administration.*)

Health and Safety Legislation

Many federal and state laws protect the health and safety of employees in the workplace. Regulations that affect food service departments in health care organizations are discussed in detail in chapters 13 and 14. However, the most far-reaching federal law that affects the health and safety of U.S. workers is briefly described below.

Occupational Safety and Health Act of 1970

Under the Occupational Safety and Health Act, employers are required to provide employees with "employment and a place of employment which are free from recognized hazards that are causing or are likely to cause death or serious physical harm." Employers also are required to obey all safety and health standards established by the Occupational Safety

173

and Health Administration (OSHA). One such standard deals with bloodborne pathogens. The OSHA standards are enforced through on-site inspections, and employers found to be in violation are subject to fines and other penalties. (The OSHA standards related specifically to the food service department also will be discussed in chapters 13 and 14.)

Immigration Reform Legislation

Federal legislation affects all U.S. employers. It has specific impact on those employers who employ or seek to employ citizens of countries other than the United States. The body of law that covers employment of immigrant (or alien) workers in the United States is described in the following subsection.

Immigration Reform and Control Act of 1986

The Immigration Reform and Control Act of 1986 (IRCA) went into effect on November 6, 1986. Its purpose is to stop the unlawful employment of unauthorized aliens in the United States. The act requires employers to verify the citizenship status and employment eligibility of all employees hired after June 1, 1987, as well as all current employees hired after November 6, 1986. To comply with this law, employers must request all new employees to supply proof of their identity and employment eligibility. Proof may be in the form of a valid driver's license, a social security card, or an unexpired reentry permit, among others. They also must complete a Form I-9 certifying that they are eligible for employment.

The IRCA imposes substantial civil and criminal penalties on employers who knowingly violate this law. In addition, the law makes it illegal to discriminate against any individual other than unauthorized aliens on the basis of national origin or status as a citizen or an "intending citizen." All areas of human resource management are covered, including hiring, recruitment, referral, and discharge. A separate enforcement procedure has been established to handle discrimination violations. However, any alleged discrimination that is covered under Title VII of the Civil Rights Act of 1964 would still be addressed under the provisions of that act.

In addition to national legislation, state and local governments enact their own employment laws. Usually, these are modeled on the federal law.

☐ Role of the Human Resource Department

Most organizations today have some form of human resource department. In large organizations especially (those with more than 200 employees), this department will be a separate, discrete entity whose role is to perform unique functions. In some organizations, the human resource department may be called the personnel department or employee relations department.

Health care human resource departments are charged with four major areas of responsibility:

• Recruitment and employment activities
• Performance evaluation policies and procedures
• Compensation and benefits administration
• Labor relations

Specific responsibilities of the department vary from one organization to another, depending in part on the organization's structure and number of people it employs. For example, in a large teaching hospital, the human resource department might be responsible for the initial screening and interviewing of potential employees. In addition, it might be active in developing standards for evaluating employee performance, maintaining employee records, and operating employee training and orientation programs. In most health care organizations, the human resource department is directly responsible for administering the compensation and benefits program, managing the overall employment process, and overseeing labor relations.

Functions of the human resource department revolve around recruitment and retention of competent employees to staff the organization. Responsibility for successfully performing these functions generally is shared with department and unit managers. Human resource specialists advise, counsel, and assist health care managers from all departments in a variety of activities related to employee management. For example, human resource specialists may perform the following functions:

- Recruit new employees and offer advice on hiring decisions
- Help determine what new employees should be paid
- Set up standards for evaluating the performance of current employees
- Help initiate disciplinary procedures
- Handle employee grievances
- Resolve benefit issues
- Interpret personnel policies and procedures
- Coordinate the negotiation and implementation of labor contracts

In health care as in other businesses, the human resource department acts as a communications link between employees and their managers. As a trusted employee advocate, a human resource representative is available to help resolve employee issues and problems. For example, an employee may wish to discuss a work-related issue, such as perceived discrimination, or a personal problem that affects work performance, such as stress or chemical dependency. In this capacity, the representative works to resolve the issue or problem by taking appropriate action.

Another key function of a human resource department is to ensure fair treatment to all employees. Accomplishment of this priority depends on having the support and cooperation of management, administration, and the board of directors. The department also is responsible for ensuring compliance with federal, state, and local laws regulating employment, prohibiting discrimination, and promoting equal employment opportunities for protected classes, such as women, minorities, and persons with disabilities. If the organization is required by law to have an affirmative action plan, the human resource department is responsible for its development and implementation.

The food service director must work closely with human resource specialists to keep the nutrition and food service department in compliance with the law and with the institution's personnel policies and procedures. In addition, the director should make sure that his or her department's employee performance records contain all information required by law. In managing conflict resolution, the director must carefully follow human resource policies on disciplinary, probation, and grievance procedures. Finally, the director should discuss special problems—for example, claims of sexual harassment within the department—with representatives of the human resource department. In addition, the organization's legal affairs staff may need to be consulted at times to ensure nondiscrimination.

☐ Recruitment and Hiring

The food service director may share responsibility for recruiting and hiring new employees with the human resource department. No matter where this responsibility falls, nine basic steps are almost always followed in the process of recruiting and hiring employees (sometimes referred to here as the employment process):

1. Prepare the personnel requisition.
2. Recruit qualified applicants.
3. Take applications.
4. Screen applicants.
5. Interview applicants.
6. Check references.
7. Make the final hiring decision.
8. Arrange for a physical examination and drug screen, if applicable.
9. Conduct a new employee orientation program.

The operation of a food service department is like the operation of any business organization in that its success depends on the skills and commitment of its human resources—the people who do the work. For this reason, it is extremely important that the recruitment and hiring process be conducted with careful adherence to the letter and spirit of the law. Hiring employees who lack the skill, experience, and incentive to perform their jobs contributes to an organization's turnover rate. Turnover is expensive because the process involved in recruiting, hiring, and training new employees draws on a number of resources including time, energy, staff, money, and materials. During this process, the department's productivity can fall, and so can employee morale. Therefore, excessive repetition of this cycle should be guarded against.

The legislation described at the beginning of this chapter is intended to ensure that employers conduct the employment process fairly. To avoid illegal discrimination against applicants on the basis of sex, age, race, color, religion, or national origin, and to refrain from asking illegal questions on application forms and during interviews, managers who take part in this process must remember one critical fact: Their organizations can be sued by unsuccessful applicants who claim unfair treatment or discrimination.

Preparing a Personnel Requisition

A food service department's operating budget specifies how many full-time equivalent (FTE) employees it may employ. A position becomes vacant when an employee resigns or is dismissed, or when a new position is added because of increased work load. At this point, the food service director should start the recruitment and hiring process to avoid problems associated with understaffing.

The first step is to fill out a *personnel requisition.* The official title of the vacant position, the pay grade, job description, qualifications and experience required, and any other information needed by the human resource department should be completed on this form. The director then signs the request and, if applicable, submits it to his or her immediate supervisor for approval.

Once approved, the personnel requisition is sent to the human resource department, where it is checked for accuracy and completeness. In large organizations, the requisition is handled by an employment manager; in small facilities, it may be handled by the director of the human resource department or by one of the department's clerical assistants. The next step is recruitment.

Recruiting Qualified Applicants

Recruitment is the process of identifying and attracting qualified potential employees. Usually, the human resource department is directly responsible for recruiting applicants from inside and outside the organization. However, qualified candidates can be recommended or referred by members of the food service staff or by outside referral sources (for example, another health care facility).

In filling job openings, many organizations have a policy of hiring from within the organization. This policy encourages employees' commitment and allows them to advance within the organization. Also, such a policy may be part of the organization's contractual agreement with an organized labor union. With a policy of *internal recruiting,* the vacancy must be publicized in-house prior to seeking outside applicants. For a certain length of time as specified by policy, job openings are routinely posted on bulletin boards in the human resource department, in staff lounges, and/or other designated posting places in the facility.

Once internal candidates have been given the chance to apply, the department begins the *external recruiting* process. One source for potential external applicants is current staff members who may recommend people they know. Government and private employment agencies are another source. Colleges with food service programs and dietitian training programs have placement offices that are eager to help students and graduates find jobs. Advertisements can be run in local and out-of-town newspapers and in food service industry publications.

Advertisements should briefly describe the duties and responsibilities of the position as well as the qualifications required. Such information should be taken from a current job specification that corresponds to the official job description for the position. For a new position, a job description and job specifications must be developed by the appropriate team. (Job descriptions and specifications are discussed in chapter 6.) All recruitment activities must comply with equal employment opportunity law as outlined earlier in this chapter.

Taking Applications

Each external applicant should fill out a written employment application. Internal candidates should fill out whatever forms are required by the institution's personnel policies and procedures. Application forms should ask only for job-related information needed to determine an applicant's qualifications for the position. Forms should be supplied or approved by the human resource department to ensure compliance with EEOC guidelines, immigration regulations, and affirmative action program requirements.

No application may ask questions that violate the legal rights of an applicant. For example, employers may not ask—on written application forms or during personal interviews—whether an applicant has ever been arrested or has organizational affiliations that do not relate directly to the position applied for. Civil rights laws forbid employers from asking questions related to age, race, religion, or national origin. Questions related to disabilities or medical conditions also may not be asked as part of the hiring process. Applicants may not be asked about their familial status or whether they plan to have children. However, questions about age, medical condition, marital status, and number of dependents may be asked *after* an applicant officially has been hired. This is because such information is needed on applications for the health and life insurance coverage offered to new employees as part of their employee benefits.

Screening Applicants

The sequence of activities in the screening stage may vary. Many times, unqualified applicants are screened out, or eliminated, when they inquire about the position by telephone or mail prior to their filling out an application. Furthermore, the human resource representative may either screen out unqualified applicants soon after they apply or wait until all potential candidates have filled out applications and then eliminate those whose skills, training, or experience do not match requirements for the position.

If the position requires special skills, such as typing, computer literacy, or experience using technical office equipment, the human resource department may test the applicants to determine whether their skills meet the criteria specified for the job. Some organizations may administer intelligence, personality, and aptitude tests as well. However, test results cannot be used for purposes of discrimination. In addition, these tests must be standardized and proved to be ethnically and sexually unbiased by independent testing authorities. The use of all such tests must be coordinated and monitored by professionals trained in their administration and fair interpretation.

The food service director may further screen qualified applicants to determine which individuals will be interviewed. Interviewing is time-consuming and costly and should be reserved for the best-qualified applicants. There is no magic formula for the number of candidates who should be interviewed, but enough people should be seen to ensure that the best candidate available is offered the job.

Interviewing Applicants

After unqualified applicants have been screened out, interviews with potential employees are scheduled by the human resource department. In some organizations, the employment manager interviews the candidates before the food service manager does. In others, the food service director or a designee may be the only person who actually interviews the candidates. An organization's personnel procedures dictate who has this responsibility.

Interviewing is not an exact science. Interviewers have responsibility for treating candidates fairly, cordially, and professionally. They must make every effort to suspend negative judgment of candidates based on appearance or language and conduct the interview with an open mind. Interviewers should remember, too, that the candidates are judging them as well. The interviewer must dress professionally and give the candidate a positive impression of the job and the organization.

The interview should be a positive experience for both managers and prospective employees. A well-conducted interview is the first step in establishing a constructive and professional relationship with new employees and in creating goodwill with those who are not hired. Unsuccessful applicants may be qualified for future openings or may recommend the organization to others who may be interested in applying for future openings.

Well before the scheduled time for the interview, certain preparatory steps should be taken. These are listed below:

1. The human resource department should give the interviewer copies of all information available on individual candidates. The information must include application forms, screening notes, letters of reference, resumes, and applicable test results.
2. The interviewer should review the job description for the vacant position, making notes on the specific qualifications required and ranking them in importance.
3. The interviewer should write an interview plan that includes direct questions intended to elicit information on each candidate's qualifications as compared with the qualifications shown on the job description.
4. Next, the interviewer should thoroughly review all candidate information supplied by the human resource department, looking for points of compatibility between the candidate and the position requirements.
5. The interviewer should compile a list of open-ended questions designed to reveal or clarify information about the candidate's education and training, work history, and career goals. Questions about the candidate's salary expectations also should be planned. Open-ended questions require more than yes-or-no answers and give the applicant a chance to demonstrate his or her knowledge, experience, and ability to communicate, whereas yes-or-no questions do not.
6. The interviewer should reserve a private setting in which to conduct the interview. Interruptions from phone calls and would-be visitors interfere with privacy, making it difficult for both candidate and interviewer to give their full attention to the interview.
7. The interviewer should set aside enough time to make sure that all questions planned are asked of the candidate and that the candidate has enough time to ask questions he or she has about the job and the organization.

Following are some questions that might be asked of candidates for food service jobs:

- Why did you choose food service as a field of work?
- What type of position are you most interested in? Why?
- What qualifications do you have that would make you a success in this job?
- What are your strengths and weaknesses as a food service worker?
- What hours of work do you prefer? Why? Could you work overtime in case of an emergency?
- What did you like and dislike about your previous job? Why?
- What did you do in your last job?
- Why did you leave your last job?
- What do you enjoy doing most in food service?
- Do you work better in a group or alone? Please explain.
- What do you know about food service in a health care operation?

During the interview, certain steps establish an atmosphere conducive to conducting an effective session. Interviewers can follow these steps as outlined below. The interviewer should:

1. Greet the candidate cordially while shaking the candidate's hand, identifying himself or herself, and telling the candidate what position he or she holds. Then ask the candidate what name he or she prefers to be addressed by.

2. Describe how the interview will proceed so that the candidate knows what to expect. Ask whether the candidate minds if the interviewer takes notes during the interview. Notes are extremely valuable for making evaluations and comparisons of candidates after the interview process. However, note taking can make some candidates apprehensive. In addition, interview notes may be examined as part of legal proceedings if an unsuccessful candidate later sues the organization for discrimination. Therefore, interview notes must contain only objective and relevant comments.

3. First, ask general questions about training and work history, but questions already answered on the application form should not be repeated unless clarification or additional information is needed. For example, the interviewer might ask, "I notice that you left your previous job for personal reasons after just six months there. Can you tell me why you stayed at that job for such a short time?" Because most interviewers make the mistake of talking too much, the interviewer should be careful to allow the candidate to answer all questions completely and to be given enough time to ask questions in turn.

4. After the candidate's educational background and work history have been explored fully, describe the position and give the candidate a copy of the job description.

5. Ask a series of open-ended questions to see whether the candidate understands what the position involves and to see whether he or she has the skills and knowledge needed to perform the job.

6. Encourage the candidate to ask questions about the job itself, about the organization, about wage levels and work schedules, about the employment benefits available, and about opportunities for advancement or promotion.

7. Once the candidate has been given every opportunity to ask questions and seems satisfied with the information provided, move the interview toward conclusion. Tell the candidate what will happen next and when he or she may expect to hear a decision. Be friendly and positive, but be careful not to give the impression that the candidate definitely will be offered the job. It is especially important not to create false hopes for candidates who did not perform well in the interview or who obviously are much less qualified for the position than other candidates being considered. Disappointed candidates may feel that they have been treated unfairly when they are not offered employment.

8. Express sincere appreciation for the interest the candidate has shown in working for the organization.

After the interview, the interviewer should take the following additional steps. He or she should:

1. Review the notes taken during the interview immediately, adding missing information and noting final impressions of the candidate. Make a preliminary notation on the candidate's qualifications and a preliminary ranking compared with other candidates. For example: "Mary Johnson appears to be very well qualified for the job. She has four years' experience and a steady work record. One of the top three candidates so far." In making such appraisals, consciously try to overcome biases based on the candidate's personal qualities and physical characteristics.

2. After all candidates have been interviewed, review all notes and preliminary rankings again. Then rank the candidates a final time according to their skills, knowledge, and experience. The rankings also should take into account the candidates' degree of interest, usually expressed during the interview by the number of questions candidates ask and

by their general attitudes toward the interview process and the position being offered. An enthusiastic candidate with two years' experience may make a better employee than a disinterested candidate with five years' experience. Such decisions are always based on the experience and judgment of the interviewer.

3. Decide which candidate seems to be best suited for the job. At this point, it may be appropriate to seek the advice of the human resource department, especially if one of its representatives also interviewed candidates. For professional positions, it is customary to conduct more than one interview with one or more candidates before a decision can be made.

4. Inform the human resource department of the decision to offer a particular candidate the position.

Checking References

After the decision to offer the job is made, a human resource representative is informed so that the chosen candidate's references can be checked. The reference check involves contacting at least the candidate's most recent employer by telephone or letter. Often other former employers are contacted as well. The educational credentials of professional employees also should be verified at this time.

Because employers are sensitive to the legal liability associated with supplying potentially damaging information about former employees to prospective new employers, many organizations have a personnel policy that forbids disclosure of employee information beyond dates of employment, job titles, and final salaries or wages. If the candidate has given written consent to do so, the human resource representative also may contact the candidate's former supervisor directly. This person may be asked to describe the candidate's work habits and attendance record. If there is any doubt about the candidate's work record or personal integrity, the human resource representative may contact all previous employers, confirm the candidate's personal references, or check the candidate's record with legal authorities.

In checking references, employers must avoid questions that are prohibited under the federal Privacy Act and the Fair Credit Reporting Act. It is for this reason that most organizations have a personnel policy that requires the human resource department, instead of the interviewing department manager, to check the references of potential employees. Human resource specialists usually are fully aware of what questions may and may not be asked in the employment process.

Making the Final Hiring Decision

The final decision to hire a new employee is one of the most important any manager will make. Hiring unqualified or uncooperative employees can waste training dollars and damage department morale. The wrong decision also may cost the organization hundreds or thousands of dollars. The employment process is expensive because it requires a great deal of the manager's and the human resource department's time. Advertisements in publications and fees charged by private employment agencies and recruitment firms are increasingly expensive.

Therefore, the hiring decision must be based on careful screening of all candidates available, a fair and well-thought-out interview, and thorough reference checking. The hiring decision should never be rushed, and it should never be based on superficial first impressions or personal biases.

Once the final hiring decision has been made and it is agreed that the best-qualified candidate has been found, the human resource department representative and the food service director jointly decide what starting salary or wage the candidate should be offered. The starting salary is based on the wage or salary range for the position and on the candidate's work experience and educational training.

The human resource representative then contacts the candidate (by letter or telephone) to offer the position at the salary assigned. In some organizations, the employing manager may make the actual job offer. However, again because human resource specialists are trained to address sensitive legal issues that surround the employment process, the trend is toward having them make job offer contacts with candidates. One important area of concern is that the offer of employment be made in such a way that the candidate is not led to misconstrue the offer to be an employment contract.

Making the job offer includes giving the candidate specific information about the starting salary or wage, anticipated date of employment, official job title, and other information about employment with the organization. Other information might include details about qualifying for health benefits and vacation time. Often the candidate may ask for some time to think about the offer. Setting a definite time for a follow-up contact for a final decision prevents delays in filling the position.

If the candidate accepts the offer, the human resource representative arranges for the new employee to undergo a physical examination. If the candidate decides not to accept the position, the representative notifies the food service director so that a second candidate can be chosen and the cycle repeated.

The application forms, test scores, interview notes, reference check notes, and any other information on unsuccessful candidates should be filed in the human resource department. Such materials will be extremely valuable in the event that unsuccessful candidates take legal action against the organization. (However, this material can become a double-edged sword if records reveal that the organization failed to follow its own policies and procedures, for example, to check references.) In addition, the files may be a source of information on potential candidates in recruitment efforts to fill future openings for similar positions. The files should include clear statements indicating the reasons the candidates were not hired. The application forms and other information gathered on successful candidates should be kept as part of the permanent personnel records, discussed later in this chapter.

Arranging for a Physical Examination

Prior to the implementation of the Americans with Disabilities Act of 1992, employees were usually given a preemployment physical before a job offer was made. Because organizations must be careful not to discriminate against disabled individuals, most now make a preliminary job offer pending completion of a postoffer medical examination, agility evaluation, or other testing. Upon the applicant's acceptance of the initial job offer, the human resources department schedules the candidate for a physical examination to be performed by a physician, nurse, or nurse practitioner, who should be given a copy of the candidate's job description.

The examination is intended to determine whether the new employee can meet the physical demands of the job or needs reasonable accommodations, to detect health conditions that might pose a risk to the employee if he or she were placed in a specific job or area, and to protect the organization's customers and staff from exposure to potentially infectious illnesses. This step is especially important for food service workers because of the danger of spreading communicable diseases through food handling and because much of the work involved is physically taxing. During the preplacement examination, the employee generally is asked to provide a cardiopulmonary history and to take a tuberculin skin test.

Screening for illegal or controlled drug usage has been implemented by many health care organizations. Drug screens are meant to combat absenteeism, accidents, work-related injuries, equipment damage, and inefficient performance due to substance abuse among employees. Screening for substance abuse also can help employers control the cost of health care and worker's compensation. Employers may deny employment to individuals who are using illegal or controlled substances at the time of a preemployment screen, but applicants with prior addictions are covered under the ADA.

Organizations that decide to use drug screening must use a nationally approved laboratory and follow strict protocols for chain of custody to ensure the validity of the test results. Confidentiality is of critical importance and is generally ensured through minimal handling of the specimen as outlined in the organization's human resource policy and procedure. The manager of the food service department should become familiar with the policy and procedures of the organization to ensure compliance.

Conducting a New Employee Orientation Program

The first few days on the job are crucial for new employees. Not only must they be introduced to the job, other employees, and the organization, but their future performance may depend on the attitudes and impressions they form during these first days. Therefore, well-organized orientation procedures are needed to help new employees quickly become productive members of the staff.

Orientation to the Organization

In many medium- and large-size health care organizations, the human resource department is responsible for explaining the organization's personnel policies, regulations, and employee benefit programs. During general orientation sessions, new employees fill out tax withholding statements for the Internal Revenue Service and application forms for health insurance, life insurance, and other group benefits.

Also during this time, new employees may be given a guided tour of the facility. This inspires pride in the organization and helps the employee understand his or her role. A brief history of the organization and an introduction to the organization's mission and goals also are common elements of employee orientation programs. The new employee may be given a copy of the organization's employee handbook at this time. (The employee handbook will be discussed later in this chapter.)

In smaller health care facilities, the food service director may be responsible for conducting general orientation for new employees as well as their orientation to the food service department. When this is the case, the director should make every effort to make the general orientation an interesting and thorough introduction to the operation of the organization as a whole. Specific training for work tasks should be conducted only after the general orientation session.

Orientation to the Food Service Department

The new employee's introduction to the food service department should be warm and friendly. The director and any other department managers who will work with the new employee should set aside time to welcome and introduce him or her to others in the department. People should be introduced by name and a brief description of their duties given. Such introductions will make it easier for the new member to understand who does what in the department.

After all introductions have been made, the person who will supervise the employee directly should begin the gradual process of easing the new person into department operations and his or her specific job requirements. By conveying a sincere interest in making the orientation and training period a pleasant experience, the supervisor supports a new employee's eagerness to do the job well, be accepted by coworkers and supervisors, and overcome being nervous in a new situation.

The supervisor should not cover too much information at once, reassuring the new worker that additional information will be given gradually throughout the orientation period. Information overload may cause a new employee to become confused and even more apprehensive. The new employee should be given a copy of the department's procedures handbook and be allowed enough time to read it thoroughly before beginning work.

The next section of this chapter will discuss in detail some methods for training new employees to perform their jobs. However, it first may be helpful to offer guidelines for a typical orientation and training program for a production worker. Managers should keep in mind that these guidelines would not be suitable for orienting professional or managerial employees. For example, an orientation and training program for registered dietitians and other nutrition professionals should be arranged on an individual basis so as to be suited to the various levels of experience and knowledge such professionals would have.

The following guidelines cover the first five days (one workweek) of a new employee's orientation as a food service production worker in a hospital:

- *Day 1:* The supervisor explains the general departmental routine and where the new employee's job fits in; shows the employee the general work area, the employees' lounge, and the employees' locker room; assigns the new employee to an experienced employee whose duties are identical or similar to those the new employee will perform; and gives the new hire a copy of the department procedures handbook. The new employee spends the rest of day 1 observing and working with the experienced employee.

- *Day 2:* The supervisor checks with the new employee to see whether he or she has questions about yesterday's activities; clarifies any task or departmental routine; and reaffirms a friendly and supportive atmosphere by offering encouragement and helpful suggestions rather than criticism. The new employee spends the rest of day 2 working with and observing the mentor employee perform tasks the new employee eventually will perform.

- *Day 3:* The new employee spends more time working independently. The supervisor observes his or her job behavior and corrects or clarifies work performance as necessary.

- *Day 4:* The new employee continues to work independently, but the supervisor and coworkers remain available to answer questions and offer advice. The supervisor begins to review the job description as well as key points of departmental policies—especially those on infection control, disaster planning, fire safety, and hazardous substance handling—offering the new member opportunity to raise questions and clarify points as necessary (for example, fine points of the department's or organization's personnel policies such as employee benefits, grievance procedures, and performance evaluation).

- *Day 5:* The new employee assumes job tasks independently. The supervisor may apprise the employee of training opportunities in specific production procedures and techniques once the employee has adjusted to his or her new work setting.

☐ Training

Employee training is one of a food service director's most important responsibilities. A continuous, well-organized training program for all levels of employees increases productivity, quality level, safety consciousness, and department morale. New employees may require a complete training regimen. Experienced employees may need training in new or updated production methods, equipment, and approaches to handling set job tasks. Most new employee training is conducted one on one, whereas experienced food service employees usually are taught new or updated skills and concepts during in-service group training sessions.

The department director responsible for the performance and training of unit managers and nonmanagerial employees in a hospital setting has access to more resources than ever. Many hospital human resource departments now employ training specialists (sometimes called education coordinators) who serve as instructors or advisers in helping facilities plan their training programs. These specialists coordinate department-level in-service programs or design individual training plans for all levels of department employees.

Nonprofessional employees in the food service department have varied educational and social backgrounds. Some may lack skill in food service work per se upon being hired. Despite the differences in abilities, social backgrounds, and basic skill levels (for example, in math and reading), it is essential that all food service employees receive adequate training. Part of that training is understanding the responsibility of the food service department to provide safe, nutritious, and high-quality food to customers.

Training for physically or mentally challenged employees must be conducted on the basis of any accommodations needed by these individuals. For example, if an employee were learning disabled, training would require verbal instructions and demonstrations. If modifications were made to equipment to enable a physically challenged worker to complete a task, it might be necessary to train other staff to use the modified equipment.

In the United States, billions of dollars are invested annually in job training. This level of investment makes it incumbent on managers to ensure the highest return possible. Training can pay for itself many times over when an employee is consistently and adequately trained from day one. Training programs should be planned and designed with specific and objective outcomes for knowledge or skill enhancement in mind. Planning and determining objectives are discussed later in this section.

Understanding the Instructor's Role

The instructor, a key to successful training, must maintain a positive attitude toward the work to be learned and toward the employees who must be trained to perform it. To facilitate the learning process, the instructor must first earn employees' respect and confidence by demonstrating his or her skills, explaining convincingly why tasks are performed in particular ways, and showing fairness and patience. The instructor also should be careful to gauge the employees' knowledge beforehand so as to avoid unnecessary training as well as training for which they may be inadequately prepared. For example, training in use of new cook–chill or cook–freeze procedures is futile unless employees understand the importance of maintaining the structural and textural integrity of the food prepared with these systems. Assessing an employee's knowledge can be accomplished through observation or written pretesting. For example, if training involved the proper method of steaming vegetables, the employee could be asked to demonstrate the technique. A written pretest should ask questions regarding the key concepts the trainer wishes the employee to learn. For example, a pretest on proper food handling should ask specific questions regarding holding temperatures and proper labeling of the product.

The instructor also must understand basic principles of training adults. Some of these include the following:

- The desire to learn must come from the learner.
- People learn at different rates.
- All training does not progress smoothly but in up-and-down cycles.
- If treated with disrespect, adults resist taking part in activities.
- Learners become discouraged when they reach a plateau in their skill levels.
- Adults come to the learning situation with a great deal of life experience and want to contribute actively.
- A certain amount of apprehensiveness is a natural part of learning.
- Adults require practical outcomes from their learning experience.
- A whole task should be demonstrated before it is broken down into its component parts for learning purposes.
- Poor training methods hinder learning.
- Adults learn more efficiently in well-timed training periods that last no longer than an hour without a break.
- The reasoning behind every element of the skill being taught must be explained to help employees understand the whole process.
- Learners need to be told how well they are doing as the learning progresses.

Although, as stated above, a positive attitude is important, instructors should not expect maximum skills to be attained by the end of the training session. Full learning of tasks requires on-the-job practice.

Conducting Individual Training Programs

In many food service departments, individualized training of new nonprofessional employees is delegated to experienced employees who perform identical or similar jobs. The employee selected for this task should know how to teach, so the manager must work with this person to plan step-by-step how the new employee is to be trained. This way, common errors made by inexperienced trainers can be circumvented. Some of these errors include the following:

- Trying to teach too much at one time
- Describing how to perform a task without first demonstrating it
- Lacking patience
- Failing to give and receive feedback as the learning progresses
- Failing to prepare adequately
- Forgetting, overlooking, or inadequately explaining key points

The director or manager who delegates training responsibility must check periodically to ensure that training is proceeding appropriately. Any shortcomings in the process must be addressed so that both employee trainer and manager can learn from mistakes.

The step-by-step plan worked out between manager and designated trainer must be designed carefully for maximum benefit to the new employee. Following are some basic guidelines for training new nonprofessional food service employees:

1. Use the new employee's job description to plan which tasks and skills need to be taught.
2. Outline a step-by-step procedure for teaching each task or skill. The goal of each training session should be stated and communicated to the trainee.
3. Set aside a specific time for each training session so that interruptions are kept to a minimum.
4. Gather and arrange all supplies, utensils, equipment, and teaching aids before the session begins. The workplace should be set up just as the employee will be expected to keep it.
5. Prepare for each session by first learning what the new employee already knows about the task.
6. Demonstrate each task before teaching it. Explain each step completely and clearly, stressing and repeating key points and demonstrating acceptable shortcuts that make the task easier, faster, or more effective.
7. Ask and invite questions at each juncture of the demonstration to ensure the trainee's comprehension.
8. Give the trainee ample opportunity to perform the task and explain its steps along the way while observing and correcting errors patiently. Have the trainee repeat the task until it is clear that he or she understands it fully.
9. Allow the trainee to practice the task independently after all safety procedures have been learned fully. However, remain close at hand to answer questions and provide feedback or help if needed.
10. Withdraw direct supervision gradually as the trainee becomes proficient at the task.
11. Acknowledge the trainee's progress and congratulate him or her upon successful completion of the assigned task.
12. Discuss the schedule for additional training and set reasonable goals for learning related tasks.

Conducting Group In-Service Training Programs

An in-service training program is essential for maintaining an efficient and cost-effective food service department. Continuing education enables employees to grow in their jobs by learning new techniques or gaining new knowledge that will help them become more productive and increase job satisfaction and ownership. Well-organized group training sessions are the primary method of conducting in-service training. They are an efficient means of communicating vital information in a structured training environment. Most states require official in-service training programs for health care providers.

Program Planning and Scheduling

Once staff needs have been assessed, the topics for in-service training can be rated by importance, and the employees who require training can be identified. A successful program is based on employee needs: What problems, issues, or changes need to be explained? What attitudes, knowledge, and skills will help employees do their jobs effectively, now and in the future? Some topics may be relevant to the work of the whole department (for example, safety procedures). Other topics apply to only a few employees (for example, salad preparation techniques). A firm schedule for training sessions must be established several months in advance. The date, time, and subject of each session should be stated on the schedule and made available to all employees.

The food service director and/or education coordinator should plan the entire year's in-service program in conjunction with the organization's annual business plan activities. The program should take into consideration overall organizational requirements and legislative and regulatory agency requirements. For example, programs may cover disaster planning, fire and safety procedures, infection control, OSHA regulations, or quality assurance and quality control procedures.

Because most food service employees work in shifts, two or more sessions on each topic need to be planned. Work schedules and work loads should always be considered when designing training schedules. Whenever the work volume does not allow enough time to schedule group meetings during the workday, sessions should be scheduled at the end of the workday or between two overlapping shifts. Personnel policies should be followed to determine whether hourly employees are paid overtime for attending sessions outside their regular working hours.

The topic to be presented for each in-service meeting should be defined narrowly so that the subject can be covered adequately. Most sessions conducted during the regular workday should be short (20 to 40 minutes) because employees may be too fatigued to learn effectively.

Behavioral objectives should be developed with a method to evaluate the results of training. Objectives and results can be identified by asking two basic questions: What do the employees need to know? How can the results of training be evaluated?

A *behavioral objective* states in specific terms what the outcome of the training should be and how it is to be measured. Behavioral objectives should be based on the kind of material to be learned. Should it be a skills objective, an attitude objective, or a knowledge objective?

A *skills objective* involves teaching some kind of manipulative skill, in psychology called a *psychomotor skill*. The level of psychomotor skill can be easily measured. An example of a skills objective could be the following: At the end of training, the employee will be able to disassemble the dishmachine, clean it, and reassemble it correctly 100 percent of the time.

Attitude objectives involve developing in participants new or modified feelings (attitudes) toward the topic covered in the training session. (Such emotional components are called *affects* in the terminology of psychology.) Attitude objectives also involve individual interests, values, and feelings of appreciation. The level of accomplishment in fulfilling attitude objectives is difficult to measure because personal emotions and beliefs are intangible and elude assessment. An example of an attitude objective could be the following: At the end of training, the employee will have an increased appreciation of the need to practice good guest relations when serving patients and other customers.

A *knowledge objective* involves teaching intellectual skills (called *cognitive skills* in the language of psychology). The level of knowledge or understanding gained through in-service training is relatively easy to test and observe. An example of a knowledge objective could be the following: At the end of training, the employee will be able to calculate the composition of a 1,200-calorie, low-fat diet correctly 100 percent of the time.

No matter what skills or attitudes are being taught, all behavioral objectives should accomplish five things:

1. State the action to be accomplished.
2. State what the action is directed toward.

3. Describe how the action is to be accomplished.
4. State how accomplishment of the action is to be measured.
5. Include clarifications of the preceding components as necessary.

After the type of objective has been determined, the behavioral change or changes being sought as the goal of the training should be determined. This can be done by asking one of the following questions: What can the employees now do that they could not do before? What do they now understand that they did not understand before? What do they now know that they did not know before? What will they now do that they would not do before?

Evaluating In-Service Training Sessions

To determine whether the desired outcome has been achieved at an in-service meeting, a method must be devised to evaluate its end results. Tests, reports, demonstrations, and so forth can measure the level of employee competency. In some cases, posttraining follow-up may indicate that some individuals need individual training to achieve the level of competency required.

Once the outcome of training and an evaluation method are determined, a task analysis is completed. A *task analysis* is a written description outlining the main steps of a specific work activity in order of occurrence. Figure 8-1 is an example of a task analysis. The task analysis may be supported by notes on the main points to be emphasized in the training. These materials also are used as the basis for the instructor's plans for the training session.

If the session's instructor is from outside the department or the organization, a department representative must contact him or her well in advance to explain what skills or concepts are to be taught. The representative also should offer help in setting up demonstrations and/or obtaining audiovisual equipment.

Figure 8-1.   Example of a Task Analysis for a Food Service Department Training Session

TASK ANALYSIS

Position: Dining room cashier
Task: Cash transactions
Frequency: For each cash customer
Equipment: 190 Cash Register cash drawer
Contact: Cafe manager or head cashier

Important Steps in Job	Key Points
1. Tally each food item on the tray.	Tally each item under the proper food category.
2. Push subtotal button.	–
3. Push the tax button.	–
4. Push total button.	Be sure the tax has been added.
5. Check the amount on the indicator.	Be sure it agrees with the amount of sale.
6. Tell the customer the amount.	Speak clearly.
7. Take the money from the customer.	Hold the palm of your hand upward.
8. Punch value received.	Be sure to punch value in correctly.
9. Place the money in drawer.	Be sure to place in appropriate value category.
10. Punch the change indicator button.	Check the indicator for the amount of change to be returned to the customer.
11. Count bills back to customer.	Tell the customer to pick up change from counter. Start with ones, fives, tens, and so on.
12. Close cash drawer.	Do not lock cash drawer.
13. Give receipt to customer.	Do not drop it.
14. Say thank you.	Smile.

Identifying In-Service Training Topics and Resources

As a result of the employee needs analysis for in-service training, a number of issues or themes may surface. Some possible topics for a continuing education program for the food service staff include:

- Standards for personal hygiene
- Advances in food-handling procedures
- Changes in cleaning techniques and procedures
- Operation and maintenance of new equipment
- Current fire safety and disaster procedures
- The importance of energy conservation
- Future operational changes in the department and in the organization
- Basic concepts of nutrition
- Procedures for preparing and serving foods for modified diets
- Changes in personnel policies
- Meeting the needs of special patient populations (for example, the elderly and the physically or mentally challenged)
- Safety precautions related to equipment, hazardous chemicals, cuts, burns, and falls

It may be useful to maintain a list of people who demonstrate interest in teaching in-service training sessions in their areas of expertise. Speakers and instructors from the community may be employed by state and local public health agencies, universities, and technical colleges. Potential speakers also may be identified at meetings of professional organizations serving the food service and health care fields or through national speakers' bureaus. Staff members from other departments in the organization as well as from nearby health care organizations are additional resources.

Training materials are available from a number of sources and in varying formats, including videotapes, filmstrips, slides, and printed materials. Trainers should prescreen all materials before renting or purchasing them to ensure their appropriateness for the training planned. Screening further ensures that the department's training dollars are being put to good use.

Program Implementation

The instructor for a particular in-service training session should prepare a detailed instruction plan based on the objectives previously identified. A *lesson plan,* a written blueprint of how a lesson is to be conducted, describes key points to be covered and how they are to be taught (for example, by demonstration or discussion) and lists all materials needed to conduct the lesson. Lesson materials may include printed handouts, wall charts, audiovisual materials, equipment, and supplies, among others. The lesson plan also should include written questions to be discussed with the group. The instructor should be sure that the elements in the lesson plan can be covered adequately in the amount of time scheduled.

Well before the session is scheduled to begin, the instructor should check whether all audiovisual equipment needed is available and in good working order. Similarly, he or she should have any posters, charts, handouts, and other printed materials prepared in advance. Such materials should be well organized and neatly prepared. Posters and charts should be large enough to be seen from all areas of the training room.

The session should start on schedule. At the beginning of the session, the instructor should introduce him- or herself to the group if necessary. Next, other members of the group should introduce themselves in the event they are not known by name to all present.

The session should begin with an overview of the topics to be discussed and/or demonstrated. Any supplementary teaching aids should be set up or passed out when appropriate. The instructor should involve members of the group in as many demonstrations and role-playing activities as possible, asking questions all along so as to encourage further discussion and involvement.

At the end of the session, the subject should be summarized, with time allowed for any additional questions to further ensure that all key points have been covered adequately and are understood by all participants. Finally, the group should be asked to give specific examples of how the skills and concepts learned in the session can be applied to the everyday work of the food service department.

Program Evaluation

Measuring the outcome of in-service training and evaluating the overall program are important to the training process. Employee performance should be assessed on an ongoing basis to determine the need for further training or retraining. Employees' skills can be tested and measured immediately before and shortly after a program to determine its effectiveness. On-the-job performance tests and observations, interviews, questionnaires, and department records also serve as indicators. Department accident and event reports, as well as quality control assessments, are reliable gauges of job-related skills and attitudes and, therefore, of the merits of the department's training program.

An instructor's training skills also can be evaluated by asking questions about how well the instructor knew the material and how well the material was presented. Were the teaching aids helpful and interesting? Was the class discussion informative? Did the instructor answer all questions thoroughly and respectfully?

Participants can be asked to complete written evaluation forms at the end of each training session. Survey questions might include the following:

- Will information from this session help you to improve your job skills?
- What did you learn that will help you in your work?
- Was this subject interesting to you?
- Was this session worthwhile?
- Did the session contain enough practical information, or was it too theoretical?
- Was the session long enough? Too long?
- How could the session have been better?
- What subjects would you like to learn more about in future sessions?
- Was the learning environment comfortable physically and socially (too crowded or too warm)?

Maintaining Records of Individual and Group In-Service Training Programs

Records of individual and group training efforts must be maintained by the food service department. Employees should sign attendance sheets for each training session they attend. A monthly report showing the number of sessions conducted and the level of staff attendance can be a valuable part of the department's quality program. Such records may be examined by JCAHO surveyors as well as by state regulatory agents.

☐ Performance Evaluation Systems

The level of success attained by a business organization is directly related to the level of performance attained by its employees. Therefore, managers must be thoroughly familiar with the job-related activities and abilities of each employee they supervise. A system for regular and fair evaluation of individual employee performance is instrumental to the success of the department and the organization in a number of ways. A performance evaluation system tracks progress in the development of job skills while identifying and correcting substandard performance. It further serves as a basis for recognizing and rewarding employee achievements through promotions, salary increases, and other incentives. In providing a means of giving verbal and written feedback on individual employee performance, an evaluation system benefits the overall functioning of the department and the organization as well as promotes employees' well-being,

189

job satisfaction, and sense of ownership in their work. Finally, equitable and well-prepared evaluations given constantly can improve working relations and communications among employees and between employees and their supervisors. All of these pluses ultimately boost morale and productivity while minimizing costly employee absenteeism and turnover.

In most medium- and large-size organizations, the performance evaluation system is administered by the human resource department. However, the food service director or manager still has direct responsibility for rating employees according to objective performance standards. These standards usually are developed by the director, who follows procedures established by the human resource department. Generally, the performance evaluation process includes two components: a written evaluation and a verbal review. Regular increases in employee salaries or wages are based in large part on their performance evaluations. (Compensation and benefits will be discussed later in this chapter.) In addition to determining salary increases, performance reviews can identify areas where training and coaching can improve performance.

Developing and Using the Performance Evaluation Form

Fair performance standards must be developed before a fair performance evaluation can be made. Performance standards are based on the responsibilities outlined in the job description. Each performance standard should reflect a required work-related behavior and should be clearly stated in written form. The standard should cite specific task-related activities that can be measured or observed.

General factors that should be evaluated by written performance standards include the following:

- Quality of work performed
- Quantity of work performed
- Employee's working relationships with coworkers and superiors
- Employee's attendance record
- Employee's work habits

An employee's attitudes also affect overall performance but are difficult to rate. How an employee behaves toward other employees and how well he or she accepts supervision provide observable attitude indicators that can be rated.

The rating scale for each performance standard should follow the system developed by the human resource department. In most systems, the rating scale is based on descriptive terms that correspond to the points on a scale. Figure 8-2 lists examples of performance standards and shows a commonly used rating scale.

Several errors often occur during the evaluation process. One is the *halo effect,* the tendency on the part of certain supervisors to let very good or very poor performance in one task affect the evaluation of other unrelated tasks. Some supervisors also make the mistake of consistently giving too-lenient or too-severe ratings. Others tend to make the overall evaluation task easier for themselves by giving everyone in similar jobs average ratings instead of ratings based on individual performance. Another common problem is the *recency error.* Here, the supervisor mistakenly judges a whole review period's performance on the basis of the employee's most recent behavior. Because most employees are rated only once or twice a year, much of the employee's work performance could be misevaluated if only recent performance were considered.

To avoid such problems, use of a rating scale based on descriptive gradations (such as those given in figure 8-2) is helpful. Scales based on general terms such as *outstanding, superior, average,* and *poor* should be avoided because they make it too easy to give average ratings to every employee's performance on every standard. In addition, supervisors can avoid the natural tendency to be influenced by recency error if they make evaluation an ongoing part of everyday department management. Ongoing review is the basis for performance coaching,

Figure 8-2. Excerpt from a Performance Evaluation Form for a Food Service Employee

Department: _____   Date: _____

Job Title: _____   Evaluator: _____

Circle the number on the rating scale that most accurately describes this employee's performance.

Performance Standard	Rating				
	Always	Almost Always	Sometimes	Rarely	Never
Accurately measures and/or weighs ingredients according to instructions in recipes or on boxes.	4	3	2	1	0
Requisitions food, stores food items for next day, checks and properly stores issues.	4	3	2	1	0
Pulls recipes, computer sheets, and menus for next day's work before going off duty.	4	3	2	1	0
Keeps work area clean and in sanitary condition.	4	3	2	1	0
Cooperates with fellow employees and willingly assists where and when needed.	4	3	2	1	0
Reports to work on time and in uniform.	4	3	2	1	0

which is covered later in this section. Notes on individual work performance and coaching sessions could be made regularly—monthly, for example—and then used as the basis for performance evaluation at the end of the review period.

The human resource department's policy on scheduling regular performance evaluations should be followed. Many organizations have a system of annual review and performance appraisal, whereas others may follow a schedule of quarterly or semiannual reviews. Informal ratings of new employees are sometimes made monthly during the training and/or probationary periods of their employment.

Conducting Verbal Performance Reviews

The second component in the individual evaluation process is the review conference held between the employee and his or her direct supervisor. Individual conferences should be scheduled well in advance so that employees have enough time to prepare questions and comments. The reviewer should also schedule enough time for a thorough and unrushed private discussion of each employee's past and future performance. Conferences should be conducted in a positive and cooperative manner. Once areas of good performance have been covered, the supervisor should offer constructive suggestions for improvement. Finally, employee and supervisor can reach agreement as to what steps are needed to improve specific areas of performance, along with a timetable for reaching the desired outcomes. Following up on the mutually agreed upon steps is part of coaching performance for positive outcomes (discussed in the next section).

It is very important that the reviewer remain open-minded throughout the evaluation process by respecting and noting the employee's opinions. The employee also should be given opportunity to include written responses to the evaluation, to be included with the documents filed in the human resource department.

Once the conference is over, both employee and supervisor should sign the evaluation form. In some organizations, the next level of management also may be required to review and approve completed evaluation forms. A copy of the form should be made for the supervisor's files and for the employee. The original form, with all the necessary signatures, should be placed in the employee's permanent personnel file, which usually is kept in the human resource department. In many organizations, a representative of the human resource department may check that the evaluation form has been completed according to accepted personnel policies.

Coaching for Peak Performance

In addition to the regular written and verbal employee reviews, managers should make informal, day-to-day observations of employee performance, accomplishments, or problems. Unlike performance reviews, which are retrospective and infrequent, coaching requires concurrent ongoing performance monitoring and feedback for improvement. Regular feedback, or coaching, is basic to effective employee management and can prevent minor work-related problems from becoming major performance problems.

A positive approach to performance improvement, coaching provides individualized direction, information, and support on a daily basis. As a "performance coach," the manager is committed to the employee's development and to helping the employee reach full potential. A participative management style fosters a constructive environment in which coaching can be used to improve individual, team, and department performance. The effective manager will provide both opportunity for employees to become involved and the necessary learning through performance coaching. Effective coaching helps people trust their instincts and take responsibility for the organization's success.

The first step in performance coaching is to diagnose performance deficiencies and their causes. Performance gaps exist when employees are not meeting goals or expectations agreed on with their manager. To identify performance deficiencies, employees must be observed over time. A number of causes may contribute to less-than-satisfactory performance. Some of these are:

- Lack of ability or knowledge to accomplish assigned tasks
- Lack of interest in doing the job
- Absence of opportunity to grow and advance that creates feelings of helplessness within the employee
- Lack of clearly defined departmental goals
- Employee uncertainty about what is expected of him or her
- Absence of feedback on how well the employee is performing
- No rewards for high performance
- No negative consequences for poor performance
- Lack of resources to do the job
- Limitations or misunderstandings created by cultural differences

In diagnosing a problem, the first question the manager must ask is whether the employee knows what is expected and has the requisite skills to do the job. If not, the manager as coach must arrange for employee training as outlined earlier in this chapter.

Lack of information or skills is the most common reason for poor performance or goal accomplishment. Causes ascribed to other reasons will make the coaching session even more complex. When coaching, the manager must remain focused on measurable behaviors that can be identified and shared with the employee. *Measurable performance behaviors* are behaviors that can be assessed in comparison to established standards for performance. For example, the supervisor could make a statement like the following in a coaching session: "The standard for preparing and delivering late trays is 15 minutes. However, when you work this station, more than 50 percent of the trays are delivered to patients after 30 minutes. The delay causes a backlog of trays and results in unhappy patients and nurses." Coaching can be divided into three segments: creating the game plan, conducting the coaching session, and following up to ensure success and provide positive feedback.

Create a Game Plan

Coaching takes time because of the preparation involved and the commitment to involve the employee in making performance-related decisions. The following steps will help create a game plan for discussing performance problems with employees:

1. Identify the behavior or habit that is nonproductive or contrary to policy, quality, or customer service.
2. Decide how the behavior affects the manager, work unit, fellow employees, or customers.
3. Determine why the behavior has this effect on those mentioned.
4. Determine how the behavior should change and the benefits those changes will bring about.

These steps will help the manager stay focused on the behavior in question and keep judgments about the employee from concealing the issue. The game plan must be flexible and capable of being changed as the employee's perceptions and needs change. Flexibility also is necessary for determining what actions should be taken to correct undesirable behavior.

Conduct the Coaching Session

Coaching sessions require use of effective communication skills on the manager's part. The coaching action plan shown in figure 8-3 may be helpful in providing written documentation of the coaching session. Typically, a coaching session has six steps:

1. *Describe performance in terms of specific behaviors.* Inform the employee of observations of what he or she did or said inappropriately. Describe how the inappropriate behavior affects the manager, the organization, the department, the team, and the employee. Pause to allow feedback from the employee.
2. *Obtain agreement from the employee on the information presented in step 1.* An employee who disagrees with or cannot understand the implications of the offending behavior is less likely to move toward changing it.
3. *Discuss solutions that can be implemented to resolve the performance problem.* Solutions should be mutually agreed on and should involve the employee in the decision-making process to arrive at resolution.
4. *Agree on an action plan to be implemented for correcting the situation.* Summarize the information shared in the coaching session to ensure that both parties understand the behavior that led to the problem and the agreement on how improvement will occur.
5. *Establish a time line for the action plan.* Having a time frame in which to assess the employee's progress helps keep the action plan and both parties' efforts focused.

Figure 8-3. Example of a Coaching Action Plan

Coaching Action Plan		
Employee:		
Job Title:	Date:	
Current Behavior:		
Expected Behavior:		
Action Step	**Completion Date**	**Follow-up**

6. *Acknowledge the employee's achievement in correcting the behavior and in turn his or her performance.* The manager should document this improvement for the next performance evaluation.

When describing employee performance, it is important to remain objective and to give examples of actual behaviors. Avoid the following approaches:

- Labeling employee behavior (for example, "unprofessional" or "childish").
- Using absolutes or exaggerations for behavior that was observed only once or twice (for example, "You *always* do that"). These comments increase the potential for employee resistance.
- Judging the employee as "good," "better," or "worse"; such value judgments imply that the manager is always right and inhibits open discussion of the problem.
- Using someone else's words or implying that the problem is due to another person's observations (for example, "Jim says you often return from lunch late").

Coaching is a positive approach the manager can use continuously to provide information about expectations, observed performance, and skill development as well as to provide praise and improve self-esteem. Managers and supervisors should have regular meetings with individual employees who report to them. The length of these meetings will depend on the nature of the problem, the complexity of the work, and the responsibility charged to the employee. Coaching should not be confused with discipline, which may be necessary if efforts to improve performance are not successful. (Disciplinary policies and procedures will be covered later in this chapter.) Training and coaching employees to achieve peak performance allows the manager to delegate work effectively.

Follow Up Coaching Efforts

Consistent follow-up with employees demonstrates the manager's support and commitment to improving their performance and helping them to be successful in their jobs. Unfortunately, this step is frequently overlooked by managers. However, without follow-up it is difficult to sustain improvement and assist with future growth. The amount of follow-up should be based on the individual skill levels and needs of the employees. For example, an employee who has difficulty greeting and assisting customers in the cafeteria may need to frequently discuss his or her comfort level with public contact and suggestions for how to answer customers' questions as well as receive praise for success from the manager. A star performer who is being asked to create a quality control checklist for the first time may need follow-up to ensure that the assignment has been completed successfully.

☐ Personnel Records

Every organization is required to keep certain kinds of records on each employee. Official personnel records are usually maintained by the human resource department. Individual departments may keep records on their own employees as well. Generally speaking, department personnel records are less formal than the human resource files. Department records may contain managers' notations on an employee's work performance, coaching action plans, attendance records, copies of vacation requests, notes on scheduling availability, and so forth. The official personnel files should contain the following information for each employee:

- Complete name, home address, telephone number, social security number, and name of the nearest relative
- Job title or classification and rate of pay (hourly, weekly, or monthly)
- Reports of initial and periodic physical examinations
- Promotion records (start date, changes in job classification, pay increases)
- All records from the hiring process (application form, interview notes, records of education, references)

- Records on initial training
- Records of attendance (including vacation days, holidays, and sick days)
- Records of regular and overtime hours worked (for hourly employees only)
- Safety records (accident reports, worker's compensation claims)
- Information on benefits (health insurance, life insurance, pension plan, savings plans, and so forth)
- Records of performance evaluations (written evaluation forms signed by employee and supervisor, special awards and notes of commendation, and written comments on performance made outside the formal evaluation process)
- Records of disciplinary actions, grievances, or complaints
- Termination date and acceptability for reemployment, when appropriate

Keeping records of all disciplinary actions and dismissal procedures is absolutely necessary. Complete documentation of work-related problems will be needed if a former employee takes legal action against the organization for any reason. Because of the confidential nature of personnel records, they should be stored in a place that is inaccessible to unauthorized employees. All managers should have a locked drawer or filing cabinet for personnel files kept in the department.

□ Personnel Policies and Procedures

Most human resource departments in health care organizations develop and administer general *policies* on how employment issues are to be handled. In turn, formal, written personnel *procedures* based on general policies are adopted. Step-by-step procedures are valuable tools for managers' use in administering policies consistently and fairly. Policies and procedures that are understood by all employees and followed by all managers protect everyone from potentially unfair treatment. In addition, they help protect the organization from lawsuits, union and employee grievances, and accusations of illegal discrimination.

Comprehensive organizational policies should cover at least the following basic employment-related topics:

- Work hours
- Overtime
- Pay periods
- Physical examinations
- Termination
- Performance evaluation
- Promotions and job postings
- Holidays and holiday pay
- Vacations
- Training and educational opportunities
- Personal leaves (maternity, bereavement, family, medical, nonmedical, and military)
- Employee grievances
- Disciplinary and corrective actions
- Tardiness and absenteeism
- Sexual harassment

The organization's personnel policies usually are written and distributed in an employee handbook, which is given routinely to all new employees and updated regularly. When a personnel policy changes significantly, the change is publicized through memorandums, posters, and other appropriate means. New policies often emerge from topics covered during in-service training sessions.

Every manager is responsible for applying the organization's personnel policies uniformly and consistently to all employees. Personnel policies on employee discipline, promotions, dismissals, and so on must be followed closely to avoid liability risk to the organization as a result of failure to follow its own policies. For example, an organization whose policy on termination stated that an employee would be given a written warning and placed on probation before being dismissed could be sued by an employee who was terminated without warning, even if the termination was justifiable. In addition to legal problems, consistent failure to follow its policies and procedures can expose a facility to charges of favoritism and/or discrimination. Employee morale problems might be created as well.

Developing a Food Service Department Employee Handbook

An employee handbook that clearly sets down policies and procedures to be followed in the food service department is a useful training and management tool. This handbook could be used as the basis for training new employees and as a handy reference for experienced food service workers. The handbook, which should be reviewed annually by the department director and updated as necessary, can include at least the following information:

- A department flowchart
- Dress code requirements
- Hygienic standards (for example, personal grooming and hand washing)
- Work schedules
- Policy on smoking in the workplace
- Right-to-know information on hazardous substances used in the workplace (for example, kitchen cleaning agents; see chapter 14)
- Infection control standards (based on JCAHO standards; see chapter 13)
- Safety policies (for example, fire and disaster planning)
- Relationships between the food service department and other departments

Maintaining Positive Approach to Corrective Action

Most employees accept policies and procedures as a necessary condition of working, and they expect the rules to be enforced fairly and evenhandedly. Employee morale suffers when certain employees are permitted to violate policies and procedures, which promotes favoritism. More important, employee safety may be at risk if policies and procedures are violated. For example, violation of safety procedures can cause equipment damage and endanger workers, for which the organization might be held accountable. This is especially true in the food service department, where fire safety and safe food-handling procedures are doubly crucial. For these reasons, prompt and fair disciplinary action is a necessary element of managing employees.

When disciplinary action must be taken, the appropriate manager should do so immediately. However, the facility's formal written disciplinary procedures must be followed assiduously to ensure that the employees involved are treated fairly and lawfully. Most important, situations requiring disciplinary action should be regarded as teaching opportunities rather than as excuses to impose punishment.

As a form of discipline, corrective rather than punitive action is more appropriate for the work setting. With a corrective approach, acceptable behavior is encouraged based on known standards, policies, and procedures whereas unacceptable behavior is discouraged on the basis of its being inefficient, unfair, and/or potentially dangerous. Often employees respond reasonably to what should be the first—and hopefully the last—step in disciplinary action: a verbal reprimand. Actual penalties such as fines, suspensions, and dismissals should be rare events.

Although violations of procedure should be dealt with immediately, they should not be addressed hastily or in anger. Before taking action, the manager should thoroughly investigate the situation and determine whether the employee understood that he or she was violating a policy. If it becomes necessary to reprimand the employee, the manager should do so in private and with diplomacy. The disciplinary action should fit the seriousness of the offense, with the manager having considered fully the circumstance, implication, and effect of the infraction beforehand. An extreme example would be the difference between an employee observed serving him- or herself a meal from the patient tray line versus an employee discovered loading a box of steaks into a car. The employee who consumed food without paying for it would likely receive a verbal reprimand with an explanation of how his or her actions constitute theft. The employee who stole the steaks, on the other hand, would likely be dismissed.

The primary purpose of a disciplinary action is to prevent the violation from recurring. For repeat violations, most employers use a system of progressive discipline under which the penalty becomes more severe with each repeat violation.

The first step in disciplinary action should be a verbal reprimand. A second violation would incur a written reprimand to be placed in the employee's permanent personnel record for a predetermined time. With a third offense, a written warning delineating the potential consequences of future violations would be issued to the offending employee. If the problem is not resolved, the manager might issue another written warning to the effect that a subsequent violation will result in dismissal or demotion (the reassignment of an employee to a job with less responsibility and a lower pay scale). Although demotion is sometimes used as a disciplinary action, it has severe drawbacks. For one thing, the demoted employee could become a demoralizing element within the work force. Also, he or she might do damage to supplies or equipment or otherwise sabotage operations. Employee transfers to other work groups as a disciplinary action usually have the same effects.

With few exceptions, dismissal is appropriate only for the most serious or habitual offenses. For example, some personnel policies require the immediate suspension and possible dismissal of any employee who uses or sells illegal drugs anywhere on the worksite premises.

Whenever dismissal is the only solution to an ongoing personnel problem, such as repeat complaints from other employees or patients, the supervisor must follow the organization's procedures exactly to avoid potential liability consequences for the organization. Employee offenses must be thoroughly documented in writing, as must each step in the progressive chain of disciplinary action. This evidence must be recorded in the employee's permanent personnel record. The human resource department should be consulted prior to actual dismissal to make sure that all necessary documentation has been prepared.

No matter how severe or how minor the department's disciplinary problems, two principles must be borne in mind: consistency of enforcement and objectivity of approach. Every time a violation occurs, disciplinary action must be taken. Without relentless enforcement of policy and procedure in the workplace, employee morale and security can disintegrate, with employees eventually losing respect for their managers. Consistency, however, does not mean rigidity. Each case must be addressed individually and complete information gathered before action is taken.

As for objectivity of approach, disciplinary decisions must be fact based, not gossip or rumor based. That is, an employee must be given opportunity to present his or her side. As mentioned earlier, it cannot be assumed that an employee *knowingly* violated a policy or procedure. In remaining objective, a manager must exercise unbiased discretion in listening to the employee's side. As shown in the discussion on communication, objectivity is best maintained by separating the message from the messenger; that is, by suppressing personal bias in efforts to resolve a disciplinary problem.

Following Grievance Procedures

Employees have the right to register complaints and to have them considered with fairness and objectivity. A written procedure for conducting grievance hearings should be established whether employees are union members or not. However, under collective-bargaining agreements between employers and unions, grievance procedures are always made part of the labor contract. Usually, the union steward is responsible for helping union members prepare and present grievances to management. A sound and fair grievance procedure permits union and nonunion employees alike to express their complaints without fear of reprisal or job loss.

Steps in a grievance procedure may vary among organizations, but most follow a pattern. Again, it is vital that managers follow to the letter procedures dictated by organizational policy. In a *nonunionized* hospital, the procedure typically begins when an employee brings a complaint or employment-related problem to his or her immediate supervisor. Usually, the supervisor is able to settle the problem at this stage by either granting or denying the grievance. A written record of the decision and of any action taken should be kept in the employee's personnel record.

If the problem cannot be resolved by the supervisor's and employee's joint efforts and the supervisor denies the grievance, the employee can take it to the next level of management. In most cases, the employee's supervisor will have informed his or her own supervisor of the situation so that the grievance will come as no surprise to the next higher authority, usually a department director. If dissatisfied by the decision on this level, the employee may take the grievance higher up, eventually to the topmost authority—in most hospitals the chief executive officer (CEO). Meanwhile, the human resource director may have been consulted at any point for advice on solving the problem. In a nonunion setting, the CEO's decision is final.

In a *unionized* hospital, a grievance procedure follows similar steps except that a union steward or other union representative would assist the employee through all stages. A union business agent would participate in arriving at a final agreement on the solution if the problem was brought to top-level management. A matter that cannot be settled by the CEO and the union agent may be submitted for arbitration (discussed later in this chapter). *Conciliation,* the act of bringing in a person from outside the organization to reconcile opposing parties, is an alternative to arbitration. The conciliator would attempt to help the parties find a common ground for agreeing on a solution to the problem.

The grievance procedure is reviewed at regular intervals by the human resource department to make certain that it is progressing in a satisfactory manner. However, it should be the goal of every manager to handle as many employee grievances as possible within the department. To deal successfully with employee complaints, managers must listen carefully to the facts and deal calmly with the emotions involved. Anger and snap judgments must be avoided, despite pressure to make a decision immediately. The manager should communicate the reasoning behind his or her decision whether to take action on the employee's grievance. Responding to complaints fairly and quickly encourages employees to speak openly about department problems. Productivity and morale may be improved greatly as a result.

Conducting Exit Interviews

Employees leave jobs voluntarily for any number of reasons: to take new jobs for better pay or career advancement, to retire, or to relocate to other parts of the country, for example. Inevitably, some employees are dismissed because of poor job performance, chronic absenteeism, or other serious problems. In today's changing business climate, employee cutbacks and layoffs have also become common.

Many human resource departments routinely conduct *exit interviews* with employees shortly before they leave the organization. During an exit interview, the outgoing employee is advised of his or her right to continued medical and life insurance coverage or to receive vacation or severance pay. This is also an opportunity to discuss why the employee is leaving the organization, the quality of supervision and training received, the adequacy of advancement opportunities, benefits and incentives, and other related topics.

The information disclosed during exit interviews can be valuable to department managers, including human resource managers. For example, managers may learn where problems lie in their training programs and management skills. Or light may be shed on shortcomings in the compensation and benefits structure or in working conditions.

Reducing Employee Turnover

Whenever an employee leaves a job—either voluntarily or involuntarily—it costs the organization money, time, goodwill, and other resources. The more skilled the employee, the higher the replacement cost. The rate at which employees leave their jobs—called employee *turnover*—can be determined by using a simple formula. The rate of turnover equals the total number of separations per year divided by the average number of employees on the payroll and multiplied by 100. Or:

$$\text{Turnover rate } (\%) = \frac{\text{Number of separations per year}}{\text{Average number of payroll employees}} \times 100$$

For obvious economic reasons, it is to the organization's advantage to keep the turnover rate as low as possible. Furthermore, because high turnover endangers employee morale and reduces productivity, managers should try to identify the causes of high turnover and, when possible, take action to improve the conditions that led to the unacceptable levels. It is difficult to define which levels of turnover are acceptable and which are not: Turnover rates are affected by the geographic location of the organization as well as by the availability of other employment opportunities in the area. For example, an annual turnover rate of about 10 percent might be acceptable in a large urban area on the West Coast but would be considered unusually high in a rural community in the South.

High rates of turnover frequently are caused by errors in the employment process, specifically, hiring the wrong person for the job. Managers can help correct this situation by taking more time to analyze the employee qualities for specific jobs before screening, interviewing, and selecting employees. Other reasons for high turnover rates include the following:

- Poor employee orientation procedures
- Insufficient training of new employees
- Lack of retraining opportunities for current employees
- Poor supervision and management of employees
- Lack of consistency and objectivity in enforcing policies and procedures, which can lead to favoritism
- Failure to appreciate and recognize employee achievements

Reducing Absenteeism

High levels of employee absenteeism often are tied to the same factors that cause high turnover. Although employees miss work for any number of personal reasons (such as illness and family emergencies), unacceptable surges in absenteeism usually signal work-related problems such as poor working conditions (inefficient systems or outdated equipment), slumping morale (due to favoritism or lack of incentive, for example), and inadequate supervision (supervisor apathy or poor interpersonal skills). Thus, a manager who notices excessive absenteeism should first look within the environment for clues and then take steps to improve the situation. An employee attitude survey or a culture audit (described in chapter 4) would be a useful tool in this respect.

The rate of absenteeism can be determined by using another simple formula. The rate of absenteeism equals the number of workdays lost per pay period divided by the average number of employees multiplied by the number of days worked, and then multiplied by 100. Or:

$$\text{Absenteeism rate } (\%) = \frac{\text{Number of workdays lost per pay period}}{\text{Average number of employees} \times \text{number of days worked} \times 100}$$

Unusual levels of absenteeism among employees also may signal potentially serious personal problems that should be investigated. The most frequent reason given for missing work is illness, but illness may be an excuse to cover up serious chronic problems such as alcoholism, substance abuse, or debilitating physical or mental conditions. If a manager suspects that an employee's attendance and work performance are negatively affected by such problems, he or she should refer the employee to the organization's employee assistance program if one is available. (An *employee assistance program,* or EAP, is an occupational health service offered by an employer. Its purpose is to help workers solve or deal with personal problems that affect their work performance.)

The manager should never attempt to diagnose a suspected problem, openly accuse the employee, or give advice on sensitive subjects such as alcoholism or chemical dependency. If the organization has no EAP, the manager should strongly recommend that the employee seek qualified professional assistance to identify a possible problem.

☐ Compensation and Benefits Administration

The human resource department is responsible for establishing and maintaining an organization's compensation and benefits program. An equitable and competitive program is essential to the organization's ability to attract and retain competent and qualified employees. The compensation system is the mechanism by which the human resource department sets salary and wage rates for new employees, approves increases for current employees, maintains and updates wage and salary schedules and job classification schedules, authorizes position changes, and authorizes creation of new positions.

The employee benefits component of the compensation program includes a number of traditional "perks" as well as more innovative ones. Traditional benefits commonly include vacation and holiday pay, health insurance, life insurance, short-term and long-term disability insurance, and pension plans. More and more organizations are offering dental coverage (including orthodontics), vision coverage, profit sharing, and gain sharing. Limited coverage for holistic or alternative healing methods are not unheard of in some institutions.

Managers outside the human resource department play a role in compensation administration when they recommend salary or wage adjustments for individual employees, when they recommend changes in the pay scale for positions under their management, and when they recommend salaries or wages for new or newly promoted employees.

Role of the Human Resource Department in Compensation Administration

Compensation programs of all but the smallest health care organizations are directly administered by the human resource department. Typically, human resource managers develop and maintain programs through a series of ongoing activities, including the following:

- Formulating and regularly updating a job description for every position
- Evaluating each position and ranking it according to standard factors such as educational level required, degree of job responsibility, level of skill needed, number of employees supervised, amount of experience required, and so forth
- Assigning each position to a wage grade on the basis of the position's rank in comparison to all other positions in the institution
- Establishing a pay scale for each wage grade
- Conducting regular (usually annual) wage surveys of comparable employers in the same geographic area
- Using the results of wage surveys to adjust pay scales so that the organization remains competitive in its labor market
- Reviewing and approving the salary and wage adjustments recommended by managers on the basis of individual employee performance reviews
- Reviewing and approving the salary and wage adjustments recommended by managers for employees who have been promoted or assigned to newly created positions
- Reviewing and approving salaries or wages recommended by managers for new employees

- Taking part in negotiations to determine compensation agreements for unionized employees

Role of the Food Service Director in Compensation Administration

The food service director must work within the compensation program set up by the organization's human resource department. Although position pay scales within the department are determined by human resources or by a compensation committee, the food service director may suggest changes in pay scales when the responsibilities of individual positions are increased or decreased or when the director becomes aware that salaries or wages are no longer competitive.

The food service director determines the salaries or wages of individual food service workers, within the limits of the compensation system. Most positions are compensated by a range of pay. For example, the position of food service assistant might be assigned to job grade C, which has a pay scale that ranges from $4.90 per hour to $5.60 per hour. When a new food service assistant is hired, the director decides whether to pay the new employee at the bottom of the range, the middle, or the top. The new employee's starting wage is based on his or her level of experience or training. Therefore, a new employee with three years' experience as a food service assistant would be considered very well qualified and be offered a salary at least at the middle of the range for that position.

Performance evaluations have a direct influence on the pay increases awarded employees. Generally, the process of performance evaluation culminates in the reviewer's recommendation for a pay increase based on the employee's work performance. Here again, the food service director works within the limits of the overall compensation system. In many organizations, the human resource department determines a range of pay increases for current employees. This range is based on the organization's current level of profits (for-profit health care facilities) or current level of assets (not-for-profit facilities) and current economic conditions.

Most employers of nonunionized workers use a system of merit increases for rewarding employee performance as determined during the performance evaluation process. *Merit increases* are intended to reward some employees more than others on the basis of their overall productivity and quality of work. For example, employees who were rated by their supervisors as "outstanding" in all aspects of their work might receive a higher raise (merit increase) than employees who were rated as "acceptable."

The merit increase system is based on the idea that employees will work harder if they know they will be rewarded monetarily for their increased effort. However, as shown in chapter 2, many other factors play a role in worker motivation, and merit pay increases may or may not result in increased productivity. Effectiveness of the merit increase system is also affected by the fact that due to current economic conditions, health care providers have been forced to limit their compensation spending. As a result, the difference between consistently "outstanding" performance and "acceptable" performance might mean a differential of only one or two percentage points in merit increases. For the merit increase system to surely boost employee productivity, pay differences based on performance differences must be more than marginal. Unfortunately, many health care organizations no doubt will be unable to meet this demand in the foreseeable future.

Benefits Administration

As shown, monetary compensation is one element of the compensation package. Benefits are the other. A competitive benefits program is key to attracting and retaining qualified employees, but it has little effect on employee performance because the benefits offered are tied to employee status. In other words, all full-time employees are covered by the same benefits, but certain benefits (such as the amount of life insurance coverage) may be linked to salary level.

Large employers may offer a full range of benefits, whereas the benefits offered by small employers usually are more modest. Several kinds of benefits may make up a compensation package. One is pay for time not actually worked—vacations, sick leaves, paid holidays, and unemployment compensation. Insurance benefits, extremely important to most employees, include medical coverage for the employee and (sometimes) the employee's spouse and dependents; life insurance; disability insurance; dental insurance; and (sometimes) vision insurance. Retirement benefits may include a private pension plan administered by the employer. Social security is also considered a retirement benefit because employers make contributions to the fund on behalf of their employees. (Employees are required to make contributions as well.) Another kind of benefit is employee services such as employee credit unions and tuition reimbursement programs.

Benefits provision is costly for U.S. employers, estimated by authorities to equal more than one-third of the average employee's annual salary. Employee benefits have become a major expense during the past 15 years or so because of rising health insurance premiums, increased social security payments, and changes in the way pension plans are administered.

Because of the economic pressures in the health care industry, human resource departments are continually reviewing and revising benefits plans in terms of their cost, relevance, and value. As a result, the food service director is often called on to explain benefit changes to food service workers.

☐ Labor Relations

In 1974, health care employees became a class of workers covered by the federal laws that govern collective bargaining between unions and management in the private sector. (*Collective bargaining* is the activity engaged in when representatives of an employee's organization, association, or union and representatives of the employer's management negotiate wages, hours, and other conditions of employment. Prior to 1974, the collective-bargaining activities of health care workers were covered by state law. However, when health care came under federal jurisdiction by authority of the Health Care Amendments to the National Labor Relations Act (the Taft–Hartley Act) in 1974, union organization activities in hospitals increased significantly. Today, it is not uncommon for hospitals to have one or more bargaining units or even for the entire work force, except for supervisors and administrators, to be unionized.

The human resource department is responsible for interpreting and applying the provisions of a labor contract between the health care organization and the union. Problems with enforcing the contract or with the work of individual employees covered by the contract are handled according to a strict grievance procedure dictated by the terms of the contract. When grievances involving union employees cannot be settled within the organization, a special form of negotiation is required as set forth in the union contract. *Binding arbitration* is the process by which an impartial outside party is called in to settle a labor dispute. The *arbitrator* is an expert in labor law hired by the organization and the union to analyze the labor contract, listen to both sides of the issue, and make a decision on the validity of the grievance. The arbitrator's decision is *binding* in that both the organization and the union must abide by it. The system of binding arbitration prevents any kind of strike during the period covered by the labor contract.

☐ Summary

Human resource management deals with the organization's most important resource—its workers. Many aspects of human resource management are covered by federal, state, and local laws and regulations that are intended to protect the rights of employees and employers.

Human resource management involves the same management functions (organizing, planning, controlling, leading) and skills (technical, administrative, interpersonal, and the like) discussed in earlier chapters. The work of the organization's employees is *organized* through the use of job descriptions, which in turn are used as the basis for formulating the compensation program. Employee activities are *planned,* and the plans are carried out by qualified employees recruited and hired to do the work. Training also depends on planning for the human resource needs of specific activities within the organization. Employee performance and productivity are *controlled* through systematic performance evaluations. *Leadership* and communication skills are required in every aspect of recruiting, screening, interviewing, and hiring new employees. These skills are also required in handling personnel problems and in making valid employee evaluations based on performance merit. Productivity, leadership, and employee motivation are also required for effective human resource management.

☐ Bibliography

The Americans with Disabilities Act is here to stay. *FoodService Director* 5(8):10, Aug. 1992.

Americans with Disabilities Act of 1990: EEOC Technical Assistance Manual. Chicago: Commerce Clearing House, 1992.

Anderson, S. Subtle sexual harassment: what is your responsibility? *The Bottom Line* 7(5):18–23, Oct.–Nov. 1992.

Elliott, C., and Kaiser, G. How to stop sexual harassment. *Credit Union Management,* Apr. 1984.

Elliott, C., and Kaiser, G. Sexual harassment hurts productivity. *Modern Healthcare,* Sept. 1982.

Equal Employment Opportunity Commission. *Guidelines on Employee Selection Procedure.* Washington, DC: U.S. Government Printing Office, 1979.

Eubanks, P. Hospitals begin to implement worker drug-testing programs. *Hospitals* 66(20):38–41, Oct. 1992.

Feinberg, M. R. Sexual and ethnic harassment. *Restaurant Business,* June 1, 1981.

Haas, S. A. Coaching: developing key players. *Journal of Nursing Administration* 22(6):54–58, June 1992.

Hersey, P., and Blanchard, K. *Management of Organizational Behavior: Utilizing Human Resources.* 4th ed. Englewood Cliffs, NJ: Prentice-Hall, 1982.

Lundstrom, R. Prepare now for ADA's effects. *Healthcare Foodservice* 2(3):1, 11, Sept.–Oct. 1992.

Madri, J. R. Directing the interview. *Credit Union Management,* Mar. 1984.

Miller, M. F. *Detecting Training Needs: A Guide for Supervisors and Managers.* Washington, DC: U.S. Government Printing Office, 1983.

Mosley, D. C., Megginson, L. C., and Pietri, P. *Supervisory Management: The Art of Working with and through People.* Cincinnati: South-Western, 1985.

Mullineaux, J. Sexual harassment: what it is and what you should do about it. *Food Management* 27(8):56–63, Aug. 1992.

Owen, L. J., Rose, J. C., Wrase, D. J., and Revland, A. *Dietary Lesson Plans for Healthcare Facilities.* Rev. ed. Rochester, MN: Learning Resources, Rochester Methodist Hospital, 1981.

Pointer, D. D., and Metzger, N. *The National Labor Relations Act: A Guidebook for Health Care Facility Administration.* Chapters 7 and 8. New York City: Spectrum, 1975.

Puckett, R. P. *Dietary Manager's Independent Study Course.* Gainesville, FL: Department of Independent Study by Correspondence, University of Florida, 1985.

Puckett, R. P. Training: a how to do it. In: J. C. Rose, editor. *Handbook for Health Care Food Service Management.* Rockville, MD: Aspen, 1984.

Scholtes, P. R. *The Team Handbook.* Madison, WI: Joiner Associates, 1982.

Stokes, A. Avoid asking illegal questions during pre-employment interviews. *Food Service Marketing* 6(9):27–28, Sept. 1981.

Your rights under the family and medical leave act of 1993. *Federal Register* 58(106):31837–39, June 1993.

Nutrition Management

☐ Introduction

In 1983, significant changes in nutrition management began to occur when Medicare reimbursement to hospitals changed from a cost-based to a service-based structure. Under the new prospective payment system (PPS), payment rates to Medicare providers for most inpatient services are established in advance, with providers paid on the basis of these prospective rates regardless of the actual costs of service provision.

Along with PPS came an era of increased competition among health care providers. To survive in this new reimbursement environment, hospitals must scrutinize closely every department's level of clinical productivity and competence, including that of the nutrition and food service department. In addition to careful planning, monitoring, and evaluation of departmental productivity and competence, the department's quality assessment and control programs and its marketing efforts must be seen as essential components of the organization's success.

Environmental trends in health care affect the nutrition manager's role and responsibilities just as they affect those of other food service functions. With the continuing escalation of health care costs and demands for shorter lengths of stay, assessing and improving patients' nutrition status becomes even more crucial. Early nutrition intervention has been identified as a preferred preventive measure for high-risk populations such as women, children, and the elderly. For the elderly in particular—a population already shown to be on a growth curve—improvement in quality of life and minimization of the chronic need for health care is a decided priority. It is within this context of assessment and intervention that the role of nutrition specialists takes on added significance.

Shorter lengths of stay also will increase the number of individuals served by alternative health care delivery systems such as nutrition management. Despite this projection, the dietitian has yet to be "legitimized" by the federal government and other third-party payers as a necessary adjunct to the home health team. It is through the support of dietitians that the nutrition needs of home health patients can be assessed and a plan developed to eliminate or minimize patient readmissions. The dietitian plays a major role in long-term care facilities, in both the nutrition care of residents and the smooth operation of facilities' kitchens.

Another environmental trend discussed earlier in the book, one that affects the nutrition specialist, is the average consumer's heightened awareness of the nutrition–health ratio. Although selecting healthier foods over nutritionally inferior ones has not yet become a consistent routine, today's health care consumers are asking more questions and requesting more products to meet their nutrition needs.

This chapter will examine the dual role of the nutrition manager in health care operations: service manager and service provider. The first part of the chapter discusses management of nutrition services with an emphasis on requirements unique to the planning, organizing, leading, and controlling functions of management. The second segment presents information relevant to providing nutrition services to various customer types. These services include screening for nutrition risks, assessing nutrition status, developing a nutrition care plan (critical care paths, patient education, discharge planning), and documenting nutrition care.

☐ Managing Nutrition Services

The nutrition manager is responsible for managing human and other resources to accomplish the objective of delivering high-quality and cost-effective nutrition care. The nutrition manager's roles encompass the following activities and skills:

- Ensuring compliance with JCAHO and other regulatory bodies
- Maintaining open lines of effective oral and written communication
- Providing leadership as a liaison with medical, nursing, and allied health professionals
- Developing standards of care
- Developing long-range plans and implementing objectives
- Developing departmental policies and procedures
- Applying clinical nutrition training, knowledge, and expertise
- Overseeing staff development, evaluation, job descriptions, and counseling
- Keeping abreast of departmental productivity, budget, and other control measures
- Assisting in marketing of the organization's nutrition services
- Monitoring department operations such as patient tray system, food spoilage and inventory, vendor relations, menu planning, and so forth

Some responsibilities within each of the four management functions (planning, organizing, leading, and controlling) require unique application of skills. These responsibilities will be reviewed here in detail.

Planning

As already shown, a manager must develop departmental goals and objectives that are consistent with those of the larger organization. Planning affords assessment of future needs of the organization's patient mix and determination of changes needed in staffing and services. Nutrition care planning assesses the current patient care process and the need for changes based on the evolving standards of practice for the community. Adapting to change includes modifying policies and procedures and standards of nutrition care.

Planning efforts include investigating and developing new business opportunities to enhance the distribution of nutrition information and to increase the department's revenue flow. Responding to changes in the patient mix may necessitate dietitians relocating to an outpatient setting, implementing educational classes for the elderly, or meeting the community's need for better nutrition education by conducting grocery store tours. (Review chapter 5 for details of the planning function related to writing policies and procedures and developing business plans for new business opportunities.)

Policies and Procedures

Policies and procedures and standards of care must be maintained to provide effective nutrition services to customers. Policies and procedures should cover at least the following areas:

- Nutrition screening including priority ratings
- Nutrition assessment

- Nutrition care plans
- Documentation protocols
- Instruction and counseling
- Education (specific for each type of class offered)
- Specialized nutrition support (such as enteral and parenteral nutrition)
- Discharge planning and referral
- Intervention for patients NPO (nothing by mouth) or on clear liquids for extended periods
- Standards of nutrition care
- Nourishments and between-meal supplemental feedings
- Education for drug–nutrient interactions
- Requirements and protocol for student rotations
- Approved diet manual
- Outpatient education
- Nutrition analysis of patient or resident menus
- Community education programs
- Performing calorie counts

Policies and procedures should be updated as needed (at least annually). Usually, the policies and procedures related to nutrition care will require medical staff approval, as will the diet manual used by the facility. The approved diet manual must be made available on all patient units as a reference for physicians and nursing and other medical personnel.

Policies and procedures that describe responsibilities for interdisciplinary roles should be approved by the affected department. For example, because the policy related to drug–nutrient interactions involves both the pharmacy and nursing services, these departments should be involved in the development and approval process for this policy. In addition, each department will need to provide copies of the policies to its staff.

Marketing and Program Development

Today's hospitals face the challenge of maintaining the quality of care provided to patients while simultaneously striving to deliver cost-effective, patient-centered care. Prospective pricing has been adopted by other third-party payers, such as state-administered Medicaid programs and private insurers. Overall, prospective pricing rewards hospitals that reduce their costs.

Patient-focused health care organizations conduct market research to identify customer preferences. As a result of these efforts to identify consumer wants and needs, many institutions have added the following departments: public relations, planning and development, and marketing. Health care providers continue to identify new markets for the services they offer and to propose new services for larger or redefined consumer groups. For example, many hospitals have initiated programs specifically designed to meet women's health care needs.

To accommodate the needs of a unique marketing niche, dietitians and food service directors can offer personal expertise as well as actual nutrition and food services. Planning, then, as a key to program development and marketing, can help boost wellness or health promotion as one area that lends itself to nutrition program development and marketing. Nutrition services are an integral part of these programs, which generally involve screening, education, and specific interventions if the screening identifies a need. Many chronic diseases have been attributed to controllable life-style patterns or habits.

New areas that the nutrition manager may need to include in planning include skilled nursing and rehabilitation units within the hospital, especially beneficial to the patient and the institutions with Medicare reimbursement guidelines. The patient is able to stay in the same facility and continue to receive care from the same individuals. At the same time, the facility can maximize reimbursement for the patient's length of stay because patients who meet the parameters for long-term or rehabilitation care are granted a longer length of stay and higher reimbursement levels under Medicare.

Other areas in the nutrition and food service department could be developed into new programs and services to be offered inside and outside the hospital. Examples include:

- Inpatient gourmet meal service
- On-site bakeries for patients, visitors, and staff
- Room service for inpatients and visitors
- Storefront nutrition assessment facilities
- Outpatient weight reduction programs
- Nutrition education publications and programs

Changes in health care will continue, not only in the ways in which care is provided, but also in the ways services are marketed to consumers. Patient-centered, cost-effective care will remain a driving force. Thus, services must be designed around the opinions and perceptions of patients, medical staff, and public.

Nutrition and food service departments must determine strategies to promote patient satisfaction and enhance the reputation of the facility and the department. Improving hospitality services, providing patients what they want to eat when they want to eat it, and offering good basic nutrition information should promote a facility's favorable public image. Upon discharge, patients tell their families and friends about the quality of food and service they received while hospitalized. In some cases, these word-of-mouth reports influence the choices of potential patients.

All nutrition and food service employees are responsible for providing and promoting appropriate quality of care for the patient. This can be accomplished best when all employees work toward a common mission and goal. The nutrition manager is responsible for marketing nutrition services to patients, physicians, other health care providers, and administrators of their facilities. (Refer to chapter 3 for ways in which the nutrition manager can incorporate marketing into the department's planning functions.)

Organizing and Staffing

Organization and staffing functions include creating the structure needed to provide nutrition services and recruiting, retaining, and developing the staff necessary to implement these services. Staffing of the nutrition management unit of the food service department mandates hiring clinically competent people who can be trained to provide high-quality patient care.

Depending on the size and organizational structure of the institution, the nutrition staff may include all of the staff members shown in figure 9-1 or only registered dietitians and nutrition assistants. For example, in a small health care institution, patient nutrition services might be managed by a registered dietitian, with nutrition assistants and aides processing diet changes or serving meal trays.

In a major organization such as the one illustrated in figure 9-1, several levels of employees might fulfill specific duties in the nutrition care of patients. The nutrition team might include registered dietitians, dietetic technicians, nutrition managers, nutrition hosts and hostesses, and nutrition assistants and aides. (In many institutions, nutrition assistants and aides are called clerks. Their functions are basically the same even though the job titles are different.) Each team member has specific responsibilities in the patient's care, but responsibilities merge to serve all of the patient's needs as delineated in table 9-1.

Role Responsibilities

The *nutrition manager* monitors day-to-day nutrition care activities and usually supervises patient nutrition hosts/hostesses, assistants, and aides. In large organizations the nutrition manager usually is a registered dietitian. In the smaller or extended care facilities, this person may be a dietetic technician with management skills or a certified dietary manager (CDM). Many facilities are adopting a flatter organizational structure, requiring the nutrition manager to assume additional management responsibilities. This is especially true in medium-size facilities where the manager may be responsible for patient service and nutrition management. (See figure 9-2.)

The *registered dietitian* (RD) functions as the team leader and is responsible for developing nutrition care plans, performing nutrition assessments, counseling patients, formulating educational materials, and performing research. Dietitians often function either as a nutrition specialist

Figure 9-1. Clinical Nutrition Staff for a Major Medical Center

Table 9-1. Nutrition Management Team

Title	Qualifications[a]	Responsibilities
Nutrition manager	Registered dietitian, registered dietetic technician, or certified dietary manager	Plans, organizes, staffs, directs day-to-day nutrition care, supervises, and provides leadership
Dietitian	Registered dietitian and/or state licensed if applicable	Team leader, nutrition care plans, assessments, counseling, education, research
Dietetic technician	Registered dietetic technician or nonregistered equivalent with a degree in nutrition	Patient screening, counseling, menu editing, education
Nutrition assistants, aides, or clerks	High school diploma or equivalent	Process patient menus, diet order changes, nourishment orders, late tray requests
Nutrition host or hostess	High school diploma or equivalent	Serves trays and nourishments, assists with menu selection, stock units

[a]Qualifications will vary depending on size of facility.

Figure 9-2. Organizational Chart—Medium-Size Facility

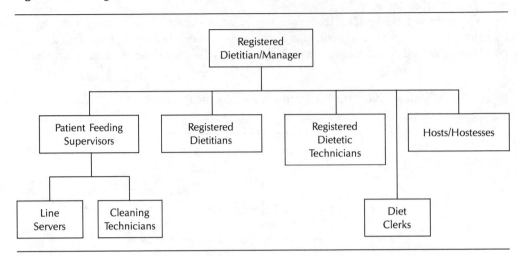

or as an administrative or management specialist. Whether the dietitian selects nutrition or management as an area of focus, he or she may be employed in hospitals, extended care facilities, fitness centers, outpatient clinics, weight management clinics, home health care, food and nutrition product or equipment sales, or with food service management companies. The dietitian who selects health care as an area of employment must have management abilities, whether his or her focus is in the nutrition or administrative area. To provide effective quality nutrition services, dietitians must network and work with colleagues in the community. Employment in health care nutrition may be full-time, part-time, or on a consultant basis.

The *dietetic technician* works with the dietitian to provide nutrition care services to patients. The registered dietetic technician (DTR) is technically skilled in nutrition care and has an associate's degree from a program approved by The American Dietetic Association (ADA). In addition, the dietetic technician must pass a registration examination administered by the Commission on Dietetic Registration. The DTR is often responsible for conducting nutrition screening, menu editing, planning between-meal feedings, and nutrition counseling. The role of the DTR varies significantly depending on the size of the organization. In smaller facilities, the DTR may have supervisory responsibilities, in addition to the nutrition care of patients.

Patient nutrition assistants and aides process patient menus, diet order changes, nourishment orders, and late tray requests. In some facilities, especially with decentralized meal service, these positions may assume the roles outlined for the nutrition host or hostess. In other facilities, they may assume duties strictly within the department and are referred to as diet clerks.

The *nutrition host or hostess* serves trays and nourishments to patients and may be involved in some food preparation. He or she also answers simple questions about the menu and the services the food service department offers. Nutrition hosts and hostesses work directly with the nursing staff.

Both nutrition assistants and hosts may have completed an approved dietary manager's course or simply be high school (or equivalent) graduates. These individuals are generally supervised by the nutrition manager in institutions that employ a large nutrition staff or by the director in institutions with small nutrition staffs.

All members of the nutrition team have an influence on, and a responsibility to, the patient. They need to know and practice good guest-relations skills, which include being friendly and polite to patients and greeting them by name. Members of the team need to be knowledgeable enough to answer questions about the hospital, provide guidance as needed, and promote a positive impression of the facility.

At all times, the team must protect the patient's right to confidentiality. Confidentiality should be stressed in training programs for team members, and the policy should be reviewed at least annually. Some organizations are requiring staff to sign confidentiality statements.

The nutrition staff interacts with many other health care providers in the hospital, including physicians, nurses, unit secretaries, pharmacists, therapists, and medical records personnel. Registered dietitians (or, in some institutions, skilled and experienced dietetic technicians) may be asked to communicate individual nutrition histories and care plans at patient care conferences, on rounds, during family conferences, and in other situations.

Nutrition managers also may be involved in outpatient and community services. Outpatient services will continue to grow in importance with decreased lengths of stay and the increased number of patients seen in outpatient clinics. There are many advantages to instructing patients in an outpatient setting. The dietitian is notified of the need for an instruction in adequate time to provide the patient and/or family members with the details needed for success. Early discharge may result in the patient not being emotionally prepared to accept drastic changes in his or her life-style as it relates to food. The registered dietitian can provide more relaxed and informative diet instruction if the patient can be scheduled to return at a later date.

Patient-Centered Care

In the past several years, special interest has been placed on developing patient-centered care units to replace traditional nursing units. The principle behind such units is to centralize staff to the units, thus minimizing the number of caregivers who interact with the patient. This allows the caregivers to provide a better continuation of care and increases the patient's comfort level. The patient and family become familiar with caregivers and can expect to see them on a daily basis.

Patient-centered care units have implications for nutrition care and food service delivery. Duties typically provided by the dietetic technician, or hostess, may be assumed by unit staff. For example, a patient care assistant may be responsible for conducting nutrition screening. A support person assigned specifically to the unit may assume the responsibilities of passing trays, assisting with menu selection, producing and delivering between-meal feedings, and preparing late trays. The nutrition manager will have to consider the number of duties to be assumed by these personnel and adjust staff accordingly. He or she also will have to assist with monitoring the activities of these persons to ensure that the patient receives the appropriate level of care.

Leading

Providing leadership to the nutrition staff is a central function in that the nutrition manager must direct the staff to goal accomplishment (as discussed in chapter 2). As always, interpersonal skills and technical expertise are critical.

A high level of trust in the manager is necessary for managers to create a vision that leads the nutrition staff to goal accomplishment. Trust in the leader's knowledge is especially important among professional staff whose members need less direction on a daily basis and may prefer to work in self-directed teams. However, the need for less direction does not imply that structure and control mechanisms are not necessary. Providing structure allows the manager to spend less time on direct supervision and more time on the important function of planning and organizing for the future.

In many health care facilities, the nutrition manager's leadership responsibilities also include serving as a mentor and providing direction for students. Student education programs may include internships for dietitians or practical experience in conjunction with programs for dietitians and/or dietetic technicians. The nutrition manager and the facility both benefit from providing direction and leadership to students. While in the facility, these individuals can assist with the nutrition care of patients and serve as a resource for future recruiting efforts.

In larger institutions, the nutrition manager may be involved with research within the facility. This may include supervision of the dietitians involved in coordinating and directing a specific research project.

As always, providing leadership means communicating effectively as outlined in chapter 7. The nutrition manager plays a significant role in establishing interdepartmental relationships among the medical staff, nursing services, and the pharmacy, for example. Many of the policies and procedures related to the nutrition care of the patient require cooperation and input from these various departments.

Controlling

Responsibilities assigned the nutrition manager (evaluation and control, for example) ensure that standards, policies and procedures, and budgets are followed as delineated by the leadership function. Control mechanisms provide structure for evaluation and monitoring to assess performance.

In that fiscal responsibilities continue as an overriding concern of food service managers, the nutrition manager must create and monitor the department's budget and establish standards for monitoring staff productivity. The nutrition manager can improve the fiscal situation by creating and marketing new programs that will provide revenue as discussed in the planning section. Information on determining needs and monitoring other financial indicators are presented in chapter 11.

Another controlling function of the nutrition manager includes quality improvement and assessment, that is, responsibility for ensuring that the standards of care and policies and procedures related to patient care are followed as outlined. These standards are reviewed in chapter 4.

Measuring Productivity of the Nutrition Staff

Cost containment in nutrition management is focused on the best utilization of the professional staff, as assessed here by the productivity of the nutrition staff. Three aspects must be considered in the productivity review: determination of the time spent to provide services, assessment of whether the skill level of the dietitian is appropriately utilized, and establishment of the benefit or outcome of nutrition intervention.

First, the *amount of time spent on each task* performed by the RD and DTR should be carefully determined. This is best accomplished by asking the professional to keep accurate records of the patients he or she sees, the amount of time spent, and the type of activity completed. This can be facilitated by creating a department-specific form with the most common tasks listed or by using one of the many accepted forms created by the ADA or other professional organizations. Both the *Handbook for Clinical Nutrition Services Management* by Schiller, Gilbride, and O'Sullivan and resources available through ADA can be used for this purpose. This type of record allows the manager to assess the time spent on various tasks as a portion of the whole, as illustrated in figure 9-3.

The second consideration in establishing cost-effective nutrition services is to ensure that the job responsibility is matched to the appropriate skill level of individuals on the team. For example, the dietitian should perform more complex nutrition intervention activities while dietetic technicians are available to conduct assessments and diet instructions. The dietitian and dietetic technician need not be utilized to perform the initial screening of patients for existing or potential nutritional risk. This task is easily performed by a nutrition assistant or hostess with a carefully designed screening protocol.

The third aspect the nutrition manager should consider when assessing the cost efficiency of staff utilization is determining the benefits associated with the nutrition intervention offered. Quality assessment must be accomplished to determine whether patient outcome is improved by providing the service. Cost–benefit analysis is a method commonly used to assess whether the benefit of a particular product or program is greater than the cost of providing it. Although this technique works effectively for services with a direct charge attached, it is less effective in evaluating nutrition-related programs.

Figure 9-3. Proportion of Registered Dietitian's Time Spent on Various Tasks

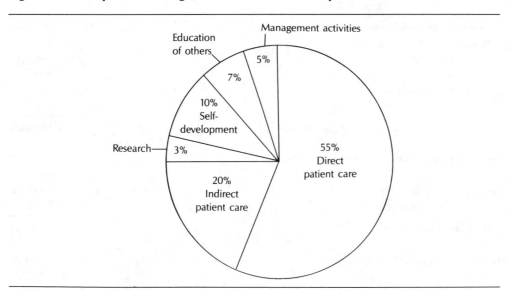

Nutrition intervention should provide a positive outcome for the patient and improve the quality of life. Many nutrition intervention programs, especially future programs, will be designed to prevent long-term illnesses and to keep individuals from using the health care system unnecessarily. To measure the benefit of these types of programs, a cost-effective analysis (CEA) will be needed. Conducting a CEA also identifies the cost of the service or program in monetary terms. The benefits, such as decreased length of stay or improved quality of life, are identified as outcomes for the patient and the organization.

Designing a Nutrition Services Payment System

Services that could be provided for a fee by the nutrition and food service department include computerized nutrient analysis, computerized menu planning, inpatient and outpatient nutrition counseling, weight reduction counseling, and other specialized nutrition programs. However, before these services are developed for distribution, a market analysis must be completed to determine whether the customer is willing to pay for them. Before the nutrition manager can initiate a charge directly for nutrition services, he or she will need to determine how dietitians spend their time and the dollar value of their services. The costs involved in providing the services and the price to be charged for them can then be determined realistically. All costs involved in providing the service must be included in determining total cost per unit of service. In that a portion of all bills will be uncollectible even though the service has been provided, a provision for bad debts must be included in the overall cost. An example of such a cost calculation is illustrated in figure 9-4.

Maximizing Reimbursement for Services

Nutrition services payment systems must be created with a clear vision of health care reform and the future direction for reimbursement. Currently, reimbursement systems work in one of two ways. With the fee-for-service model, the payer controls the price for the service and determines which services are necessary for the covered individual. The second model is used by Medicare PPSs and health maintenance organizations (HMOs). These managed care organizations provide capitated payments for the care of the covered individual and do not determine what services should be included in the bundled care.

The existing methods used to determine fees for nutrition services are based on the fee-for-service model. Increasingly, however, fee for service is being replaced by managed care.

Figure 9-4. Cost Calculation for the Services of a Registered Dietitian

Total Number of Work Hours per Year[a]	2,080 hours
Less: vacation time (10 days)	(80)
holidays (8 days)	(64)
sick leave (8 days)	(64)
education leave (8 days)	(64)
nonproductive time[b]	(312)
Actual Number of Work Hours Available per Year	1,496 hours
Approximate Number of Units of Service per Year[c]	600
Average Yearly Salary	$22,500
Plus: fringe benefits[d]	5,625
Total Yearly Compensation	$28,125
Salary per Hour ($28,125 ÷ 1,496)	$18.80
Labor Cost per Unit of Service (2.5 hours × $18.80)	$47.00
Yearly Indirect Costs[e]	$18,000
Indirect Cost per Unit of Service ($18,000 ÷ 600)	$30.00
Labor Cost per Unit of Service	$47.00
Indirect Cost per Unit of Service	30.00
Profit (12 percent of labor and indirect costs)	9.24
Total Cost per Unit of Service	$86.24

[a]The number of work hours per year is based on a 40-hour workweek.

[b]Nonproductive time accounts for approximately 15 percent of the total work hours and includes coffee breaks, time spent waiting, and so forth.

[c]The standard amount of time allowed per patient referral, or unit of service (as determined by work analysis; includes evaluating the order, securing counseling materials, and performing counseling, charting, etc.), is 2.5 hours. 1,496 hours ÷ 2.5 = 598, or for the sake of computation 600 units of service per year.

[d]Fringe benefits are assumed to equal 25 percent of the average salary and include insurance benefits, social security payments made by the employer, and so forth.

[e]Indirect costs include expenses for telephone service, postage, copying service, general overhead, allowances for uncollectibles, and administrative expenses.

Source: Based on J. C. Rose. Hospital Food and Nutrition Focus 2(3), Nov. 1985.

Because of this trend and the known positive effect of nutrition care on patient outcome, identifying nutrition intervention as a quality-of-care issue is appropriate.

Using cost-effectiveness analysis, the nutrition manager must prove that nutrition intervention, rather than being an add-on cost, can replace more costly interventions and provide a positive outcome to the patient. With the cost of health care continuing to rise, it is not likely that managed care providers will indiscriminately pay for nutrition services. The positive benefits must be well documented. However, on the opposite end of the spectrum, if adequate nutrition is not occurring, the provider in question will have difficulties with regulatory issues. The American Dietetic Association continues to support efforts to establish the appropriate role of nutrition intervention in treatment and prevention of disease as it relates to health care reform.

☐ Providing Nutrition Services

The goal of the nutrition team is to fulfill the nutrition needs of the patient or client. The nutrition services offered in health care institutions generally include screening for nutrition risk, assessment of nutrition status, development of a nutrition care plan, discharge planning, nutrition counseling, and evaluation of adequacy of and adherence to each patient's diet order. Nutrition services are the responsibility of registered dietitians, registered dietetic technicians, and other nutrition care workers within the department. Malnutrition in hospitals continues to receive attention from both the community and physicians and other medical professionals. In their role as nutrition experts, clinical dietitians play an important part in solving malnutrition and other nutrition-related problems and in providing cost-effective nutrition services. Related activities include:

- Working in partnership with the nutrition support team to provide total parenteral nutrition (TPN) or enteral feedings to patients who are at high nutrition risk (such as burn and protein- or calorie-deficient patients)
- Identifying malnutrition, which is considered a secondary diagnosis or a comorbidity or comortality factor
- Identifying patients who frequently return to the hospital because of disease complications
- Investigating average length of stay for the 10 most frequently admitted DRGs and determining whether nutrition intervention might be beneficial in decreasing average length of stay

Nutrition service professionals can contribute to department visibility in a number of ways. For example:

- Becoming nutrition experts
- Implementing programs to encourage public acceptance of the need for nutrition services
- Providing educational programs in the community and for the hospital staff
- Integrating health and fitness with wholesome food and education in community outreach programs
- Providing quality services to the aging population through home care
- Seeking physician referrals for nutrition analysis and counseling
- Using computerized information systems to perform nutrition analyses for patients, thereby enhancing the quality of nutrition services
- Developing contractual agreements for providing services to extended care facilities, halfway houses, day care centers, correctional institutions, and other organizations outside the hospital

Some of these service applications are briefly described in the following subsections.

Nutrition Risk Screening

The first step in establishing nutritional needs is to develop and administer a screening protocol for all patients or residents entering the facility. Screening protocols should outline parameters to be evaluated for diagnosing any existing or potential nutrition risk. A first-level screen may simply be review by age, diagnosis, and type of diet (parameters will vary from one facility to another). Some general screening guidelines are included in figure 9-5.

A more in-depth screen would include patient height, weight, recent unintentional weight loss, percent of usual body weight, percent of ideal body weight, and albumin level. During the second-level screening, usually conducted by the dietetic technician, questions on intake, digestion, or elimination problems may be asked. If the patient is on a special diet, the DTR should ensure that the patient has been instructed on the diet. General guidelines for a secondary screen are outlined in figure 9-6. Composite nutrition screening information may be recorded on a form similar to the one in figure 9-7 (p. 218) and kept in the nutrition department for reference during the patient's stay.

Figure 9-5. Form Used in Initial Screening for Nutrition Risk

All patients screened within 36 hours of admission

A. All diagnoses
B. Diet prescriptions
C. Age

Refer to RD for
Secondary Screening

Diagnoses

- Cachexia
- Cardiomyopathy
- End stage cardiac disease
- Eating disorders:
  - Compulsive overeaters
  - Anorexics
  - Bulimics
- Malnutrition, PCM
- Marasmus, Kwashiorkor
- Weight loss
- Malabsorption

Diet

- Enteral
- Parenteral
- NPO past 7 days

Other

- Rehab (2NA)
- CCA

Refer to Tech for
Secondary Screening[a]

Diagnoses

- Aides
- Bowel obstruction
- Burns (2nd and 3rd degree)
- Post-CABG
- Cancer
- CVA, intracranial bleed
- COPD, bronchitis, emphysema, respiratory distress
- CHF
- Crohn's disease
- Dehydration
- DKA, diabetes
- Fever of unknown origin
- Fistulas
- Hyperemesis
- Ileitis
- Liver disease
- Pancreatitis
- Pneumonia
- Post-gastrectomy
- Sepsis
- Short bowel syndrome
- Sternal wound infection
- Trauma
- Ulcerative colitis

Diet Prescriptions

All patients on modified diets except: general, soft, NAS, mechanical soft, high fiber, fractured jaw, full and clear liquids, or any combination of above.

Age

< 18 years
> 75 years

[a]Patients not referred for secondary nutritional screening are rescreened within 7–10 days.
Source: Reprinted with permission of All Saints Health System, Fort Worth, TX.

Figure 9-6. Form Used in Secondary Nutrition Screening

Completed within 72 hours of admission

---

1. Anthropometrics: height, weight, weight history
2. Factors affecting po intake: appetite, chewing or swallowing problems, food allergies or intolerances
3. Gastrointestinal complaints: nausea, vomiting, diarrhea, constipation
4. Discussion of modified diet prior to admission, if any
5. Provision of between-meal nourishments, diet consistency modifications, and discussion of additional menu options as needed
6. Obtain food preferences on diabetic and low-protein diets, and as necessary on others

---

Refer to RD

Unresolved eating problems—reevaluation by tech within 72 hours

---

Unintentional weight loss:
> 5% UBW in 1 month
< 7.5% UBW in 3 months
Serum Albumin < 3.0 mg/dl
Patients on TPN/EN
Patients who request or require the clinical dietitian's expertise in education/assistance with a modified diet

---

1. Poor appetite for one month prior PTA, unresolved
2. Poor appetite since admission, unresolved
3. Initiation of TPN/EN
4. Patients who request or require clinical dietitian's expertise in education/assistance with modified diet
5. Two or more of the following: chewing, swallowing, nausea, vomiting, diarrhea, constipation

---

Refer to clinical dietitian for nutrition assessment

Dietetic technician to follow as indicated

Source: Reprinted with permission of All Saints Health System, Fort Worth, TX.

Nutrition Status Assessment

In most health care facilities, physicians work with a dietitian, a dietetic technician, or a nurse to provide nutrition care for their patients. However, basic nutrition services are provided as standard protocol and do not require a physician's order (for example, screening patients for nutrition risk, providing assessment, and implementing between-meal feedings).

Nutrition assessment should not be performed only when there is an obvious problem. Patients or residents determined to be at nutrition risk through screening should be assessed by the registered dietitian or registered dietetic technician. The purpose of the assessment is to evaluate the patient's current nutrition status.

The procedure for nutrition assessment varies depending on the availability of staff and the needs of the patient or resident. The evaluation may be relatively simple for a patient in apparent overall good health. A more thorough assessment should be carried out for patients who have chronic debilitating medical problems, acute illnesses, or injuries that increase their nutrition needs or hinder their food intake.

The parameters reviewed will depend on the standard of care specific to the diagnosis. Generally, a nutrition status assessment involves evaluating adequacy of the patient's nutrition on the basis of food intake records, assessing relevant physical measurements, and analyzing laboratory test results. Information obtained from the patient or a family member may include:

- Patient's past and present eating habits
- Patient's food intolerances, if any
- Patient's lifestyle (including physical, psychological, socioeconomic, psychosocial, and religious background)
- Any handicapping conditions that might affect the patient's food intake and mobility (energy needs)
- Patient's weight history and current height and weight

Figure 9-7. Composite Nutrition Screening Form

Name: _____   Date/Time: _____

Room: _____ Age: _____ Sex: _____   Height: _____ Weight: _____

Medical Record #: _____   UBW: _____ IBW: _____ % IBW: _____

Diagnosis: _____   % Weight Change: _____ /_____

Current Diet: _____   Serum Albumin: _____ g/dl   (_____)
                                                                                          date

Has patient experienced any of the following?	Yes	No
• Recent unintentional weight loss (specify) _____		
• Poor appetite (specify) _____		
• Difficulty chewing and/or swallowing _____		
• Persistent nausea and/or vomiting _____		
• Diarrhea or constipation _____		
• Any food allergies/intolerances _____		
• Are you familiar with your present diet _____		

Comments: _____

_____

Plan of Action:

_____ Refer to dietitian

_____ Dietetic technician to follow as indicated. Will follow up for resolution of above-stated nutrition problems within 72 hours.

_____ Screening parameters are within normal limits and do not warrant nutritional intervention at this time. Will reevaluate within 10 days.

_____

_____

_____

_____

_____   _____
        (signature)   (date)

Source: Reprinted with permission of All Saints Health System, Fort Worth, TX.

Some of this information may be available from the medical record. The information gathered should be summarized, evaluated, and then recorded in the patient's medical chart.

Nutrition information should be evaluated to identify poor nutrient intake or significant weight loss or gain. If the patient's nutrient intake seems inadequate or the relationship between weight and height is not within normal limits, further assessment should be done. A comprehensive physical examination should include checking the patient's eyes, mucous membranes, hair, and skin for obvious signs of malnutrition. Table 9-2 lists malnutrition indicators.

Laboratory analysis may be necessary to determine serum or blood levels of various nutrients, and the reason for any abnormal values should be identified. Abnormal laboratory values that correlate with poor intake of a particular nutrient warrant changes in food intake. For example, if the serum protein or serum albumin level is low and the patient's dietary intake

Table 9-2. Physical Signs Indicative of Malnutrition

Body Area	Normal Appearance	Signs Associated with Malnutrition
Hair	Shiny; firm; not easily plucked	Lack of natural shine, dull and dry; thin and sparse; fine, silky, and straight; color changes (flag sign); easily plucked
Face	Skin color uniform; smooth, pink, healthy appearance; not swollen	Skin color loss (depigmentation); skin dark over cheeks and under eyes (malar and supraorbital pigmentation); lumpiness or flakiness of skin of nose and mouth; swollen face; enlarged parotid glands; scaling of skin around nostrils (nasolabial seborrhea)
Eyes	Bright, clear, shiny; no sores at corners of eyelids; membranes healthy pink and moist; no prominent blood vessels or mound of tissue or sclera	Pale eye membranes (pale conjunctivae); redness of membranes (conjunctival infection); Bitot's spots; redness and fissuring of eyelid corners (angular palpebritis); dryness of eye membranes (conjunctival xerosis); dull appearance of cornea (corneal xerosis); soft cornea (keratomalacia); scar on cornea; ring of fine blood vessels around cornea (circumcorneal injection)
Lips	Smooth, not chapped or swollen	Redness and swelling of mouth or lips (cheilosis), especially at corners of mouth (angular fissures and scars)
Tongue	Deep red in appearance, not swollen or smooth	Swelling; scarlet and raw tongue; magenta (purplish color) tongue; smooth tongue; swollen sores; hyperemic and hypertrophic papillae; and atrophic papillae
Teeth	No cavities, no pain, bright	Missing or erupting abnormally; gray or black spots (fluorosis); cavities (caries)
Gums	Healthy, red, not bleeding, not swollen	Spongy and bleed easily; recession of gums
Glands	Face not swollen	Thyroid enlargement (front of neck); parotid enlargement (cheeks become swollen)
Skin	No signs of rashes, swellings, dark or light spots	Dryness of skin (xerosis); sandpaper feel of skin (follicular hyperkeratosis); flakiness of skin; skin swollen and dark; red swollen pigmentation of exposed areas (pellagrous dermatosis); excessive lightness or darkness of skin (dyspigmentation); black and blue marks due to skin bleeding (petechiae); lack of fat under skin
Nails	Firm, pink	Spoon-shaped nails (koilonychia); brittle, ridged nails
Muscular and skeletal systems	Good muscle tone, some fat under skin, ability to walk or run without pain	Wasted appearance of muscles; baby's skull bones thin and soft (craniotabes); round swelling of front and side of head (frontal and parietal bossing); swelling of ends of bones (epiphyseal enlargement); small bumps on both sides of chest wall (on ribs); beading of ribs; baby's soft spot on head not hardened at proper time (persistently open anterior fontanelle); knock-knees or bowlegs; bleeding into muscle (musculoskeletal hemorrhages); inability to get up or walk properly
Cardio-vascular system	Normal heart rate and rhythm, no murmurs or abnormal rhythms, normal blood pressure for age	Rapid heart rate (above 100 tachycardia); enlarged heart; abnormal rhythm; elevated blood pressure
Gastro-intestinal system	No palpable organs or masses (in children, however, liver edge may be palpable)	Liver enlargement; enlargement of spleen (usually indicates other associated diseases)
Nervous system	Psychological stability, normal reflexes	Mental irritability and confusion; burning and tingling of hands and feet (paresthesia); loss of position and vibratory sense; weakness and tenderness of muscles (may result in inability to walk); decrease and loss of ankle and knee reflexes

Source: Adapted from G. Christakis, editor. Nutritional assessment in health programs. *American Journal of Public Health* 63(11), 1973 (supp.).

of protein is low, increasing protein intake might be advisable, along with adding high-protein supplements. Nutrition status should be reevaluated at appropriate intervals according to the patient's medical condition.

In extended care facilities such as nursing homes, residents' food intake patterns can be changed gradually and low intake can be overlooked. These patients' food intake should be noted daily and their weight should be monitored regularly. Laboratory tests should be done whenever there is significant change in the patient's food intake or weight. An assessment should be completed by a consulting dietitian and a care plan developed for the certified dietary manager or other staff members to follow. These care plans should be updated with each visit from the dietitian and the dietitian notified should significant changes occur between visits.

Assessments of patients on hospital skilled nursing units and rehabilitation units generally are more time-consuming for the dietitian. Frequently, these patients have more eating, swallowing, digestion, and elimination difficulties than other patients. Regulations provide specific guidelines for conducting team conferences and patient–family conferences. Guidelines also specify the type and frequency of assessments and documentation of care plans expected. The dietitian attends family conferences with other health care professionals. Generally, team conferences are held once a week and the dietitian must be present to provide input and to update the patient's overall care plan.

The Nutrition Care Plan

When nutrition assessment indicates that a patient is at risk, a nutrition care plan should outline what nutrition care is needed and how it is to be provided. Results of the nutrition assessment and the nutrition care plan should be charted in the patient's medical record and communicated to the physician. Although the physician will use the medical record, it may be necessary to place a sticker on the record to call the physician's attention to the nutrition note. The medical record then serves as:

- A means of communication among all members of the treatment team
- A resource to be used in treating the patient's illness
- A means of providing continuing patient care in different health care settings
- An important tool in utilization management and quality assessment programs
- A constant and valuable source of information for research and educational and statistical studies
- Proof of services provided (to be used for reimbursement documentation)
- A document that can afford legal protection to the health care facility, its employees, and its patients

The nutrition care plan is based on the standards of care for specific disease entities. Standards for nutritional care are guidelines that outline the acceptable level of intervention or care for a particular diagnosis. These standards are based on the latest available scientific information and the best demonstrated practice of nutrition care. Care plans should follow the standards of care but be individualized to each patient's needs.

Critical Paths

Critical paths, another term for standards of care, are interdisciplinary mapping standards for particular diagnoses and are used to direct care of the patient from admission to discharge. Nutrition care plans should be based on critical paths. For example, the care plan for a cardiac patient would specifically state when nutrition education should begin. The dietitian developing a care plan should record when the instruction is to occur and document in the medical record when it is complete.

The use of critical paths allows the patient's care team to anticipate the patient's needs and to be prepared in advance. Critical paths also serve as valuable thresholds to identify when a patient is not responding to treatment as expected and to provide the team with the information needed to pursue other avenues of treatment. Critical paths provide objective measurements in assessing quality of care because the care to be given for a delineated set of parameters is clearly stated and any exceptions can be detected readily. Although the critical path identifies standards for patient care, individualized treatment is not ruled out; deviations should be documented, along with the appropriate rationale.

Nutrition Education

Nutrition education should be provided to the patient or family as determined by the organization's policy. Some organizations may require a physician's order prior to providing nutrition education, but once the determination is made for nutrition education, the dietitian or dietetic technician contacts the unit staff to assess the patient's schedule.

Nutrition education is based on the patient's life-style and current eating habits as disclosed by a food history. Food tolerances also must be considered in developing diet patterns for patients. As stated earlier, due to shorter lengths of stay and the fact that news of their medical condition and prescribed life-style changes may require an adjustment period, inpatient instructions may be less effective. If possible, the patient should be scheduled for an outpatient return visit for the diet instruction or clarification.

Nutrition education should be tailored to the patient's needs, education level, diagnosis, and life-style. For example, a diabetic patient who works a night shift should not be prescribed a meal pattern that accommodates the lifestyle of a day-shift worker.

Discharge Planning

Discharge planning should begin with the initial screen or assessment. Potential nutrition needs and risk factors should be evaluated and steps taken to ensure adequate nutrition intervention. The dietitian should complete a discharge summary and send information regarding the patient's nutrition needs to extended care facilities. If the patient will need assistance from home care or a community agency, these services should be arranged for prior to discharge. Arrangement for such services is usually done through the organization's social work department.

Discharge planning may include arranging for the patient to leave the hospital on a tube feeding or on total parenteral nutrition. Written discharge instructions may be necessary for the patient, family member, or organization to which the patient is being discharged. As mentioned earlier, the patient may need to be scheduled for outpatient diet instruction or for a follow-up to an inpatient instruction. Immediately, the dietitian should carefully review the medical records of patients readmitted to assess whether a lack of nutrition intervention or an inadequate care plan led to the readmission.

Documentation of Nutrition Care

It is up to the individual facility to authorize specific staff members to make entries into medical records. If a full-time registered dietitian is not available on a regular basis, dietetic technicians or nutrition assistants may be authorized to record pertinent information about the nutrition care plan.

Accurate documentation of nutrition services provided to patients is vital to hospital systems for utilization management, quality control, and assessment and reimbursement. Basically, services are documented in the same way, and by the same staff members, as nutrition assessments and care plans. In addition to descriptions of the nutrition assessments, care plans, and services provided, the medical record should reflect periodic evaluations and revisions of the plan based on the overall effectiveness of the patient's treatment.

The frequency with which nutrition services are recorded depends on the patient's condition and the institution's policies. For example, daily progress notes might be required for a critically ill patient or a patient whose condition is rapidly improving or deteriorating. A hospital policy might mandate a progress note each time a nutrition care plan is revised or reviewed, in which case a statement of the new plan or review findings would be included. Documentation is important for quality management because changes in status, especially incremental improvements, can be useful in justifying nutrition intervention.

The actual format used for writing progress notes depends on the policies of the individual organization. Whatever the format, information should be as clear and concise as possible without omitting pertinent details. Usually, either source-oriented medical records (SOMRs) or problem-oriented medical records (POMRs) are used.

In the *source-oriented format,* entries are structured according to the source of information, with entries included in order of occurrence. Nutrition care information should be included in the appropriately designated section of the medical record. In some organizations the designated section may be the physician progress notes, whereas in others a separate section is identified for ancillary departments. Entries are written in brief paragraph form; sentence fragments or key phrases are acceptable. The entry is signed with the name and title of the person writing it, the month, day, year, and time of day.

The *problem-oriented format* focuses on the patient's problems, personal profile, plans for care and education, assessment of progress, and results. An initial data base consisting of the patient's medical and social history is gathered in which problems are listed and assigned a number. The initial treatment of these problems is recorded and progress notes are added as they pertain to specific problems in the problem list. An approach referred to as SOAP is used for each progress note, *SOAP* being the acronym for the elements of information in each progress note:

- Subjective information: what the patient or family says
- Objective information: what the facts relate to the patient's progress, such as laboratory values, results of diagnostic tests, changes in weight, observations and examinations by health professionals, and nutrient intake calculated from diet history
- Assessment: what the data mean
- Plan: recommendation of what should be done for the patient

More information on recording nutrition information in medical records is available in an American Hospital Association technical advisory bulletin entitled *Recording Nutrition Information in Medical Records.* Figure 9-8 provides illustrations of nutrition care documentation in both the SOMR and POMR (SOAP) formats.

☐ Summary

The role of the nutrition manager is similar to that of other health care managers. Planning includes creating policies and procedures for providing nutrition care, writing goals and objectives consistent with those of the department, and developing and marketing new programs. Organization of the nutrition section of the food service department depends on the size of the facility and patient types. The nutrition team generally consists of some configuration of nutrition managers, registered dietitians, dietetic technicians, nutrition assistants and aides (or clerks), and/or hosts and hostesses.

The nutrition manager must develop and utilize leadership skills that motivate the staff toward the department's and organization's vision. Financial expertise on the manager's part has become increasingly important with the demand for cost-effective services. The nutrition manager must seek to prove the necessity of nutrition intervention in health care delivery through the measurement of positive patient outcomes.

Patient nutrition services include screening to determine nutrition risk, assessment, education, and discharge planning. All of these are accomplished through the use of care plans and may be based on interdisciplinary critical paths. In addition, the nutrition staff may provide intervention through enteral or parenteral feeding. Regardless of what nutrition intervention or treatment is provided, the care must be fully documented in the appropriate section of the patient's medical record. Documentation entries must be made by the person performing the treatment.

Figure 9-8. Example of SOMR and POMR (SOAP) Formats for Nutrition Care Documentation

Mr. Allen is concerned about feeding himself. He is unable to see what is on the tray and has minimal use of his right hand. His appetite is good and he currently weighs 160 pounds.

Dietetic service will arrange the dishes appropriately on the tray. Self-feeding devices will be included. A plate waste study will be performed for three days, and the nutrient intake will then be evaluated. Nurses will provide encouragement and supervision during mealtime.

Joan Smith, R.D.
Consultant Dietitian

Date: _____ Time: _____

S – Patient wants to feed himself, even though he has minimal use of right hand and is blind.

O – Patient attempts to feed himself and asks questions about arrangement of foods on tray.

A – Appetite is good; weight is 160 pounds.

P – Dietetic services uses self-feeding devices and appropriate tray arrangement; plate waste study for three days enables evaluation of nutrient intake; nurses encourage intake; nurse and/or dietitian supervises patient during mealtime.

Joan Smith, R.D.
Consultant Dietitian

Date: _____ Time: _____

☐ Bibliography

All Saints Health System, Nutrition and Food Service Policy and Procedure Manual. Fort Worth: All Saints Health Care, 1992.

American Hospital Association. *Recording Nutrition Information in Medical Records [Management Advisory].* Chicago: AHA, 1990.

Folz, M. B., and Stephens, G. Marketing: food and nutrition service. *Hospital Administration Currents* 29(2):7–12, 1985.

Hill, M. *Managed Care and Case Management: Clinical Systems for Cost/Quality Outcomes.* South Natick, MA: The Center for Case Management, 1992.

Lanz, S. J. *Introduction to the Profession of Dietetics.* Philadelphia: Lea and Febiger, 1983.

Moffitt, K. Roles/responsibilities of clinical nutrition managers in health care facilities. Unpublished thesis, Texas Woman's University, Denton, 1987.

Pricing clinical services, part 1. *Hospital Food and Nutrition Focus* 2(3):1–9, Nov. 1985.

Schiller, M. R., Gilbride, J. A., and Maillet, J. O. *Handbook for Clinical Nutrition Services Management.* Gaithersburg, MD: Aspen Publishers, 1991.

Shands Hospital at the University of Florida. *Guide to Normal Nutrition and Diet Modification.* 3rd ed. Gainesville, FL: Shands Hospital, 1983.

Smith, P. E., and Smith, A. E. Can nutrition services affect hospital costs under PPS? *Journal of Healthcare Financial Management Association,* July 1985.

Splett, P. L. Effectiveness and cost effectiveness of nutrition care: a critical analysis with recommendations. A supplement to the *Journal of The American Dietetic Association,* Nov. 1991.

Ward, M. *Marketing Strategies: A Resource for Registered Dietitians.* Johnson City, NY: Marcia Ward, 1984.

Management
Information Systems

☐ Introduction

The complexities faced by today's health care food service managers make it necessary to implement methods for producing precise, sophisticated information. This need has led to the development of management information systems (MIS), a network of people, procedures, and equipment used to gather and process data to provide routine information to managers and/or decision makers. Its techniques include selecting, storing, processing, and retrieving operational data. In so doing, the MIS supports the food service department's functional units, such as marketing, purchasing, production, meal service, and financial management by providing routine reports about these units. The reports are used by management to support decision making, with a focus on operational efficiency.

This chapter will discuss concepts of information—what it is and how it differs from data, the value of information, and features of an effective MIS. The tasks that go into information production (developing, implementing, and operating an MIS) will be described, as will the four elements that comprise an MIS: input, processing, output, and feedback. After examining MIS methodology, such as manual systems and computer-assisted systems, the chapter will outline a six-stage process of developing a computerized MIS from a manual system:

1. Investigating the current system
2. Analyzing the current system
3. Designing the MIS
4. Implementing the MIS
5. Maintaining the MIS
6. Reviewing the MIS

Based on information in this chapter, a food service manager can facilitate development of an MIS that is capable of generating any number of information-bearing instruments (for example, reports, cost analyses, electronic spreadsheets). Furthermore, the system built will be tailored to specific needs of the department.

☐ Information Concepts

Information is one of a health care food service operation's most valuable resources. Current environmental pressures such as cost containment mandates, changing patient demographics, and work force diversity require that the department's MIS produce accurate information in a timely fashion. Developing, implementing, and operating an MIS is probably one of the most time-consuming tasks faced by a food service manager. Although the terms *information* and *data* frequently are used interchangeably, they are not to be confused with one another in discussing an MIS.

Distinguishing Data from Information

Data consist of raw facts about the transactions that occur during the course of providing goods and services to customers. The check total for a single cafeteria customer is an example of one unit of data (or datum). If a health care food service manager were to sort through all single or unit transactions (that is, all data) generated by the cafeteria, he or she would be unable to carry out other managerial responsibilities. Therefore, data must be transformed into a more accessible form; that form is information. *Information* is the product that results from sorting, processing, and combining data to produce a collection of facts that has value beyond the value of the individual, separate facts. Thus, a manager would find the *total weekly cafeteria sales* to be more valuable than individual check totals.

Measuring the Value of Information

The value of information is directly linked to how it helps a food service manager achieve the operation's goals and objectives. That value typically is measured in terms of money or time. In monetary terms, value equals either increased revenues or decreased expenses. In terms of time, the value of information might be measured by how much less time is spent on making a decision. According to his book *Principles of Information Systems: A Managerial Approach,* author R. M. Stair says that information should have certain characteristics before it can be deemed valuable to managers. In most cases, it must be accurate, complete, economical, flexible, reliable, simple, timely, and verifiable to qualify as valuable.

Characterizing an Effective MIS

Information, as indicated above, can only result from very carefully designed systems. Although MIS design varies from operation to operation, certain characteristics are common among effective systems. In the book *Computer Systems for Foodservice Operations,* Kasavana lists these five features:

1. The MIS provides a means by which to achieve organizational goals and objectives.
2. The MIS treats information as an important resource and is responsible for its proper handling, flow, and distribution.
3. The MIS enables improved integration of operations, communications, and coordination.
4. The MIS will interface people and equipment in relationships designed to free personnel to fulfill jobs requiring human capabilities.
5. The MIS will store large volumes of transactional data to support planning, decision making, and analytical activities.

☐ Elements of an MIS

In addition to the characteristics enumerated above, an effective MIS design meets the specific needs of an individual food service operation. Although this tailoring requires a variety of approaches and designs, all effective systems typically evolve from four interrelated elements or components: input, processing, output, and feedback. These components are illustrated in figure 10-1 and detailed in the following sections.

Figure 10-1. Four Elements of an MIS

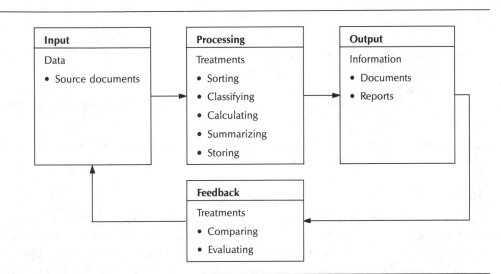

Input

Input involves the capturing and gathering of raw data for each business transaction. In producing monthly checks for a cafeteria's vendors, for example, the dollar value of each delivery by each vendor during the month must be arrived at before checks can be calculated by accounts payable or printed. Input can take many forms but is usually supported in writing by a source document. A *source document* provides a permanent record of an individual transaction. In an MIS designed to produce vendor checks, then, an invoice provided by the vendor at the point of delivery would serve as the source document. Source documents for the operation's marketing unit could include cafeteria customer surveys or records of patient interviews.

The typical health care food service operation collects volumes of source documents during the course of business. This creates numerous problems for handling, storing, and retrieving original source documents. Due to advances in MIS technology, certain aspects of the MIS are available in a paperless, electronic format. But before this format can be implemented successfully, the accuracy and security of data must be assessed, which occurs in data processing.

Processing

Processing involves the actions or treatments required to convert data into useful information. Processing usually involves sorting and classifying data into categories, performing calculations, summarizing results, and storing both data and information for further processing. In the accounts payable example described above, data manipulation involves determining the dollar value of all purchases made from individual vendors, as documented by invoices, to determine what is owed each vendor.

Further coding of data may occur by classifying each purchase by type of commodity (such as produce, meat, dairy product, chemicals, or paper supplies). This allows the system not only to produce checks for vendors but also to generate information that allows the food service director to monitor the dollar value of different categories of purchases.

Data-processing functions are similar for all the various units of a food service operation—such as marketing, purchasing, inventory control, and meal service. According to Stair, all processing elements have a number of characteristics in common, including:

- A large volume of input data
- A large volume of output

227

- Numerous users affected by the system
- A need for efficient processing
- Large-volume storage requirements
- Fast input and output capabilities
- Low computational complexity
- A high degree of repetition in processing
- A high potential for problems related to security
- A severe negative impact on the organization if the processing element breaks down or fails to operate correctly

Each of these characteristics must be considered when developing the MIS and particularly when designing the system's processing element.

Output

In an MIS, *output* involves producing information, usually in the form of report documents, that is appropriately relevant for the food service operation and its decision makers. Other outputs may include vendor checks, reports of purchases by food category, and analyses of patient food costs for the administration's use. The MIS can produce reports required by local, state, or federal agencies—for example, sales tax reports for cafeteria operations. Three broad report categories are described briefly below.

Types of Reports

The reports output by an MIS can be classified as scheduled, demand, or exception reports. *Scheduled* reports are produced periodically based on a set schedule (daily, weekly, or monthly). For example, the food service manager might receive a weekly report of sales for each revenue-producing food unit in the health care operation. Or, an inventory report might be produced on a monthly basis so that the value of each category of food inventory can be monitored.

Demand reports, on the other hand, are developed and produced to provide specific information requested by a manager. In other words, these reports are not generated on a routine basis. Thus, a manager who needed to know total sales for a specific menu item during the year would rely on the information generated by a demand report.

Exception reports are produced when a situation occurs outside the parameters set by management and require manager action. For example, an exception report could be generated automatically to report all vending food items that fall below a certain level of sales activity. In this case, the manager might want to consider replacing the item with a more popular product. If none of the food items offered by the vending operation fall below the minimum sales level, no exception report need be generated.

Design and Development of Reports

The purpose of MIS reports is to help managers in their planning, decision making, and controlling functions as they relate to various department operations. According to Stair, the guidelines that should be followed in designing and developing effective reports include:

- Tailoring each report to satisfy specific user needs
- Spending time and effort on producing only those reports that are necessary and will be used
- Paying attention to report content and layout
- Utilizing exception reporting
- Producing all reports in a timely fashion

Feedback

Another function of the MIS is to provide feedback so as to make managers aware of the level of performance within their operations. *Feedback* enables food service managers to take preventive and corrective action. For instance, an MIS report might indicate that the inventory levels of specific chemicals and cleaning supplies are too low, thus prompting the manager to place an order with the appropriate vendor. Upon delivery of supplies, the data generated by this transaction (invoices, bill of receipts, for example) are input into the system.

☐ Information Management

A variety of methods can help managers generate information from operational data. In some cases, the manager can process data mentally, for example, by estimating the appropriate menu price based on cost data. Other informal information systems, such as oral communication during training sessions, have been used with some success. Because of the volume of data generated by most health care food service operations, formal systems for data processing and transformation have become commonplace.

Manual Systems

Originally, a food service operation's MIS relied on repetitive manual procedures, whereby input was provided for each transaction by means of a source document, usually in paper format. Each transaction was then posted by hand and calculations performed either by hand or by means of a calculator. Reports were handwritten or typed up individually. At best, manual systems could generate elementary outputs on meal equivalents, customer counts and sales, labor hours and costs, food and supply costs, and personnel records.

Computer-Assisted Systems

Although manual systems are still used in some health care food service operations, as the complexity of operations increases, so too does the demand for an MIS that can provide more information with more accuracy and within a shorter time than can be generated by traditional manual systems. Undoubtedly, the most important advancement in collecting, maintaining, and processing data has been the development of computers. Once available data are entered (input) into the computer, the data can be stored, retrieved, and processed rapidly and accurately as many times as needed to meet the operation's information needs. More and more facilities that formerly depended on manual systems are now converting to computerized MIS.

Converting from a manual to a computerized system requires a great deal of time and expense. Therefore, the conversion process should yield concrete benefits for a facility's operations. Again according to Stair, benefits include:

- *A higher degree of accuracy:* With manual systems, because more than one employee might be responsible for reviewing reports for accuracy, inaccurate reporting may occur due to faulty cross-checking. With computerized systems, accuracy can be checked not only by employees but by the computerized system as well.
- *Timeliness of documentation and reporting:* Manual systems can take days, weeks, or months to produce even the most routine reports. Computerized systems can significantly reduce this time. This can prove to be a valuable attribute in data processing for functions such as payroll or nutrient analysis of menus.
- *Service expansion and enhancement:* Manual systems may not afford the rapidity with which operations need to meet their customers' expectations. Computerized systems that link functions (such as customer orders and inventory) can facilitate improved customer service.
- *Labor efficiency:* Manual systems are extremely labor-intensive. Computerized systems can substantially reduce clerical labor requirements. This is the case when data are used for multiple purposes. For instance, after cost data have been entered and stored by the computer, they can be processed into information for financial statements, variance reports, and menu pricing.

- *Data and information integrity:* Only information that is accurate, current, and relevant can be of value to the operation. Because manual systems have no parameters for information discrimination, systems with inherent check-and-error prompts are a decided advantage.

Note that computerization of a manual information system does not guarantee improved MIS performance. If the basis on which the manual system was built is flawed, computerization will only serve to magnify rather than diminish an operation's problems—and those of its MIS. A successful computer-assisted system can evolve only from an effective manual system.

☐ Development of Computerized MIS

Computers were first utilized in the industrial sector to produce payroll and personnel records, purchasing and inventory control, assembly line schedules, productivity reports, and job costing reports. Introduction and acceptance of computerization by the food service sector has been a slower realization, traceable to the early 1960s when Computer Assisted Menu Planning (CAMP) was designed by Balintfy and Nebel.

As an outgrowth of this early effort, a number of systems now enhance managers' control of food service operations. As a result, the past few years have seen an increase in use of computerized MIS in health care food service operations.

A variety of formal and informal approaches serve to develop computerized MIS for health care food service operations, with steps for systems development varying from one operation to the next. The model described here is based on the work of Gordon, Necco, and Tsai.

Step 1: Investigate the Current System

Computers can process information rapidly and store vast amounts of data. They are useful for almost all food service operations but do not present a cure for every management problem. Before implementing a computerized MIS, the food service director should spend time and effort to justify the expenses involved and to weigh them against anticipated benefits of conversion.

Usually, systems investigation is the first step in this investigation process, whose purpose is to determine whether information generated by the existing system satisfies and supports the goals and objectives of the operation. Major functions of the current system must be evaluated to determine if improvements are possible and, if so, what effect they might have on the department's revenues and expenses. Specifically, this step attempts to answer the following questions:

- What problems might an MIS solve?
- What new opportunities might an MIS provide?
- What new software or hardware will be required?
- Will the computer's presence increase or reduce the department's personnel requirements?
- What data bases and operational procedures will need to be developed?
- What costs will be involved?
- Where will the financial resources come from to develop the MIS?
- If the system is to be used by clinical nutrition staff, who will absorb the costs of nutrition services?

Step 2: Analyze the System

The existing system's ability to satisfy the information needs of managers and decision makers must be determined. Emphasis is on determining the problems and limitations of the existing system and, at the same time, identifying its strengths. Typically, this is accomplished by direct observation, structured interviews of managers and users, and questionnaires.

Step 3: Design the System

Although design of a computerized MIS often focuses on computer selection, it should be pointed out that computers constitute only part of the MIS. The purpose of systems design is to develop the best possible system that helps the operation achieve its goals and objectives and at the same time overcomes some problems of the existing systems. If this involves converting a manual system to a computerized MIS, major investments may be necessary.

A computerized MIS consists of software, hardware, data bases, telecommunications, personnel, and procedures. A common mistake made in the design of a computerized MIS is the selection of hardware without consideration of software capabilities. Selection of software is the most critical decision and must occur prior to selection of all other system components.

Software

Software consists of specific instructions given the computer. These instructions enable the computer to transform data into information, which ideally results in increased profits, decreased costs, and/or improved customer service.

Microcomputers use two types of software: systems software and applications software. *Systems software* is designed to support the overall computer system by controlling and enhancing the capabilities of the hardware and application software, rather than performing a specific function. *Applications software* programs are designed to solve specific user-oriented problems. Examples of application software are word-processing systems, data-base management systems, and decision support systems including electronic spreadsheets. Because of the important nature of applications software, outside discussion is warranted. Characteristics that must be considered when matching software to a specific business application include the source, scope, and function of the software.

Source

Source refers to the degree to which the manager is involved in design of the software and/or development of the instructions provided to the hardware. Most software can be classified as customized, full-featured, or generic.

In health care food service operations, many early users of computer technology found it necessary to design and develop customized software. This type of software was written specifically for their operations, and the managers were actively involved in determining the functions to be performed by the software. Many times, the written reports generated by the existing manual system were used as the basis for the design of the computer-generated reports. This resulted in software that generated reports tailored to meet the specific needs of a specific operation. However, many operations do not have the resources necessary to develop their own systems. In addition, errors or bugs in these types of systems usually had to be caught and corrected after the system had been implemented.

An alternative to customized software is full-featured software. A wide variety of full-featured software systems has been developed for use by health care food service operations. Systems have been developed by over 200 companies to perform functions ranging from inventory and purchasing control to nutrient analysis of both menus and intake of individual patients.

Full-featured software generally is less expensive than customized software and usually has been widely tested and sold. This software can be seen through demonstrations at trade shows or by previewing program copies. With so many choices available, guidelines for evaluating these programs must be developed for the food service director who is considering the purchase of full-featured software. See Fowler's proposed methodology for evaluating full-featured food service software in *Effective Computer Management in Food and Nutrition Services.*

An economical alternative to customized and full-featured software is generic software. A variety of generic programs can be purchased at retail software stores or from mail-order houses at a cost of $300 or less. Generic software programs include word processing that handles word applications, electronic spreadsheets for mathematical applications, data-base management that equates to an electronic filing system, and graphics to display information in graph form. These general purpose programs can be modeled to meet a variety of needs for a specific food service operation. Many operations choose to supplement their full-featured systems with generic software.

Scope

The *scope* of software refers to the range of applications or functions that can be performed by the software. Software is either single application or integrated in its orientation. Single-application software is designed to handle one specific function. Three common single-application software packages are word processing, data-base managers, and electronic spreadsheets. Single-application programs also are available to support such functions as inventory control and nutrient analysis. These systems generally are easier to evaluate and less expensive than integrated systems. However, they may be less efficient because each application requires that the same data be entered before being used by the program.

In most food service operations, some of the same data are used for numerous applications. Data about an individual food item might be used in ordering, receiving, issuing, recipes, production, sales control, and nutrient analysis. Integrated food service software allows for easy transfer of data directly from one application to another. The data are entered only once. Thereafter, the data can be used to provide information for planning and control purposes for a variety of functions with a minimum of user interaction.

Function

Function refers to the specific job or tasks that can be accomplished with the software. Software designed for health care food service operations perform a wide variety of functions, including:

- Point-of-sale record keeping and sales analysis
- Menu planning and cost analysis
- Inventory and purchasing control
- Maintenance of purchasing and receiving records
- Recording production schedules
- Production control and forecasting
- Labor productivity and payroll records
- Financial management
- Clinical nutrition care

An excellent discussion of the inputs, outputs, and capabilities of most of these functions is provided in *Foodservice in Institutions,* revised in 1988 by Harger, Shugart, and Payne-Palacio.

Selection

When determining what to purchase, there are literally tens of thousands of application software packages to choose from. In their book *Microcomputers: Business and Personal Applications,* Burns and Eubanks recommend the following procedure for selecting software:

- Define the application to be computerized.
- Develop a list of available software.
- Gather information about available packages.
- Narrow down the list of possible choices.
- Obtain hands-on demonstrations.
- Perform a final evaluation.
- Make a decision.

Hardware

Once software has been selected, hardware that can run the software must be identified. The computers used in health care operations vary from microcomputers used at individual workstations to large mainframes used for major organizational data-processing functions. The following discussion focuses on characteristics of the microcomputer because of its prevalent use by health care food service managers.

Components

Microcomputers consist of basic hardware components to perform input, processing, and output activities. Input devices include such formats as keyboards and optical scanners. Processing devices include the central processing unit (CPU), memory, and storage. The most common output devices are printers and displays on computer screens. Microcomputers, available in a variety of formats based on their anticipated use, include desktop computers, transportable computers, laptop computers, and hand-held computers.

Desirable Characteristics

Selection of equipment is a major decision. Hardware features that should be considered include CPU speed, types of input and output devices, primary storage capacity, secondary storage capacity, and number of workstations supported. Expandability of the system is an important feature, and expansion products can be used to increase the power, enlarge the storage space, and customize the computer for special functions. Additional features to consider are warranties, user-support services, and maintenance contracts that may be provided by computer vendors.

Data Bases

Once the food service operation has selected the software and hardware components, a data base must be designed. A *data base* consists of an organized collection of raw facts. These facts can be about the operation's customers, employees, food items in inventory, and many others. Most managers believe that the data base is one of the most valuable components of a computerized MIS, and in fact a great deal of time and effort must be contributed to data-base design and development. Some vendors may provide data about their products in a format that can be used by computerized systems, thus minimizing the time required to develop the data base. For example, data concerning the nutritional composition of frozen entrees could be provided on a diskette for use during analyses of the nutritional adequacy of menus offered to patients.

Telecommunications

Telecommunications allow the health care operation to link discrete computer systems to create networks. Local-area networks (LANs) can connect computer equipment within the department or within a single building for purposes of resource sharing and information dissemination. With capability for connecting a variety of computer systems and supporting electronic mail, LANs must be supported by both network software and specially designed application software. Specific features of LANs and their application in food service operations are described by Shrock and Shrock in *Effective Computer Management in Food and Nutrition Services*.

Personnel

Perhaps the most important component of a computerized information system are the people who manage, run, program, and maintain the system. Personnel requirements for support of the computerized MIS must be carefully assessed: Will a computerized MIS mean adding new employees to realize project objectives? Will the nature of projects dictate whether tasks are modified or changed altogether? System design also must consider user needs and expectations. System users include managers, decision makers, employees, and other individuals who access the systems to carry out the department's work.

Procedures

The last MIS design component to consider is the body of procedures that detail how the systems are to be operated. *Procedures* include strategies, policies, methods, and rules for operation of the system. Procedures must be developed to define when reports are to be generated, who has access to the data base, and contingency measures to be taken in case of a disaster or system malfunction.

Step 4: Implement the System

Upon conclusion of the system design stage, specifications for each of the six basic components of the computerized MIS should have been developed. These specifications dictate which software, hardware, data bases, telecommunications systems, and personnel should be acquired. Acquisitions are made by following the health care operation's purchasing and hiring policies. Operating procedures for the computerized MIS, as discussed previously, must be made available to all users. Then implementation can take place.

Preparation of Users, Site, and Data

Prior to implementation, preparation of users, site, and data must be accomplished. Preparation may involve nothing more than promoting the new computerized MIS so as to minimize resistance to change; even so, this step generally involves training user personnel so as to ensure that they get the most from the new system. Training may be conducted by the software vendor, an outside contracted source, or even departmental personnel who have received in-depth training. In any case, on-line tutorials that accompany some software also can be useful.

The site selected for hardware placement must be carefully considered. The location must have a power supply that is relatively free from power surges, and the equipment should be located in a relatively clean environment, free from temperature extremes. Additional furniture may be needed to promote efficiency and ensure the comfort of users.

All data that previously have been maintained manually must be converted and saved in a format that the MIS can access. This conversion-and-save process is a very time-consuming task, and the food service director may elect to hire temporary, part-time data-entry clerks.

Installation, Testing, and Start-Up

The hardware and software must be installed on-site so that system testing can occur. Each system application program must be tested with data so that potential problems can be identified and circumvented prior to system start-up. There are several approaches to start-up, but when several applications are to be computerized, the preferred method is to keep things simple by starting up one application at a time. Once the new application is performing as expected, another application can be implemented.

Step 5: Maintain the System

The purpose of system maintenance is to keep the computerized MIS operating as efficiently, effectively, and error free as possible. This step involves monitoring and modifying the MIS to make it more useful and valuable to users. Maintenance may be required to resolve major problems or to make minor modifications. Given that most computerized MIS require substantial maintenance, the quantity and availability of maintenance support is an important factor to consider when comparing vendors of full-featured programs.

Step 6: Review the System

The final step of systems development is the process of evaluating all systems components to make sure that they are operating as intended. All six components are subject to review. This means that applications software, hardware, telecommunications systems, data bases (containing all facts used by the system), personnel (either full-time or part-time) who work with the system, and the procedures that provide guidelines for system operations must be evaluated, troubleshot, and adjusted as necessary. System review should take place on a regular scheduled basis, with backup provisions made to guard against loss of data.

Software Review

Because of the critical role software plays in computerized MIS, its performance should be reviewed carefully. For instance, a problem would arise if the system were designed to value inventory by means of average cost method and the operation specified the standard cost method. Problems identified during this process may require modification of customized or full-featured programs. Usually, this is best done by the program developers. However, in the case of generic software, most problems can be resolved by users.

Hardware and Telecommunications Review

Existing equipment, hardware, and telecommunications systems must be evaluated based on their efficiency and effectiveness. As new input and output devices (such as bar-code readers and high-speed printers) become available on the market, their potential benefit to food service operations should be assessed. Vendor demonstrations and presentations in-house should be encouraged.

Data-Base Review

Data-base review is critical because this component "houses" the raw facts that feed the computerized MIS. The data bases of a food service operation should be evaluated for accuracy of data, speed of retrieval, and storage capacity. The product data provided by vendors should be checked for accuracy. Errors for characteristics such as price, size, and packaging should be corrected prior to implementation and use of the data base.

Personnel

Personnel review, an evaluation of the staff responsible for operating the computerized MIS, should focus on number of staff and their skill levels. Capability of existing staff to handle a new application program should be determined prior to implementation of additional applications. This can be accomplished by means of reviewing continuing education credits and administering written and skill exercises.

Procedures

As with any other procedure developed by a health care food service operation, procedures that support the computerized MIS should undergo routine review and be revised as necessary. This ensures meeting the changing needs of the department, the health care operation, and regulatory mandates. As new equipment and/or software is added, procedures must be developed so that they will be operated properly. For example, when a bar-code reader is purchased for inventory control purposes, operational procedures must be developed and implemented.

☐ Summary

The health care industry operates in an extremely dynamic business environment. As a result, the operations of all units of a health care facility—including the food service department—are affected. There is increased pressure for food service department decision makers to make not only more decisions but more qualitative decisions in less time. This environmental mandate has resulted in the implementation of management information systems (MIS) that are designed specifically for health care food service operations.

This chapter introduced and described several key concepts related to MIS. The four basic elements of an MIS (input, processing, output, and feedback) were identified and discussed. Even though many traditional manual systems incorporate all four elements, they have been judged by many food service directors to be inadequate for their needs.

To design an effective health care food service MIS, a systematic approach that investigates and analyzes the current manual system must be taken. Once problems are identified in the existing system, the new system should be designed to meet the information needs of decision makers in a more timely and more efficient manner. Design considerations encompass specifying software, hardware, data-base, telecommunications, personnel, and procedure needs. A wide variety of computer software has been developed specifically for health care food service operations, among them full-feature and generic software. After system implementation has been accomplished, the system components should be maintained regularly and reviewed routinely. If these steps are followed, the full potential of the computerized MIS can be realized by the food service department.

☐ Bibliography

Alexander, J. Selecting and acquiring a computer system for the food and nutrition services department. In: F. A. Kaud, editor. *Effective Computer Management in Food and Nutrition Services*. Rockville, MD: Aspen Publishers, 1989.

American Hospital Association. Hospital Computer Systems Planning: Preparation of Request for Proposal. Chicago: AHA, 1980.

Burns, J. R., and Eubanks, D. N. *Microcomputers: Business and Personal Applications*. St. Paul, MN: West Publishing, 1988.

Chaban, J. *Practical Foodservice Spreadsheets with Lotus 1-2-3*. 2nd ed. New York City: Van Nostrand Reinhold, 1993.

Coltman, M. M. *Hospitality Industry Purchasing*. New York City: Van Nostrand Reinhold, 1990.

Computers in Food and Nutrition Services: Promises and Prospects. Report of the Tenth Ross Roundtable on Medical Issues. Columbus, OH: Ross Laboratories, 1990.

Computers: what is new in hardware and software. *Hospital Food & Nutrition Focus* 7(5):3–4, Jan. 1991.

Dougherty, D. Avoiding common computer management mistakes. *Hospital Food & Nutrition Focus* 9(2):2–3, Oct. 1992.

Fowler, K. D. Evaluating food service software. In: F. A. Kaud, editor. *Effective Computer Management in Food and Nutrition Services*. Rockville, MD: Aspen Publishers, 1989.

Gordon, C. L., Necco, C. R., and Tsai, N. W. Toward a standard systems development life cycle. *Journal of Systems Management* 38(8):24–27, Aug. 1987.

Grossbauer, S. Manage them or they manage you: service contracts. *FoodService Director* 5(9):170, Sept. 1992.

Grossbauer, S. To get a grip on the budget: how to use spreadsheets. *FoodService Director* 5(8):170, Aug. 1992.

Hard, R. CEOs link IS visions to hospital strategic plans. *Hospitals* 66(23):42–46, Dec. 1992.

Harger, V. F., Shugart, G. S., and Payne-Palacio, J., editors. *Foodservice in Institutions*. 6th ed. New York: Macmillan Publishing Company, 1988.

Herlong, J. E. The good news about computers. *Restaurants USA* 12(9):15–19, Oct. 1992.

How to handle the hard facts. *Healthcare Foodservice* 2(3):6–7, Sept.–Oct. 1992.

Kasavana, M. L. *Computer Systems for Foodservice Operations*. New York City: Van Nostrand Reinhold, 1984.

Kasavana, M. L., and Cahill, J. J. *Managing Computers in the Hospitality Industry*. 2nd ed. East Lansing, MI: Educational Institute of the American Hotel & Motel Association, 1992.

Kaud, F. A., editor. *Effective Computer Management in Food and Nutrition Services*. Rockville, MD: Aspen Publishers, 1989.

Matthews, M. E., and Norback, J. P. A new way of thinking about computers and information processing in hospital food services. In: J. C. Rose, editor. *Handbook for Health Care Food Service Management*. Rockville, MD: Aspen Publishers, 1984.

Microcomputers: some successful uses. *Hospital Food & Nutrition Focus* 1(9):1–6, 1985.

Pellegrino, T. W. *Selecting a Computer-Assisted System for Volume Food Service.* Chicago: American Hospital Publishing, 1986. [Out of print.]

Sawyer, C. A. Computer-assisted management: role delineation for entry-level positions in foodservice management. *Journal of The American Dietetic Association* 87(1):75–77, Jan. 1987.

Shrock, J. R., and Shrock, J. M. Local area network systems. In: F. A. Kaud, editor. *Effective Computer Management in Food and Nutrition Services.* Rockville, MD: Aspen Publishers, 1989.

Spears, M. C. *Foodservice Organizations: A Managerial and Systems Approach.* 2nd ed. New York City: Macmillan Publishing, 1991.

Stair, R. M. *Principles of Information Systems: A Managerial Approach.* Boston: Boyd & Fraser Publishing Company, 1992.

Waller, A. The use of computer technology in nutrition and food services. *Hospital Materiel Management Quarterly* 7(3):50–60, 1986.

Youngwirth, J. The evolution of computers in dietetics: a review. *Journal of The American Dietetic Association* 82(1):62, Jan. 1983.

Financial Management

☐ Introduction

The changing trends and focus within the health care industry have definite implications for health care facilities' individual departments, which are responding in various ways. At the departmental level—including the food service department—there is increased emphasis on cost-effectiveness, cost efficiency, and cost containment. To control costs and adapt to changes, food service department managers and their staffs must know where and how costs originate. They must be able to predict how costs will be affected by economic conditions and changing levels of service delivery. Executive decisions about resource allocation require skill and insight backed by appropriate financial information. Financial management, then, is concerned with accessing information that helps managers make financial decisions whose ultimate purpose is to provide high-quality nutrition and food services while maximizing revenues and minimizing costs.

To assist health care managers in meeting this challenge, their institutions' accounting and finance departments generate and distribute a variety of reports. Although these reports can be useful in directing department operations, many times they fail to provide the detail necessary to fully evaluate a department's performance. In some cases, managers may not receive reports soon enough to pinpoint areas where corrective actions are needed. For this reason, a sound system of financial control and management is essential for the operation of an efficient and effective food service department.

Financial management is a significant part of the management information system (MIS) discussed in chapter 10. Inputs to the financial MIS are source documents such as invoices, deposit records, and cash register tapes that evidence a business transaction having taken place. These business transactions must be recorded and summarized by completing the processing steps of the accounting cycle. As a result, output can be produced in the form of financial statements and other management reports. Feedback includes the analysis and interpretation of information as presented in the financial statements and reports. As with other MIS, the system can be supported by manual or computerized methods.

This chapter will discuss the food service manager's role in financial management and the process of financial management using a five-part model. The focus of the discussion is on managerial accounting and, to a lesser degree, on finance and its relationship to the overall financial management system of a health care food service operation.

☐ Financial Management Systems Model for Health Care Food Service Operations

The ability of an operation's financial management system to satisfy the information needs of food service managers and decision makers can be evaluated by analyzing the current manual system (as discussed in chapter 10). As the basic operating device of systems analysis, the model is effective in representing the elements of an actual system. A model is always less complex than reality but a good model has sufficient detail to approximate major characteristics of the actual system. Therefore, models that incorporate desirable elements can be useful in systems evaluation.

Hoover's prototype, a financial management systems model for health care food service operations, consists of five essential elements. They are:

1. Control
2. Input
3. Processing
4. Output
5. Feedback

The model is illustrated in figure 11-1, which also shows the components of each element. Note that the processing element is further divided into three standard accounting cycle steps: journalizing, posting, and making adjustments. Each element in the model is connected by lines with arrows that depict the flow of financial information within the system.

Figure 11-1.   Financial Management Systems Model for Health Care Food Service Operations

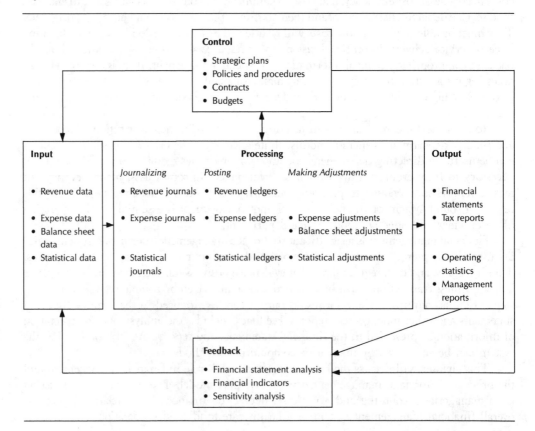

This chapter is organized around the five elements in Hoover's model. Only those components of each element that are considered critical for financial management of most health care food service operations will be discussed in detail. Appropriate references will be identified for those financial management concepts not fully developed in this chapter.

☐ Control Element

The control element helps management ensure that planned goals and objectives are accomplished with the most efficient and effective use of the organization's resources. The control element is closely linked to the planning function as described in chapter 5. Planning establishes the organization's goals and objectives, develops strategies for meeting them, and develops standards of performance. The control element of the financial management system incorporates these organizational plans and standards to provide guidance for food service operations. Normally, these plans and standards are established or reviewed on an annual basis. Actions involved in the other four elements of the financial management system generally are based on the operation's accounting period.

Components of the control element include strategic plans, policies and procedures, contracts, and budgets. Information from these control documents influences the choices made in the input element and interacts with the actions in the processing element. A very important function of this control is that it provides standards on which results are evaluated in the feedback element.

Characteristics of Effective Control

No matter what type of control element an organization designs, this element should have certain characteristics that ensure its effectiveness. For example:

- The control element should be an extension of the planning process, as described in chapter 5. The element implements plans and standards, such as policies and procedures regarding the generation of financial statements or the definition of an accounting period.
- The control element should provide accurate and up-to-date information about the organization's plans and standards.
- The control element should be flexible enough to deal with changes in the business environment inside and outside the organization.

Without these three features—plan orientation, accuracy/currentness, and flexibility—the control element (and, consequently, the other four elements) will be weak.

Activities of Control

Except for small organizations, most health care operations have managers who specialize in performing the functions of the control element. Called controllers (or comptrollers), their role is to assist line managers, such as the food service director, with the processes of the control element. The controller is also responsible for organizing the overall control system and for gathering and distributing the information related to each process. In most health care operations, the food service director will need to implement an information system at the departmental level to supplement the information provided by the controller. Almost all managers take some part in the control process by virtue of their involvement developing plans and establishing standards.

Developing Plans

As described in chapter 5, plans identify the possible courses of action the food service department might take to achieve its goals and objectives. The types of plans that provide

241

guidance to the financial management system include both strategic and operational plans. *Strategic plans* represent the health care operation's "game plan" for optimizing achievement of goals and objectives. These plans involve the allocation of large amounts of operation resources, including those of the food service department. *Operational plans,* more specifically *policies and procedures,* specify methods and steps to be followed when dealing with the department's financial resources.

Establishing Standards

Standards can be defined as the predetermined targets against which future performance will be measured. Standards must be based, at least in part, on the formal goals of the organization. They also should be similar to the organization's objectives in that the objectives and standards for performance should all be stated in measurable terms as described in chapter 5.

Standards measure the quality and quantity of organizational output, the cost of producing that output, and the time needed to produce it. For example, food service department standards can be set for the number of trays assembled per minute, the number of meals prepared and served per labor hour, and the total meal cost per patient.

Standards for the organization and for units and departments within the organization are based on several factors. As mentioned earlier, standards should be based generally on the overall goals of the organization, which usually are identified and developed during the strategic planning process. In health care organizations, the standards set and followed by individual departments are directly affected by government regulations. In addition, most hospitals and many other health care operations in the United States voluntarily follow the standards published by the Joint Commission on Accreditation of Healthcare Organizations (JCAHO).

Essential Components of Control

The components of the control element for the financial management system of most health care food service operations include strategic plans, policies and procedures, contracts, and budgets. Each component is important in that it provides guidance for the system and specifies the standards against which the operation's performance will be compared.

Strategic Plans

The development of strategic plans was detailed in chapter 5 and only need be revisited here briefly in the context of a health care operation's financial management system. Strategic plans typically involve substantial resource allocation. The financial resources to support these plans must be either obtained from outside the food service department or redirected from internal sources. In either case, this type of plan commits the operation to a series of financial actions over an extended period of time. The ultimate results of well-conceived strategic plans are provision of goods and services that satisfy customer wants and needs *and* increased revenues and/or decreased expenses.

Policies and Procedures

Responsible financial management depends on written statements of the organization's goals and of the department's objectives, along with detailed written procedures for reaching those goals and objectives. (Developing and writing goals, objectives, and procedures was discussed in chapter 5.) Financial management policies and procedures must cover a variety of issues including record keeping, cash control, separation of duties, accounts receivable and payable, payroll, fixed assets, financial analysis tools, and various procurement issues. For a fuller discussion of these topics, refer to either Sneed and Kresse's book, *Understanding Foodservice Financial Management,* or Schmidgall's book entitled *Hospitality Industry Managerial Accounting.* Because of the critical nature of record keeping and cash control, however, and their relationship to the financial management system, a brief discussion is provided below.

Record Keeping

A system of records and reports facilitates timely documentation, evaluation, and control of departmental activities and expenses. Although many acceptable systems are available for keeping records, it is essential that record-keeping procedures be sufficiently standardized to permit comparison of the department's actual expenses with expenses allowable under the operating budget. In addition, standardized procedures are valuable for comparing the food service department's financial data with those of other departments within and outside the institution. Especially during difficult economic times, the challenge of containing costs while providing needed services requires that all health care managers place a high priority on their function as financial managers and controllers.

Cash Control

The handling of cash in the food service department requires very carefully designed procedures. Basic controls that should be incorporated into cash-handling procedures include the following:

- All cash should be collected frequently from cash registers and cashiers. Cash receipts should be deposited in a safe by a supervisor specifically charged with this responsibility.
- Cash receipts should be deposited in a bank daily.
- Cash receipts recorded on the cash register should be matched with the cash on hand at frequent, specified intervals by a person other than the cashier. (One good practice is to make unannounced audits and to withhold from the cashier the beginning and ending register readings.)
- An electronic register that provides sales data on specific items or groups of items should be used whenever possible. Because of their greater capacity for providing information for analysis and control, electronic registers are especially useful for large food service operations.
- Catering income should be controlled through appropriate documentation of orders and charges, along with proper handling of receipts.

Revenue from all sources must be accounted for by using reporting techniques approved by the health care operation.

Contracts

A contract is a control document that describes the terms of an agreement between two (or more) parties. Most health care operations specify who within the organization is authorized to enter into a contractual agreement. Food service managers should become familiar with and carefully follow this policy.

A health care food service operation may enter into a variety of contracts. In purchasing, for example, contracts might delineate group purchasing or prime vendor agreements. Specialized service agreements may address pest control or hood cleaning and maintenance by outside firms. Unions that represent food service employees require contracts that specify the terms under which employees will work. Finally, some health care operations contract a portion or all of the services related to food and nutrition care to contract management companies. Each type of contract affects the food service department's financial management system.

Budgets

One essential part of the control element is the plan that dictates how the organization's financial resources will be allocated to units or departments within the organization. The financial resources of a health care operation include cash on hand, supply inventories, the value of property and equipment owned, investments, and the expected earned revenue from current business activities. The *budget* is the organization's primary tool for this purpose and is the foundation of most control elements.

Financial management relies on the development and use of one or more budgets that estimate the organization's proposed expenses for a given financial period and its proposed means for meeting those expenses. Budgets are almost always based on dollar values. Non-monetary budgets are expressed in nonfinancial terms; for example, labor hours or units of output. Budgets provide managers with the basis for allocating resources, setting standards, evaluating performance, and controlling costs.

Types of Budgets

Most health care operations have four types of budgets. The *operating budget* forecasts the level of service to be provided and projects the costs necessary to support this level of service. The *capital budget* finances major improvements or purchases—for example, physical facilities, equipment, or property—during the period covered by the budget. The *cash budget* represents management's best estimate of cash income and cash expenditures (or outlays) over a specified period. The purpose of the cash budget is to ensure that the organization will have enough cash to meet its financial obligations when they come due. The operating budget for the food service department is only part of the institution's overall operating budget. Other department-level managers submit budgets for their departments, and top-level managers prepare a final budget called a *master budget* for the whole operation. Often a facility's financial controller coordinates the budget preparation process among department heads and top-level managers to make sure that the final budget reflects the operation's established goals.

All of these budgets are used by top-level managers in health care institutions, although the operating and capital budgets are the most important ones in the financial management of a food service department. The operating budget describes the organization's or department's plan for operations during a specified period of time—usually a fiscal year, or a period of 12 months used for accounting purposes that does not necessarily coincide with the calendar year. The operating budget includes forecasts of both revenues and expenses. The revenue budget shows all income from normal operations that can be expected for the upcoming fiscal year. Similarly, the expense budget shows all anticipated expenses for the fiscal year. Often the revenue and expense budgets are combined on one form.

The operating budget is more than an operating plan for the upcoming year in that it also provides a standard for comparing actual performance with performance forecasts. This comparison is key to the feedback element.

The annual operating budget for the food service department works as a financial plan for allocation of the department's resources, which include labor, food, supplies, and equipment. The budget also serves as an organizational plan for meeting the department's objectives and representing a forecast of the department's activities for the upcoming year; for example, the number of meals to be served, the number of nutrition assessments to be performed, and the number of patient visits to be made. In preparing for these anticipated activities, the food service director draws up employee work schedules, purchases food and supplies, and arranges for the preparation of foods to meet the anticipated demand for specific menu items. As will be discussed later in this chapter, the annual operating budget is also used by the food service director as the primary feedback tool to evaluate department operations.

Budget Planning and Preparation

Generally, the process of budget preparation and approval in most organizations follows certain prescribed steps. In health care operations, these are as follows:

1. Department or operating unit directors prepare estimates of revenues and expenses for the upcoming fiscal year and develop budget proposals based on those estimates.
2. The directors submit their budget proposals to their division heads for approval. Each division head may or may not require the director to revise the proposed budget.
3. The division head combines the proposals from various reporting directors. For example, in some large hospitals, the food service director receives proposed budgets from the assistant director for nutrition care services and the assistant director for food

production. In this case, the director combines the proposals to prepare an overall budget for food and nutrition services.

4. Each division's proposed budget is submitted to a top-level manager such as the chief executive officer (CEO) or the chief financial officer (CFO). The proposals are submitted to a budget committee of top-level managers, including the CEO and the CFO.
5. Either the top-level manager or the budget committee reviews each department's proposal, corrects any inconsistencies, and deletes any duplicate information.
6. The controller or CFO evaluates the combined proposed budget and prepares the final budget for the organization.
7. The CEO examines the final budget and approves it or requests further revisions.
8. The board of directors reviews and approves the final budget.
9. The final budget is communicated to the various department and operating unit managers throughout the organization.

The degree of the department manager's responsibility and authority in budget preparation varies with the size and type of health care operation. However, almost all food service directors are responsible for preparing proposed operating budgets. The basic steps in this preparation process are as follows:

1. Set a timetable for the budget preparation process.
2. Examine the department's objectives for the upcoming fiscal year.
3. Analyze the financial feasibility of departmental objectives.
4. Obtain information from members of the food service staff on factors that may affect the upcoming budget—for example, current food and supply costs.
5. Review historical data on units of service (meals served, nutrition assessments made, and so forth) and costs from previous years.
6. Estimate the number of units of service for the upcoming fiscal year.
7. Estimate operating expenses for the upcoming fiscal year.
8. Determine statistical indicators for the upcoming fiscal year.
9. Calculate productivity indicators for the upcoming fiscal year.
10. Prepare a proposed operating budget that shows all financial information required for the upcoming year's financial planning and control.

In setting a timetable for budget preparation (step 1), the food service director must devise a timetable for budget planning activities that corresponds to the operation's overall timetable as determined by the CFO. Adequate time should allow for considering and formulating operational decisions that will affect the financial health of the food service department and the operation as a whole. A budget developed under a time pressure may not be accurate or insightful enough to adequately guide operational decisions for the upcoming year.

Examining the department's objectives for the upcoming fiscal year (step 2) must be undertaken before the operating budget can be planned, prepared, and submitted for approval. Furthermore, clear and specific objectives covering the extent and quality of service to be provided must have been established. Setting goals and objectives is an important part of the planning process that must be performed before control activities (such as budget preparation) start.

Departmental objectives must be compatible with, and contribute to, the health care operation's goals and the objectives of the other departments within the operation. For example, if the health care operation's goals were to expand outpatient services and to extend community services, then the food service department would need to plan for providing meals and developing appropriate educational programs for outpatients.

In analyzing the financial feasibility of objectives (step 3), the director should consider conducting specific programs and offering specific services identified in the department's objectives. The food service director must analyze the objectives in terms of departmental and institutional financial limitations. The resources needed to provide such services and the costs associated with each service eventually must be allocated to appropriate areas in the operating budget. If the potential revenues to be gained from the planned services are lower than the anticipated costs of supplying the services, the director must reexamine the department's objectives or identify additional sources of financial support for the services before an operating budget can be proposed.

When obtaining information from the food service staff (step 4), the director should ask for specific information on food service operations from appropriate staff members who may have insight on costs related to labor, food, supplies, equipment, and other related costs. Staff also may be able to provide valuable information on potential increases or decreases in the number of units of service forecast for various units within the department (for example, the employee cafeteria).

Reviewing historical data, step 5 of the budget preparation process, involves the director in performing the vital function of reviewing data on the department's past performance. Most operating budgets are based on the preceding fiscal year's operating budget, a practice called *incremental budgeting*. Changes in the business environment and the country's economic environment, the preceding year's performance, and proposed changes in service are incorporated into the former budget to arrive at a new proposed budget. To arrive at accurate forecasts of future activities and projected costs, the historical data used in budget preparation must be reliable.

There are two exceptions to the practice of basing upcoming budgets solely on the preceding year's budget. The first approach, *flexible budgeting,* is developed for various levels of activity or service. In a fixed budget, estimated revenues and expenses are estimated based on one level of service, generally expressed as patient days and outpatient visits. The flexible budget, in contrast, is usually prepared for levels of service at both higher and lower levels than the original estimate. The levels commonly reflected in flexible budgets are 90, 100, and 110 percent of the estimated level of service. Although this budgeting approach requires more preparation and maintenance time, it enables the food service manager to adjust expenditures in relation to actual levels of service.

The second budgeting approach, which disregards the previous year's budget completely, is referred to as *zero-based budgeting,* also called *project-based budgeting.* Zero-based budgets require justification for each type of expenditure. Although a detailed discussion of this budgeting system is beyond the scope of this manual, it is relevant to note that some health care operations have adopted this budgetary system. In the *Handbook for Health Care Food Service Management,* Faisal A. Kaud discusses in detail the preparation of project-based budgets.

In step 6, estimating number of units of service, after the preliminary gathering and analysis of background data have been completed, the food service director should be ready to start the process of making actual estimates of how many units of service the department will be expected to provide during the upcoming year. The number of patient days (for inpatients) expected by the health care operation determines the number of patient meals the department will need to serve. In an operation that provides outpatient services, the number of clinic visits determines the level of activity in the outpatient nutrition program. Obviously, this information on the expected volume of service, usually provided by the finance department, directly affects the department's expense estimates.

Step 7 in budget preparation, estimating operating expenses, involves projecting operating expenses for the upcoming fiscal year. Operating expenses, which are based directly on the number of service units projected, include expenses for staff salaries and benefits, food and supplies, and other unit-of-service-based costs. Other expenses include expenses for office supplies, menus, laundry, maintenance, telephone service, depreciation of equipment, and so forth.

When determining statistical indicators (step 8), the food service director calculates various statistical indicators and the unit costs per meal. Salary and benefit expenses per meal, food expenses per meal, supply expenses per meal, and other expenses per meal are determined. Total operating expenses per meal, net cost per meal, and net cost per patient day also are calculated.

Step 9, calculating productivity indicators, involves the calculation of productivity indicators for the upcoming fiscal year. Productivity indicators demonstrate the number of meals served per hour paid to the employee as well as the number of meals served per hour worked by the employee (the first indicator takes into account actual costs for vacation days, sick days, and holidays). The number of meals served per patient day is also an indicator of the food service department's productivity.

In the final step of budget preparation, preparing the proposed operating budget, the food service director uses all the financial information gathered in the nine preceding steps to prepare a formal operating budget proposal. The following data are needed to complete the food service department's operating budget:

- Forecast numbers of patient days and outpatient clinic visits
- Forecast numbers of patient meals, cafeteria meals, stipend meals, meals for special functions, and other nonpatient meals
- Total wage, salary, and benefit expenses for food service employees
- Total expenses for patient and nonpatient meals
- Total supply expenses
- Total of all other direct expenses

After the proposed budget has been approved by the organization's top-level managers, the budget will serve as an invaluable tool in the ongoing management of the department's performance. Figure 11-2 shows a section of an annual operating budget for a food service department.

The main objective in preparing an operating budget is to formulate a carefully delineated plan for making management decisions and controlling the department's activities throughout the upcoming year. For this reason, the annual budget is broken down into 12 monthly schedules. Having an operating budget that shows monthly estimates of units of service and expenses allows the food service director to identify financial problems as they come up. In addition, the director can maintain an accurate record of the department's actual performance for monthly comparisons with the budgeted forecasts of its performance. Monthly budget review also allows the director to determine whether the department's objectives are being met and, if not, to take corrective action.

Capital budgeting is the process of planning for major expenditures, called *capital expenditures*. Health care operations define the criteria that must be met for an item to be classified as a capital expenditure. Generally, these criteria specify that the item is not consumable and that the cost level and usable time period of the item are defined. Capital expenditures include new or replacement equipment or furnishings, renovation projects, and the purchase of new facilities.

Unlike operating budgets, which generally deal with the next 12-month period, capital budgets are prepared for multiple-year periods, up to five years. According to Sneed and Kresse (1989), the following information must be provided by the food service director for each capital expenditure:

- Description of the item requested
- Indication of whether the item is new, a replacement, or an improvement
- Unit cost of the item
- Total costs for the request
- Justification for the expenditure
- Salvage value of the item, if applicable
- Indication of whether the request is urgent, essential, economically desirable, or generally desirable

The decision about capital expenditures is made based on the results of a variety of capital investment analysis techniques. (These techniques are discussed in *Understanding Food-service Financial Management* by Sneed and Kresse.)

247

Figure 11-2. Excerpt from Annual Food Service Department Operating Budget

	January Total			February Total			Annual Total		
	Patient	Nonpatient	Total	Patient	Nonpatient	Total	Patient	Nonpatient	Total
1. Patient Days									
2. Patient days	2,250		2,250	2,050		2,050	27,500		27,500
3. Clinic visits		4,000	4,000		4,100	4,100		50,000	50,000
4. Meal Count									
5. Patient meals	6,300		6,300	5,740		5,740	77,000		77,000
6. Cafeteria meals		3,500	3,500		3,250	3,250		40,975	40,975
7. Stipend meals		500	500		475	475		6,650	6,650
8. Special-function meals		750	750		700	700		9,000	9,000
9. Other meals		0	0		0	0		0	0
10. Total meals	6,300	4,750	11,050	5,740	4,425	10,165	77,000	56,625	133,625
11. Operating Expenses									
12. Salary and benefit expenses	$6,010	$2,563	$8,573	$5,476	$2,387	$7,863	$73,458	$30,550	$104,008
13. Food expenses	6,151	4,145	10,296	5,604	3,861	9,465	75,175	49,411	124,586
14. Supply expenses	901	669	1,570	821	623	1,444	11,011	7,973	18,984
15. Other expenses	392	161	553	358	150	508	4,797	1,920	6,717
16. Total operating expenses	$13,454	$7,538	$20,992	$12,259	$7,021	$19,280	$164,441	$89,854	$254,295
17. Less: cash receipts	0	8,000	8,000	0	7,400	7,400	0	95,750	95,750
18. Net dietary expenses	$13,454	$(462)	$12,992	$12,259	$(379)	$11,880	$164,441	$(5,896)	$158,545
19. Statistical Indicators/Unit Cost per Meal									
20. Salary and benefit expenses	$0.9540	$0.5396	$0.7758	$0.9540	$0.5394	$0.7735	$0.9540	$0.5395	$0.7784
21. Food expenses	0.9763	0.8726	0.9318	0.9763	0.8726	0.9311	0.9763	0.8726	0.9324
22. Supply expenses	0.1430	0.1408	0.1421	0.1430	0.1408	0.1421	0.1430	0.1408	0.1421
23. Other expenses	0.0623	0.0339	0.0500	0.0624	0.0339	0.0500	0.0623	0.0339	0.0503
24. Total operating expenses	$2.1356	$1.5869	$1.8997	$2.1357	$1.5867	$1.8967	$2.1356	$1.5868	$1.9032
25. Less: cash receipts	0	1.6842	0.7240	0	1.6723	0.7280	0	1.6909	0.7166
26. Net cost per meal	$2.1356	$(0.0973)	$1.1757	$2.1357	$(0.0856)	$1.1687	$2.1356	$(0.1041)	$1.1865
27. Net cost per patient day	$5.98		$5.77	$5.98		$5.80	$5.98		$5.70
28. Productivity Indicators									
29. Meals per hour—paid	5.00	8.80	6.14	4.97	8.30	6.02	4.97	8.78	6.09
30. Meals per hour—worked	4.03	7.09	4.95	4.01	6.69	4.85	4.01	7.08	4.91
31. Meals per patient day	2.8		2.8	2.8		2.8	2.8		

Relationship of Control Element to Other System Elements

As indicated earlier, components of the control element are usually developed or reviewed annually, and the remaining four elements of the financial management system are affected by the plans and standards of the control element. Functions of the input, processing, output, and feedback elements occur during the course of the operation's accounting period, usually on a monthly basis. The first three elements (inputs, processing, and outputs) are necessary to carry out the financial accounting aspect of financial management. These elements will be discussed in the following sections in relation to the typical accounting cycle of a health care food service operation.

☐ Input Element

The input element includes the basic data that are available to be converted by the processing element, primarily by means of accounting cycle functions, to produce outputs of the system. Outputs of the financial management system are usually in the form of reports. Therefore, the type of reports needed by the food service manager for financial management purposes determines the type of data that must be collected.

Characteristics of Input

The quality of reports generated by the financial management system is directly related to the quality of data used in their preparation. Therefore, the food service manager must develop methods for data collection that ensure data accuracy.

Essential Components of Input

Several kinds of data must be compiled and recorded on a daily, weekly, or monthly basis by the food service department. As mentioned, these data usually are in the form of source documents and are used as the basis for the department's period ending reports. The four categories of data—revenue data, expense data, balance sheet data, and statistical data—are discussed below.

Revenue Data

Revenues are payments received by the food service operation for providing services to patients and nonpatients. Chargeable and/or reimbursable patient services provided by the department were identified in chapter 9. The methods for collecting and reporting these data must be coordinated with the health care operation's patient charge system. An example of a source document for patient revenue is shown in figure 11-3.

Nonpatient revenues usually come in the form of cash receipts or sales on account. The majority of cash receipts are composed of cafeteria sales and sales from vending machine operations. Sales on account include charges for catering special events and for stocking food and beverages at various locations in the health care operation.

Effective mechanisms must be developed for collecting and documenting data about each class of nonpatient revenue produced by the department. For example, data about cafeteria revenue are usually documented by a cashier's report, which is produced either manually or by a computerized point-of-sale (POS) cash register system. The amount of data provided by the cashier's report varies but at a minimum should include the number of customers served, total sales, and appropriate sales tax data. (See figure 11-4.) Typical source documents for sales on account include catering meal counts and charge records.

Expense Data

Most health care food service operations classify their direct expenses in four categories: food, labor, supply, and other costs. In some cases, indirect expenses are also allocated to

249

Figure 11-3. Patient Revenue Source Document

ABC FOODSERVICE DEPARTMENT
FROZEN MEAL REVENUE REPORT
FOR THE MONTH OF: JULY

ITEM DESCRIPTION	… 30	31	TOTAL COUNT	ITEM COST	SELLING PRICE	GROSS MARGIN	% GROSS REVENUE	ITEM REVENUE	GROSS REVENUE
MACARONI IN CHEESE SAUCE	1	1	27	$2.30	$2.75	$0.45	5.34%	$74.25	$12.15
SPAGHETI AND MEATBALLS	3		42	$2.90	$3.30	$0.40	7.38%	$138.60	$16.80
LASAGNA WITH MEAT SAUCE		4	46	$3.10	$3.60	$0.50	10.11%	$165.60	$23.00
SWEDISH MEATBALLS	2	4	24	$3.12	$3.60	$0.48	5.06%	$86.40	$11.52
CHEESE MANICOTTI	2		24	$3.14	$3.65	$0.51	5.38%	$87.60	$12.24
BEEF STROGANOFF	3		52	$3.22	$3.70	$0.48	10.97%	$192.40	$24.96
SALISBURY STEAK	2		36	$3.34	$3.80	$0.46	7.28%	$136.80	$16.56
BEEF POT ROAST	2	2	41	$3.40	$3.85	$0.45	8.11%	$157.85	$18.45
CHICKEN IN BARBECUE SAUCE			31	$3.49	$3.90	$0.41	5.59%	$120.90	$12.71
CHICKEN IN DIJON SAUCE	2		45	$3.53	$3.95	$0.42	8.31%	$177.75	$18.90
TURKEY TETRAZZINI		4	38	$3.61	$4.00	$0.39	6.51%	$152.00	$14.82
VEAL & BEEF PARMIGIANA	2	3	31	$3.63	$4.00	$0.37	5.04%	$124.00	$11.47
SEAFOOD NEWBURG		2	22	$3.78	$4.15	$0.37	3.58%	$91.30	$8.14
STUFFED FILLET OF SOLE		3	28	$3.92	$4.30	$0.38	4.68%	$120.40	$10.64
CHICKEN NEW ENGLAND	2		40	$4.12	$4.50	$0.38	6.68%	$180.00	$15.20
TOTAL	25	23	527				100.00%	$2,005.85	$227.56

	ITEM REVENUE	GROSS REVENUE
BUDGET	$1,750.00	$210.00
VARIANCE	$255.85	$17.56
% VARIANCE	14.62%	8.36%

Figure 11-4. Cashier's Report

Cashier: _____ Date: _____

1. Ending reading: _____

2. Beginning reading: _____

3. Total sales + tax: _____

4. Less charge sales: _____

5. Subtotal: _____

6. Less overrings: _____

7. Total cash sales: _____

8. Actual cash turn-in: _____

9. Cash (+) over; (−) under _____

10. Receipt number: _____

11. Cash turned in:

    Currency: $ 1 _____

                $ 5 _____

                $ 10 _____

                $ 20 _____

    Coin: _____

    Other: _____

    Subtotal: _____

    Less cash bank: _____

    Total: _____

    Verified by: _____

    Business office cashier: _____

the department. As is true for revenue data, methods for documenting each class of expense data must be implemented.

Food Cost Data

Purchasing, food issues, and transfer records are used to document food costs. Purchasing transactions are usually documented by means of invoices that accompany deliveries or by bills issued by the vendor. The actual food issued to the production units of the food service department can be documented by means of requisitions prepared by production employees or produced by computerized systems. Other aspects of food costs that should not be overlooked are the cost of food transferred to patient floors and other units of the operation. A count of all food items transferred should be recorded on a form similar to the one illustrated in figure 11-5. Systems must be developed so that food cost source documents can be collected and made available to the processing elements of the financial management system.

Figure 11-5. Food Transfers

ABC FOODSERVICE DEPARTMENT
NOURISHMENT COST REPORT   1NW   ACCT: 1626
FOR THE MONTH OF: JULY   PATIENT DAYS: 825

ITEM DESCRIPTION	ITEM COST	1	2	3	4	5	6	7	25	26	27	28	29	30	31	TOTAL COUNT	TOTAL COST
APPLE JUICE	$0.14	14	15	15	10	10	10	10	14	14	10	10	10	10	8	359	$50.26
CRANBERRY JUICE	$0.34	10							10					6		81	$27.54
GRAPEFRUIT JUICE	$0.14	14	4	4	10	10			14	10	10	10	10		10	251	$35.14
PINEAPPLE JUICE	$0.29															0	$0.00
PRUNE JUICE	$0.34						6		10					10		36	$12.24
TOMATO JUICE	$0.21															0	$0.00
NECTARS	$0.33															0	$0.00
ORANGE JUICE	$0.14								5							5	$0.70
ORANGE JUICE (QT)	$1.10	3	4	2	3	3	2		3	3	3	3	2	2		67	$73.70
GATORADE	$1.13															0	$0.00
COKE	$0.35	6		6					12							62	$21.70
DIET COKE	$0.35															0	$0.00
TAB	$0.35															0	$0.00
SEVEN UP	$0.35	3							2			6		2	4	32	$11.20
DIET SEVEN UP	$0.33															0	$0.00
DR. PEPPER	$0.35										6					6	$2.10
DIET DR. PEPPER	$0.35															0	$0.00
GINGERALE	$0.35															0	$0.00
SKIM MILK	$0.15															0	$0.00
WHOLE MILK	$0.15	10							10		10	10	6	6	3	146	$21.90
CHOCOLATE MILK	$0.15														3	3	$0.45
BUTTERMILK	$0.15															0	$0.00
ICE CREAM	$0.12		6										6			23	$2.76

TOTAL NOURISHMENT COST :	$259.69
NOURISHMENT COST/PD :	$0.31
BUDGET :	$0.26
VARIANCE :	$0.05

Labor Cost Data

Payroll records are a convenient source of data on labor costs. The hours worked and the costs associated with the work are usually documented by a time card system. Smaller operations may still use manual systems, in which case the department is involved in collecting labor cost data. However, this is one of the most commonly computerized functions in health care operations. With these types of systems, the food service manager may merely need to review the data that will be used by the payroll system to determine labor costs. In addition to the costs of wages and salaries, the cost of providing benefits, both optional and required by law, must also be determined.

Supply Cost Data

Supplies include dishware, glassware, serviceware, kitchen utensils, disposable paper products, cleaning compounds and equipment, printed forms and other office supplies, and small equipment. Procedures for documenting costs for such supplies are the same as those for food supply documentation. Invoices documenting purchases are the most common type of source document used by the processing element to determine supply costs.

Other Direct Cost Data

Most food service operations incur costs for products and services that do not fall in the categories of costs discussed previously. Examples include repairs and maintenance, laundry services, pest control, telephone, and postage. These costs can be traced directly back to the food service department based on the existence of a variety of source documents.

Allocated Cost Data

The final category of costs are those generated by the health care operation and/or food service department but for which no source document exists. For instance, the food service department is usually one of the largest consumers of energy. However, unless the department has separate utility meters, the cost data for energy are not available and cannot be collected. These costs may be allocated to the various departments in the operation. (This practice is discussed in the section on the processing element.)

Balance Sheet Data

A *balance sheet* is a financial report that illustrates the food service operation's financial condition on a particular date. It shows what the operation's assets are and how they are balanced against its liabilities. Assets include all items owned by the organization that have financial value. These items include actual cash on hand, accounts receivable, the value of inventory and supplies, and so forth. Liabilities, the opposite of assets, include the organization's current operating expenses as well as its long-term debt.

Because the balance sheet may not be as valuable to a department manager as the revenue expense statement, it may not be generated on a routine basis by the operating departments. However, when it is generated, the required asset data include cash on hand, beginning inventory, accounts receivable, value of equipment and furnishings, and accumulated depreciation. Data about the operation's liabilities include accounts payable, wages payable, and taxes payable. These data are used by the processing element to generate the balance sheet.

Statistical Data

Statistical data are necessary for the production of nonfinancial reports, which are components of the output of the financial management system that generally focus on the food service operation's productivity. *Productivity* can be defined as the relationship of the amount of resources used to the amount of products or services produced, or the relationship between inputs and outputs of the food service department. Overall, productivity is a valuable index of the department's efficiency and performance. To determine the department's level of productivity, labor hours data (the input) and volume of service data (the output) must be provided.

Labor Hours Data

As mentioned earlier, the same system that provides labor cost data usually is capable of providing data about the labor hours that were paid for by the department during a specific period. The system must be capable of providing data about regular productive hours, overtime, and nonproductive hours (hours paid but not worked as in the case of holiday or sick pay). These data are either provided by means of a time card system or tracked by a computerized system. Regardless of the method used, labor hours data are a necessary input so that further analysis of the department's productivity can be performed.

Volume of Service Data

All health care operations should keep a daily record of the volume of services provided to customers. This includes a count of the number of meals served to patients and nonpatients. The most accurate method of collecting volume data is to count the number of trays prepared for each meal and to keep a record of the total number counted for each day. (See figure 11-6.)

The nonpatient meal count can be broken down into subcounts, such as meals for staff members, meals for employees, meals for special functions, catered meals, and so forth. The methods used for determining the number of nonpatient meals served each day vary among operations, depending on whether an operation follows a cash payment system or whether employees purchase monthly meal tickets. Stipend meals (meals provided free of charge to special groups, for example, interns) also are taken into account. A common method for determining the number of nonpatient meals requires the operation to track and report total cash sales (the method is described in the processing section of this chapter).

☐ Processing Element

All the actions necessary to convert inputs (the data collected during the accounting period) into outputs are included in the processing element which, as discussed in this manual, focuses on the processes of managerial accounting. Although the function of financial accounting to provide historical information according to strict accounting procedures is important, usually this function is the responsibility of the accounting department. The food service director is more likely to need and use information that results from managerial accounting processes. This approach to accounting focuses on providing information upon which future decisions may be made. Although both approaches to accounting generally use the same data, managerial accounting is much more flexible in its approach to the handling and processing of data than is the structured approach of financial accounting.

Characteristics of Processing

The processing element of a food service operation may be simple or complex, depending on the amount of specific information required. However, this element must produce accurate and timely reports. To accomplish this objective, the actions of this element must be based on standardized managerial accounting procedures as defined by the operation, so that the information from the food service department's reports can be compared to current and future performance.

Although manual systems can be designed to provide basic information, this is best accomplished on either a full-featured computer system or a specific type of generic software such as an electronic spreadsheet. Accuracy of information can be increased and the time required to process data decreased with computerized systems. In addition, once data are entered, they are available to be used in an infinite number of reports.

Activities of Processing

Three classes of data (revenue, expense, and statistical) must first be processed by means of journalizing, a process that records each transaction in the journal designated for that specific

Figure 11-6. Daily Meal Census

Department of Nutrition and Food Services
Daily Meal Count
Month of _____

Date	Patient Meals				Guest trays	Cafeteria Meals			Special Function	Totals
	C	Tray line	Late trays	Totals		B	L	D		
01										
02										
03										
04										
05										
06										
07										
08										
09										
10										
11										
12										
13										
14										
15										
16										
17										
18										
19										
20										
21										
22										
23										
24										
25										
26										
27										
28										
29										
30										
31										
Total:										

class of data. At the end of the accounting period, each journal must be totaled and the information recorded in the appropriate ledger. The final process, making adjustments, includes the end of period mathematical matching of revenues and expenses, recording changes in balances of assets and liabilities, and calculating and matching statistical information such as labor hours and volume of services.

Essential Components of Processing

Financial management requires that revenues, expenses, and operating statistics be recorded and analyzed on a regular basis throughout the fiscal period. These factors should be reported on a monthly operating statement (described in the output section of this chapter) that summarizes the cost of providing services to patients and other customers. Journalizing, posting, and making adjustments are the processes by which this is accomplished.

Journalizing

Journalizing is the process of recording in chronological order each activity or transaction that occurs during an accounting period. Data about each activity should be recorded in the appropriate transaction journal. Transaction journals consist of either manual worksheets or electronic spreadsheets designed for a specific type of data. The transaction journals typically maintained by a health care food service operation to record revenues include a cash receipts journal and a sales journal. In general, expenses are recorded in purchase registers, and operating statistics are recorded in journals reserved for labor hours and volume of service. A departmental payroll journal is optional based on whether this function is centralized for the entire health care operation.

Revenue Journals

Revenue generated by the food service department generally results in the collection of cash from the customer at the point of service or charges made to the customer. The amount of cash collected and its source (patients, nonpatients, staff, and so on) should be recorded in the cash receipts journal. For example, the amount of daily cafeteria and vending sales should be recorded separately based on appropriate source documents. Source documents for other types of cash transactions should be collected and recorded by type of transaction in the cash receipts journal. This separation by type of transaction allows the food service manager to monitor not only cash sales but also the level of cash generated by each type of service.

A record should be made in the sales journal of any sales transaction for which the customer will be billed. Again, the specific source of this type of revenue should be identified to allow for tracking and analysis.

Expense Journals

Expenses of the food service operation are generally composed of consumables such as food and supplies, services that are generally classified as other expenses, and labor. The purpose of the purchase register is to monitor all purchases for food, supplies, and other expenses purchased on account. In addition to recording total costs, it is advisable to break down food costs into categories according to food group such as meat, fish, poultry, and eggs; dairy products; frozen goods; fresh produce; bakery goods; groceries; and beverages. (See figure 11-7.) Supply costs also might be kept and information reported by type of commodity, such as paper supplies and cleaning supplies. Cost breakdowns such as these enable the manager, during the course of the feedback processes, to further scrutinize costs for month-to-month fluctuations that may require corrective action.

Sometimes it is desirable to calculate food costs more frequently than once a month. If day-to-day figures are needed, the form shown in figure 11-8 can be prepared manually or generated by an electronic spreadsheet. However, the value of these data should be considered in relation to the time and effort required to record and report them. Also taken into account

Figure 11-7. Food Purchases Register

ABC FOODSERVICE DEPARTMENT
FOOD PURCHASES REGISTER   SUPPLIER: XYZ QUALITY FOODS
FOR THE MONTH OF: JULY

INVOICE DATE	INVOICE NUMBER	MEAT/FISH POULTRY	FROZEN	PRODUCE	EGG/MILK DAIRY	BAKERY	GROCERY	BEVERAGE	INVOICE TOTAL
7-02-89	32448	$185.97					$606.70		$792.67
7-08-89	32575	$93.79	$156.12				$274.05		$523.96
7-11-89	32560						$238.98		$238.98
7-16-89	32507					$674.86	$248.12		$922.98
7-23-89	32542	$201.31					$218.41		$419.72
7-30-89	32634		$104.21				$249.26		$353.47
VENDOR CATEGORY TOTAL		$481.07	$260.33	$0.00	$0.00	$674.86	$1,835.52	$0.00	$3,251.78
TOT PURCH/CATEGORY		$25,997.00	$8,092.00	$5,450.00	$10,912.00	$1,592.00	$20,705.00	$5,705.00	$78,453.00
% OF TOT PURCH/CATEGORY		1.85%	3.22%	0.00%	0.00%	42.39%	8.87%	0.00%	4.14%

Figure 11-8. Form for Calculating Daily Food Costs (by Month)

DAILY FOOD COSTS								
					Month: _____ Year: _____			
	Total Purchases				**Issues from Storeroom**	**Net Food Cost**		
						Today	**To Date**	
Day **(1)**	**To Kitchen** **(2)**	**To Storeroom** **(3)**	**Cost Today** **(4)**	**Cost to Date** **(5)**	**(6)**	**(2 + 6)** **(7)**	**Actual** **(8)**	**Budgeted** **(9)**
1								
2								
3								
4								
5								
6								
7								
8								
9								
10								
11								
12								
13								
14								
15								
16								
17								
18								
19								
20								
⋮								
31								
Total								

is the fact that daily cost calculations are even less accurate than weekly or monthly cost figures because of variations in purchasing and use patterns. However, the daily food cost record does reflect the approximate cost per day. In addition, it provides data for calculating monthly total purchase and cost figures during the posting process. Computer-assisted inventory and accounting systems can provide weekly or even daily food cost data with relative ease and at reasonable expense.

If the payroll system is unable to provide departmental labor cost data, a form such as the one illustrated in figure 11-9 can be used. In some cases, operations may prefer reporting by week or by pay period. Either alternative reporting period offers the advantage of supplying data based on a fixed number of days, thus simplifying the comparison of costs. However, monthly reporting has the advantage of relating labor costs to other expenses reported and summarized by the month.

Statistical Journals

Operating statistical journals contain a listing of the daily transactions related to both labor hours used and volume of services delivered. The form shown in figure 11-9 not only provides for tracking labor costs, it also provides a convenient record for tracking regular productive and overtime hours worked (both are necessary for productivity calculations). In addition, this form can be used to track sick days taken and vacation days and holidays used. Such a form can be implemented by departments with both manual and computerized operations.

After the labor hours (inputs of the system) have been recorded in the operating statistical journal, volume of services (outputs of the system) must be recorded. As with the revenue journals, entries should be classified and recorded according to type of service.

Posting

At the end of the accounting period, the transactions recorded in the journals must be summarized, a process usually accomplished by totaling the transactions for each journal maintained by the operation. For manual financial management systems, this involves adding up all transactions to determine the total for a journal. If the journal has been maintained on an electronic spreadsheet, the total is available as soon as the last entry has been completed.

Each revenue, expense, and statistical journal must be summarized as described above. For instance, the cash revenue generated by the operation during the accounting period is determined by adding up all the cash revenue–producing transactions that have been recorded in the cash receipts journal. The total cost of food purchases for the month can be calculated by adding up all food purchasing transactions, based on invoices from suppliers, during the accounting period. The two journals for operating statistics (labor hours and volume of services) also must be summarized similarly. At the end of this process, the transaction journal totals are transferred to the *general ledger,* which contains a separate section for each type of transaction monitored by the operation.

Making Adjustments

The final step in the processing element is making adjustments to the general ledger entries. This step is necessary primarily to match the expenses that were necessary to generate the revenues during the accounting period. The types of end-of-period adjusting entries made by health care food service operations include:

- Food inventory adjustments
- Supply inventory adjustments
- Labor cost adjustments
- Allocation for indirect costs
- Depreciation adjustments
- Meal equivalent calculations
- Full-time equivalent (FTE) calculations

Figure 11-9. Labor Cost Analysis Form

LABOR TIME AND COST RECORD

Date: _____
Number of Working Days: _____

Employee Classification and Number	Total Hours					Total Pay ($)			
	Productive[a]		Nonproductive[b]			Productive		Nonproductive	Fringe Benefits[c]
	Regular	Overtime	Sick	Vacation	Holiday	Regular	Overtime		
Tray-Line Employees (701)									
Smith	112	11	8		8	346.00	53.00	52.00	91.00
Johnson	104	–	4		8	338.00	–	39.00	84.50
...									
First Cook (900)									
Jensen	160	–	–	12	–	880.00	–	66.00	220.00
Monthly Total									
Daily Average									

[a]Productive hours are those hours worked, including overtime.
[b]Nonproductive hours are hours paid (sick, vacation, holiday, and so on) but not worked.
[c]Fringe benefits vary from 10 to 34 percent of total pay and may include unemployment insurance, other insurance (such as health, life, dental), meals, uniforms, education and recreation pay, parking fees, and employer's share of social security.

Expenses

The food inventory adjustment is necessary to determine the amount of food actually consumed (versus the amount purchased) during the month. The data needed to determine food inventory adjustments are the total cost of foods purchased during the month and the value of physical inventories at the beginning and end of the month. The following steps represent one method for calculating the total cost of food used in a month:

1. Start with the value of the beginning inventory (including food in storage and food used in the kitchen).
2. Add the total value of purchases made (the total of invoices) during the month.
3. Subtract the value of the inventory at the end of the month (total of the physical inventory and the stock in the kitchen) to arrive at the total cost of the food used during the month.

The value of kitchen inventory may be deleted from the calculation if the amount is fairly small or has high turnover, or if calculating its value is too time-consuming. Other methods for determining raw food costs can be used, but time expended as well as method accuracy should be considered. The supply cost adjustment also can be determined by calculating beginning inventory, monthly purchases, and closing inventory.

For many health care operations, the accounting period begins on the first day of the month and ends on the last day of the same month. However, many of these same operations pay their employees biweekly. In such cases where the end of the accounting periods and the end of the pay periods do not coincide, an adjustment must be made to the labor costs or salaries paid. Again, the principle is to identify the costs, in this case the labor costs, that were associated with generating revenues and providing services during the accounting period. Depending on what payroll system is in place, this may be a cumbersome task. The food service manager should work with the payroll manager to determine the best method for identifying actual labor costs for the accounting period.

As pointed out in the input section of this chapter, a number of costs are generated by health care operations that benefit the food service operation. In addition, some costs are generated by the food service department for which no source document exists—in which case an allocation of costs may be made to the department. For example, the housekeeping department may clean the various dining areas located throughout the health care operation. In such a case, no source document is available to be processed, but the costs of the housekeeping department may be distributed or allocated among the users of its services. The basis commonly used is the square footage cleaned for each user as a percentage of total square footage cleaned. If such costs are allocated to the food service department, the manager should evaluate the appropriateness of the basis for allocation.

The final adjusting entry related to expenses is for depreciation. *Depreciation* is the decrease in value of equipment and furnishings over a period of time. There is no source document for depreciation. Depreciation expense is the depreciation of equipment and furnishings for a specific accounting period. Accumulated depreciation is the total depreciation of a piece of equipment since its purchase and installation. These adjustments must be made so that the depreciation expense can be reflected on the revenue and expense statement and the accumulated depreciation total reported on the balance sheet.

Operating Statistics

As described earlier, the actual volume of services provided to customers should be tracked and recorded in the appropriate journal. In the case of patient meals, this has been described as a relatively easy process of counting the number of trays sent to patients. However, for the cafeteria, each customer, representing a single transaction, does not necessarily purchase a full meal. Therefore, a method must be developed for translating cafeteria sales.

The most appropriate method for determining the number of meals served in a cash payment cafeteria requires calculating the average selling price for a full noon meal (including meat, potato, vegetable, salad, beverage, and dessert). When a selective menu is offered, the average price of each meal component (for example, the entree, vegetable, salad, or dessert) should be used in the calculation of the average number of meals. Once the average selling price of a meal has been determined, the total cash sales can be divided by the average price per meal to determine the daily meal equivalent, or the average number of meals served per day for record-keeping purposes.

☐ Output Element

As a result of activities of the processing element, end-of-period reports are generated. This activity represents a primary function of the financial management system. These reports not only provide valuable information about current operations but also are compared to standards by the techniques available in the feedback element.

Characteristics of Output

To determine whether the standards set during the control process are being met, performance must be measured. Written reports on the department's work status and financial position are essential parts of the output element. The preparation of monthly reports ensures that standards and budgetary guidelines are followed and that the department's financial health is maintained. However, the food service manager needs to make sure that the reports are clear, concise, accurate, and complete.

Essential Components of Output

Most health care food service operations use their revenue, expense, balance sheet, and statistical data to generate four classes of end-of-period reports. These include financial statements, tax reports, operating statistics reports, and other reports that combine financial and nonfinancial information. The reports generated by the output element are utilized by both food service and upper-level management.

Financial Statements

Successful financial management requires a system of records and reports that generates financial information in the most efficient and usable way possible. Few health care operations can afford to prepare more financial records and reports than needed to keep managers informed of the operation's fiscal status. For this reason, the food service department's financial record-keeping system should concentrate on information of value for evaluating, allocating, and controlling the department's expenses.

The adjusted and extended figures developed by the processing element are used to create the operation's financial statements. Some operations may find the periodic generation of the balance sheet to be beneficial. By far the most valuable financial statement is the revenue-and-expense statement (also known as the profit-and-loss statement or income statement).

The CFO often develops monthly revenue-and-expense statements for each department. Formal revenue-and-expense statements are prepared by the operation's finance department on the basis of data supplied by the accounting department and the food service department. The report's degree of sophistication depends on whether the health care operation is for-profit or not-for-profit and on its financial policies.

Most food service directors produce their own version of the revenue-and-expense statement, which provides more detail and is available in a more timely manner. If an electronic spreadsheet is utilized, this report is available immediately following the last entry. A simple format for a monthly revenue-and-expense statement is shown in figure 11-10. (The analysis of this statement is discussed in the feedback section later in this chapter.)

Figure 11-10. Format for Monthly Revenue-and-Expense Statement

Food Revenues $ _____

Cost of Food

Purchases $ _____

Less: inventory   (_____)

Net food costs $ _____

Cost of Labor

Salaries/wages $ _____

Benefits   _____

Total labor costs $ _____

Operating Costs

Office rent $ _____

Laundry   _____

Maintenance   _____

Telephone   _____

Postage   _____

Utilities   _____

Depreciation   _____

Equipment   _____

Total operating costs $ _____

Total Expenses $ _____

Operating Profit (Loss) $ _____

(Revenues minus total expenses)

Tax Reports

As indicated in the input discussion, sales tax data should be recorded on the cashier's report. In most operations, once the cash from operations and the cashier's report are turned in to the health care operation's cashier, the food service department no longer is responsible for tracking these data. If this is not the case, the department must develop a system to support the requirements of the taxing authority. In a for-profit operation, tax reports used for income tax purposes also will be necessary as an output of the financial management system.

Operating Statistics Reports

The operating statistics report combines information about labor hours and volume of service to determine the food service department's level of productivity. Productivity can be calculated simply by dividing the amount of input by the amount of output. For example, dividing the number of labor hours worked (input) by the number of meals served (output) provides a meaningful indicator of productivity. Other productivity measures that can be provided in this type of report include:

- The number of patient trays served per patient day
- The number of labor minutes per patient meal
- The number of labor minutes per nonpatient meal equivalent
- The amount of revenue produced per full-time equivalent employee assigned to nonpatient meal service
- The number of customer transactions performed per each FTE assigned to nonpatient meal service
- The total number of food service employee work hours per patient day
- The total number of food service employee work minutes per unit of service

Other Reports

Other reports to be generated by the department vary based on the information needs of both food service and upper-level management. Usually, these types of reports do not require the collection data not already described in the input section of this chapter. The purpose of these reports is to combine critical financial and nonfinancial information. The monthly operating statement and the monthly performance report are the most common report of this type.

Monthly Operating Statements

After all individual cost categories have been determined for the month, it is helpful for the food service director to prepare a summary form that includes all important operational data for the department. The food service operating statement shown in figure 11-11 is an example of a comprehensive and useful monthly summary. Not only does it identify performance in the areas of volume of service, costs, and productivity, it also provides a means for comparing current costs against budget targets from one month to the next (as described in the feedback section of this chapter). In addition to its value to managers in the food service department, this report may be shared with appropriate facility administrators.

Monthly Performance Reports

The monthly operating statement does an excellent job of identifying the different categories of costs per meal equivalent (as calculated by the method already described). However, this figure only indicates the average cost of all meals served. The director also should be concerned with the costs per meal for each group served, patient or nonpatient. Therefore, a method is needed to allocate costs efficiently and accurately. The monthly performance report provides a mechanism for accomplishing this objective.

Figure 11-11. Sample Monthly Operating Statement

		January Total	
	Actual	Budget	Variance
1. **Patient Days**			
2. Patient days	2,192	2,250	–2.6%
3. Clinic visits	4,132	4,000	+3.3%
4. **Meal Count**			
5. Patient meals	6,136	6,300	–2.6%
6. Cafeteria meals	3,539	3,500	+1.1%
7. Stipend meals	493	500	–1.5%
8. Special-function meals	728	750	–2.9%
9. Other meals	0	0	–
10. Total meals	10,896	11,050	–1.4%
11. **Operating Expenses**			
12. Salary and benefit expenses	$ 8,839	$ 8,573	+3.1%
13. Food expenses	10,698	10,296	+3.9%
14. Supply expenses	1,606	1,570	+2.3%
15. Other expenses	533	553	–3.6%
16. Total operating expenses	$21,676	$20,992	+3.3%
17. Less: cash receipts	(8,080)	(8,000)	+1.0%
18. Net dietary expenses	$13,596	$12,992	+4.6%
19. **Statistical Indicators/Unit Cost per Meal**			
20. Salary and benefit expenses	$0.81	$0.78	+4.6%
21. Food expenses	0.98	0.93	+5.7%
22. Supply expenses	0.15	0.14	+6.2%
23. Other expenses	0.05	0.05	–
24. Total operating expenses	$1.99	$1.90	+4.9%
25. Less: cash receipts	(0.74)	(0.72)	+2.7%
26. Net cost per meal	$1.25	$1.18	+6.3%
27. Net cost per patient day	$6.20	$5.77	+7.4%
28. **Productivity Indicators**			
29. Meals per hour–paid	5.88	6.14	–4.3%
30. Meals per hour–worked	4.74	4.95	–4.2%
31. Meals per patient day	2.83	2.80	+1.2%

The monthly performance report shown in figure 11-12 incorporates the American Society for Hospital Food Service Administrators (ASHFSA) system for allocating costs to patient and nonpatient activities. The first step is to allocate any costs that can be directly linked to either patient or nonpatient services. For example, some employees spend their work time exclusively in the nonpatient areas; therefore, their labor costs would be attributed to nonpatient services.

The remaining costs should be allocated based on patient and nonpatient meal count information. A ratio of the two types of meals served should be determined and the costs assigned accordingly. For example, if 60 percent of the meals prepared by the department are served to nonpatients, 60 percent of the food costs should be allocated to nonpatient services. If cost allocations have been made properly, the true costs of patient and nonpatient meals will be indicated on the monthly performance report. Further analysis of this report will be discussed in the feedback section below.

☐ Feedback Element

The feedback element involves any process that compares the operation's actual performance, as documented in output reports, with standards of performance, as established in control

Figure 11-12. Example of a Monthly Performance Form

MONTHLY FOOD SERVICE PERFORMANCE REPORT

Hospital: _____
Period: _____
Prepared by: _____

Meal Count		Current Week	Percentage of Total (7)	YTD Meals
Patient meals	(1)		%	
Cafeteria meals	(2)		%	
Free meals	(3)		%	
Special-function meals	(4)		%	
Other meals	(5)		%	
Total meals	(6)		%	

Labor Cost		Patient Service	Nonpatient Service	Total Labor	YTD Labor
Patient service direct	(8)	$	$	$	$
Nonpatient service direct	(9)				
Allocated labor	(10)				
Total labor cost	(11)	$	$	$	$
Total labor hours	(12)				
Total full-time equivalents					

Food and Supply Costs

Food Costs

	Meat, Fish and Poultry	Fresh Produce	Frozen	Groceries	Milk and Dairy	Bakery	Total Food	YTD Food
Beginning inventory (13)	$	$	$	$	$	$	$	$
Purchases (14)								
Ending inventory (15)								
Gross cost (16)	$	$	$	$	$	$	$	$
Percentage (17)	%	%	%	%	%	%	%	%

Less nourishments (18)
Less transfers (19)
Net food cost (20) $

Supply Costs

	Cleaning Supplies	Dis-posables	China, Silver, and Utensils	Other	Total Supplies	YTD Supplies
	$	$	$	$	$	$
	$	$	$	$	$	$
	%	%	%	%	%	%

Less transfers (19a)
Net supply cost (21) $

Figure 11-12. *Continued*

Net food cost × _____ % Patient meals and nourishments = Patient food cost = (22) $ _____ Net supply cost × _____ % Patient meals = Patient supply cost (23) $ _____

Recap

Remarks		Patient Costs					Nonpatient Costs				
		This Period	Cost per Meal	Budget Cost per Meal	YTD Total	YTD Cost per Meal	This Period	Cost per Meal	Budget Cost per Meal	YTD Total	YTD Cost per Meal
	Labor (24)	$	$	$	$	$	$	$	$	$	$
	Food (25)										
	Supplies (26)										
	Total (27)	$	$	$	$	$	$	$	$	$	$
	Less revenue received (28)										
	Net cost (29)	$	$	$	$	$	$	$	$	$	$

Patient meals/labor hour _____ (30) Nonpatient meals/labor hour _____ (31)

267

documents. Information generated by the feedback element can be utilized to evaluate the financial and operational performance of various components of the system and to identify potential problems and/or opportunities.

Characteristics of Feedback

The feedback element should be objective, based on fair observations of actual data, activities, and conditions and not on the opinions of individuals. If the observations reveal discrepancies between the organization's actual performance and its planned performance, goals and objectives should be reevaluated to assess where any discrepancies lie. The planning process may need to be adjusted in consideration of the organization's actual performance.

Activities of Feedback

The feedback element involves determining how effectively and efficiently the various units and departments have used observation resources. This involves comparing performance with standards, taking corrective actions, and communicating results.

Comparing Performance with Standards

Once the operation's performance has been measured objectively and documented by one of the output reports, performance should be compared with the standards established in the control element of the financial management systems model. (For example, the actual revenue generated by the catering unit may not meet budgeted revenue.) Many reasons may explain why performance failed to meet standards, and it is the food service director's responsibility to uncover those reasons and decide what needs to be done to correct the inconsistency.

Taking Corrective Action

Prior to taking steps to reconcile performance with standards, all relevant information must be analyzed. The following actions, or decisions not to act, may be appropriate:

- Actual performance may be only slightly higher or lower than the standard requires. In such cases, no action may be needed, although the director must use valid information to determine which differences between performance and standard are significant and which are not.
- It may be found that standards were unrealistically high or low, in which case the appropriate action would be to change the standards to reflect the realities of the work situation.
- If the problem is determined to lie with individual work performance, the director should judge whether employees need retraining or job counseling.
- Shortcomings in work performance may be the result of equipment problems. In such cases, equipment should be repaired or maintenance procedures improved.
- If inadequate performance is the result of poor supervision, inefficient procedures, or inadequate staffing, the director should take immediate and specific steps to identify and correct these causes.

Communicating Results

Finally, at the end of the accounting period, the information generated by the feedback element is recycled back to the initial elements to provide a basis for the next accounting period. Feedback results also may be shared with other managers in the food service department, and with appropriate health care facility administrators.

Essential Components of Feedback

As illustrated by the financial management systems model in figure 11-1, three key feedback processes are at work. These are financial statement analysis, financial indicators, and sensitivity analysis.

Financial Statement Analysis

As a result of the accounting processes of journalizing, posting, and making adjustments, a variety of financial statements (discussed in the output section) can be produced by the financial management system. Although mere production of these statements is beneficial, their full value is realized by applying any number of financial statement analysis techniques. Among these are trend analysis, ratio analysis, common size statements, and variance analysis. *Trend analysis* allows the food service manager to compare either financial or nonfinancial results from several accounting periods. Trend analyses are particularly valuable when represented graphically. *Ratio analysis* involves determining the mathematical relationship between two items from any of the output reports. *Common size statements* report each line item from any of the financial statements as a percentage. Because *variance analysis*, which reports significant differences between actual and projected outcomes, is a particularly powerful method, a thorough discussion as it applies to the monthly operating report (see figure 11-11) is provided in this chapter. Discussion of the other techniques mentioned can be found in *Understanding Foodservice Financial Management* by Sneed and Kresse or *Hospitality Management Accounting* by Coltman.

By preparing monthly operating statements, the food service director is able to monitor overall departmental performance and determine which activities, if any, need to be adjusted to meet budget targets. This involves the three steps of the feedback element:

1. Comparing actual operations data with budget forecasts
2. Evaluating actual operations data according to an adjusted operating budget
3. Reviewing operating procedures, standards, and expenses

The remainder of this section will use figure 11-11 as the basis for discussion of the monthly operating statement as a feedback tool for the food service department. (Much of the material in this discussion is based on Faisal A. Kaud's *Financial Management of the Hospital Food Service Department;* see the bibliography at the end of this chapter.)

Step 1: Comparing operations data with budget forecasts. The five main sections of the monthly operating statement coincide with the sections of the food service department's annual operating budget. The sections are patient days, meal count, operating expenses, statistical indicators/unit cost per meal, and productivity indicators.

The patient days section (lines 1 through 3) represents the overall level of business activity in the department during the month of January. The operating statement shows that the number of actual patient days was 2.6 percent below the budgeted level. The lower number of patient days indicates that comparably lower expenses for the month are needed to keep costs within the month's budget guidelines and eventually for the entire fiscal year. The number of clinic visits, however, was 3.3 percent above the budgeted level. This slight increase in activity over estimated levels for the month could affect the budgeted expenses associated with the nutrition outpatient clinic if the upward trend continued into later months.

The meal count section (lines 4 through 10) shows the actual number of meals served in January to all of the department's customers, including patients and nonpatients. The food service director should note that the number of patient meals, stipend meals, and special-function meals were lower than budgeted: 2.6, 1.5, and 2.9 percent, respectively. However, the number of cafeteria meals served was 1.1 percent higher than budgeted. Overall, the total number of meals served by the department was 1.4 percent lower than anticipated. If the trend continued into later months, an adjustment in the budget for later months in the fiscal year might be justified.

Lines 11 through 18 indicate the operating expenses for salaries and benefits, food, supplies, and other expenses. In January, the actual expenses for salaries and benefits were 3.1 percent higher than allowed for in the budget; actual food expenses were 3.9 percent higher; and supply expenses were 2.3 percent higher than anticipated. The other expenses category showed a 3.6 percent decrease over budgeted figures. Total operating expenses were 3.3 percent higher than budgeted. In addition, higher-than-budgeted cash receipts can be credited to improved cafeteria sales. Overall, the net expenses for the food service department in the month of January were 4.6 percent over budget.

The section on statistical indicators/unit cost per meal (lines 19 through 27) also shows that expenses and unit costs were significantly over budget. In addition, the section on productivity indicators (lines 28 through 31) suggests that the department's performance was below the targeted level. Changes in productivity statistics may indicate the need to change operating procedures or staffing levels. When such indicators are calculated on a regular monthly basis and analyzed promptly, the director can make appropriate changes before the department's long-term financial goals are negatively affected. The number of meals served per patient day was slightly higher than budgeted.

The preceding step in the financial review of January operations highlights the variances between actual performance and budgeted performance. Next, the food service director needs to perform a more thorough analysis of the financial data to determine strengths and weaknesses in the department's performance.

Step 2: Evaluating operations data according to a revised budget. To evaluate performance for the month of January, the budget must be adjusted to show the estimated cost at the actual level of patient days and the actual level of patient and nonpatient meals served. To accomplish this evaluation, the number of patient days and the number of total meals served are adjusted on the budget to correspond to the actual data for the month. These two indicators are recorded in the revised budget. (See figure 11-13.) To determine the amount of budgeted resources needed to supply the services listed under operating expenses, the revised budget column is determined according to the method illustrated in figure 11-14.

The revised budget amounts are recorded in the revised budget column of figure 11-13. Because the revised budget and the actual levels of expenses and statistical indicators are now based on the same financial data, the food service director can make more meaningful comparisons. The variance column shows that actual expenses were higher than budgeted expenses in every category. From this evaluation, the variance in the actual net cost per patient meal from the budgeted net cost is significant at 5.9 percent. In addition, the productivity indicators demonstrate that more labor hours than budgeted were used to produce fewer meals than budgeted.

The evaluation makes it clear that the food service department's operating expenses are above the levels authorized in the operating budget. It is also clear that the level of productivity is lower than is required by the operating budget. Variances occurred in several categories of operating expenses: salary and benefits, food, supply, and other expenses. At this point, the food service director must identify the reasons for the unacceptably high operating costs and prepare a plan for taking corrective action.

Step 3: Reviewing operating procedures, standards, and expenses. To identify problems in food service operations that may be behind the unacceptable expense levels, the director will need to review the department's operating procedures and standards. In the category of food and supply costs, the following factors (discussed in detail in later chapters) should be examined:

- Physical inventory
- Invoice records
- Invoice payments
- Receiving and storage procedures
- Purchasing specifications
- Production requisitions
- Menu plans

Factors to be considered in the category of labor cost include labor time and work schedules. The efficiency of labor utilization can be evaluated more precisely by calculating productivity statistics each month and by comparing them with those for past months or with statistics from other operations.

Figure 11-13. Sample Monthly Operating Statement and Revised Budget

	January Total			Percentage of Total Operating Expense Variance	Cash Receipts Variance Applied on Basis of Percentage Variance	Adjusted Variance
	Actual	Revised Budget	Variance			
2. Patient days	2,192	2,192	0			
10. Total meals	10,896	10,896	0			
11. Operating Expenses						
12. Salary and benefit expenses	$ 8,839	$ 8,499	+ $340	+4.0%	+35%	$ 82	$258
13. Food expenses	10,698	10,133	+ 565	+5.6%	+58%	136	429
14. Supply expenses	1,606	1,525	+ 81	+5.3%	+ 8%	19	62
15. Other expenses	533	545	- 12	-2.2%	- 1%	(2)	(10)
16. Total operating expenses	$21,676	$20,702	+ $974	+4.7%	100%	$235	$739
17. Less: cash receipts	(8,080)	(7,845)	+ 235	+3.0%			
18. Net dietary expenses	$13,596	$12,857	+ $739	+5.7%			
26. Net cost per meal	$1.25	$1.18	+ $0.07	+5.9%			
27. Net cost per patient day	$6.20	$5.87	+ $0.33	+5.6%			
28. Productivity Indicators						
29. Meals per hour—paid	5.88	6.14	-0.26	-4.3%			
30. Meals per hour—worked	4.74	4.95	-0.21	-4.2%			
31. Meals per patient day	2.83	2.80	+0.03	+1.2%			

271

Figure 11-14. Method for Calculating Revised Operating Expenses

Operating Expenses	Meals Served		Budget Unit Cost ($)		Revised Budget ($)
12. Salary and benefit expenses	10,896	×	0.78	=	8,499
13. Food expenses	10,896	×	0.93	=	10,133
14. Supply expenses	10,896	×	0.14	=	1,525
15. Other expenses	10,896	×	0.05	=	545
16. Total operating expenses					20,702
17. Less: cash receipts	10,896	×	0.72	=	(7,845)
18. Net dietary expenses					12,857
26. Net cost per meal	12,857	÷	10,896	=	$1.18
27. Net cost per patient day	12,857	÷	2,192	=	$5.87

The category of other expenses also should be examined. However, other expenses include fixed payments that are made periodically without regard to level of activity. The variance between actual other expenses and budgeted other expenses may reflect an error in the original budget.

In large part, the director's ability to perform such operational reviews depends on adequate financial record keeping and reporting, which is composed of the input, processing, and output elements. When performance is analyzed regularly during the actual budget period, estimates of expected performance for upcoming months can be adjusted as necessary to match actual performance. It should be kept in mind that projections can only be estimates of performance in that the business and economic climates of health care institutions can change quickly. As a result, the best projections may turn out to be too high or too low. Revising projections for upcoming months in the fiscal year does not reduce the budget's value as a basis for financial management and control. Rather, it indicates that the food service director is keeping track of operational performance and general business trends.

When a variance (or a significant difference) occurs between the forecasts in the operating budget and the data on actual performance, the manager must follow the steps in the control process (determining the problem, identifying its cause, and taking appropriate corrective action) to correct the inconsistency.

Financial Indicators

Financial indicators are financial statement analysis techniques that support decision making based on volume planning. They attempt to answer questions that cannot be answered by analyzing the financial statements. For example, the revenue-and-expense statement cannot determine what level of revenue is necessary to produce a desired profit. However, the techniques of contribution margin and break-even analysis will address these and other cost–volume–profit issues. These techniques as applied to the financial management of food service operations are discussed by Coltman in *Hospitality Management Accounting*.

Sensitivity Analysis

The last major component of the feedback element is sensitivity analysis. This technique can best be supported by an electronic spreadsheet to provide a means for testing the impact of changes. For instance, to learn what effect a 5 percent increase in cafeteria revenue would have on net income, the food service manager could apply the technique of sensitivity analysis, which uses data and calculations already established in the processing element. When changes in the input are proposed, the recalculation function of the electronic spreadsheet provides almost-instantaneous feedback. This technique once again illustrates the benefits of computerized financial management systems for all elements of the financial management system.

☐ Summary

Under the current health care environment, informed financial management is critical to the viability of health care organizations. The current health care financial management focus is on predicting costs before they are incurred. This proactive management approach requires departmental information, including food service information.

In the midst of changes that will continue to occur in the health care industry, the food service manager has emerged as the controller of significant and valuable resources, accountable for their efficient allocation. Thus, financial management has become one of the primary responsibilities of the food service manager. To meet the departmental and organizational needs for financial information, food service managers may find it necessary to develop and implement comprehensive financial management systems, such as the model described in this chapter.

☐ Bibliography

Accounting for cost and quality. *Hospitals* 66(19):38, Oct. 1992.

American Society for Hospital Food Service Administrators. *Determination and Allocation of Food Service Costs.* Chicago: American Hospital Association, 1976. [Out of print.]

American Society for Hospital Food Service Administrators. *Hospital Food Service Management Review.* Chicago: American Hospital Publishing, 1980. [Out of print.]

Anderson, H. J. The new finance department: CQI triggers big changes in role. *Hospitals* 66(19):40–43, Oct. 1992.

Coltman, M. M. *Cost Control for the Hospitality Industry.* 2nd ed. New York City: Van Nostrand Reinhold, 1989.

Coltman, M. M. *Hospitality Management Accounting.* 5th ed. New York City: Van Nostrand Reinhold, 1993.

Elerding, W. T. Auditing food and nutrition services. *Internal Auditing* 5(4):86–91, Spring 1990.

Griffin, R. W. *Management.* 2nd ed. Boston: Houghton Mifflin, 1987.

Hoover, L. C. A comprehensive financial management systems model for the health care foodservice industry. Dissertation, Texas Woman's University, Denton, 1990.

Kaud, F. A. Budgeting: a comparative analysis of techniques and systems. In: J. C. Rose, editor. *Handbook for Health Care Food Service Management.* Chapter 13. Rockville, MD: Aspen, 1984.

Kaud, F. A. *Financial Management of the Hospital Food Service Department.* Chicago: American Hospital Publishing, 1983. [Out of print.]

Keiser, J. *Controlling and Analyzing Costs in Food Service Operations.* 2nd ed. New York City: John Wiley and Sons, 1989.

Kis, G. M. J., and Bodenger, G. Cost management information improves financial performance. *Healthcare Financial Management* 43(5):36–48, May 1989.

Lesure, J. D. The breakeven point. *Restaurant Hospitality* 67(1):134, Jan. 1983.

McCool, A. C., and Garand, M. M. Computer technology in institution foodservice. *Journal of The American Dietetic Association* 86(1):48–56, Jan. 1986.

Megginson, L., Mosley, D., and Pietri, P., Jr. *Management: Concepts and Applications.* New York City: Harper and Row, 1986.

Moncarz, E. S., and O'Brien, W. G. The powerful & versatile spreadsheet. *The Bottomline* 5(4):16–21, Aug.–Sept. 1990.

Moncarz, E. S., and Portocarrero, N. J. *Financial Accounting for Hospitality Management.* New York City: Van Nostrand Reinhold, 1986.

Nyp, R. G., and Angermeier, I. Financial plan charts a hospital's course for success. *Healthcare Financial Management* 44(5):30–36, May 1990.

Schmidgall, R. S. *Hospitality Industry Managerial Accounting.* East Lansing, MI: Educational Institute of the American Hotel & Motel Association, 1990.

Schmidgall, R. S., and Andrew, W. P. *Financial Management in the Hospitality Industry.* East Lansing, MI: Educational Institute of the American Hotel & Motel Association, 1993.

Slavinski, G. Basic systems analysis for hospitality management. *The Bottomline* 7(3):14–17,45, June–July 1992.

Sneed, J., and Kresse, K. H. *Understanding Foodservice Financial Management.* Rockville, MD: Aspen, 1989.

Stokes, J. *Cost Effective Quality Food Service: An Institution Guide.* 2nd ed. Germantown, MD: Aspen, 1983.

Tarras, J. *Practical Guide to Hospitality Finance.* New York City: Van Nostrand Reinhold, 1991.

Part Two

Operation of the Food Service Department

Environmental Issues
and Waste Management

☐ Introduction

Food service directors or managers are expected to know about issues that will affect the cost and efficiency of their operations. Environmental issues such as the disposal of solid biological waste and hazardous waste (including medical waste and hazardous chemicals); air pollution; energy conservation; water quality and quantity; and the cost and availability of natural resources are some of the issues predicted to influence health care food service operations during the next 10 years. Hospitals are being challenged by the public to take a more active role in addressing environmental concerns within the community. As a result, many hospitals now provide leadership in developing strategic environmental programs that extend into the community.

This chapter will present an overview of environmental issues; suggest waste management strategies that can be implemented in health care food service departments; emphasize the importance of top-management support and employee involvement in developing and implementing various waste management programs; and identify environmental issues to be monitored. Specifically, the chapter will discuss solid waste management strategies—waste source reduction, composting, and recycling. Two methods of identifying a facility's waste stream, waste stream analysis and waste auditing, will be described. Next, the chapter will examine hazardous waste management in a nutrition and food service operation, with specific emphasis on hazardous chemicals waste, storage, and disposal.

Guidelines for energy use and conservation via an energy management program will be presented, using a five-step model, after which air pollution and water conservation will be examined in light of current legislation. All these will be tied into comprehensive environmental issues as they affect a food service department director's responsibilities.

☐ Solid Waste Management

Solid waste, specifically municipal solid waste (MSW), is the most visible evidence of the limited concerns individuals have regarding the disposal of renewable resources. Solid waste disposal is currently one of the most costly environmental problems affecting not only the food service department but every department in a health care facility. The Environmental Protection Agency (EPA) defines *municipal solid waste* as "waste such as durable goods, containers and packaging, food scraps, yard trimmings, and miscellaneous inorganic waste from residential, commercial, institutional and industrial sources." Thus, all the waste generated in food service operations, excluding chemicals, is MSW. Increased disposal fees, landfill shortages, government regulations, and consumer demands for a safer environment are cited as priorities that require immediate action on the part of health care food service facilities.

The national average cost per ton for disposal of MSW was $35.95 in October 1993. The cost ranged from an average of $15.47 per ton in the western region of the United States to $64.94 per ton in the northeastern region. Tipping fees (the costs of transporting and discarding MSW at transfer stations or landfills) increased approximately 5.9 percent during 1992 and are expected to continue to escalate as stricter government regulations associated with Subtitle D of the Resource Conservation and Recovery Act are enforced, as local and state governments develop their solid waste management plans, and as the cost and difficulties of siting new landfills increase.

Approximately 50 to 65 percent of the waste (weight and volume) generated in commercial and noncommercial food service operations is food waste. Paperboard and corrugated cardboard are two materials that contributed most to the volume of packaging waste. Other packaging materials found in health care food service waste include tin, plastic, aluminum, glass, and styrofoam. Some factors influencing the volume of each type of material disposed of include type of serviceware (reusable or disposable) used for service of patient and nonpatient meals; type of production system; availability of volume reduction equipment such as compactors, pulpers, and disposals; accuracy of forecasts and production and service controls, such as use or disposal of leftover food; portion control; and reuse of plastic and glass containers after sanitization. The waste management industry estimates that from 0.5 to 1.5 pound of total waste is generated per meal served depending on the type of food service operation. Research at noncommercial food service facilities found an average of 0.39 to 0.61 pound/meal or 0.002 to 0.03 cubic yards/meal total waste (production, service, and packaging). Table 12-1 compares composition of waste generated in two noncommercial operations.

The volume of packaging waste can be reduced by approximately 50 percent if corrugated cardboard boxes are collapsed and tin cans are crushed. In that most health care operations are charged on the basis of dumpster capacity and waste disposal pickup frequency, their waste disposal costs would be reduced if waste volume were decreased. However, the cost of waste management equipment (such as compactors and balers) and labor costs must be analyzed and compared with waste-hauling expenses.

An integrated waste management system designed to decrease the quantity of waste to be disposed of is recommended. According to the U.S. Environmental Protection Agency, the

Table 12-1. Percentage Volume of Materials Disposed of by Two Noncommercial Food Service Operations

Material	College/University Study[a] (%)	School Study[b] (%)
Cardboard	44.6	27.5
Food waste from production and service	21.3	22.9
Paper	13.1	8.4
Paperboard	8.6	23.4[c]
Plastic (including film)	7.5	4.0
Metal (including tin and aluminum)	4.3	6.8
Miscellaneous (including wood, glass, and so on)	0.6	7.0

Note: Volume is uncollapsed because facility had no compactor.
[a]University food service operation is a centralized conventional food production system serving an average of 3,300 meals per day. Data are based on a 14-day waste stream analysis excluding liquid waste.
[b]School data are based on analysis of average waste generated for 10 days in six schools serving an average of 4,500 lunches per day.
[c]Gabletop milk cartons comprised greatest percentage of waste.

term *integrated system* refers to "complementary uses of a variety of waste management practices to safely and effectively handle the municipal solid waste stream with the least adverse impact on human health and the environment." In such a system, renewable natural resources are not disposed of as waste but are reused, recycled, and composted. Incineration is one option for reducing volume of waste while capturing energy. In an integrated system, burying waste in landfills should be the last alternative. Figure 12-1 illustrates the components and order of preference of an integrated solid waste management system. A brief discussion and examples of source reduction and reuse (recycling and composting) is presented in the following sections because these are options that food service directors can implement. The food service director will need to assess the feasibility of combusting packaging materials if the health care facility has an incinerator. Because of its water content, food waste usually is not combusted.

Source Reduction

Reducing the amount of waste generated, or *source reduction,* is a preventive approach that eliminates the need to determine the most cost-effective method of waste disposal. Source reduction also conserves natural resources and enhances preservation of the environment. Examples of reuse and source reduction efforts that have been implemented in health care food service operations are:

- Working cooperatively with manufacturers and distributors to reduce packaging materials
- Purchasing reusable products or products packaged in reusable containers or having products delivered in reusable containers rather than in cardboard boxes
- Purchasing cleaning products in more concentrated form
- Purchasing products in bulk form rather than in smaller packages
- Reducing the quantity of disposables used
- Evaluating which packaging material generated the largest volume of waste (for example, purchasing products such as sauces and salad dressings in individual portion packages rather than in bulk containers, such as polyethylene pouches or tin cans)

Figure 12-1. Integrated Solid Waste Management System

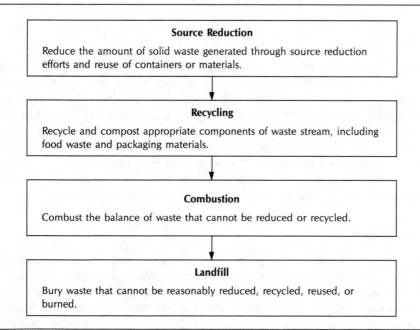

- Using sanitized glass or plastic containers for product storage
- Evaluating accuracy of production forecast to minimize quantity of leftovers
- Serving condiments and beverages from dispensers rather than in single-service containers
- Minimizing waste potential through careful menu planning
- Introducing a reusable mug program in cash operations where discounts are given to employees who use the mug when purchasing beverages
- Donating leftover food from catered events to homeless shelters, schools, long-term care facilities, or other social programs (However, food service directors must obtain prior approval from health departments so as to ensure compliance with sanitation codes and must consult their organizations' legal counsel to avoid risk liability.)

How effective each of these approaches is depends on several factors. Some of these are the organizational culture; the extent of commitment and involvement on the part of managers, employees, and customer/recipients; and the education, training, and motivation of food service providers.

Recycling

Food service directors have found that *recycling* can be an effective alternative to solid waste management, although it is not without problems. For example, recycling efforts have not been successful in areas where markets for recyclable materials are limited or nonexistent. Prior to initiating a recycling program, a food service manager must contact a local waste hauler to learn whether the company offers its customers a recycling option. Many major waste management companies have developed programs whereby they provide special dumpsters for recyclable materials. Some haulers may require that materials be separated and stored in a separate dumpster, whereas others allow facilities to commingle their recyclables. If commingling is an option, food service directors should work to negotiate a new contract with the hauler that includes a recycling option—including training employees on what types of materials to separate and how to separate them. If plastics are to be recycled, employees will need to learn which types of plastic containers can be placed in recycling bins. If an operation is located in an area where recycling is not available, the next option is to identify buy-back centers, which accept or purchase recyclable materials.

Composting

Composting, as it relates to food service waste management, is the process of separating organic waste (that is, food and other organic waste from production and service areas including plate waste, napkins, paper, paperboard, and cardboard) from other waste so that the organic waste is stored and eventually used as fertilizer or land conditioner. Composting has been implemented successfully in operations located in close proximity to a commercial compost facility. The food service director must first assess the financial feasibility of composting and the availability of storage space for holding waste prior to pickup. Approximately 50 to 60 percent of waste generated in food service operations is organic (or biological). Removal of organic waste from trash sent to landfills could significantly decrease waste-hauling expenses.

Waste Stream Analysis

If recycling appears to be a feasible option, the next step is to become familiar with the *waste stream,* that is, the type and quantity of waste generated throughout the food service operation. Two methods can help make this determination: waste stream analysis and waste auditing. A *waste stream analysis* involves the simultaneous collection, separation, and determination of volume and weight of all waste generated and disposed of in all production and service areas for a certain period (such as five days or one week). Wastes are sorted by type of packaging material (corrugated cardboard, plastic [high-density polyethylene (HDPE), low-density polyethylene (LDPE), film], paper, or food). The weight and volume of each material collected is recorded at different times throughout the day. The total weight and volume is then computed per day and per week.

A *waste audit,* whose data, although similar to those obtained from a waste stream analysis, are not as detailed, is easier and less labor-intensive and can provide the essential information for planning a recycling program. Conducting a waste audit involves assessing the type of waste generated (including hazardous waste, discussed later in this chapter) in each area of the operation (receiving, food production, service areas, dishwashing, sanitation and pest control, office, and so on). Information is recorded on a recycling form, such as the one shown in figure 12-2, or on similar forms developed by food service suppliers. When conducting a waste audit, department managers must use a separate sheet for each major category of waste (cardboard, plastic, and so on).

A practical way to collect this information is to investigate waste generated in a given area or during a specific activity. For example, to assess quantity and type of waste generated in the production area, an employee would collect the waste containers, sort the waste, and record its weight and volume throughout an entire day. The number of days this information is collected will depend on variability in menu offerings, type of production system, market form of food, product acceptability, and effectiveness of control measures.

Information collected should result in a profile of food waste and in identification of major reasons for waste. The profile can be used by the director in identifying alternatives for decreasing and disposing of waste and determining which materials can be recycled.

The information also can be used to evaluate the economics of recycling, that is, disposal costs and savings to be realized vis-à-vis waste volume. (See figure 12-3.) Other worksheets can facilitate planning a recycling program that includes selection of materials storage containers, materials transportation options, and baler or crusher options. (See figures 12-4, 12-5, and 12-6, respectively.) In addition, the logistics of how recyclable materials will be collected, sorted (if required by hauler or buy-back center), and stored must be well delineated. Again, the need for waste reduction/processing equipment—compactors, balers, pulpers, crushers, and the like—should be evaluated. Sanitation remains an issue throughout the process, including waste storage. If other departments in the health care facility have implemented recycling programs, consult their managers to learn from their experience and then coordinate efforts where feasible. Volunteer to participate or invite a food service representative to work on the institution's recycling or waste management team.

Factors Influencing Success

Several factors will affect the success of a recycling program. Probably the two most critical internal factors are management support and motivated, educated employees and guests. Management should initiate recycling education and incentive programs that stress the role played by employees in a program's success. Employee involvement and feedback, along with a team approach throughout program planning and implementation, are essential. External factors that influence the long-term success of recycling as a cost-effective component of waste management include a continuous source of supply of recyclable materials, a significant volume of recyclable materials, and adequate end-use markets for recycled products that support sufficient market value for such materials. Food service operators should purchase as many products made from recycled material as is economically feasible.

☐ Hazardous Waste Management

Handling and disposing of hazardous waste presents unique challenges to the health care industry. Even though hazardous materials comprise only 10 to 15 percent of hospital waste, waste management procedures have become more complex and costly following enactment of the

Figure 12-2. Recycling Materials Flow Plan Worksheet

Department: _____

Instructions

Complete a recycling flow plan(s) for each area of the food service department. Identify location(s) of the recyclables in each area at location 1. Move the materials from location 1 to location 2, 3, and so on until it is picked up by the recycler/waste hauler. At each location in the flow procedure, identify the container(s) to be used and who will be handling the materials. Handle materials as few times as possible.

Location 1 — Source of Materials	List recyclables to be collected at this location. Move recyclables to storage locations 2 and 3.
	A. _____
	B. _____
	C. _____
	D. _____
	E. _____
	F. _____

Collection Container(s)	Instructions	List employees collecting material.
A. _____	A. _____	A. _____
B. _____	B. _____	B. _____
C. _____	C. _____	C. _____
D. _____	D. _____	D. _____
E. _____	E. _____	E. _____
F. _____	F. _____	F. _____

Location 2 — Temporary Storage	List containers to be used for storage or moving of each recyclable listed above.	List employees picking up materials.
	A. _____	A. _____
	B. _____	B. _____
	C. _____	C. _____
	D. _____	D. _____
	E. _____	E. _____
	F. _____	F. _____

Location 3 — Recycling Center or Roll-Off Unit	List containers to be used for storage or moving of each recyclable listed above.	List employees picking up materials.
	A. _____	A. _____
	B. _____	B. _____
	C. _____	C. _____
	D. _____	D. _____
	E. _____	E. _____
	F. _____	F. _____

Source: Reprinted, with permission, from *Recycling in Hotels and Motels*, by Jo Townsend, University of Florida, Energy Extension Service, Gainesville, FL, 1993.

Figure 12-3. The Economics of Recycling: A Worksheet

Volume Data

What type of waste disposal container is in use? _____
How many refuse containers are being used? _____

1. Determine the present volume of waste that you are disposing of.
   How many pickups per month do you have? _____
   Estimate the number of tons per month from waste volume. _____
   (Calculate this by multiplying the waste capacity of the container by a factor
   that corresponds to the number of tons that container typically holds.)

2. Estimate the potential volume of recyclable materials.
   Estimate percentage of extractable recyclables. _____ %
   Estimate the tons/month. _____ tons of _____ (material 1)
   Estimate the tons/month. _____ tons of _____ (material 2)

3. Calculate the waste volume left after recycling.
   Estimate the number of tons/month left after recycling. _____
   (Subtract line 2 from line 1.)
   How many pickups/month will you have? _____
   (This will be reduced in proportion to the percentage of material recycled.)

Waste Disposal Cost Data

4. Determine your present monthly waste removal costs.
   (If no invoice is available, you can estimate.)
   What is the pickup charge each time? $ _____
   Multiply the pickup charge by the number of pickups per month (#1). $ _____
   What is the landfill "tipping" fee per ton? $ _____
   Multiply the tipping fee times the estimated number of tons per month. $ _____
   Are you paying monthly container rental or lease fees? $ _____
   Add up your total current monthly waste disposal costs. $ _____
                                                      $ _____

5. Determine your waste removal cost/ton (#4 divided by #1). $ _____

6. Estimate your waste removal costs after recycling. $ _____
   Pickup charges $_____ times number of pickups _____ = $ _____
   Tipping fee $_____ times number of tons _____ = $ _____
   Monthly equipment rental or lease fee = $ _____
   Add up your total current monthly disposal costs after recycling. $ _____

7. Monthly waste disposal costs you avoided (#4 minus #6). $ _____
   (Calculate your savings by subtracting your disposal costs after recycling
   from your total current waste disposal costs.)

8. Annual avoided waste disposal costs (#7 times 12). $ _____

9. Calculate the recycling program start-up investments.
   Recycling containers, boxes, or carts. $ _____
   Recycling equipment, balers, compactors. $ _____
   Cost of training program or internal publicity. $ _____
   Other. $ _____
   Total start-up investment for recycling program. $ _____

10. Estimated revenues from recyclables. $ _____
    From your estimate of the volume of recyclable materials (#2)
    _____ tons of _____ (material 1) times $_____/ton = $ _____
    _____ tons of _____ (material 2) times $_____/ton = $ _____
    (We recommend you use a conservative market price for these recyclables.)
    Your total monthly revenues from sale of recyclables. $ _____
    Your total annual revenues from sale of recyclables. $ _____
    (Multiply the monthly revenues by 12 to get annual revenues.)

Summary of Savings

11. Annual avoided waste disposal costs (from line #8). $ + _____
    Your total annual revenues from sale of recyclables. $ + _____
    Total annual savings. = $ _____
    Total 5-year savings (multiply annual savings by five). = $ _____
    Total start-up investment for recycling program (line #9). = $ _____

12. Net estimated 5-year profit on recycling program. $ _____

Source: Reprinted with the permission of the Public Utilities Department, Jacksonville, FL, 1991.

Figure 12-4. Selection of Waste Materials Storage Containers: A Worksheet

Company	Cost of purchasing roll-off containers	Cost of leasing roll-off containers	Length of lease	Size of compartments	Choice of container color?	Are compartments labeled?	Who is responsible for repairs?	Who is responsible for cleaning containers?	Location requirements concrete or pavement
1.									
Phone #									
2.									
Phone #									
3.									
Phone #									
4.									
Phone #									
5.									
Phone #									
6.									
Phone #									
7.									
Phone #									

Source: Reprinted, with permission, from *Recycling in Hotels and Motels*, by Jo Townsend, University of Florida, Energy Extension Service, Gainesville, FL, 1993.

Figure 12-5. Selection of Waste Materials Transportation Options: A Worksheet

Transporting recyclable materials to an intermediate processor or materials recovery center is usually done by a waste hauler or recycling center. Careful research needs to be done before signing contracts.

Company	Charges for transporting a leased or purchased roll-off	Fees for picking up materials in smaller containers	Add-on charges such as franchise fees or gas surcharges?	Hours of pickup	How often are materials picked up?	How much notice is required for pickup?	Length of Contract	Provide Weight Records	How often are containers cleaned?
1.									
Phone #									
2.									
Phone #									
3.									
Phone #									
4.									
Phone #									
5.									
Phone #									

Source: Reprinted, with permission, from *Recycling in Hotels and Motels*, by Jo Townsend, University of Florida, Energy Extension Service, Gainesville, FL, 1993.

Figure 12-6. Selection of Waste Baler or Crusher Options: A Worksheet

Company Name	Model #	Bale Size	Cost	Delivery and Installation	Warranty	Equipment Features
1. Phone #						
2. Phone #						
3. Phone #						
4. Phone #						
5. Phone #						

Source: Reprinted, with permission, from *Recycling in Hotels and Motels,* by Jo Townsend, University of Florida, Energy Extension Service, Gainesville, FL, 1993.

Medical Waste Track Act of 1988 (MWTA), an amendment to the Resource Conservation and Recovery Act (RCRA). The cost of hazardous waste disposal is three to five times more per ton than for other types of waste generated. Hazardous materials include infectious waste; diagnostic equipment batteries; laboratory solvents and acids; therapeutic radioactive chemicals; and chemicals used for cleaning and sanitizing equipment, surfaces, serviceware, utensils, and so on.

Medical waste disposal has been a very sensitive public issue since 1987 when hypodermic syringes, containers of blood, and other medical effluvia washed ashore on East Coast beaches. After enactment of MWTA, the EPA issued "Standards for the Tracking and Management of Medical Waste" (40 CFR 259). These standards provide health care facilities and other operations generating medical waste with definitions and procedures for disposal, transportation, incineration, and management of this type of waste. In general, the food service department is not directly affected by these regulations, what with its limited (if any) contact with medical waste. Nonetheless, managers should be familiar with their organization's policies and procedures regarding medical waste. Either the food service director or a department representative should participate on the facility's infection control committee or continuous quality improvement team and provide input regarding service of meals to patients in isolation and the handling of soiled serviceware and leftover food (in most instances, isolated trays are handled the same as other medical waste). The director should see to it that policies and procedures for handling and disposing of infectious waste are communicated to all food service employees.

Food service departments are more influenced by hazardous chemicals, defined by the Occupational Safety and Health Administration (OSHA) as "any chemical which is a physical hazard or health hazard." Hazardous chemicals require the director to implement specific policies and procedures for purchasing, storing, handling, and disposing of all chemical compounds used in the operation. In addition, OSHA standards (known as Hazardous Communication Standards; also referred to as the "right to know") mandate all employers to provide information to their employees concerning hazardous chemicals through an established hazardous communication program. In turn, manufacturers and importers of chemicals are mandated to assess the hazard potential of those chemicals they produce or import, information that is communicated to end users on material safety data sheets (MSDSs). Part of a sample MSDS is shown in figure 12-7.

When ordering chemicals (for example, detergents and other cleaning compounds), the purchasing agent should request MSDSs for products for which no MSDSs are already on file at the facility. Multiple copies of each MSDS are helpful so that a copy is available in the work area where the chemical is used as well as being on hand for use in developing training materials and instructional guides for using a particular chemical. (The recommended content of a training program and the food service director's responsibilities related to OSHA's Hazardous Communication are discussed in chapter 14.) Some distributors of cleaning supplies have developed training materials and MSDS manuals for their products. In addition to cleaning and sanitizing chemicals, the food service director should be familiar with and have on file MSDSs for chemicals used by exterminators. (Storage of chemicals is discussed in chapter 13.)

The food service manager will need to work with facility maintenance or the waste hauler to determine how to dispose of empty chemical containers. In most instances, these should be disposed of following the same procedure as for other hazardous waste. Chemical containers should never be rinsed and used to store food.

☐ Energy Utilization and Conservation

Despite legislation and consumer pressure, energy conservation programs have not been a priority among food service directors. Even though the energy crisis of the late 1970s is a fading memory for most directors, the United States still faces serious energy problems, not the least of which is increasing energy cost. This problem is anticipated to intensify if the Clinton administration imposes taxes on energy use. This section will review energy conservation practices that can be implemented to contain energy costs and preserve endangered natural resources. Much of this material is summarized from resources published during the late 1970s and early 1980s because current references on the topic are limited.

Figure 12-7. Material Safety Data Sheet (Excerpt)

Material Safety Data Sheet May be used to comply with OSHA's Hazard Communication Standard, 29 CFR 1910.1200. Standard must be consulted for specific requirements.	U.S. Department of Labor Occupational Safety and Health Administration (Non-Mandatory Form) Form Approved OMB No. 1218-0072
IDENTITY *(As Used on Label and List)* High Alkline Oven Extra Strong Degreaser Cleaner/Degreaser	Note: Blank spaces are not permitted. If any item is not applicable, or no information is available, the space must be marked to indicate that.

Section I

Manufacturer's Name Chemicals Unlimited	Emergency Telephone Number 1-800-000-1234
Address *(Number, Street, City, State, and ZIP Code)* Tanktown, USA. 00001	Telephone Number for Information 1-123-000-4567
	Date Prepared February 31, 1989
	Signature of Preparer *(optional)*

Section II — Hazardous Ingredients/Identity Information

Hazardous Components (Specific Chemical Identity; Common Name(s))	OSHA PEL	ACGIH TLV	Other Limits Recommended	% (optional)
Sodium Hydroxide (Caustic Soda) 1310-73-2	2		2 C	5
Butoxyethanol (Butyl Cellosolve) 111-76-2	240		120	10
(Skin) — This product contains no other component considerd				
hazardous according to the criteria of 29 CFR				
1910.1200.				

Section III — Physical/Chemical Characteristics

Boiling Point 212°F	Specific Gravity (H₂O = 1) 1.05-1.08
Vapor Pressure (mm Hg.) N/A	Melting Point N/A
Vapor Density (AIR = 1) N/A	Evaporation Rate (Butyl Acetate = 1) N/A
Solubility in Water 99%	
Appearance and Odor Opaque red/purple liquid: slight glycol ether odor.	

Section IV — Fire and Explosion Hazard Data

Flash Point (Method Used) N/A	Flammable Limits N/A	LEL N/A	UEL N/A
Extinguishing Media N/A			
Special Fire Fighting Procedures Product does not support combustion.			
Unusual Fire and Explosion Hazards None			

(Reproduce locally)   OSHA 174, Sept. 1985

Source: U.S. Department of Labor, Occupational Safety and Health Administration, Sept. 1985.

There are several key areas in which effective energy management practices can eliminate wasteful energy use, including the design of the operation and the selection, use, and maintenance of food service equipment. Furthermore, proper equipment operation and ventilation systems can reduce energy costs and improve employee productivity and comfort.

Energy Management Program

Five key steps dictate the design of an energy management program as delineated in figure 12-8. The first step, establish an energy management team, assigns primary management responsibility to a team member whose knowledge of and commitment to conserving energy is outstanding. In smaller operations the food service director may be given this responsibility. An energy conservation "subteam" may be composed of members from each functional area of the operation (for example, inventory control or food purchasing). The larger team should identify its goals and objectives, determine methods to collect information needed to develop the energy management program, and establish a realistic time period for developing and implementing the program. A time frame for initial evaluation also may be set at this point. To begin with, the team leader should obtain essential information—for example,

Figure 12-8. Energy Management Program

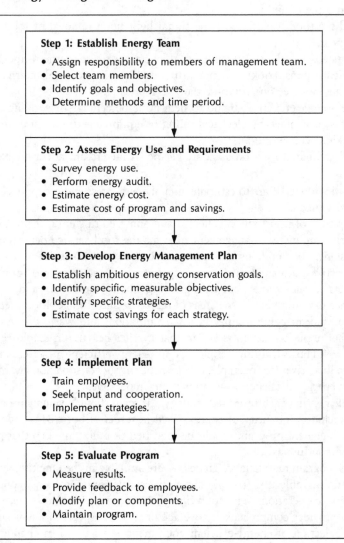

Step 1: Establish Energy Team

- Assign responsibility to members of management team.
- Select team members.
- Identify goals and objectives.
- Determine methods and time period.

Step 2: Assess Energy Use and Requirements

- Survey energy use.
- Perform energy audit.
- Estimate energy cost.
- Estimate cost of program and savings.

Step 3: Develop Energy Management Plan

- Establish ambitious energy conservation goals.
- Identify specific, measurable objectives.
- Identify specific strategies.
- Estimate cost savings for each strategy.

Step 4: Implement Plan

- Train employees.
- Seek input and cooperation.
- Implement strategies.

Step 5: Evaluate Program

- Measure results.
- Provide feedback to employees.
- Modify plan or components.
- Maintain program.

documentation of current energy costs and method of determining them, anticipated increases in energy costs due to planned facility expansion or rate increases, and addition of energy-intense equipment in the food service department.

The second step, assess energy use and requirements, will provide the team with information essential to develop the energy plan. For example, during a walk-through survey of the cafeteria and floor/pantry units, team members should identify potential energy-loss areas and energy requirements for each piece of equipment. The Food Service Energy Management Survey, developed by the research and development committee of the American Society of Hospital Food Service Administrators in 1979 (see figure 12-9), although dated, may be useful in identifying areas on which to focus the team's initial efforts. An energy equipment survey form, such as the one shown in figure 12-10 (p. 294), should be completed during the walk-through to assess energy requirements for major pieces of equipment and refrigerated units. During the walk-through, employee practices and work methods, as they relate to energy conservation, should be observed and recorded.

Sometimes detailed information is required on the amount of energy needed to produce specific recipes. The following method, described by F. Romanelli in a 1979 issue of *Hospitals,* can still be used for electrical equipment:

1. Record the "on" time of the thermostat signal light immediately after placing food item into the equipment.
2. Record the total "on" time of the signal light upon removal of food product from equipment.
3. Repeat steps 1 and 2 throughout five duplications for the same recipe using identical ingredients, pans, cooking temperature, and initial and final internal temperature.
4. Calculate average "on" time for the five replications.
5. Divide average "on" time by 60 to determine percentage of cooking time in hours.
6. Multiply percentage by electrical rating of equipment to obtain estimated kilowatt hour (kwh) consumption.
7. Record estimated kwh on standard recipe (if meters are not available).

The final activities in step 2 are to estimate annual energy cost and compute cost of program and anticipated savings.

Based on results of information collected and analyzed in step 2, the team can move on to step 3, develop an energy management plan for the food service department. This step involves establishment of ambitious, realistic energy conservation goals; identification of specific, measurable objectives; determination of specific strategies; and estimation of cost savings for each strategy. Strategies should focus on improving employee practices and on the operation and maintenance of equipment in the areas of receiving and storage; food preparation; heating, ventilation, and air-conditioning (HVAC); sanitation; and waste disposal.

Step 4, plan implementation, is key in that it relies heavily on employee participation and cooperation. Thus, training employees in energy-efficient practices and providing implementation incentives (for example, department energy conservation awards or employee suggestions for energy efficiency innovations) are imperative.

After implementing each proposed strategy, the team should evaluate program effectiveness (step 5), including quantity of energy saved in terms of both BTUs and energy costs. The energy management program should be modified or maintained so that program goals can be attained continuously.

Numerous program maintenance guidelines are available in the literature and from equipment manufacturers. Table 12-2 (p. 295) summarizes some common energy conservation practices in food service operations. The book *Energy Management in Foodservice* by Unklesbay and Unklesbay provides comprehensive coverage of various aspects of energy utilization and conservation. (Selection of energy-efficient equipment is discussed in chapter 21.)

Figure 12-9. Food Service Energy Management Survey

Instructions:

Questions have been divided into seven categories and points assigned to each question. Circle the points for each question if you can answer "yes" at least 90 percent of the time. Do not circle point value for a question answered with "no" or "not applicable."

At end of each section, total the circled points and record on the survey summary sheet. Record the points in each section that were not applicable for specific design of your operation.

Question	Points if Yes	Not Applicable
Category 1 – Lighting		
1. Has a lighting survey been completed?	2	
2. Is sunlight used (and overhead lights turned off) during the day?	1	
3. Has lighting in storerooms and aisles been reduced to one-half of the tray line?	2	
4. Are lights turned off in the cafeterias when not in use?	2	
5. Have iridescent bulbs been replaced with fluorescent?	2	
6. Have rheostats been placed in large lighting usage areas?	1	
7. Are lights cleaned at least monthly?	1	
Total Points for Category		
Category 2 – Heating, Ventilation, Air-Conditioning		
1. Can heat requirements be controlled by area of the kitchen?	3	
2. Is heat-generating equipment placed so that heat can provide employee comfort?	2	
3. Are ventilation hoods designed to recirculate heat?	5	
4. Are filter hood screens cleaned weekly?	2	
5. Are hoods thermostatically controlled?	4	
6. Are hoods covering all ovens, grills, dishwashers, kettles, and steamers?	2	
7. Can air-conditioning be adjusted in the kitchen?	3	
Total Points for Category		
Category 3 – Serving Area		
1. Are serving wells individually controlled?	1	
2. Are all serving wells covered when on?	3	
3. Is water in the serving wells (up to 50% saving over dry)?	3	
4. Is warmup time for all hot wells, platewarmers, etc., controlled to 15 min. or less?	3	
5. Are serving wells turned off 10 min. before the end of the serving period?	1	
6. Are compressor filters on carbonated beverage and juice machines cleaned weekly?	1	
7. Are warmers individually controlled?	1	
8. Are refrigeration units cleaned and free of ice?		
Total Points for Category		
Category 4 – Refrigeration		
1. Are compressor screens cleaned weekly?	1	
2. Are thermostats set at maximum acceptable temperatures?	1	
3. Do all walk-in doors have automatic closers?	1	
4. Are food items unboxed before storage so energy is not used to cool cardboard boxes?	2	
5. Are issues designed so that all items needed for a meal are collected at the same time to reduce door openings?	4	
6. Do all items being refrigerated require refrigeration?	3	
7. Are frozen items defrosted in the refrigerator?	1	
Total Points for Category		

291

continued on next page

Figure 12-9. *Continued*

Question	Points if Yes	Not Applicable
Category 5 – Sanitation		
1. Has dish machine temperature been lowered to the minimum 140° wash, 180° rinse (160° if chlorine booster)?	3	
2. Are machines operated at least at 80% capacity?	4	
3. Is a chemical rinse used in pot washing instead of 180°?	3	
4. Are the number of dishes rewashed below 1%?	3	
5. Are drain valves, overflow valves, and washarms clear and leak free?	2	
6. Is the machine turned off between batches?	2	
7. Is a steam instead of electric booster being used?	2	
8. Are dishes being done in 2 hours per meal or less?	2	

Total Points for Category

Category 6 – Production		
Steam		
1. Are all steam lines insulated?	2	
2. Are covers used when steam kettles are in use?	2	
3. Are gaskets and seals tight to prevent steam losses?	2	
4. Are kettles or steamers filled at least 60% before start?	2	
5. Are steam lines delimed at least every 6 months?	2	
6. Is hot water added to kettles to reduce energy demand?	1	
7. Are pressure steamers used in place of pressureless ones?	2	
8. Are small kettles available for saucemaking instead of using the stovetop?	1	
Ovens		
1. Are preheat times limited to maximum of 15 min.?	3	
2. Are ovens loaded during warmup where food quality is not affected?	2	
3. Are ovens used at full capacity?	4	
4. Are ovens turned off between meals?	4	
5. Is a thermometer with external gauge used to check roasts?	2	
6. Are oven timers used?	1	
7. Is the fuel–air ratio on gas ovens checked and/or adjusted at least monthly?	2	
8. Are ovens used at night (for roasting meat) at lower temperatures to take advantage of nonpeak energy charges?	5	
9. Are oven doors left closed during baking and roasting?	4	
10. Are ovens not used to hold food after preparation?	2	
11. Are oven thermostats checked weekly?	2	
12. Are sheet pans double-stacked where possible (e.g., bacon) to increase capacity?	2	
13. Are potatoes baked without foil wrapping?	2	
14. Are casserole dishes baked uncovered?	2	
Grills and Griddles		
1. Are preheat times limited to 15 min.?	3	
2. Are charbroilers turned to medium after briquets are hot?	2	
3. Are briquets clean?	1	
4. Are griddles cleaned after every use?	2	
5. Are grills turned off during employee breaks?	3	
6. Are the lowest cooking temperatures possible used?	3	
7. Is maximum surface area used to decrease heat loss to air?	1	
8. Are ovens used instead of grills where possible?	1	
9. Is only that portion of the grill being used heated?	2	
10. On gas units, does the flame tip touch the heating plate?	1	
Stoves		
1. Are preheat times limited to a maximum of 20 min.?	3	
2. Are kettles and pots larger than burners?	1	

Figure 12-9. *Continued*

Question	Points if Yes	Not Applicable
3. Has foil been placed under range burners to reflect heat?	1	
4. Are only the units being used on?	3	
5. Are kettles covered with tight-fitting lids?	2	
6. Are ranges banked together to allow better insulation?	2	

Total Points for Category

Category 7 – Management of Facility

Question	Points if Yes	Not Applicable
1. Are all external doors closed when heating or air conditioners are being used?	4	
2. Are all windows closed when heat or air-conditioning is on?	4	
3. Has gas pressure been checked and compared to equipment demand?	2	
4. Does steam line provide the correct equipment steam pressure?	3	
5. Has a schedule of preheat times, cooking temperatures, and turnoff times been developed and implemented?	4	
6. Are energy areas balanced so that energy demands are constant (ovens turned off when dish machine is operating, etc.)	5	
7. Have the food service energy demands been balanced with those of other departments so when the peak demand for the hospital is high, the energy demands by food service are low?	5	
8. Has your push on energy control been scheduled to coincide with the hospital's peak month of energy usage?	5	
9. Does the food service administrator and all supervisors know when the hospital's peak demand for energy is?	2	
10. Are new equipment purchases evaluated for reducing energy?	4	

Total Points for Category

ASHFSA Energy Management Survey Summary

Category	Possible Points (A)	Points Earned (B)	Points Not Appl. (C)	% (A or B − C) × 100
1	11			
2	21			
3	14			
4	13			
5	21			
6	82			
7	38			
TOTAL	200			

Interpreting the Results:

Scores below 50 indicate a high potential for cost savings through effective energy management. Scores above 140 indicate that additional effort to conserve energy may not produce a high return on time spent. Initial energy management efforts should focus on the area(s) in which you scored less than 50 percent.

Note: This survey was developed by the Research and Development Committee of the American Society of Hospital Food Service Administrators (ASHFSA) in 1979. Although this survey may be outdated and is no longer available from ASHFSA, it remains a helpful model for designing food service energy management surveys.

Figure 12-10. Energy Equipment Survey Form

Location _____

Equipment	Number	Electricity Requirement								Gas Equipment Rated Input				Comments
		Amperes[a]	Volts[a]	Kilowatts × (kw)[b]	Hours operated per day	Days operated per week	KWH per week[c]	1000 BTU per week[d]	BTU[a] per hour	Cubic feet[e] per hour	Hours operated per day	Cubic feet[f] per week	1000 BTU[g] per week	

[a] Information found on name plate.

[b] Kilowatt—multiply amperage by voltage divided by 1000 [AMP × Volts ÷ 1000]. If horsepower unit appears on name plate, multiply by .746 for kilowatts. If wattage appears on name plate, divide by 1000 for kilowatts.

[c] Kilowatt-hours per week—measure of energy use per week. Kilowatt × hours per day × number days per week. This information can be used to determine energy cost. Multiply kilowatt-hours per week by cost per kilowatt to determine energy cost.

[d] One thousand BTUs per week. $1000 \text{ BTU} = \dfrac{\text{Kw-hr} \times 3412}{1000}$

[e] Cubic feet per hour. $\dfrac{\text{BTU per hour}}{1000}$

[f] Cubic feet per week = hours per week × days operated per week × cubic feet per hour.

[g] One thousand BTUs consumed per week = $\dfrac{\text{cubic feet} \times 1000}{1000}$

Note: There is some variance in BTU content of different types of gas but this figure will provide satisfactory results for this analysis.

This information can be used to determine energy cost. Cubic feet × cost by unit = $ _____. If billing is in therms, divide total cubic feet by 100 for number of therms.

Table 12-2. Energy Conservation Practices

Area	Conservation Practice
Food Preparation	• Cook in largest volume possible. • Cook at lowest temperature that still gives satisfactory results. • Reduce excess heat loss by carefully monitoring preheat times, cooking temperatures, and maintenance checks. • Reduce peak loading. Examples: Use high-energy-demand equipment sequentially rather than simultaneously, if possible. Schedule energy-intense cooking, such as baking and roasting, during nonpeak demand time. • Heat only portion of griddle to be used. • Use hot top water for cooking, whenever possible, except in localities where water contains concentrates of heavy metals.
Refrigeration	• Open doors as seldom as possible. • Allow hot foods to cool briefly in accordance to safe food-handling practices [see chapter 13]. • Clean condenser frequently. • Keep thermometers properly calibrated.
Lighting	• Turn off lights when not in use. • Install timing mechanisms, dimmers, or automatic photocell devices. • Color-code light control panels and switches according to a predetermined schedule of when lights should be turned on or off. • Compare the efficiencies of various types of lamps in terms of wattage, lifetime, and illumination when replacing light bulbs. • Replace incandescent lamps with high intensity.
HVAC	• Lower thermostat to 68°F in winter; raise to 78°F in summer. • Adjust duct registers to give the most efficient airflow within a room and balanced airflow between kitchen and service area if located adjacent to each other. • Stagger start-up time for individual HVAC unit to reduce demand for kilowatt-hour usage on your system and to eliminate unnecessary cooling or heating during hours before operation opens.
Sanitation	• Turn off exhaust fan when not required. • Fill dishwasher to capacity. • Hot water booster should be located within five feet of a dishwasher to avoid heat loss in the pipes. • Install a spring-operated valve on your kitchen and restroom faucets to save water. • Repair leaking faucets. • Implement effective maintenance program.

Source: Federal Energy Administration, Office of Energy Conservation and the Environment. *Guide to Energy Conservation for Food Service.* (041-018-00127-1.) Washington, DC: U.S. Government Printing Office, Jan. 1977.

☐ Air Pollution

For decades now, concerns about air pollution have commanded national and international attention. *Air pollution* is defined as the presence of substances in the air in an amount sufficient to interfere directly or indirectly with human comfort, safety, and health. Most pollutants emerge from activities associated with human comfort and a life-style oriented to conveniences and possessions. Widely recognized pollutants are products of combustion and include carbon monoxide, sulfur and nitrogen oxides, hydrocarbons, and other particulates. These pollutants have been linked to environmental concerns such as global warming (the greenhouse effect), ozone depletion, and acid rain.

Clean Air Legislation

The first Clean Air Act (Public Law 88-206), passed in 1963, established a national program to control community air pollution. Subsequent legislation has included the Air Quality Act of 1967, which identified geographic areas with significant problems and designated air quality control regions and the 1970, 1977, and, most recently, 1990 amendments to the Clean Air Act. The goal of the 1990 amendments is to remove two-thirds of U.S. air pollutants by 2005. The act also contains regulations that will directly affect food service operations, in that it contains mandates affecting the production and usage of chlorofluorocarbons (CFCs) and hydrochlorofluorocarbons (HCFCs). The control provisions of the act are to be superseded by those of an amended Montreal Protocol, whenever the Protocol is more restrictive. The act includes a requirement for the EPA to prepare comprehensive regulations for various issues related to CFC and HCFC such as service, use, and disposal of CFCs and HCFCs including recovery and recycling. These regulations will directly influence the type of refrigerants used in refrigeration and air-conditioning systems in the food service industry.

Production of chlorofluorocarbons R-11, R-12, R-113, R-114, and R-115 was to be phased out as of year-end 1993, and HCFCs will be banned by 2030. The phaseout and recovery and recycling components of the bill have already affected the design of refrigeration systems and air-conditioning units and the servicing of existing units. As of this writing, the cost of CFC R-12 is projected to triple within the next five years. Increased cost of coolants, investment in recovery systems, service contracts, and/or replacement of older refrigerators will affect food service budgets. When selecting new refrigeration equipment, food service directors must determine the type of refrigerant used, its efficiency, and the expected date it is scheduled to be phased out. Maintenance of refrigeration equipment will become more critical as refrigerant replacement cost increases.

Stricter emission standards for selected pieces of production equipment (such as charbroilers and fryers) have already been adopted in metropolitan areas that fail to meet EPA's air quality standards. When renovating production areas, it is important to check with the state and local air quality office to identify specific regulations that would dictate the type and quantity of emissions allowed from an operation.

☐ Water Conservation

Another valuable natural resource too often taken for granted by food service employees and consumers is *water*. The contamination of groundwater due to industrial wastes, human and animal feces, and other wastes; landfill leachate (ash); and fertilizer and pesticides is even more prevalent today. In addition, excessive levels of lead and other heavy metals have been found in municipal water supplies.

Clean Water Legislation

The Clean Air Act, as it is known today, was originally enacted in 1972 as the federal Water Pollution Control Act. Amendments to the original act were passed in 1977, 1981, and 1987 (the 1987 amendment is formally referred to as the Water Quality Act of 1987). The Clean Water Act is intended to improve the quality of water for human consumption through the elimination of pollution discharges into navigable rivers and to assist in the establishment of public water treatment facilities. To facilitate attainment of the goals of the act, two separate standards have been established: receiving water quality standards and effluent standards.

Selected food service operations have been affected by these standards in that providers that exceed effluent standards are subject to fines. In most instances, the source of the problem was the garbage disposal, in which cases operations were forced to discontinue using their garbage disposals. Also, where strainers have been added to pipes discharging water from warewashing equipment, operations have had to identify alternative methods for collecting and disposing of food waste and scraps and trimmings from food preparation. Consultation with representatives from local wastewater (sewage) treatment plants or the director of facilities management will assist in determining local water conservation regulations.

The availability of safe water in sufficient quantity to meet competing demands in health care operations and within the community will significantly influence operational decisions. Food service department areas that require large quantities of water include warewashing, ice machines, food preparation, drinking water, sanitation, and cooling and heating. Water conservation programs patterned after the energy management plan described earlier in this section should identify specific strategies for each of the above areas. Following are some simple commonsense suggestions:

- Repair leaking faucets.
- Do not leave water dripping from faucets.
- Thaw frozen foods in the refrigerator rather than under running water.
- Wash only full loads of dishes.
- Evaluate water consumption requirements when selecting warewashing equipment.
- Serve water only on request at catered meals.
- Evaluate feasibility of installing water-saving devices in sinks and toilets.

The goal of a water conservation program is to preserve the water supply for the most critical needs within the health care operation and the larger community.

☐ Summary

Each of the environmental issues—solid waste, hazardous waste, air pollution, energy conservation, and water quality—affects not only operational practices but also the costs of providing high-quality products and services to guests. Each waste management alternative carries with it pros and cons that must be assessed in terms of costs, effectiveness, storage capacity, and environmental impact. Because no one strategy will work for all food service operations, managers must look to the long term in selecting viable, cost-effective alternatives to waste management for their food service operations. Otherwise, the quality of life valued by most Americans will be threatened.

☐ Bibliography

Boss, D., and King, P. SFM's waste management survey. *Food Management* 28(3):42,44, Mar. 1993.

Calmbacher, C. W. Diagnosis pending for medical waste. *Environmental Protection* 4(5):22–23, 25–26, May 1993.

Casper, C. The greening of food service distribution. *Institution Distribution* 28(12):32–36, 41–42, Oct. 1992.

Chernicak, M. J. MSDs enhance training experience. *Environmental Protection* 3(4):20–21, May 1992.

Colorado Hospital Association. *Colorado Hospitals and the Environment: A Guide to Developing and Operating Effective Environmental Programs.* Denver: CHA, 1992.

Commonwealth Edison. *How to Reduce Your Energy Costs.* 2nd ed. Chicago: Commonwealth Edison, 1992.

Cummings, L. Food service solid waste wars: the solid waste audit. *The Consultant* 24(4):37–38, Fall 1991.

Cummings, L. E., and Cummings, W. T. Food service and solid waste policies: a view in three dimensions. *Hospitality Research Journal* 14(2):163–71, July 1991.

Federal Energy Administration, Office of Energy Conservation and the Environment. *Guide to Energy Conservation for Food Service.* (041-018-00127-1.) Washington, DC: U.S. Government Printing Office, Jan. 1977.

Flores, R., and Hayter, R. *Questions and Answers on Refrigerant Replacement.* (Publication No. 2-91-2M.) Manhattan, KS: Kansas State University, Cooperative Extension Service, Feb. 1991.

Frumkin, P. A little education at work goes a long way toward saving water. *The Consultant* 24(4):29, Fall 1991.

Gilkey, H. T. The coming refrigerant shortage. *Heating/Piping/Air Conditioning* 63(4):41–46, Apr. 1991.

Hagland, M. A greener image: hospitals take on environmental challenges of the '90s. *Hospitals* 67(1):17–24, Jan. 5, 1993.

Hankinson, M. G. The greening of food and beverage operations: management practice and the law. *Hospitality and Tourism Educator* 4(4):4, 9–14, Aug. 1992.

Hirshfeld, J. Maintaining refrigerators and freezers: coolant solutions. *Foodservice Director* 5(9):144, Sept. 15, 1992.

Hollingsworth, M. D., Shanklin, C. W., Gench, B., and Hinson, M. Composition of waste generated in six selected school foodservice operations. *School Food Service Research Review* 16(2):125–30, Fall 1992.

Jaffe, W. F., Almanza, B. A., and Min, C-H. J. Solid waste disposal: independent food service practice. *FIU Hospitality Review* 11(1):69–77, 1993.

King, P., and Pennacchia, M. High cost of garbage. *Food Management* 24(1)96–106, 108, Jan. 1990.

Miller, K. C. *A Profile of Energy Use in Restaurants (Tampa Bay Area).* Report to the Florida Energy Office; Energy Extension Services. IFAS. Gainesville, FL: University of Florida, Jan. 1992.

National Restaurant Association. *Utility Billing and Energy Surveys.* Chicago: TVRA, 1977.

Romanelli, F. Study shows how to measure energy use, costs, in food service. *Hospitals* 53(3):77–78, 91, Feb. 1, 1979.

Shanklin, C. W. Solid waste management: how will you respond to the challenge? *Journal of The American Dietetic Association* 91(6):663–64, June 1991.

Shanklin, C. W., and Hoover, L. Position of the American Dietetic Association: environmental issues. *Journal of The American Dietetic Association* 93(5):589–91, May 1993.

Spencer, R., and Tracy, K. Turning food waste into humus: the composting solution. *Foodservice Director* 5(10):46, Oct. 15, 1992.

Thompson, P. K. Saving water can save you money. *Restaurants USA* 12(4):10–11, Apr. 1992.

Unklesbay, N., and Unklesbay, K. *Energy Management in Foodservice.* Westport, CT: AVI Publishing Company, 1982.

U.S. Department of Labor, Occupational Safety and Health Administration. Hazardous communication. *Federal Register* 48(228):53280–348, 1983.

U.S. Environmental Protection Agency, Office of Solid Waste. *The Solid Waste Dilemma: An Agenda for Action. Final Report of the Municipal Solid Waste Task Force.* (EPA/530/SW-89-019.) Washington, DC: U.S. Government Printing Office, Feb. 1989.

Weinstein, J. Greening of the giants. *Restaurants and Institutions* 102(19):146–50, 152, 156, Oct. 15, 1992.

Chapter 13

Sanitation

□ Introduction

Food service directors have a responsibility to ensure that their operations serve food that is safe and free of contamination. The most frequently reported causes of food-borne illnesses are improper cooling of food, a lapse of 12 or more hours between preparation and consumption, infected persons handling food, inadequate reheating, improper hot holding of food products, contaminated prepared food and raw ingredients, and contaminated food preparation surfaces. Other causes include food from unsafe sources, improper cleaning of equipment and utensils, and cross-contamination of raw and cooked food. These causes illustrate that the majority of food-borne illness can be prevented if food sanitation practices and temperature controls are an integral component of a continuous quality improvement program.

Health care food service operations should take particular caution to prevent food-borne illness caused by microbial (biological), chemical, or physical hazards. Certain consumers are among the high-risk populations for contracting food-borne illness, whereas healthy individuals are at less risk. *At-risk groups* are composed of immune-compromised persons who cannot tolerate even small levels of microorganisms. At-risk groups include infants, fragile elderly, pregnant women, inpatients, malnourished individuals, and individuals with controlled physical and metabolic disorders such as diabetes and high blood pressure.

Control must be established throughout an operation. Employees should be trained on proper food handling and sanitation practices. The importance of monitoring food-handling practices must be stressed to all supervisors. Purchasing of food from reputable suppliers is essential in controlling food contamination and providing high-quality products.

Food service operations are being encouraged to implement the Hazardous Analysis Critical Control Points (HACCP) system, which was originally developed by the Pillsbury Company for the National Aeronautics and Space Administration. The HACCP system serves two functions: control of food-borne illness and monitoring of food for time–temperature abuse. Adherence to HACCP standards should result in decreased incidence of food-borne illness and in improved quality.

The food service director's responsibilities include the following:

- To provide clean and properly equipped storage and work areas that meet state and local health department standards

- To purchase wholesome food from sources that meet the standards developed by regulatory agencies and to receive and store such foods under conditions that maintain their wholesomeness and minimize the risk of contamination by microorganisms, insects, rodents, and toxic substances
- To develop written policies and procedures for maintaining the staff's personal hygiene and for preparing and serving food safely on a daily basis
- To develop written policies and procedures for cleaning and sanitizing equipment, utensils, and work areas
- To dispose of waste materials according to accepted sanitation principles and local health department regulations
- To develop programs for training and supervising employees to ensure implementation of policies and procedures established by the department and approved by the facility's administration

To implement an effective sanitation program, all managers and employees must understand causes and preventive methods for protecting food from biological, chemical, and physical hazards that can result in food-borne illness. Each operation should have established procedures that minimize risk, monitor time-temperature and cross-contamination, and initiate HACCP practices. Maintaining a clean physical plant and conducting frequent self-inspections are essential components of this effort.

This chapter will address how food service directors can help their operations protect workers and consumers against food-borne illness due to contaminated food, equipment, or work surfaces that come into contact with food. Additionally, this chapter will provide information for establishing and maintaining a sanitation program for training employees. The hazardous analysis critical control process (HACCP) will be used as a model for establishing a sanitation management program for a food service operation.

Food-borne pathogens that cause illness will be described so that managers can help guard against food-borne infections (for example, salmonellosis); food-borne intoxications (for example, staphylococci contamination); and food-borne, toxin-mediated infections (for example, *Clostridium perfringes*). Common emerging pathogens in the United States will be described, along with safeguards for suppressing them.

Chemical hazards common to the food service workplace will be described, among them insecticides, pesticides, and herbicides. Physical hazards inherent in products and packaging will be cited, as will methods for identifying critical control points along the flow of food in an operation.

Sanitary food handling—including a recommended technique for proper hand washing by food-handling personnel—will be addressed. Recommendations for safe food purchasing, storage, preparation, display, and service will be made, and environmental sanitation techniques (cleaning and sanitizing methods) and equipment storage techniques will be explored.

☐ Microbial Hazards

Microbial (biological) hazards cause the greatest number of food-borne illness outbreaks and are the most difficult to control because they involve microorganisms. *Microorganisms* are very small living creatures that multiply rapidly given the right environment. These microorganisms are classified into four major groups: bacteria, viruses, parasites, and fungi (specifically, yeasts and molds). Familiarity with each of these organisms and how they can lead to food-borne illness is essential to a food service director.

Bacteria

Of all microorganisms in a food service, bacteria are most abundant. A *bacterium* is a small single-cell organism that, like all living organisms, requires nutrients and other environmental factors such as proper pH and temperature to survive.

Bacteria cause food-borne illness in one of two ways—as pathogens or as toxins released by the bacteria. Some bacteria are pathogens or infectious disease–causing agents. Pathogens obtain their nutrients from potentially hazardous foods—meat, eggs, dairy products—and reproduce rapidly in favorable temperatures. Other bacteria in and of themselves do not cause food-borne illness, but the toxins they release as waste and decomposed material into food products cause illness when eaten by humans. Examples of pathogens include *Salmonella, Listeria monocytogenes,* and *Clostridium perfringens. Bacillus cereus* and *Clostridium botulinum* are examples of bacteria that produce toxins. Features of bacteria are described in the following subsections.

Mobility

Bacteria have been described as "notorious hitchhikers" due to their attachment to humans. Bacteria can be found in the hair; on the skin; on scars; under fingernails; on clothing; and in the mucous membranes in the nose, mouth, and throats of every individual. They are present in the intestinal tracts of humans and animals; and are transported from place to place by the air, other human beings, water, food products, rodents, insects, and other animals. Because bacteria are everywhere, they frequently end up on human hands and, if proper hygiene and food-handling practices are not followed, will end up in food products served to an operation's clients, employees, and visitors.

Growth and Reproduction

Bacteria grow by increasing their numbers through cell division rather than by increasing the size of individual cells. Thus, one cell becomes two, two become four, four become eight, and so forth. The rate at which growth occurs varies among different kinds of bacteria. Also, their growth is affected by environmental temperature, moisture levels, available food sources, oxygen levels, acidity or alkalinity of the environment, presence or absence of inhibitors, and the length of time available for reproduction.

Temperature

Bacteria grow over a wide range of temperatures. Even though the majority grow best between 60° and 120°F (15° and 49°C), some grow at even higher temperatures—the 110° to 150°F (43° to 65°C) range. Others live and multiply under refrigeration. By varying the temperature of the environment, bacterial growth can be increased, inhibited, or stopped altogether. Therefore, the growth of most bacteria can be inhibited—although not totally stopped—by reducing the temperature of foods to 45°F (7°C) or lower. This fact makes quick cooling and adequate refrigeration an important means for preventing food-borne illness caused by bacteria. Bacterial growth can be stopped completely by raising food temperature to a point at which pathogenic (disease-causing) bacteria are destroyed (a process called *pasteurization*) or to a point at which all bacteria are killed (a process called *sterilization*). At temperatures above 120°F (49°C), many bacteria begin to die or are injured; more are killed as food temperatures are increased. Because most bacteria are destroyed at 140°F (60°C), that temperature is recommended as a minimum temperature for cooking and holding foods. (Figure 13-1 illustrates the effect of temperature on bacterial growth in food.) However, optimum standards for acceptable food temperatures should be determined by individual health care institutions. Contamination usually occurs between preparation and serving, so it is important that total time between preparation and service be limited to two hours. Food held longer than two hours must be immediately refrigerated at 40°F or below, or heated to at least 140°F. Otherwise, the food must be discarded. Some bacteria develop a heat-resistant form as they grow, posing another hazard. In this form, called a *spore,* the organism's capacity to survive under unfavorable conditions is increased. Spores are so resistant to the effects of heat that very high temperatures, such as those used for canning low-acid foods (240°F or 115°C), are required for their destruction.

Figure 13-1. Effect of Temperature on Bacterial Growth in Food

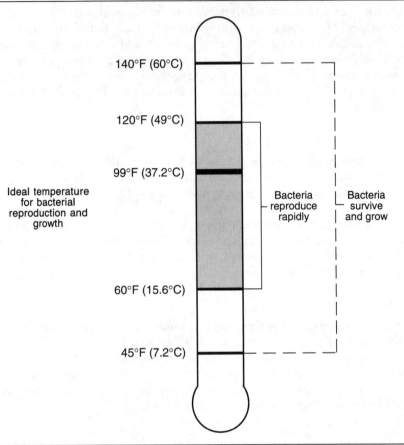

Source: Reprinted, with permission, from *Applied Foodservice Sanitation: A Certification Coursebook.* 4th ed.; published by The Educational Foundation of the National Restaurant Association, copyright 1992 by The Educational Foundation of the National Restaurant Association.

Moisture

In general, bacteria need water to grow. The amount of water available to bacteria is decreased in the presence of high concentrations of sugar or salt. This fact explains some of the preservative effects of sugar and salt solutions. Similarly, when foods are frozen, no water is available to support bacterial growth. The drying of food also reduces the moisture content to levels that cannot support the growth of most bacteria, although spores may survive the drying process.

Food

Like all living organisms, bacteria need food to fulfill their energy needs and to provide the building blocks of their physical structure. Various bacteria have markedly different food requirements: some can grow on glucose, ammonium salts, water, and certain mineral ions. Others require complex foods including vitamins, minerals, and proteins. The bacteria that cause food-borne illnesses thrive in many of the foods humans eat, especially in foods that contain proteins such as milk, milk products, eggs, meat, poultry, fish, and shellfish.

Oxygen

Some bacteria will grow only if oxygen is present, whereas others will grow only in the absence of oxygen. Many can grow under either condition.

Acidity and Alkalinity

Slightly acid (sour), neutral, and slightly alkaline (bitter) foods can support the growth of bacteria that cause food-borne illnesses. Such food materials include those of animal origin (such as meat, poultry, seafood, eggs, and milk) and low-acid vegetables (such as corn, peas, beets, and beans). Acids such as vinegar are used in food preservation to slow down bacterial growth and, in some cases, can be used in food preparation to inhibit bacterial growth. For example, commercial mayonnaise is acidic enough to suppress bacterial growth in salad mixtures when it is added early in the preparation process. Acidity also increases the sensitivity of bacteria to heat. For example, low-acid vegetables must be treated at a higher temperature and for a longer time in the canning process than is required for high-acid fruits.

Inhibitors

Many naturally occurring or manufactured chemicals, called *inhibitors,* can be used to prevent or slow down bacterial growth. For example, sodium nitrite (which is used in the curing of bacon, ham, and sausage) is effective in preventing the growth of *Clostridium botulinum* (the bacteria that cause botulism) even at low levels of concentration.

Time

Bacterial multiplication takes place over time. How rapidly bacteria grow depends on environmental conditions, including those factors already described. In food service operations, the objective is to keep foods at the recommended temperatures and under sanitary conditions for the recommended periods of time to prevent bacterial growth. Foods requiring refrigeration after preparation must be cooled rapidly to an internal temperature of 45°F (7°C) or lower. Large quantities of such foods need to be cooled in shallow pans, under quick-chilling refrigeration, or by cold-water circulation around the food container. The cooling time needed to reach 45°F (7°C) should be no more than four hours. On the other hand, cold foods should be heated as rapidly as possible to an internal temperature of 165°F (74°C) or higher and should be held at that temperature for no more than two hours.

Viruses

Viruses, another type of microorganism, are defined as noncellular organisms consisting of nucleic acids and protein that reproduce in host cells. They are the smallest and perhaps the simplest form of life and are a concern of food service managers because, unlike bacteria, viruses do not multiply outside a living cell in food products and are not complete cells. Once viruses enter a living cell, they force the cell to stop its life processes and assist in producing more viruses.

Sources of food-borne outbreak or water-borne viral disease include contaminated water supply, food handled by an infected employee who failed to follow correct personal hygiene practices, and, if eaten raw, molluscan shellfish (oysters, mussels, and clams) harvested from polluted water. The virus is found in urine and feces of infected persons and in contaminated water.

Two viruses of particular concern to the food service operation are hepatitis A and the Norwalk virus (discussed later in this chapter under emerging pathogens). These viruses are known to cause food-borne illness through poor personal hygiene practices.

Foods most often implicated in outbreaks caused by hepatitis A are prepared salads, raw or slightly cooked oysters, and items from salad bars. Any food not cooked prior to serving and handled by an infected person who practices poor personal hygiene can cause food-borne illness. To help control outbreaks, management should insist that all employees wash their hands thoroughly and often with hot water and soap, especially after toileting. As further assurance, shellfish should be purchased only from safe, certified sources.

Parasites

Parasites are tiny organisms that must live in or on a specific host to survive. Trichinosis and anisakiasis are two food-borne illnesses caused by parasites. Trichinosis is caused by ingesting undercooked pork or wild game infested with the larvae of *Trichinella spiralis*.

When humans eat undercooked, infected meat, trichinosis can result. Hogs contract the disease by consuming infested, uncooked garbage. Because most commercial pork producers no longer feed garbage to hogs, trichinosis is much less prevalent today than earlier in the century.

Heating pork to an internal temperature of 137°F (58°C) destroys the parasite, although at this temperature pork is very rare and pink and is not very palatable. Current recommendations for cooking pork to an internal temperature of 170°F (77°C) provide an ample margin of safety and yield juicy, tender meat. Processing at the temperatures used for ready-to-eat hams and canned hams also renders the meat free from potential contamination. Frozen storage at 5°F (−15°C) or lower for 20 days also will destroy the organism that causes trichinosis.

Another potential source of larvae is cross-contamination from equipment used first to grind pork infested with the parasite, and then to grind other raw meat. Pork should be cooked to an internal temperature of 150°F (65.6°C) or 170°F (76.7°C) if cooked in the microwave.

Equipment used to grind raw pork should be thoroughly washed, rinsed, and sanitized before grinding additional ingredients. The larvae can be killed if pork products less than six inches thick are stored at 5°F (−15°C) for 30 days, −10°F (−23.3°C) for 20 days, or −30°F (−34.4°C) for 12 days.

Anisakiasis is caused by the anisakis roundworm, which is found in some finfish. Foods that potentially could contain this parasite include raw fish such as sushi, ceviche, salmon, herring, and lightly cooked fish fillets.

Control measures include purchasing all fish products from reliable suppliers, obtaining guarantees that products have been properly frozen (−31°F or −25°C or lower for 15 hours), and cooking fish to an internal temperature of 140°F (60°C). (Parasites in fish products can survive the acidity of marinades.)

Fungi

Yeasts, single-celled organisms that reproduce by budding, are another organism that can cause illness in humans and result in food spoilage. (However, yeasts are also very useful in the fermentation of wines and the leavening of bakery products.) *Budding* is the process by which a small part of the parent breaks off to form a new organism that is exactly like the parent. Yeasts are responsible for a few diseases in humans, although there is no evidence to support that these diseases are transmitted by food or that yeasts occurring naturally in food are harmful to humans. Because yeasts cause spoilage of many types of food, their growth should be controlled.

Most yeasts grow best at room temperature, but some grow at the freezing point. Yeast growth is retarded or stopped at temperatures above 100°F (38°C). Yeasts require moisture and food sources such as sugars and acids for growth — a fact that explains the abundant growth of yeasts in carbohydrate foods and in acidic liquids such as vinegar and wine. Yeast-based spoilage can be controlled by following adequate cleaning and sanitizing procedures that kill the cells readily at temperatures above the boiling point of water (212°F or 100°C).

Molds are multicelled organisms that usually reproduce by spore formation. Mold spores are extremely small and very light. As a result, they can be spread quite easily by air currents, insects, and animals. Under favorable conditions, spores actively produce a fuzzy, filamentous growth on the surface of foods and other substances. Some molds are useful in the manufacture of foods, although many molds spoil foods and, under some conditions, can develop highly poisonous by-products called *mycotoxins.* Molds can grow over a wide range of conditions: moist or dry, acid or nonacid, high or low salt or sugar content, and at almost any temperature above freezing. Mold spores and vegetative growth can be destroyed easily by heat. However, constant care is needed to keep work surfaces, containers, and equipment free from mold to prevent contamination of food products.

☐ Food-Borne Illnesses

Thousands of cases of food-borne illness are reported to the U.S. Public Health Service every year. In addition, many thousands of cases go unreported. Food-borne illnesses are characterized by various degrees of upset stomach, nausea, vomiting, diarrhea, intestinal cramps, and fever. These illnesses are usually classified as either food-borne infections; food-borne intoxications; or food-borne, toxin-mediated infections. Physical and chemical hazards also can result in food-borne illnesses.

Food-Borne Infections

Food-borne infections are defined as diseases resulting from eating foods containing harmful living organisms. They are caused by the growth and activity of the infectious agent itself—bacterium, virus, or parasitic organism—in the human digestive tract. Because illness results from the activity of large numbers of cells, the time lapse between ingestion of the contaminated food and onset of symptoms may be 8 to 72 hours. During the hours before symptoms appear, the organisms actively multiply in the digestive tract.

The most frequently occurring food-borne infection, salmonellosis, is caused by *Salmonella* bacteria of several different types. The bacteria are very common in the intestinal tracts and feces of humans, animals, poultry, and shellfish from polluted waters. *Salmonella* contamination occurs in a continuous cycle: The bacteria are excreted by animals, rodents, and birds and by humans who have had the illness and who may remain carriers for some time. The microorganisms are discharged into sewage and manure and can be found in contaminated soil and sewage-polluted waters. During the slaughter of food animals, equipment and employees in the packing plant can become contaminated. In addition, the food animals themselves often are contaminated during processing. Frequently, waste products from the slaughterhouse are made into animal feeds, and viable *Salmonella* can be transmitted back to farm animals and pets when animal feeds are improperly processed. Thus, bacteria can be found on fresh meat, poultry, shelled or cracked eggs, and shellfish from contaminated waters. Bacteria also can be found in foods made from these products and contaminated during preparation. The presence of *Salmonella* bacteria in food is unnoticeable because the appearance, flavor, and odor of the food usually are not altered.

Symptoms of salmonellosis vary in severity, depending on the individual's susceptibility to the infection, the total number of cells ingested, and the bacterial strains involved. Symptoms include nausea, vomiting, abdominal pain, diarrhea, headache, chills, weakness, drowsiness, and possibly fever. The illness usually lasts two or three days, but it may linger.

Salmonellosis can be avoided by reducing the possibility of food contamination during handling and processing, by adequately cooking vulnerable foods (which can be contaminated even under the best processing conditions), and by preventing the cross-contamination of foods during the preparation process. Therefore, preparation surfaces and cutting boards should be sanitized after each use. For example, after preparation of raw chicken, the area should be thoroughly cleaned before being used for any other raw or cooked food preparation. Employees should wash their hands thoroughly with soap and running water before handling any other food products.

Food-Borne Intoxications and Food-Borne, Toxin-Mediated Infections

Food-borne intoxication results from eating food that contains toxins produced by bacterial activity. These poisonous substances are not destroyed at normal cooking temperatures. Nor do they change the flavor, appearance, or odor of foods they permeate. Several kinds of bacteria are capable of producing illness-causing toxins, but only those responsible for significant outbreaks of illness in the United States are discussed here. The symptoms of food-borne intoxication, which resemble those of salmonellosis, have more rapid onset than do the symptoms associated with infections spread through food. However, the symptoms of food intoxication persist until the toxins are eliminated from the body.

Staphylococcus aureus (S. aureus) bacteria are responsible for frequent outbreaks of food-borne illness. The most common source of staphylococci contamination is the human body, where organisms are found on the skin and in the mouths, nasal passages, and throats of healthy people. Infected pimples, sinuses, and cuts also are reservoirs for the organism. Food supplies and household pets also can be sources of *S. aureus*. Toxins are produced when foods that support the growth of staphylococci are contaminated with the organism and are allowed to stand for a sufficient period at temperatures favorable for bacterial growth. Although the bacteria are killed when subjected to temperatures as low as 140°F (60°C) for 10 minutes, toxins are highly resistant to heat, cold, and chemicals. Freezing, refrigerating, or heating foods to serving temperatures does not significantly reduce the amount of toxin. The more toxin a person ingests, the greater the reaction of the body.

Foods high in protein readily support the growth of staphylococci and have been involved in many outbreaks of food poisoning. Such foods include custards; meat sauces and gravies; fresh meats; cured meats; meat products; roasted poultry and dressing; poultry, egg, and fish salads and mixtures; raw milk; puddings; and cream-filled pastries. Any food that requires a considerable amount of handling during preparation is a possible source of food poisoning, particularly if it is not kept at safe temperatures during or after preparation.

Symptoms of staphylocci infection usually occur two or three hours after consumption of the toxin-containing food. However, the time may vary from 30 minutes to six hours. Specific symptoms of staphylococcal food intoxication include nausea, vomiting, diarrhea, dehydration, cramps, and prostration.

Clostridium perfringens (C. perfringens) bacteria have been identified as the cause of numerous cases of food-borne, toxin-mediated infections in recent years. However, the apparent increase in reported outbreaks may reflect better identification techniques and increased reporting of food-borne illnesses rather than actual increases in the occurrence of contamination and illness. The foods most often involved in outbreaks of illness are meat and poultry products that have been cooked and held for long periods or that have undergone prolonged slow cooling followed by reheating to improper temperatures and further holding.

C. perfringens bacteria are commonly found in the intestinal tracts of healthy humans and animals and in soil, water, and dust. The bacteria are able to form spores that are difficult to destroy by heating alone. The growing cells in food are destroyed through cooking. However, because spores are not killed by cooking, cooking cannot be relied on to remove the threat of poisoning from these bacteria. The organisms can grow over a wide range of temperatures and are so widespread that it is impossible to reduce their incidence. Consequently, either the spore or the vegetative form should be assumed to be present in foods.

In relatively little time, under anaerobic (oxygen-free) conditions at temperatures of 60° to 120°F (15° to 49°C), large numbers can develop. An anaerobic condition is produced in meat or meat-containing liquids after air has been eliminated from the food by heating. This condition allows the surviving spores to germinate and multiply rapidly in warm foods. Large quantities of meat broths, gravies, and meat mixtures that are permitted to cool slowly provide an ideal medium for growth.

The symptoms of *C. perfringens* illness are relatively mild but include the following: abdominal cramps, diarrhea, nausea (occasionally), and fever or vomiting (rarely). Symptoms usually begin between 8 and 22 hours after eating the contaminated food, but they have been observed as early as 2 hours after eating.

Preventing food-borne, toxin-mediated infection from *C. perfringens* requires cooking high-protein foods, particularly meat and poultry, well enough to kill the vegetative forms of the organism. Prevention also involves keeping foods hot (above 140°F [60°C]) until they are eaten. In addition, promptly refrigerating foods in shallow containers for quick temperature reduction slows down multiplication of the vegetative forms of the bacteria.

Other Food-Borne Illnesses

Although the major causes of food-borne illnesses are *Salmonella, Staphylococcus aureus,* and *Clostridium perfringens,* many other microorganisms can cause serious and even life-threatening food-borne illness. Some pathogens that have resulted in food-borne illness are discussed in the following section on emerging pathogens. Other illnesses caused by microorganisms include typhoid fever; paratyphoid fever; streptococcal, *Shigellosis,* bacterial dysentery; and amoebic dysentery. Prevention of these illnesses requires high standards of personal cleanliness, good work habits, safe water supplies, and exclusion of disease carriers from food preparation jobs. Prevention also requires that foods be cooked, chilled, and held at appropriate temperatures.

Botulism is a type of food-borne intoxication that is almost always fatal. It is rarely a problem when commercially canned foods are used but a serious threat to consumers of home-canned foods. Botulism is caused by a toxin produced by various strains of *Clostridium botulinum.* These bacteria grow in low-acid foods that have not been processed at temperatures high enough to destroy the bacterial spores. Food services should purchase only commercially processed vegetables, meats, and other low-acid foods. Food service employees should *never* open or use a canned food when the can is bulging, severely dented, or leaky. Such canned goods must be discarded immediately.

☐ Emerging Pathogens

Until recently, food-borne illnesses in the United States were linked to four well-known pathogens: *Staphylococcus aureus, Salmonella spp., Clostridium perfringens,* and *Bacillus cereus.* Several other pathogens, often referred to as emerging pathogens, have been identified as important causes of food-borne illness. Examples of emerging pathogens of particular concern to food service operations include: *Campylobacter jejuni, Listeria monocytogenes,* Norwalk virus, and *enterohemorrhagic Escherichia coli* 0157:H7. These pathogens are often transmitted to the food supply through contaminated water or raw manure, carried by humans, or transferred to food products during processing.

Campylobacter jejuni

Campylobacterosis is a food-borne infection caused by the pathogen *Campylobacter jejuni.* The bacterium is a nonforming anaerobic pathogen widely found in nature. The organism is carried in the intestinal tracts of cows, pigs, sheep, and poultry, and frequently contaminates foods of animal sources. Other foods that have been found to be contaminated with *C. jejuni* include raw milk, fresh mushrooms, and raw hamburger.

Most outbreaks of campylobacteriosis are caused by underpasteurized milk or contaminated water. Food-borne outbreaks have been linked to raw or undercooked meat or poultry or these products being recontaminated after cooking by contact with *C. jejuni*–contaminated materials such as cutting boards. (See table 13-1.)

C. jejuni is sensitive to heat and temperatures below 30°C and can be easily destroyed through proper food-handling practices. The growth of this bacterium quickly declines at room temperature and more slowly at refrigerated temperature. The organism also is sensitive to acidic conditions.

Listeria monocytogenes

Although *Listeria,* a related group of bacteria, has been classified as a human pathogen for more than 60 years, the importance of food as a transmission vehicle has been identified only

Table 13-1. Emerging Pathogens

Pathogen	Infection/Illness	Source (Vehicle)	Food Implicated	Preventive/Control Measures
Campylobacter jejuni	Campylobacteriosis infection	Contaminated H_2O; domestic and wild animals (intestines); food handlers (feces)	Raw or undercooked meat and poultry; underpasteurized milk and dairy products; raw milk; raw vegetables	Purchase products from reliable sources; cook food thoroughly; pasteurization; avoid cross-contamination; time/temperature control
Listeria monocytogenes	Listeriosis	Food handlers (feces, nose and throat secretions); domestic and wild animals; water; soil and mud	Underpasteurized milk and cheese; raw vegetables; seafood; prepared ready-to-eat refrigerated foods	Use pasteurized milk and dairy products; avoid cross-contamination; thoroughly cook food; wash raw vegetables thoroughly; reheat leftovers thoroughly; time/temperature control
Norwalk virus	Norwalk	Humans (intestinal tract); domestic animals, particularly cattle	Contaminated H_2O from fecal material; raw shellfish; raw vegetables; prepared salads	Use potable water only; purchase food from reliable sources; thoroughly cook food; good personal hygiene practice followed by all food handlers
Escherichia coli 0157:H7	Hemorrhagic colitis; renal failure	Domestic animals (intestinal tract); humans (feces)	Raw and undercooked beef and other red meat; imported cheeses; unpasteurized milk; prepared ready-to-eat products	Thoroughly cooked beef and red meat; avoid cross-contamination; use only potable water; purchase food from reliable sources; food handlers practice good personal hygiene

in recent years. *Listeria monocytogenes* are the specific species of bacteria that can cause listeriosis. The source of the bacteria is most often contaminated food.

Cross-contamination can pose serious health risks. For example, if certain cheeses that have been contaminated with *Listeria monocytogenes* come in contact with raw food such as meats, poultry, fish, or raw vegetables after their package is opened, the result may be significant growth of the organism at refrigerated temperature.

Individuals most susceptible to listeriosis are persons over age 60, newborns, and patients whose immune systems are compromised by cancer, AIDS, or immunosuppressive medications such as steroids. Individuals suffering from cirrhosis, diabetes, and ulcerature colitis are more at risk. Complications including miscarriage, meningitis, septicemia, pneumonia, and endocarditis can result from serious cases of listeriosis.

Individuals in these high-risk populations are advised not to consume pâté or low-acid soft cheeses such as Mexican-style cheese, Brie, feta, bleu cheese, and Camembert. These foods have been associated with greater incidences of listeriosis. Other foods that have been found contaminated with the bacteria include raw, soil-grown vegetables, such as cabbage, celery, and lettuce; unpasteurized milk; raw meat; and poultry.

L. monocytogenes are particularly problematic in food service operations because the bacteria grow slowly at refrigeration temperatures (32° to 34°F) and on moist surfaces. Procedures to avoid cross-contamination during preparation and service should be followed by all food handlers. Because Listeria can grow on wet floors, on sponges, and in drains, food service managers should insist on clean, dry facilities.

Public health officials recommend that food-processing plants and food service operations implement the HACCP system to control transmission of Listeria during processing. Listed below are some specific recommendations for consumers and food service employees to consider in efforts to decrease risk of listeriosis and other food-borne illness.

- Monitor the temperature of food products and the length of time products are exposed to room temperature.
- Wash raw vegetables thoroughly.
- Quickly chill products.
- Thoroughly cook all food of animal origin, including eggs, and reheat leftovers thoroughly.
- Avoid cross-contamination between raw and cooked products.
- Never purchase raw or unpasteurized milk.
- Thoroughly heat refrigerated foods, including ready-to-eat meats and minimally processed foods such as sous vide products (described in chapter 1).

Compounds proved to be particularly effective in inhibiting or inactivating *L. monocytogenes* include iodine (25 ppm), acid sanitizers (130 to 200 ppm), and quaternary ammonium compounds (QUATS, at 200 ppm). Also effective is chlorine at different concentrations such as 20 ppm for water treatment and 200 ppm for cleaning walls, stainless steel equipment, and nonporous surfaces.

Norwalk Virus

Norwalk is a viral illness caused by poor personal hygiene practices among food handlers infected with the virus, which is transmitted through contaminated water supplies and human contact. Because Norwalk is a virus, it does not reproduce in food but remains viable until the food is consumed. Other foods that have been implicated in Norwalk outbreaks include raw vegetables fertilized with manure, eggs, shellfish, coleslaw, frozen foods, and manufactured ice cubes.

As with Listeria, control of Norwalk virus is difficult because the virus can withstand freezing temperatures and chlorine sanitizing solution. However, the virus is susceptible to high temperature; therefore, all food should be cooked thoroughly prior to service. Cross-contamination should be avoided. Other ways to avoid contaminating food with the Norwalk virus include ensuring proper personal hygiene among food handlers, purchasing shellfish from reliable certified sources, and using only water from a potable source.

Enterohemorrhagic Escherichia coli 0157:H7

Escherichia coli (E. Coli) 0157:H7 is a nonspore-forming, facultative bacterium, and many food-related outbreaks have been reported since the pathogen was first identified in 1982. The bacterium can cause hemorrhagic colitis (bloody diarrhea) and renal failure (hemolytic uremic symptoms). Undercooked or raw ground beef and red meat (lamb and pork) and unpasteurized milk have been implicated as transmitters of *E. coli.*

E. coli, which has also been found in prepared foods (such as mashed potatoes, cream pies, finfish, and imported cheese), differs from other *E. coli* because the organism is found in the intestinal tracts of animals used as food. Fecal contamination can occur during slaughtering. Important control measures include:

- Good food-manufacturing practices (such as avoiding cross-contamination and maintaining sanitized equipment in processing plants)
- Proper heating of meats. For example, ground beef products should be cooked to 134°F; other meats should be cooked to 134°F and held at this temperature for at least two hours or undergo thorough cooking. Leftover red meat should be reheated to at least 165°F.
- Employees should follow good hand-washing and personal hygiene practices at all times.

Other emerging pathogens include *Salmonella enteritidis* (ovarian-infecting), *Vibrio parahaemolyticus,* and *Yersinia enterocolitica.* The incidence of food-borne illness caused by these organisms is reported less frequently. Cases of food-borne disease can be significantly reduced if food handlers practice the proper food-handling and sanitation procedures discussed here and summarized in table 13-1.

□ Chemical Hazards

Chemical hazards are those dangers posed by chemical substances that contaminate food at some point along the food chain. For example, the use of agricultural chemicals such as insecticides, pesticides, and herbicides can cause food contamination. Federal regulations identify the acceptable type and quantity of these agricultural food sources. Control measures include careful and thorough rinsing of all produce prior to serving raw or cooking and purchasing of produce only from reputable, legally approved sources. Four chemical hazards are of particular concern to health care food service operations:

1. Excessive quantities of additives
2. Contamination of food products with chemicals (such as detergents, cleaning solutions, and sanitizers) used for sanitation purposes
3. Acidic food in metal-lined containers
4. Contamination of food with toxic metals

Food service managers should be especially cautious with use of additives such as monosodium glutamate (MSG), sulfiting agents, and nitrites. Adding MSG to products should be discouraged altogether if possible. The labels of prepared products should be studied closely to determine which ones contain MSG; this information should be made available to clients who express sensitivity to it. The Food and Drug Administration (FDA) prohibits the addition of sulfites to food service products. Fish, vegetables, and fruit that already contain sulfites to maintain freshness and color should be stored away from unprocessed products, especially on salad and dessert bars. Read labels and check with produce distributors to determine if sulfite has been added. Products containing nitrites should not be served if they are overbrowned or burned.

Food service managers and supervisors must familiarize themselves with the chemicals used in their operations and with the product additives approved by the FDA for food service operations. Following label instructions and storing chemicals away from food products should be routine practice.

☐ Physical Hazards

A *physical hazard* is the presence of any item that typically is not part of the food product. Examples of physical hazards that might be found in food products include metal objects (such as pins, packaging staples, and shavings from cans), pieces of broken glass, and toothpicks. These hazards can best be avoided by efficient work area layout and by employee training.

☐ Hazard Analysis Critical Control Point

Hazard analysis critical control point (HACCP) is a food safety and self-inspection process (also described as a self-control safety assurance program) that focuses on the flow of potentially hazardous foods and how they are handled throughout the operation. The National Restaurant Association has developed a similar program called Sanitary Assessment of the Food Environment (SAFE).

Although a new concept in food service operations, HACCP originated in the chemical-processing industry more than 40 years ago. The system was used by the Pillsbury Company in 1971 for developing food products for the National Aeronautics and Space Administration. Pillsbury later adopted and expanded the concept for its liability control program. The system has since been adopted by major food processors to monitor food handling and ensure zero defects.

In food service management, HACCP focuses on the flow of food through the operation, beginning with the decision of what foods to include on the menu and continuing with recipe development, food procurement, delivery and storage, preparation, holding or displaying, service, cooling, storage, and reheating. Because the potential for contamination exists at each step, the chance that a specific condition or set of conditions will lead to hazard is a considerable risk. The goal of HACCP is to identify and eliminate hazard or unacceptable contamination, be it biological, chemical, or physical. Success relies on identification of critical control points. Implementing an HACCP system involves seven steps.

Step 1: Identify and assess hazards at each step in the flow of food and develop procedures to minimize the risk at each step. By reviewing each recipe and developing a recipe flowchart such as the one shown in figure 13-2, managers and food handlers can learn what microorganisms are likely to cause food-borne illness. Sources of particular concern include raw food of animal origin (raw poultry, shell eggs, fresh seafood, dairy products, cooked rice, gravies and sauces, potato and protein salads, and raw meat) and surfaces of raw vegetables and spices and herbs. Refrigerated foods and sous vide products also should be considered potentially hazardous. In addition to recipe ingredients, other sources of potential contamination are food handlers, temperature of refrigerated and frozen storage, and food contact surfaces including equipment and utensils. It is especially important to observe food-handling practices, heating and cooling time, and temperatures. Examples of common hazardous practices in food service operations include:

- Infrequent and inadequate hand washing by food handlers
- Improper refrigerator temperatures (for example, other than 30° to 34°F)
- Rinsing raw produce in same sink where raw poultry was thawed without first sanitizing the sink
- Inadequate sanitation of slicers and food choppers between uses
- Cooling food in large stockpots in refrigerator instead of using shallow pans

Other examples are noted in table 13-2 (p. 314). Foods classified as potentially hazardous and their preparation, holding, and storage should be considered as high in risk.

Figure 13-2. HACCP Recipe Flowchart

Critical Control	Hazard	Standards	Corrective Action If Standard Not Met
		Receiving	
Receiving beef	Contamination and spoilage	Accept beef at 45°F (7.2°C) or lower; verify with thermometer	Reject delivery
		Packaging intact	Reject delivery
		No off odor or stickiness, and so on	Reject delivery
Receiving vegetables	Contamination and spoilage	Packaging intact	Reject delivery
		No cross-contamination from other foods on the truck	Reject delivery
		No signs of insect or rodent activity	Reject delivery
		Storage	
Storing raw beef	Cross-contamination of other foods	Store on lower shelf	Move to lower shelf away from other foods
	Bacterial growth and spoilage	Label, date, and use first-in-first-out (FIFO) rotation	Use first; discard if maximum time is exceeded or suspected
		Beef temperature must remain below 45°F (7.2°C)	Discard if time and temperature abused
Storing vegetables	Cross-contamination from raw potentially hazardous foods	Label, date, and use FIFO rotation	Discard product held past rotation date
		Keep above raw potentially hazardous foods	Discard contaminated, damaged, or spoiled products
		Preparation	
Trimming and cubing beef	Contamination, cross-contamination, and bacteria increase	Wash hands	Wash hands
		Clean and sanitize utensils	Wash, rinse, and sanitize utensils and cutting board
		Pull and cube one roast at a time, then refrigerate	Return excess amount to refrigerator
Washing and cutting vegetables	Contamination and cross-contamination	Wash hands	Wash hands
		Use clean and sanitized cutting board, knives, utensils	Wash, rinse, and sanitize utensils and cutting board
		Wsah vegetables in clean and sanitized vegetable sink	Clean and sanitize vegetable sink before washing vegetables
		Cooking	
Cooking stew	Bacterial survival	Cook *all* ingredients to minimum internal temperature of 165°F (73.9°C)	Continue cooking to 165°F (73.9°C)
		Verify final temperature with thermometer	Continue cooking to 165°F (73.9°C)
	Physical contamination during cooking	Keep covered, stir often	Cover
	Contamination by herbs and spices	Add spices early in cooking procedure	Continue cooking at least one-half hour after spices are added
		Measure all spices, flavor enhancers, and additives, and read labels carefully	

continued on next page

Figure 13-2. *Continued*

Critical Control	Hazard	Standards	Corrective Action If Standard Not Met
	Contamination of utensils	Use clean and sanitized utensils	Wash, rinse, and sanitize all utensils before use
	Contamination from cook's hands or mouth	Use proper tasting procedures	Discard product

Holding and Service

Critical Control	Hazard	Standards	Corrective Action If Standard Not Met
Hot holding and serving	Contamination, bacterial growth	Use clean and sanitary equipment to transfer and hold product	Wash, rinse, and sanitize equipment before transferring food product to it
		Hold stew above 140°F (60°C) in preheated holding unit, stir to maintain even temperature	Return to stove and reheat to 165°F (73.9°C)
		Keep covered	Cover
		Clean and sanitize serving equipment and utensils	Wash, rinse, and sanitize serving utensils and equipment

Cooling

Critical Control	Hazard	Standards	Corrective Action If Standard Not Met
Cooling for storage	Bacterial survival and growth	Cool rapidly in ice water bath and/or shallow pans (< 4″ deep)	Move to shallow pans
		Cool rapidly from 140°F (60°C) to 45°F (7.2°C) in four hours or less	Discard, or reheat to 165°F (73.9°C) and re-cool one time only
		Verify final temperature with a thermometer; record temperatures and times before product reaches 45°F (7.2°C) or less	If temperature is not reached in less than four hours, discard; or reheat product to 165°F (73.9°C) and re-cool one time only
	Cross-contamination	Place on top shelf	Move to top shelf
		Cover immediately after cooling	Cover
		Use clean and sanitized pans	Wash, rinse, and sanitize pans before filling them with product
		Do not stack pans	Separate pans by shelves
	Bacterial growth in time or after prolonged storage time	Label with date and time	Label with date and time or discard

Reheating

Critical Control	Hazard	Standards	Corrective Action If Standard Not Met
Reheat for service	Survival of bacterial contaminants	Heat rapidly on stove top or in oven to 165°F (73.9°C)	Reheat to 165°F (73.9°C) within two hours
		Maintain temperature at 140°F (60°C) or above; verify temperature with a thermometer	Transfer to preheated hot-holding unit to maintain 140°F (60°C) or above
		Do not mix new product into old product	Discard product
		Do not reheat or serve leftovers more than once	Discard product if any remains after being reheated

Source: Used, with permission, from *Applied Foodservice Sanitation: A Certification Coursebook.* 4th ed.; published by The Educational Foundation of the National Restaurant Association, copyright 1992 by The Educational Foundation of the National Restaurant Association.

Table 13-2. Hazardous Practices Observed in Food Service Operations

Condition/Area	Hazardous Practices

Preparation and display of potentially hazardous foods (raw poultry, raw meat, raw seafood, dairy products)	• Setting up and taking down raw and cooked items for display with either bare hands or the same pair of gloves
	• Reusing the same kale, lemon leaves, lettuce, or other vegetable garnish or decorative plastic dividers or color enhancers indiscriminately for raw and cooked foods
	• Displaying cooked foods in the same case as raw seafood, poultry, and/or meat:
	  —As to be in physical contact with one another
	  —So that drippings from raw items can flow through ice or along garnish and reach the cooked items below
	  —Without separation by baffles or in separate cases
	• Infrequent hand washing by persons who handle these foods
	• Refrigerators and cases not kept at temperatures between 30° and 34°F (±1°C)

Preparation and display of salads	• Handling salad ingredients with bare hands during preparation • Soaking vegetables in a sink previously used for thawing or washing raw poultry • Ingredients not prechilled • Slicing, chopping, and grating equipment and utensils not properly cleaned • Foods on display, particularly near top surfaces not at temperatures of 45°F (7.1°C) or below • Refrigerator temperatures higher than 40°F (4.4°C) • Infrequent hand washing
Preparation of entrees, soups, sauces, stews, and other viscous products	• Cooked food left at room temperature for several hours • Inadequate cooking of poultry, pork, and other foods that are likely to be contaminated with vegetative forms of food-borne pathogens • Temperatures of batches of meat, poultry, items containing ground meat, and stuffed items not monitored at the completion of cooking • Insufficient thawing of foods before cooking, which may contribute to inadequate cooking • Leftovers reheated to insufficiently high temperatures • Kitchen personnel handling or otherwise touching cooked foods with their bare hands • Kitchen personnel handling raw foods or eggshells either with their hands or gloves and then handling cooked foods • Table surfaces or cutting boards used for raw meat, raw poultry, raw seafood, and then (without washing or disinfecting) used for either cooked foods or foods that will not be heated subsequently • Clothes and sponges used to wipe raw-food areas or equipment

Holding of hot food	• Foods held warm, but not hot, for eight hours or longer
	• Foods not held at temperatures of 130°F (54.4°C); (140°F [60°C] to satisfy requirements in many codes) or higher, sometimes in the temperature range of 70° to 120°F (21.1° to 48.9°C) within which bacterial growth can be very rapid
	• Hot-holding units not used as designed, for example:
	  —Foods on display in baking pans or baskets that are tilted up by objects under the back end of the pans or baskets
	  —Foods in bowls while displayed in steam tables
	  —Packaged foods on edges of heating elements and on the side framing of the units
	  —Items stacked on top of other items
	• Hot-holding units not operated as intended, for example:
	  —Thermostats turned lower than recommended or necessary to hold foods at temperatures of 130°F (140°F to satisfy requirements in many codes) or higher
	  —Fans in units not turned on
	  —Glass walls removed from units
	  —Steam-table water not in

Cooling of products for storage	• Storing foods while they are being cooled in large containers, such as:
	  —Five-gallon (22.7 L) plastic buckets
	  —Stockpots
	  —Soup–kettle inserts
	  —Pans (plastic or metal) that have heights greater than 4 inches (10 cm)
	• Tightly covered containers of hot foods during initial cooling
	• Containers of foods being "cooled" while stacked on top of others
	• Refrigerator temperatures higher than 40°F (4.4°C)
	• Inadequate number of racks in refrigerators to adequately store shallow pans of foods
	• Shelf spacing in refrigerators too great to facilitate the storage of the needed number of shallow pans

Step 2: Determine critical control points (CCPs). According to the U.S. Department of Agriculture (USDA), CCPs are defined as "any point or procedure in a specific food system where loss of control may result in an unacceptable health risk." These include any operational practice or procedure at which prevention of hazard could occur and food hazards could be identified or eliminated. The following critical control points should be monitored for microbial contamination or time or temperature abuses:

- Food procurement, including source of supply and condition of food upon receipt
- Food storage, particularly refrigerator storage temperatures
- Food packaging
- Preprocessing
- Heat processing
- Food storage following heat processing
- Heat processing of precooked menu items
- Food production distribution (tray line operation and delivery)
- Food service, including display

Each type of food service production system (assembly–serve, cook–serve with limited holding, cook–serve with extended holding, cook–chill, and cook–freeze) has critical control points as illustrated in table 13-3. (A description of each of these production systems is presented in chapter 19.)

Step 3: Establish the critical limits or criteria (control procedures and CCP standards) that must be met at each identified CCP. Examples of criteria include cooling foods rapidly so they do not remain in the critical temperature zone of 70° to 120°F for longer than three hours and continue cooling foods until internal temperature is 45°F or less within six hours. Time–temperature relationships and cross-contamination are important criteria for all food products.

Step 4: Delineate responsibility of food handlers and supervisors in making observations and taking temperatures. Monitoring procedures can be devised using the recipe flowchart developed in step 1. The intent of step 4 is to identify any problems that may have occurred. Examples of problems that may be observed include improper storage of raw meat products in refrigerated storage, freezer temperature being less than 32°F, or cross-contamination from cutting boards.

Step 5: Take corrective action as needed. Corrective action on the part of employee or supervisor seeks to eliminate deficiencies identified in step 4. This may mean reheating food being held hot, chilling food in a more efficient manner to increase the rate of cooling, or discarding food. The degree of potential risk of a food-borne illness will determine the action to be taken.

Table 13-3. Critical Control Points in Food Production Systems

System	Critical Control Points
Assembly–serve	• Source of food • Storage temperature along food chain
Cook–serve	• Internal temperature and length of cooking
Cook–serve extended hold (conventional)	• Temperature of holding
Cook–chill	• Packaging • Cooling method and rate • Storage temperature • Reheating time and temperature
Cook–freeze	• Packaging • Cooking method and rate • Storage temperature • Reheating time and temperature

Step 6: Develop a record system to document HACCP. Tools toward this end may include temperature logs, flowcharts, or other techniques to monitor HACCP process. Corrective actions also should be documented.

Step 7: Verify that the HACCP system works. It is imperative that food service directors verify that known hazards have been identified, that hazard risks have been assessed accurately and rationally, and that appropriate CCPs have been identified. Furthermore, confirmation must be made that effective criteria for control have been specified, control measures are in use, and monitoring procedures are realistic and the most effective available. The verification process should also confirm that employees are actually implementing control procedures and recording only data actually observed.

Unlike approaches that focus predominately on short-term training of employees, HACCP is an ongoing self-control program that can be readily integrated into an operation's continuous quality improvement (CQI) program. However, commitment from managers and all employees is essential for it to be effective. Development and implementation require an investment of time, financial, and personal resources, but the potential to improve food safety and quality make the effort well worthwhile. Many public health departments are considering adopting HACCP for inspection of health care food service facilities.

☐ Sanitary Food Handling

The FDA developed the Model Food Service Sanitation Ordinance in 1976, since which time it has been adopted by many state and local health agencies. In addition, the Joint Commission on Accreditation of Healthcare Organizations (JCAHO) publishes standards for sanitation and safety. These revised standards became effective in January 1979 and have been updated yearly since then. The recommendations of the two organizations on the purchase; storage; preparation; and handling and holding (that is, display, service, and transport) of food and on facilities and equipment as well as on employee hygiene practices are meant to ensure provision of sanitary food in food service establishments and health care institutions. The recommendations can be used as an outline for employee orientation and continuing training in food safety.

Purchase of Food Supplies

Every effort must be made to purchase food that has been processed under safe and sanitary conditions. Toward this end, certain precautions should be considered:

- Purchases should be made only from licensed food-processing and supply sources that comply with all laws relating to food processing and labeling.
- Fluid milk and fluid milk products must be pasteurized and must meet Grade A quality standards. Dry milk products should be made only from pasteurized milk.
- Only meat and meat products inspected by the USDA or a state regulatory agency should be purchased. Poultry, poultry products, and egg products should have been inspected by the USDA as well. Fishery products inspected by the U.S. Department of Commerce (USDC) should be purchased whenever possible.
- Shellfish should be purchased from a reputable dealer that complies with the regulations of state and local agencies.
- Only clean eggs with uncracked shells or pasteurized liquid, frozen, or dried egg products should be used. Commercially prepared hard-cooked peeled eggs also could be used.
- Food products that may have been contaminated by insects, rodents, or water and foods in cans that bulge or are severely dented should not be accepted.
- All incoming food supplies should be inspected for evidence of damage to cartons, packages, or containers from filth, water, insects, or rodents. Damaged or spoiled products and frozen foods that show evidence of thawing or refreezing should be rejected.

Storage

Foods must be protected from contamination, spoilage, and other damage during storage in the dry, refrigerated, or frozen state. Guidelines for each kind of storage are provided in the following subsections.

Dry Storage

Food service directors must make every effort to comply with dry storage requirements pertaining to food supplies. These include the following:

- Food that requires no refrigeration should be stored in a clean, cool, dry storeroom that is well ventilated and adequately lighted. A temperature range between 50° and 70°F (10° to 21°C) is recommended for maintaining high quality. Containers of food, except those on pallets or dollies, should be stored at least six inches above the floor (or arranged as local ordinances require).
- Quantity lots of cases and boxed foods are more stable for handling when they are stacked in alternating patterns on dollies or pallets. Smaller lots of canned or packaged foods may be stored on metal shelves in or out of the case. A stock numbering or dating system is recommended so that all stock can be easily rotated.
- Once the original container or package of dry bulk foods (flour, sugar, cereal, beans, and so forth) has been opened, the remaining products should be emptied into good-quality plastic or metal containers with tight-fitting covers. The containers should be labeled clearly and stored on dollies or shelves that are at least six inches above the floor (or arranged as local ordinances require).
- Cleaning supplies, bleaches, insecticides, and other potentially hazardous chemicals should be labeled and stored in an area entirely separate from food and paper storage and preferably under lock and key.
- Food supplies should not be stored under exposed or unprotected water or sewer lines except for automatic fire protection sprinkler heads, which are often required by law.
- The floors, shelves, and walls of the storeroom should be kept clean and dry at all times, with cleaning scheduled at regular intervals.
- The items most frequently needed should be located near the storeroom entrance.
- Heavy packages should be stored on lower shelves.

Refrigerated Storage

Refrigerated storage standards apply not only to foods but to the refrigeration equipment as well. Some standards are:

- Enough conveniently located refrigeration facilities should be provided to ensure the proper maintenance of food at 45°F (7°C) or lower during storage. Each refrigerator should be equipped with a numerically scaled indicating thermometer, accurate to ±3°F (±1.5°C). The thermometer should be located in the warmest part of the unit and placed where it can be easily read, preferably from outside the refrigeration unit. Temperature records must be maintained. Recording thermometers accurate to ±3°F (±1.5°C) may be used in lieu of indicating thermometers.
- Perishable food should be refrigerated at 38°F (3°C) until preparation or service time.
- Potentially hazardous foods requiring refrigeration after preparation should be rapidly cooled to an internal temperature of 45°F (7°C) or lower within a cooling period of not more than four hours. Potentially hazardous foods prepared in large quantities should be rapidly cooled by using shallow pans, agitation, quick chilling, or water circulation external to the food container. Ice that has been used for cooling stored food, food containers, or food utensils must not be consumed by humans.
- In walk-in refrigerators, all foods should be covered and stored above the floor on easily cleaned metal shelves or on movable equipment. Shelves should be uncovered so as to allow full air circulation around food and facilitate shelf cleaning.

- Cooked food should be covered and positioned on shelves above raw food to avoid contamination from drippage and spills.
- Food stored in refrigerators should be covered or wrapped in labeled and dated containers. Open containers of canned food may be covered and stored in the original cans in the refrigerator for later use. Maximum recommended length of time to store open containers of canned food is two or three days.
- Dairy products should be stored separately from strong-smelling foods and fish. Fruits and vegetables should be checked daily for spoilage.
- The cleaning of refrigerated storage rooms should be scheduled at regular intervals and an established preventive maintenance program for all refrigeration equipment should be followed.

Frozen Storage

Conditions for frozen storage also apply to equipment as well as food. Some standards are:

- Frozen foods should be kept frozen and stored at a temperature of 0°F (−18°C) or lower. The freezer thermometer should be checked frequently and the temperature recorded.
- All frozen food packages should be labeled and dated and well wrapped in moistureproof and vaporproof material to prevent freezer burn.
- The shelves, walls, and floors of freezers should be kept clean at all times, with defrosting done as often as necessary to eliminate excessive frost buildup. Contents should be moved to another freezer during the defrosting process.
- Frozen foods should be thawed in a refrigerator at a temperature not higher than 45°F (7°C) or under clean potable running water at a temperature not higher than 70°F (21°C). Food thawed by the latter method should be kept in its original waterproof package. However, most frozen foods can be cooked directly from the frozen state.
- Frozen foods can be thawed in a microwave oven but only when the foods will be transferred immediately to conventional cooking equipment or when the entire uninterrupted cooking process will take place in the microwave oven.
- Thawed food should be used immediately or stored in the refrigerator for a short period before use. Refreezing of thawed foods should be avoided because of the possibility of spoilage and the loss of flavor and nutritional value.
- Partially thawed frozen foods may be safely refrozen if they still contain ice crystals, but their quality may be reduced. The quality of fruits, vegetables, and red meats usually is not as severely affected by temperature changes as that of fish, shellfish, poultry, and cooked foods.

Preparation

Food should be prepared with the least possible handling, with suitable utensils, and on surfaces that have been cleaned, rinsed, and sanitized to prevent cross-contamination. Raw fruits and vegetables should be thoroughly washed with clean water before being cooked or served. However, they should never be washed in hand sinks or dish sinks. Other guidelines are as follows:

- Washed and unwashed foods should be handled separately.
- Food service employees should wash their hands after cleaning food.
- For many potentially hazardous foods that require cooking, heating to the point that all parts of the food are heated to a temperature of at least 140°F (60°C) is sufficient. However, poultry, poultry stuffings, stuffed meats, and stuffings containing meat should be cooked to heat all parts of the food to at least 165°F (74°C), with no interruption of the cooking process. Pork and any food containing pork (for example, lard) should be cooked to heat all parts of the food to at least 150°F (65°C). Even though this

temperature is adequate to kill the organisms that cause trichinosis, a temperature of 170°F (77°C) for fresh pork is recommended to ensure the product's palatability. Rare roast beef and rare beefsteak should be cooked to an internal temperature of at least 130°F (54°C), but they must be served immediately after cooking.

- Reconstituted dry milk and dry milk products may be used in instant desserts and whipped products or for cooking and baking purposes. They should not be served as beverages or in beverages because of the potential for contamination in reconstituting and dispensing such products.

- Liquid, frozen, and dry eggs and egg products are pasteurized at temperatures high enough to destroy any pathogenic organisms that might be present. However, because of the possibility of recontaminating these products after opening, thawing, or reconstituting them, they are recommended for use primarily in cooked or baked products.

- Nondairy creaming, whitening, and whipping agents should be reconstituted on the food service premises and stored in sanitized covered containers not larger than one gallon. They should be cooled to 45°F (7°C) or lower within four hours after preparation.

- Potentially hazardous foods that have been cooked and then refrigerated should be rapidly reheated to 165°F (74°C) or higher before being served or before being placed in hot-food storage equipment. Steam tables, hot-water baths, warmers, and similar holding equipment for hot food should never be used for the rapid reheating of potentially hazardous foods.

- Numerically scaled indicating thermometers with metal stems, accurate to ±2°F (±1°C), should be provided to ensure the attainment and maintenance of proper internal cooking, holding, and refrigeration temperatures of all potentially hazardous foods.

- Separate acrylic, plastic, or rubber cutting boards that do not have holes or splints that could collect food or bacteria should be used for meat, poultry, fish, and raw fruits and vegetables. Cooked foods should not be cut on the same board as raw foods. However, nonabsorbent boards can be used for raw and cooked foods when boards are cleaned and sanitized between uses.

Display, Service, and Transport

Foods must be handled and held according to specific guidelines. The following procedures should be enforced for displaying, serving, and transporting food:

- Potentially hazardous food should be kept at an internal temperature of 45°F (7°C) or lower or at 140°F (60°C) or higher during transportation, display, and service.

- Milk and milk products for drinking purposes should be provided to the consumer in unopened commercially filled packages no larger than 1 pint in capacity. Or they should be drawn from a commercially filled container stored in a mechanically refrigerated bulk milk dispenser. If such a dispenser is unavailable and portions of less than ½ pint are required for service, the milk products may be poured from a commercially filled container no larger than ½ gallon.

- Cream and half-and-half should be provided in individual service containers or protected pour-type pitchers. Or they should be drawn from refrigerated dispensers designed for such service.

- Nondairy creaming and whitening agents should be provided in individual service containers or protected pour-type pitchers. Or they should be drawn from refrigerated dispensers.

- Condiments for self-service use can be served in individual packages, from dispensers, or from their original containers. Seasonings and dressings for self-service use can be served in the same fashion or from counters or salad bars that are protected from contamination.

- To avoid unnecessary manual contact with food, suitable dispensing utensils (for example, ladles or spoons) should be used by employees or provided to consumers who serve themselves. Between uses, dispensing utensils should be stored in the food or stored clean and dry, under running water, or in a running water dipper well.
- Food on display should be protected from contamination by being supplied in appropriate packaging; by being displayed on easily cleaned counters or serving lines; or by being protected by salad bar protector devices, display cases, or other shielding devices. Enough hot- or cold-holding equipment should be available to keep potentially hazardous food at safe temperature levels.
- Self-service consumers should not be allowed to serve themselves with soiled tableware. Beverage cups and glasses, however, may be refilled without contaminating bulk supplies.
- Once they have been served, leftover food portions should not be served again, although packaged food that is still sealed and in sound condition may be salvaged.
- Foods in original individual packages need not be overwrapped or covered unless the packages have been torn or broken.
- Ice for consumer use should be dispensed only by employees who use scoops, tongs, or other ice-dispensing utensils or through automatic self-service, ice-dispensing equipment. Between uses, utensils and receptacles must be stored in a way that protects them from contamination.
- Reuse of soiled tableware by self-service customers returning to the service area for additional food is prohibited. Reusable mugs and beverage containers are currently exempt from this requirement.
- During transportation, including transport to other locations for service, foods must be held under the conditions specified for cold or hot holding.

Surveys by Governing Agencies

A health care food service department may be surveyed by the JCAHO, state licensing agencies, and county sanitation departments, as well as other agencies. The agency surveyors follow standards that have been established under federal and state laws or by various state, county, and municipal agencies. The purpose of these surveys is to protect the health of the public by preventing and/or correcting unhealthy sanitation practices. Figure 13-3 illustrates a sample food service sanitation inspection checklist. (The JCAHO's survey procedures were discussed in detail in chapter 4.)

Health, Hygiene, and Clean Work Habits

Providing safe and sanitary food service obviously relies on the employment of healthy workers who are thoroughly trained in safe food-handling procedures, practice good personal hygiene, and perform their duties without undue fatigue. Many cases of food-borne illness can be traced to contamination by humans, so the ongoing training and supervision of food service employees should stress good health, careful personal grooming, and good work habits. The following procedures should be observed by all food service employees:

- All food handlers should undergo a health examination by a physician designated by the organization before beginning employment and at intervals specified by public health agencies and/or the institution. The medical records of employees should be maintained in a separate file from their personnel file, which should be accessible only to the immediate supervisor in case of an emergency.
- All food service employees should be clean and well groomed. Clean uniforms and/or aprons are essential. If employees are permitted to wear street clothes while on duty, the clothing should be made of washable fabric. Appropriate hair restraints (nets, hairpins) must be worn.

Figure 13-3. Example of a Sanitation Checklist

SANITATION CHECKLIST				
Checked by: _____ Date: _____				

Standard	Deficiency		Comments	Date Corrected
	No	**Yes**		
PERSONNEL				
1. Head and facial hair are covered with hairnet, cap, or other adequate restraint.				
2. Uniforms and aprons are clean and neat.				
3. Fingernails are short, clean, and unpolished.				
4. Employees are clean, neat, and well groomed.				
5. Employees are free from colds, other communicable diseases, and infected cuts or burns.				
6. Employees smoke or eat only in designated areas.				
7. Employees wash hands frequently at conveniently located hand sinks.				
8. Disposable gloves are properly used by food handlers.				
9. Medical examination schedule for employees is followed.				
10. Employees wear minimal amount of jewelry.				
RECEIVING				
1. Immediately upon receipt, food is inspected for spoilage or infestation.				
2. Nonfood supplies are immediately inspected for infestation.				
3. All food supplies are promptly moved to proper storage areas.				
4. Receiving area is clean and free of food debris, boxes, cans, or other refuse.				
5. Outside doors are equipped with self-closing devices and are kept closed.				
6. Door openings are screened or equipped with fly fans.				
DRY STORAGE				
1. Shelves are placed high enough to permit floor cleaning and to meet local ordinances.				
2. Walls, floors, and shelves are clean.				
3. All food is stored off the floor.				
4. Storage area is dry and well ventilated, and temperature is maintained lower than 70°F (21°C).				
5. Shelves are placed away from walls to permit ventilation and easy cleaning.				
6. Opened bulk-food supplies are stored in labeled plastic or metal containers with tight-fitting lids.				
7. Nonfood supplies are stored separately.				
8. Potentially harmful chemicals and cleaning supplies are stored separately.				
9. A properly functioning thermometer is kept in the area.				
10. Empty cartons and trash are removed from the area.				
11. Storage area is free from uninsulated steam and hot water pipes or other heat-producing or moisture-producing devices.				
REFRIGERATOR AND FREEZER STORAGE				
1. Walls, floors, and shelves are constructed of easily cleaned materials.				

continued on next page

Figure 13-3. *Continued*

Standard	Deficiency		Comments	Date Corrected
	No	Yes		
REFRIGERATOR AND FREEZER STORAGE (continued)				
2. Walls, floors, and shelves are free of spills and debris.				
3. Properly functioning thermometers are located in each unit.				
4. Proper temperatures are maintained: 45°F (7°C) or lower in refrigerators and 0°F (-18°C) or lower in freezers.				
5. Foods are arranged to permit air circulation.				
6. All foods are stored off the floor.				
7. Cooked foods are stored above raw foods.				
8. Foods are properly wrapped or covered.				
9. Frost buildup is kept to a minimum.				
10. Foods are dated and rotated according to standard procedures.				
FOOD PRODUCTION				
1. Floors, walls, and ceilings are clean.				
2. Ventilation hoods are provided where needed and are free from grease and dust.				
3. Adequate light fixtures are provided, guarded, and kept clean.				
4. Equipment and utensils are constructed to meet National Sanitation Foundation (NSF) standards.				
5. Equipment is placed to allow easy access for cleaning.				
6. Inside and outside surfaces of all cooking equipment and utensils are cleaned and sanitized regularly.				
7. Utensils and equipment are stored in clean, dry places at sufficient height from the floor and are protected from flies, dust, and other contaminants.				
8. Foods are stored in production areas in clean, tightly closed containers.				
9. Sanitary procedures are used for handling foods during processing.				
10. Adequate clean cloths for production and cleaning purposes are provided.				
11. Soiled towels and cloths are properly stored.				
12. Dropped items or spills are picked up or cleaned up immediately.				
13. Frozen foods are defrosted under refrigeration or in cold water—not at room temperature—in original wrapping.				
14. If recommended by local health ordinances, disposable gloves are used to handle food.				
15. After each use, preparation equipment is cleaned and sanitized.				
16. After each meal, can openers are cleaned and sanitized.				
17. Adequate garbage or trash receptacles are conveniently located, frequently emptied, and kept clean.				
18. Separate sinks are used for washing raw foods, hands, and utensils.				
19. Hot-holding equipment is used to maintain food at or higher than 140°F (60°C).				
20. Cold-holding equipment is conveniently located and kept clean.				

Figure 13-3. *Continued*

Standard	Deficiency		Comments	Date Corrected
	No	Yes		
FOOD PRODUCTION (continued)				
21. Potentially hazardous foods are not allowed to stand at room temperature longer than absolutely necessary during preparation.				
22. Metal, stem-indicating thermometers are available and are used to check food temperatures during preparation and holding.				
23. Pesticides, cleaning supplies, and other potentially hazardous chemicals are located to avoid possible contamination of foods.				
24. Disposable ware for tasting foods, as required during production, is used by employees.				
TRANSPORT				
1. Transport equipment is constructed according to NSF standards.				
2. Transport containers and carts are regularly cleaned and sanitized.				
3. Proper temperatures are maintained during transport: 45°F (7°C) or lower for cold foods and 140°F (60°C) or higher for hot foods.				
4. Transport carts and containers for food and nonfood supplies are covered or tightly closed.				
5. Cargo area for motor vehicles used for food transport is clean and free from debris and potentially hazardous materials.				
DISPLAY AND SERVICE				
1. Holding equipment and service equipment are constructed according to NSF standards.				
2. Equipment is cleaned and sanitized.				
3. Service and dining area floors and walls are clean.				
4. Tables are washed and sanitized after each use.				
5. Food on display is protected from contamination by packaging, protector devices, or other effective means.				
6. Potentially hazardous food is held at lower than 45°F (7°C) or higher than 140°F (60°C).				
7. Temperatures are checked periodically during meal service.				
8. Employees handle food with utensils or disposable gloves.				
9. Suitable dispensing equipment for trays and other tableware is used.				
10. Condiments for self-service use are protected from consumer contamination.				
11. Milk and milk products are served in unopened, commercially filled containers or from sanitary bulk dispensers.				
12. An adequate amount of tableware is provided for self-service.				
13. Leftover foods are not served again.				
14. Ice is properly dispensed by employees or through self-service equipment.				
15. Adequate means are provided for the removal of soiled tableware by consumers or employees.				

continued on next page

Figure 13-3. *Continued*

Standard	Deficiency		Comments	Date Corrected
	No	Yes		
WARE WASHING				
1. Dish-washing machines and sinks are constructed according to NSF standards.				
2. Prior to washing, tableware and utensils are scraped and flushed.				
3. Properly operating thermometers for each dishwasher compartment are provided.				
4. Proper wash and rinse temperatures during dish washing are maintained.				
5. Proper temperatures for manual ware washing are maintained.				
6. Automatic detergent and sanitizer dispensers operate properly.				
7. Liquid sanitizers, in the proper concentration, are used where necessary.				
8. All tableware and utensils are air dried after sanitizing.				
9. Employees use proper methods for handling sanitized tableware and utensils.				
10. Equipment too large for immersion is sanitized by steam and chemical sanitizers.				
11. Cleaned and sanitized tableware and utensils are properly stored.				
12. Dishwashers and sinks are thoroughly cleaned after use.				
GARBAGE, TRASH DISPOSAL, HOUSEKEEPING				
1. Adequate nonabsorbent trash and garbage containers are provided throughout the facility.				
2. Containers are emptied frequently.				
3. Containers are regularly washed and sanitized.				
4. Garbage or trash storage area is protected from insect or rodent infestation.				
5. In accordance with local ordinances, garbage and/or trash is frequently disposed.				
6. Proper storage is available for brooms, mops, and other cleaning utensils outside of food production and service areas.				
EMPLOYEE FACILITIES				
1. Adequate locker and restroom facilities are provided.				
2. Locker areas and restrooms are kept clean and free from odor.				
3. Sanitary equipment is operational and clean.				
4. Adequate supplies for rest rooms are provided.				
5. Adequate receptacles for waste materials and soiled linens are provided.				

- *Clean hands and fingernails are a must.* Food service employees should thoroughly wash their hands before and after handling food, after smoking, after using the toilet, and after using a handkerchief or tissue. Thorough and frequent handwashing is the best defense in the control of hepatitis A outbreaks. Hand sinks with hot running water must be located at the entrance to the kitchen, production area, or workstation. No other sinks (such as food preparation or three-compartment sinks) should be used for hand washing. The following six-step, double-hand-wash method is recommended for use by all employees involved in food-handling activities:
  - *Step 1:* Turn on hot, flowing water (110° to 120°F) and wet hands. (*Note:* Sufficient pressure and volume of flowing water are important in reducing high levels of organisms such as *Shigella dysenteriae.*)
  - *Step 2:* Apply an antibacterial soap to fingernail brush and onto fingers in sufficient quantity to produce a good lather. Hands and arms should be lathered up to sleeve or as far up arm as necessary to clean any exposed area. A fingernail brush is recommended to remove filth from underneath fingernails and on fingertips because fecal contamination is found there and not on palms.
  - *Step 3:* Rinse hands and brush in hot (110° to 120°F), flowing water.
  - *Step 4:* Repeat steps 1 and 2, without use of brush to ensure that all pathogens have been removed.
  - *Step 5:* Rinse hands and arms in hot, flowing water.
  - *Step 6:* Dry hands with single-use paper towels or a warm air blower. In some locales, health departments require the use of warm air blowers rather than single-use paper towels.
  The double-hand-wash method has been found to be very effective in preventing pathogen transfer.
- Employees should keep their hands away from their faces, hair, and mouths.
- In areas of the country that require it by law, employees should wear disposable gloves when preparing and serving food. Wearing gloves does not prevent cross-contamination of food and food-borne pathogens in that gloved hands touch as many contaminated surfaces and ingredients as do ungloved hands. Nonetheless, when gloves are mandated, employees should change them if they become punctured or soiled, and between handling raw and processed ingredients and food products.
- Smoking should be permitted only in designated areas away from food preparation or service areas. Again, smokers should wash hands before returning to food preparation or serving duties.
- Employees should avoid contact between their hands and fingers and food, and they should pick up serving and eating utensils only by their bases or handles.
- Spoons or other utensils used in food preparation should not be used for tasting, only separate spoons and forks (washed after each use) or disposable utensils.
- Employees should consume their meals only in designated dining areas.
- Personal belongings should be kept out of food preparation and service areas and stored in lockers located outside the food service department.
- Persons other than food service employees should be discouraged from entering the kitchen.
- All cuts should be bandaged with waterproof protectors, and employees with cuts on their hands should wear watertight disposable gloves.
- The food service department must implement and enforce procedures for ensuring that employees are protected against on-the-job injuries or diseases that could result in food contamination. Employees with open lesions, infected wounds, sore throats, or communicable disease should not be permitted to work in food preparation and service areas. An employee known to have suffered a respiratory infection should be cleared by the facility's designated physician before being allowed to return to work.
- A tuberculin (PPD) skin test should be used to screen employees for tuberculosis on a yearly basis if required by the local health department or health care organization.

- There is no scientific evidence that acquired immuneodeficiency syndrome (AIDS) or HIV infection can be transmitted through food. It cannot be spread through casual contact that occurs between employees or customers or through contaminated food. Managers should know the legal ramifications of firing or transferring an employee with AIDS or an employee who has tested HIV positive from the food service department simply because the individual handles food. Acquired immuneodeficiency syndrome is covered by the Americans with Disabilities Act, which provides civil rights protection to infected employees.

☐ Environmental Sanitation

A clean working environment is vital to good sanitation practices. Whether it is part of a new suburban facility or an older inner-city hospital, every food service department can meet basic standards of cleanliness through careful planning and management. Modern food service equipment, materials, and furnishings should be designed to be cleaned easily with hot water, detergents, and sanitizing agents. Floors should be constructed of materials that resist absorption of grease and moisture. Good sanitation also depends on having an adequate number of conveniently located sinks and floor drains to facilitate washing. Walls, ceilings, and ventilation equipment should be designed and constructed to accommodate frequent, thorough cleaning.

Sanitation features should be a major consideration in the purchase and placement of new equipment, which should be installed so that soil, food particles, and other debris that collect between pieces of equipment and surrounding walls and floors can be removed easily. Equipment cleaning must be scheduled regularly to prevent accumulation of dirt and spilled food which in turn reduces the possibility of contamination of food by microorganisms and helps in pest control.

High standards of environmental sanitation can be maintained in both modern and older facilities by meeting certain basic requirements. Some are listed below.

- All work and storage areas are kept clean and dry, well lighted, and in good order.
- Overhead pipes have either been removed or are covered by a false ceiling. Because they collect dust and might leak, such pipes are a hazard in food preparation areas and could lead to food contamination. (State and local sanitation and building codes should be complied with.)
- The walls, floors, and ceilings in all areas should be cleaned routinely.
- Ventilation hoods prevent grease buildup and moisture condensation, which can collect on walls and ceilings and drip into food or onto food preparation areas. Filters and other grease-extracting equipment are removed regularly for cleaning or replaced if they were not designed for easy cleaning in place.
- To prevent cross-contamination, kitchenware and food preparation areas are washed, rinsed, and sanitized after every use and after any interruption of operations during which contamination could occur. Manufacturers' instructions are followed for the cleaning of all equipment.
- The food-contact surfaces of grills, griddles, and similar cooking equipment and the cavities and door seals of microwave ovens are cleaned at least once a day. Deep-fat cooking equipment and filtering systems need not be cleaned daily. Surfaces that do not come into contact with food should be cleaned as often as necessary to keep the equipment free from accumulations of dust, dirt, food particles, and other debris.
- A ready supply of hot water (120° to 140°F [49° to 60°C]) is always available, and the temperature of the hot water meets the minimum requirements of state and local codes.
- Adequate lighting (at least 20 footcandles) is provided for all food preparation areas and at equipment and utensil washing stations. All lighting fixtures located over, by, or within food storage, preparation, service, and display areas are equipped with

protective shields that keep broken glass from falling into food. Areas where equipment and utensils are washed and stored are also protected from glass falling from broken light bulbs.

- Effective rodent, pest, and insect control is carried out routinely. Openings to the outdoors are protected by tight-fitting and self-closing doors, tightly closed windows, adequate screening, or controlled air currents or by other means.
- An adequate number of insectproof, rodentproof, and fireproof containers for garbage and refuse disposal are available, kept covered, and cleaned frequently. (Disposal of such materials should be in accord with local ordinances.)

Using Cleaning Compounds

The food service department uses three general types of cleaning compounds: acidic, alkaline, and neutral. It is important to use the correct cleaning compound to avoid harming food preparation surfaces or equipment being cleaned. The following recommendations should be considered:

- Acidic compounds should be used sparingly to remove lime deposits, rust, and tarnish.
- Alkaline compounds should be used to neutralize and dissolve most food deposits. These compounds can also be used for heavy cleaning.
- Neutral compounds are neither acidic nor alkaline and are frequently used to clean floors, metal surfaces such as tabletops, and pots and pans.

All cleaning compounds *must* be used as directed by their manufacturers. They should be stored separately from food, insecticides, rodenticides, and other poisons. All food service employees should be trained in the proper use of various compounds, and managers should check periodically to ensure that cleaning compounds are used appropriately.

Using Germicides and Sanitizers

The sanitation regulations of all state and local governments specify that any surface that comes into contact with food must be cleaned after every use. This requirement applies to nearly all areas in the food service department.

Germicides and *sanitizers* are chemicals that kill or retard the growth of bacteria and other microorganisms on environmental surfaces. The three most common chemicals used are chlorine, quaternary ammonium compounds (QUATS), and iodine. Chlorine is frequently combined with other chemicals and used for dish washing.

Manufacturers' directions for using these potentially harmful chemicals *must* be followed closely. Only compounds approved by the FDA for use around food should be allowed, and they should be stored away from food supplies. Instructions for mixing these chemicals with water before use should be posted.

Cleaning Equipment

Equipment should be cleaned after every use and according to manufacturers' directions, which should be posted along with schedules and work assignments for routine cleaning. Managers should conduct weekly department inspections and take immediate action to correct any problems that interfere with meeting sanitary standards.

Cleaning and Sanitizing Utensils and Serviceware

The most effective food protection program would be wasted if the dishes, equipment, and utensils that come into contact with food were improperly cleaned and sanitized. Therefore, effective cleaning procedures must be established, employees must be trained in their application, and equipment must be operated properly to achieve adequate sanitation of food production equipment and serviceware.

Mechanical Ware Washing

Dishes should be prescraped or preflushed in the prerinse section of the dishwasher. Alternatively, they could be scraped as a separate operation, with pans and dishes presoaked as needed. When dish-washing machines are available, as many pots, pans, and cooking utensils as possible should be machine washed.

Spray or immersion dishwashers must be installed properly and maintained in good repair. Likewise, automatic dispensers for detergents, wetting agents, and liquid sanitizers must be properly installed and maintained. Utensils and equipment placed in the machine must be exposed to all cycles. The following procedures also should be observed for cleaning and sanitizing all dishes and utensils that come into contact with food:

- The pressure of the final rinse water must be at least 15 pounds per square inch (psi), but no more than 25 psi in the waterline immediately adjacent to the final rinse control valve. (The data plate attached to the machine states the pressure recommended for that particular dishwasher.)
- Machine- or waterline-mounted indicating thermometers must be provided to show the water temperature of each tank in the dishwasher and the temperature of the final rinse water.
- Rinse-water tanks must be protected by baffles, curtains, or some other means to minimize entry of wash water into the rinse tank. Conveyors need to be timed to ensure adequate exposure times in wash, rinse, and drying cycles.
- Equipment and utensils should be placed in racks, trays, or baskets or on conveyors in such a way that food-contact surfaces are exposed to an unobstructed application of detergent wash and clean rinse waters and in such a way that the water can drain freely.
- When hot water is used for sanitizing, the following temperatures must be maintained:
  —*Single-tank, stationary-rack, dual-temperature machine:* wash temperature 150°F (65°C) and final rinse temperature 180°F (82°C)
  —*Single-tank, stationary-rack, single-temperature machine:* wash temperature and final rinse temperature 165°F (74°C)
  —*Single-tank conveyor machine:* wash temperature 165°F (74°C) and final rinse 180°F (82°C)
  —*Multitank conveyor machine:* wash temperature 150°F (65°C), pumped rinse 160°F (71°C), and final rinse 180°F (82°C)
  —*Single-tank pot, pan, and utensil washer (stationary or moving rack):* wash temperature 140°F (60°C) and final rinse 180°F (82°C)
- When chemicals are used for sanitizing in a single-tank, stationary-rack spray machine and glass washer, the following minimum temperatures should be maintained: wash temperature 120°F (49°C) and final rinse with chemical sanitizer 75°F (24°C) or no less than the temperature specified by the machine's manufacturer.
- All dish-washing machines must be thoroughly cleaned at least once a day or as necessary to maintain their satisfactory operating condition.
- When chemicals are used for sanitizing, they should be of a type approved by the local or state health authority. They should also be automatically dispensed in a high enough concentration and for a long enough period to provide effective bactericidal treatment (according to the manufacturer's specifications).
- After sanitization, all equipment and utensils must be air-dried. Drain boards of adequate size for handling soiled and clean tableware should be provided. Mobile dish tables can be used for these tasks.

Manual Ware Washing

The following standards should be observed for manual cleaning and sanitizing:

- A sink with at least three compartments must be used for the manual washing, rinsing, and sanitizing of utensils and equipment. The compartments should be large enough to accommodate the largest equipment and utensils. Hot and cold water sources should be provided for each compartment.
- Drain boards or easily movable dish tables of adequate size should be provided for handling soiled utensils before washing and clean utensils after sanitizing.
- Equipment and utensils should be preflushed or prescraped and, when necessary, presoaked to remove gross food particles. (*Note:* A fourth sink compartment equipped with a garbage disposal is very useful for this purpose and easily could be included in plans for facilities being renovated and for new construction.)
- Except for fixed equipment and utensils too large to be cleaned in sink compartments, the following work sequence should be followed:
  - Wash equipment and utensils in the first sink compartment with a hot detergent solution that is changed frequently to keep the compartment free from soil and grease.
  - Rinse equipment and utensils with clean hot water in the second compartment and change the water frequently.
  - Sanitize equipment and utensils in the third compartment, using one of the four following methods: (1) Immerse the equipment and utensils for at least 30 seconds in clean hot water maintained at 170°F (77°C). A heating device is needed to maintain this temperature, and a thermometer should be used to check the temperature frequently. Dish baskets should be used to immerse utensils completely. (2) Immerse the equipment and utensils for at least one minute in a clean solution that contains at least 50 parts per million (ppm) available chlorine as a hypochlorite and a temperature of at least 75°F (24°C). (3) Immerse the equipment and utensils for at least one minute in a clean solution that contains at least 12.5 ppm available iodine and has a pH no higher than 5.0 and a temperature of at least 75°F (24°C). (4) Immerse the equipment and utensils in a clean solution that contains any other chemical sanitizer approved by local and state health authorities that will provide the equivalent bactericidal effect of a 50-ppm chlorine solution at 75°F (24°C) for one minute.
  - All utensils and equipment should be air-dried after sanitizing.
- Equipment that is too large to immerse can be sanitized by treatment with clean steam, provided that the steam can be confined within the equipment. An alternative method is to rinse, spray, or swab the equipment with a chemical sanitizing solution mixed to at least twice the strength required for immersion sanitization.

Storing Equipment and Utensils

Cleaned and sanitized equipment and utensils must be stored properly to protect against contamination. The following standards should be maintained:

- Store them at least six inches above the floor in a dry, clean location in a way that protects them from contamination by splashes and dust. Stationary equipment should also be protected from contamination.
- Glasses and cups should be stored in an inverted position. Other utensils should be stored covered or inverted whenever practical. Storage containers for tableware should be designed so that only their handles are presented to the employee or consumer.

☐ Self-Evaluation of Sanitary Conditions and Practices

Ongoing self-evaluation of the food service department's sanitary conditions and practices is necessary to ensure day-to-day protection of all employees as well as all clientele served. The primary benefit of self-monitoring is that managers and employees remain aware of the advantages of maintaining a safe and sanitary operation and avoiding a serious health hazard.

The checklist in figure 13-3 can be used as a guide for developing a sanitation self-evaluation program. Local health departments also can be consulted on questions concerning food sanitation standards for specific localities.

The JCAHO's Dietetic Standards include standards for infection control that can be incorporated into the institution's program. The standards also include certain provisions for the institution's policies and procedures and for communicating them to all employees.

As part of the sanitation evaluation and control program, a department representative usually serves on the facility's overall infection control committee. The committee also reviews the food service department's policies and procedures, along with those of every other department in the facility.

☐ Summary

Food service directors must adhere to prescribed guidelines that guard against food-borne illness due to food contamination. The model suggested for the design, development, and implementation of an effective sanitation program is Hazardous Analysis Critical Control Points (HACCP), a self-evaluation system for control of food-borne illness and time–temperature abuse. The sanitation program can be incorporated into a health care food service's continuous quality improvement efforts.

The chapter described common causes of food-borne illnesses and the bacterial agents that serve as transport vehicles. Specific ways to eliminate or minimize infection were described in terms of how to purchase, store, prepare, transport, display, and serve foods. Also given were techniques for cleaning and sanitizing food service equipment, utensils, serviceware, tableware, and the larger food preparation and service areas. How to protect against the dangers posed by chemical hazards (insecticides, pesticides, and herbicides) were reviewed, as were ways to identify critical control points along the flow of food in food service operations.

The chapter closed with overviews on approaches to environmental sanitation. Specifically, the proper use of cleaning compounds; germicides and sanitizers; and agents for cleaning and sanitizing equipment, utensils, and serviceware was described. Finally, methods for proper handling and storage of clean equipment and utensils and an operation's self-evaluation of its sanitation program were given.

☐ Bibliography

Bryan, F. Application of HACCP to ready-to-eat chilled foods. *Food Technology* 44(7):70, 72, 74–77, July 1990.

Bryan, F. Hazard analysis critical control point (HACCP): systems for retail food and restaurant operations. *Journal of Food Protection* 53(11):978–83, Nov. 1990.

Cody, M. M., and Keith, M. *Food Safety for Professionals: A Reference and Study Guide.* Chicago: The American Dietetic Association, 1991.

Cox, L. J. A perspective on listeriosis. *Food Technology* 43(12):52–59, Dec. 1989.

Doyle, M. P. A new generation of food-borne pathogens. *Dairy, Food, and Environmental Sanitation* 12(8):490–93, July 1992.

Eck, L. S. HACCP: a term to remember, a procedure for safety. *Healthcare Foodservice* 21(3):29, Sept.–Oct. 1992.

Eck, L., and Ponce, H. HACCP: a food safety model. *School Food Service* 47(2):50–52, Feb. 1993.

Educational Foundation of National Restaurant Association. *Applied Foodservice Sanitation: A Certification Coursebook.* 4th ed. New York City: John Wiley & Sons, 1992.

Fabres, J. M. Prevention and control of food-borne listeriosis. *Dairy, Food, and Environmental Sanitation* 12(6):334–40, June 1992.

Fain, A. R. Control of pathogens in ready-to-eat meats. *Dairy, Food, and Environmental Sanitation* 12(9):554–58, Aug. 1992.

King, P. Implementing a HACCP program. *Food Management* 27(12):54, 56, 58, Dec. 1992.

Longree, K. *Quality Food Sanitation.* 3rd ed. New York City: Wiley (International), 1980.

Longree, K., and Blaker, G. G. *Sanitary Techniques in Foodservice.* 2nd ed. New York City: John Wiley and Sons, 1982.

Minor, L. J. *Sanitation, Safety and Environmental Standards.* Vol. 2. L. J. Minor Food Service Standards Series. Westport, CT: AVI, 1983.

National Institute for Food Service Industry. *Applied Foodservice Sanitation.* 3rd ed. Chicago: National Institute for Food Service Industry, 1985.

National Restaurant Association. *Sanitation Operations Manual.* Chicago: NRA, 1979.

Reed, G. Sanitation in food service establishments. *Dairy, Food, and Environmental Sanitation* 12(9):566–67, Aug. 1992.

Saguy, I. Simulated growth of *Listeria monocytogens* in refrigerated foods stored at variable temperatures. *Food Technology* 6(3):69–71, March 1992.

Snyder, O. P. Food safety 2000! Applying the HACCP for food safety assurance in 21st century. *Dairy, Food, and Environmental Sanitation* 10(4):197–204, Apr. 1990.

Snyder, O. P. HACCP—an industry food safety self-control program—part I. *Dairy, Food, and Environmental Sanitation* 12(1):26–27, Jan. 1992.

Snyder, O. P. HACCP—an industry food safety self-control program—part III. *Dairy, Food, and Environmental Sanitation* 12(3):164–67, Mar. 1992.

Snyder, O. P. HACCP—an industry food safety self-control program—part IV. *Dairy, Food, and Environmental Sanitation* 12(4): 291–95, Apr. 1992.

Snyder, O. P. HACCP—an industry food safety self-control program—part V. *Dairy, Food, and Environmental Sanitation* 12(5):291–95, May 1992.

Snyder, O. P. HACCP—an industry food safety self-control program—part VI. *Dairy, Food, and Environmental Sanitation* 12(6):362–65, June 1992.

Snyder, O. P. HACCP—an industry food safety self-control program—part VII. *Dairy, Food, and Environmental Sanitation* 12(8):574–77, Aug. 1992.

United States Department of Agriculture, Food Safety and Inspection Service, United States Department of Health and Human Services and Food and Drug Administration. *Preventing Food-Borne Listeria.* Washington, DC: U.S. Government Printing Office, Apr. 1992.

Safety, Security, and Disaster Planning

☐ Introduction

A primary responsibility of health care nutrition and food service managers is to help ensure maintenance of safe working conditions, equipment, and practices that promote a safety mindset among employees, staff, and vendors. The most effective way this is accomplished is through a department safety plan that complements and reinforces the larger facility's safety efforts while ensuring compliance with all federal, state, and municipal codes and standards for occupational safety and health.

A critical part of safety is the security measures that help protect food, supplies, equipment, employees, and consumers. This occurs on two levels—internally and externally. *Internal security* in food service has to do with instituting policies and procedures and controls that ensure against jeopardizing employees, consumers, food, equipment and inventory; whereas *external security* has to do with guarding against threats from outside the department. These include theft by visiting relatives, nondepartment personnel, even delivery and catering personnel.

Of course, no safety program would be complete without provisions for disaster planning. Floods, earthquakes, power outages or reductions, and massive accidents (plane crashes, for example) can pose a threat to food service operations.

This chapter will address these three areas—safety, security, and disaster planning—as they relate specifically to food service operations. The chapter will examine safe working conditions, OSHA requirements and employees' right to know with regard to hazardous chemicals in the workplace, self-inspection of safety training programs, fire safety, and first aid.

Techniques for internal and external security will be presented, along with a summary of key areas of security concern for a food service operation. The chapter will close with pointers for designing and implementing a disaster planning program. Because some events are beyond a facility's control, the chapter will discuss measures to be taken in the event of flood, earthquake, power outage or reduction, and massive casualties (for example, from plane crashes, damaging weather, or civil unrest). Throughout all such contingencies, the food service director's role and responsibilities will be clearly delineated.

☐ Safety

Safety is every employer's responsibility, not a chore left to committee action. Accidents do not just happen—something causes them. Accidents are expensive: They result in lost productivity, wasted time, overtime expenses, decreased quality of care, increased insurance premiums, increased worker's compensation claims, potential lawsuits, and—above all—human suffering. The attitudes and examples set by managers influence employees' safety practices. Thus, managers' leadership styles demonstrate their safety consciousness through how they orient and train employees in safety procedures and follow up on accidents.

In addition to safe working conditions, an effective safety program depends on several factors: established work safety procedures, thorough training and continual self-evaluation, good fire-prevention practices, and adequate first-aid training. The Occupational Safety and Health Administration (OSHA) places legal responsibility for providing a safe working environment on all employers. In practice, primary responsibility for enforcing safety rules and employee compliance in following them falls to department-level managers. The Joint Commission on Accreditation of Healthcare Organizations (JCAHO) manual describes basic safety procedures for the health care institution including the food and nutrition service department. Also, the American Hospital Association (AHA) publishes a helpful safety manual, *Safety Guide for Health Care Institutions*. In many organizations, a safety committee composed of employees is appointed or elected to work with each department director to implement a meaningful safety program.

The scope of responsibilities for the food service safety committee varies, depending on size and complexity of the department. Some committee functions include:

- Conducting a safety self-inspection to identify hazardous conditions that could result in injury to employees and customers
- Investigating all accidents or events for a previous month (or other time period determined appropriate for the operation) and recommending steps to prevent accident or event recurrence
- Documenting all accident prevention recommendations and forwarding to upper management
- Monitoring all safety training records, noting discrepancies, and recommending actions to correct discrepancies
- Following up on previous safety self-inspections to verify that corrective actions have been implemented and to identify any other problems
- Maintaining a safety committee notebook with minutes of meetings, correspondence regarding committee recommendations, and safety inspection reports
- Recommending content of safety training programs
- Conducting an audit of the safety program and identifying any areas that need modifying

Even though the committee may assume a leadership role in planning and implementing a safety program, success of the program depends on the cooperation of all employees.

Working Conditions

Before safe working policies and procedures can be developed and enforced, the basic physical safety of the food service department's facilities and equipment must be ensured. Fundamental requirements include:

- Adequate working space
- Safe clearance for aisles, doors, loading stations, and traffic areas
- Adequate lighting and ventilation
- Sufficient numbers of well-marked exits
- Guarded stairways and platforms
- Clean, dry floor surfaces free from hazards
- Suitable storage facilities for food and other supplies
- Electrical and gas equipment constructed and installed in accordance with applicable standards and codes (the National Sanitation Foundation codes, Underwriters' Laboratory codes, and National Electrical codes, as well as any state and local regulations)

- Properly grounded and insulated electrical equipment
- Guards and enclosures for potentially dangerous equipment
- Noise levels within those set by OSHA regulations
- Complete, posted operating instructions on or near every piece of equipment
- Locks that open from the inside on walk-in refrigerators and freezers
- Proper insulation or protection from heat-producing equipment, water heaters, condensing units, compressors, and water pipes
- Sharp knives that are properly stored

The regulations of federal, state, and local governments also dictate standards for safe working conditions, and government authorities are empowered to conduct inspections of health care institutions. In addition, the JCAHO bases its accreditation of individual facilities on their compliance with its published standards, as verified by periodic on-site surveys.

Occupational Safety and Health Administration

Safe and healthful working conditions were mandated by the William-Steiger Occupational Safety and Health Act of 1970, enacted by Congress in April 1971. The act established the Occupational Safety and Health Administration (OSHA) as the federal agency that administers legislation within the Department of Labor. The goal of the act is ". . . to assure, so far as possible, safe and healthful working conditions, and to preserve human resources for every working man and woman." The act covers every employee of a private commercial business with one or more employees. (Other workplaces are regulated by different federal laws and government agencies, and so their employees are not covered by OSHA regulations.) Health care institutions of all kinds fall under the jurisdiction of OSHA, although state and local governments are exempt from these standards. Individual states also have the power to establish occupational safety programs for their employees.

OSHA Record Keeping

An OSHA regulation (29 CFR 1904.2–8) requires that employers gather and record all available information about work-related accidents and illnesses that occur in the workplace. Federal regulations require employers with 11 or more employees at any time during the preceding calendar year to complete OSHA forms 100, 101, and 102, to be maintained for five years (excluding the current year). Forms 100 and 101 must be kept current to within six days. Form 102 must summarize all occupational injuries and illnesses for each calendar year and be posted in the workplace no later than February 1 each year and remain posted until March 1. The forms must be posted even if there were no injuries or illnesses during the calendar year, with zero entered on the total lines. Employers must keep records of all work-related accidents and illnesses, including those that result in any of the following:

- A fatality
- A loss of consciousness
- A lost workday or workdays
- A need for medical treatment
- An employee's transfer or termination
- A death or the hospitalization of five or more employees
- A need for employees to be advised of excessive exposure to hazardous substances

In addition, employers are required to post one full-size (10-by-16-inch) OSHA poster (OSHA 2203), or a state-approved poster where required, in the workplace. The purpose of the poster is to inform employees of their rights under OSHA regulations.

The Occupational Safety and Health Administration also encourages states to develop and operate their own OSHA-approved workplace safety and health programs, which the federal agency monitors to determine its level of commitment and effectiveness. The Occupational

Safety and Health Administration uses quarterly reports and semiannual evaluations as tools to oversee state plans, and each quarter those states having their own programs submit a summary of their enforcement and standards activities. After analyzing each state's progress toward meeting its standards and enforcement goals, OSHA conducts investigations of the performance of individual states and summarizes its findings in a comprehensive report that is submitted to the state every six months. The state is then given an opportunity to respond to the report and the recommendations.

OSHA Inspections

To determine whether a workplace is safe and healthful, OSHA officials are allowed to enter a place of business at any time for purposes of inspection. They may do so either in response to complaints filed against an employer, or as part of a random inspection. On-site inspections also are conducted when OSHA has reason to suspect imminent employee endangerment and when a fatal accident or other catastrophe has occurred at the worksite.

Certain circumstances usually surround an OSHA inspection of a food service facility, for which prior notice of the visit may or may not have been given. Upon announcing him- or herself and showing adequate identification, the compliance inspector will perform the following activities:

- Review all accident report forms on file.
- Inspect records of workplace illnesses and injuries.
- Request the name and address of the company physician or staff members trained in administering medical aid.
- Check the supplies in the first-aid kit.
- Ask questions concerning the number of people working on each shift, the number of supervisors and workers on staff, and the classification of staff members by job and gender.
- Review the department's safety training programs.
- Request that a ranking supervisor and a shop steward (if the institution is unionized) accompany him or her on the tour of the department.
- Talk with employees about safety topics.
- Point out hazards or unsafe conditions such as oil, debris, and trash in traffic and work areas.
- Check all machines, electrical equipment (including plugs) for proper grounding, ladders, tools, and storage areas.
- Note the location, application, and last testing date of each fire extinguisher.
- Report to the supervisor (and to the shop steward in unionized institutions) any unsafe actions observed among workers.
- Make written comments on all violations cited.
- Talk with individual employees previously cited for violations to determine the best way to correct the safety problems.

After the inspection, citations and penalties (if any) will be issued if the organization was found to be in violation of OSHA standards. The seriousness of the violation determines whether a fine is levied or legal action is taken.

OSHA's Hazard Communication Standard and Right-to-Know Law

The Occupational and Safety Health Administration's Hazard Communication Standard (CFR 1910.1200) was originally intended to alert manufacturing employees to the use of hazardous chemicals in the workplace. Employers were required to inform employees about the physical and health hazards involved, safe handling procedures, and emergency and first-aid procedures. In 1987, OSHA expanded the standard to include areas other than manufacturing.

Under the revised standard, chemical manufacturers and importers who produce, manufacture, or import hazardous chemicals are required to prepare technical hazard information to be used on labels and material safety data sheets (MSDSs) to accompany the hazardous chemicals. The law also defines which types of chemicals must be labeled and whether labels may be removed at any time. Employers are required to inform employees when potentially hazardous chemicals are being used in the workplace (Right-to-Know Law) and, furthermore, make the information supplied by manufacturers and importers available to employees. Also, they must establish hazard training and written communication programs (discussed below).

Materials Safety Data Sheets

Chemical manufacturers and importers must supply a materials safety data sheet (MSDS) for every hazardous chemical they produce or import. An MSDS, which must be forwarded to employers at the time of the initial shipment, must be maintained by the supervisor in the area where the chemical is to be used. The information must be written in plain English, be readily available to designated employee representatives and OSHA officials, and must include both the scientific and common names of the chemical (for example, sodium hydroxide or caustic soda). All MSDSs must contain at least the information listed in figure 14-1, with no spaces left blank.

Hazard Training Programs

As mandated by OSHA's revised standard, employers must implement a hazard training and communication program for all employees. Training should cover the following areas:

- Location and availability of the written hazard program (described in the next subsection)
- Identity of hazardous chemicals being used in the workplace
- Specific physical and health hazards of individual chemicals
- Protective measures to take when hazardous chemicals are in use
- How to read and interpret information on chemical labels and MSDSs
- Where and how to get additional information
- How to use personal protective equipment or clothing to avoid exposure to hazardous chemicals
- Symptoms of exposure including the effects of contact, inhalation, or overexposure
- First-aid measures to take in the event of contact or symptoms of overexposure
- Demonstration of first-aid procedures and identification of who can administer treatment
- What should be done in the event of a spill or other accident

The following individuals should be included in the in-service session, especially if a new chemical is involved: the user(s), the supervisor, and an individual with firsthand knowledge about the chemical (for example, the distributor's sales representative or a manufacturer's representative.) The chemical and its MSDS should be used as visual aids during the session. All in-service sessions should be documented. Employees should be retrained at least once a year on the safe use of hazardous chemicals in their work area.

Written Hazard Communication Programs

To comply with OSHA's requirement for a written program, the health care organization's food service department must address *in writing* specific issues related to hazardous chemicals in the workplace. This mandate encompasses labeling and other written forms of conveying information. A written communication program, then, should include at least four components: labeling, MSDSs, a written prospectus of the employee training program, and employees' "right to know."

Labels and other forms of written or graphic warning (for example, symbols) must be supported by a description of the labeling system used. Labeling includes the written information on in-house containers; written designation of responsible person(s) for monitoring labeling procedures and receipt of labels from manufacturers; and procedures for updating label information.

Figure 14-1. Materials Safety Data Sheet

MATERIALS SAFETY DATA SHEET

Product Name: _____ Company Name: _____

Date Issued: _____ Address: _____

Product
Identification: _____
_____

Hazardous Ingredients of
Mixture: _____
_____

Physical
Data: _____
_____

Fire and Explosion
Potential: _____
_____

Reactivity
Data: _____
_____

Spills or Leaks
Procedures: _____
_____

Health Hazard
Data: _____
_____

First Aid
Procedures: _____
_____

Special Protection
Information: _____
_____

Additional
Information: _____
_____

The *materials safety data sheet* component includes identification of person(s) responsible for obtaining and maintaining MSDSs. It also includes a description of how employees can obtain access to MSDSs and the procedures for updating or requesting them.

A *written description of the prospectus* of an employee hazard communication program should be accessible. It can be kept on file in a supervisor's office or posted prominently throughout the department.

The Occupational Safety and Health Administration's *Right-to-Know Law* described earlier must be delineated in plain English (and predominant second language if applicable) and accessible to employees. This component of the mandate includes the following disclosures:

- Employees are to have access to the hazard chemicals list for their work area (see the sample request form in figure 14-2).

Figure 14-2. Employee Chemical Information Request Form

This form is provided to assist employees in requesting information concerning the health and safety hazards of toxic substances found in the workplace.

Please print:

1. Name _____   4. Department _____

2. Job Title _____   5. Ext. _____

3. Supervisor _____

Describe briefly the toxic substance you are exposed to:

1. Trade name _____

2. Chemical name or ingredient (if known) _____

3. Manufacturer (name and address if known) _____

_____

4. Does substance have a label? _____ Yes _____ No
   If yes, copy information on label.

5. Physical form of substance: _____ Gas _____ Liquid

   _____ Dust _____ Solid

   _____ Other

6. Any other information that will identify the substance (the circumstances of exposure, other characteristics of the substance, etc.): _____

_____

_____

7. If you have specific questions, write them below. _____

_____

_____

_____   _____
Employee Signature   Personnel Signature

_____   _____
Date   Date & Time

Source: Reprinted with permission of All Saints Health System, Fort Worth, TX.

339

- Employees are to be informed of the hazards associated with chemicals contained in unlabeled pipes and where hazards are present in their work area.
- The written hazard communication program is to be accessible to all employees.
- All MSDSs are to be readily available during working hours.
- Employees must be informed of OSHA's right-to-know standard.

Open and honest communication is essential when it comes to complying with the right-to-know standard. Figures 14-3, 14-4, and 14-5 (p. 342) are examples of forms that can be used in a written hazard communication program. In addition to OSHA standards, JCAHO has certain requirements for managing hazardous materials (described in the JCAHO Hazardous Materials and Waste Management Standards).

OSHA Bloodborne Pathogen Standard

Health care organizations are responsible for the establishment and implementation of an exposure control plan that meets the OSHA Bloodborne Pathogen Standard (29 CFR 1910.1030), which

Figure 14-3. Materials Safety Data Sheet Transmittal

To: Department: _____ Date: _____

Director: _____

Chemical: _____

Reason:

_____ Updated MSDS	This updated MSDS contains new or different information on the above material. Replace the MSDS now contained in the department MSDS file with the attached MSDS. Return the old MSDS with this form.
_____ New Material	This material is to be added to your department inventory. Insert the attached MSDS in the MSDS file and return the form.
_____ Material Deleted	The above substance has been removed from the department. Remove the entry on the Department Inventory. Remove the corresponding MSDS from the MSDS file and return with this form.

	Date	By
Inventory Updated	_____	_____
MSDS Added (Deleted)	_____	_____
New Chemical Training Conducted	_____	_____

MSDS Attached ____ Yes ____ No   Return to: _____

Additional comments _____

_____

_____

_____

Source: Reprinted with permission of All Saints Health System, Fort Worth, TX.

Figure 14-4. New Employee Hazard Communication Checklist

Name: _____ Date: _____

Job Assignment: _____

Supervisor: _____

Section I

Orientation:

_____ Hospital's general safety and health rules.

_____ Hazard Communication/Right-to-Know introduction.

_____ Location and availability of the written Hazard Communication Program.

_____ Material Safety Data Sheets explained and function.

Completed by: _____ Date: _____

Section II

By New Employee's Department Manager
First Day in Work Area:

_____ Introduction to work operations where chemical and physical hazards are present—types of hazards
         encountered.
_____ Required work practices.
_____ Personal protective equipment.
_____ Emergency procedures.
_____ Detection of chemical hazards, if any.
_____ Location and availability of Hazard Communication Program.
_____ Labeling system.
_____ MSDS and location.
_____ Answer employee questions.
_____ Return completed checklist to Hazardous Materials Coordinator.

Completed by: _____ Date: _____

Employee Signature: _____ Date: _____

Hazardous Materials Coordinator: _____

Source: Reprinted with permission of All Saints Health System, Fort Worth, TX.

became effective March 6, 1992. Because the food service department is not considered an
at-risk unit, the primary component of the institution's exposure control plan that directly
affects the department is the required training. Regardless of assignment, all employees must
receive training prior to initial assignment to tasks where occupational exposure may occur.
Training for employees should include an explanation of the following concepts:

- OSHA's standard for blood-borne pathogens
- Epidemiology and symptomatology of blood-borne diseases
- Modes of transmission of blood-borne pathogens
- The institution's exposure control plan
- Procedures that might cause exposure to blood or other potentially infectious materials
  at the operation
- Control methods that will be used at the facility to control exposure to blood or other
  potentially infectious materials

- Personal protective equipment and clothing available at the facility
- Whom to contact concerning
  - Postexposure evaluation and follow-up
  - Signs and labels used at the facility
  - Hepatitis B vaccine program at the facility

Figure 14-5. Hazard Communication Checklist

	Yes	No
1. Chemical Inventory		
A. Is there a complete listing by department?	___	___
B. Are all chemicals considered (i.e., lab, maintenance, etc.)?	___	___
C. Are the quantities used listed?	___	___
D. Is the frequency of use listed?	___	___
E. Is there a procedure for updating inventory?	___	___
F. Are chemical by-products identified and treated as other chemicals?	___	___
2. Materials Safety Data Sheet		
A. Are MSDSs available for all chemicals?	___	___
B. Is there documentation of request for missing MSDSs?	___	___
C. Are files accessible to employees?	___	___
D. Is there a system for updating information?	___	___
E. Is there a statement that the employer is relying on chemical manufacturing MSDS information and is not making its own hazard determination?	___	___
3. Labeling		
A. Are all containers labeled?	___	___
B. Are all storage tanks labeled?	___	___
C. Is the responsible person for labeling designated?	___	___
D. Are labels complete with name of chemical?	___	___
E. Are labels complete with hazards of chemical? (Use manufacturers' labels when possible.)	___	___
4. Written Program		
A. Is the program in writing, with the following information?		
i. Responsibilities	___	___
ii. Labeling	___	___
iii. Shipping/Receiving	___	___
iv. Designated person to handle concerns of employees	___	___
v. Training	___	___
vi. Contractors	___	___
B. Will the written program be made available to the employees? (Where will the program be located?)	___	___
C. Is management aware of written procedures; do they know their responsibilities?	___	___
5. Training		
A. Has a training schedule been developed for supervisors?	___	___
B. Has a training schedule been developed for employees?	___	___
C. Has a training schedule been developed for managers?	___	___
D. Are trainers designated?	___	___
E. Are forms for documentation of training available?	___	___
6. Past Health Concerns		
A. Have all previous industrial health hazard concerns been addressed?	___	___
B. Are there any employee complaints about environmental conditions?	___	___

Source: Reprinted with permission of All Saints Health System, Fort Worth, TX.

The food service director or designee should be knowledgeable about the entire plan and the possible risks to the staff.

Work Safety Policies and Procedures

Once a safe working environment has been established, policies and procedures that support safe working habits must be developed by the food service director or designee, approved by the institution's administration and/or safety committee, and implemented by both management and the employees. Basic safety rules for food service workers are as follows:

- Always wear safe clothing and shoes. (Most departments require employees to wear standard uniforms and hard-toed, low-heeled, rubber-soled shoes. Heavy coats and gloves should be worn in walk-in refrigerators and freezers. Bracelets and earrings should not be worn.)
- Use ladders to reach supplies and equipment stored on high shelves.
- Use the protective guards and safety devices supplied for potentially dangerous machines and equipment, such as meat slicers.
- Use appropriate tools for opening cartons and other containers.
- Follow safe procedures for lifting heavy objects (see figure 14-6).
- Use dry pot holders or cloths to handle hot utensils.
- Maintain good housekeeping conditions in all work areas by keeping equipment clean and by properly storing equipment and supplies not in use.
- Carefully follow the established operating instructions for all tools, equipment, and machines.

The food service director and supervisory personnel are responsible for establishing and maintaining a safe working environment for all food service employees. There are a number of ways in which this can be accomplished:

- Perform regular and thorough department inspections. The sample checklist in figure 14-7 can be used as an inspection model.
- Appoint a department safety committee.
- Analyze every work-related accident and then correct any problems identified.
- Take immediate action when employees behave inappropriately (for example, engage in horseplay or in fighting), show evidence of substance abuse, or express poor attitudes toward their work.
- Train employees to be safety conscious.
- Know what to do after an on-the-job accident.
- Be sensitive to employees' work-related problems and avoid placing undue pressure on them in the workplace.

Safety Training and Self-Inspection of Safety Training Programs

The food service director and all food service managers are key people in developing a safety-minded work force. Safety training begins with a new employee's first day on the job and is reinforced by leadership style and regularly scheduled training sessions. (Posters and safety reminders are one way to help keep employees alert to safety procedures.) It must be stressed that employees should report any safety hazards immediately to get the problem corrected quickly. The entire department should be periodically inspected for safety compliance in addition to scheduled inspections of equipment by manufacturers' representatives or by the institution's maintenance supervisor. Local fire departments can assist in fire-prevention training. Regular safety training programs should include at least:

- Procedures for safely lifting heavy objects
- Procedures for handling hazardous materials
- Procedures for ensuring fire safety
- Procedures for reporting on-the-job accidents

Figure 14-6. Safe Lifting Procedure

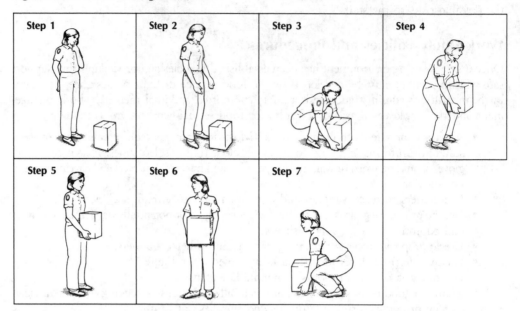

Step 1. Approach the load and size it up (weight, size, and shape). Consider your physical ability to handle the load.

Step 2. Place your feet close to the object to be lifted, 8 to 12 inches apart for good balance.

Step 3. Bend your knees to the degree that is comfortable and get a good handhold. Then, using both leg and back muscles, . . .

Step 4. Lift the load straight up, smoothly and evenly, pushing with your legs and knees. Keep the load close to your body.

Step 5. Lift the object into carrying position, making no turning or twisting movements until the lift is completed.

Step 6. Turn your body with changes of foot position after looking over your path of travel to make sure it is clear.

Step 7. Remember that setting the load down is just as important as picking it up. Using leg and back muscles, comfortably lower the load by bending your knees. When the load is securely positioned, release your grip.

Source: Adapted from R. P. Puckett. *Dietary Manager's Independent Study Course.* Gainesville, FL: Department of Independent Study, University of Florida, 1985.

A system for self-inspection of department safety programs should be conducted at regular intervals. Again, figure 14-7 can be used as a safety evaluation checklist and as a basis for developing a self-inspection program. Employees should participate in developing and enforcing the department's safety program.

Fire Safety and Prevention

The danger of fire in the food service department is always present. All employees should know and practice the department's fire-prevention and fire-response procedures, revised and reviewed annually, and those developed for the institution as a whole. The department should post its procedures and provide in-service training on how to react to different types of fires.

Electrical fires and grease fires are the two leading types of fire in the food service department. One is due to misuse or negligence with regard to electrical equipment; the other arises from grease buildup on stoves and hoods, and grills and other appliances. Employees must

Figure 14-7. Example of a Safety Checklist

SAFETY CHECKLIST				
Checked by: _____ Date: _____				
Standard	**Deficiency**		**Comments**	**Date Corrected**
	No	**Yes**		
PERSONNEL				
1. Signs prohibiting unauthorized people from entering the food service department are posted.				
2. All personnel have participated in a safety program.				
3. Personnel are lifting heavy objects properly.				
4. Authorized protection is used to prevent burns when handling hot pots and pans.				
5. Chopping, cutting, and slicing are done on cutting boards.				
6. Knives and other sharp objects are stored in a manner to prevent accidental cuts.				
7. Plastic gloves and aprons are not worn in the hot food preparation areas.				
8. Long hair is properly covered.				
9. Wearing dangling jewelry is prohibited in work areas.				
10. Only shoes with enclosed toes and low heels are worn.				
11. Step stools or step ladders are used to reach items that are stored on high shelves.				
12. Wet floor signs are used to warn personnel and customers.				
FIRE				
1. All personnel have participated in fire prevention and emergency training.				
2. All prevention instructions are posted.				
3. Department policies and procedures for fire safety are reviewed annually.				
4. Fire extinguishers are strategically placed.				
5. Fire extinguishers are clearly labeled for class of fire.				
6. Fire extinguishers are periodically checked for adequacy of pressure and chemicals.				
ELECTRICITY				
1. Routine inspection of all electrical equipment and outlets is made by the maintenance department.				
2. Food service personnel have been trained in safe use of electric powered equipment.				
3. Electric cords and plugs are in good repair.				
4. Personnel immediately report any damaged or malfunctioning electrical connections or equipment to their supervisor.				
5. All electrical equipment is properly grounded.				
6. Power to meat slicers and mixers is disconnected when the equipment is being cleaned.				
7. Equipment guards (on meat slicers and similar equipment) are in place at all times.				
FACILITIES AND EQUIPMENT				
1. There are no protrusions from walls that obstruct traffic areas.				
2. Storage drawers are kept closed.				

continued on next page

Figure 14-7. *Continued*

Standard	Deficiency		Comments	Date Corrected
	No	Yes		
FACILITIES AND EQUIPMENT (continued)				
3. Placing pots and pans on the floor in traffic areas is prohibited.				
4. Floors are regularly cleaned to prevent slips and falls in food production and refrigerated and dry storage areas.				
5. Storage areas are provided with proper shelving.				
6. Heavy items are stored on lower shelves.				
7. Cleaning supplies and other chemicals are in an area separate from food storage.				
8. Adequate lighting is provided in storage areas.				
9. Light fixtures are in good working order.				
10. Adequate lighting is provided in customer service area.				
11. Adequate lighting is provided in food production areas.				
12. Carts are provided for transport of supplies.				
13. Step stools and ladders are kept in good repair.				
14. Refrigerators and freezers are equipped with inside door release devices.				
PLUMBING				
1. Plumbing and steam and temperature gauges are regularly checked by maintenance department.				
2. Personnel have been trained in proper use of steam-heated equipment.				
3. Personnel have been trained in proper use of steam cleaning equipment.				
4. Personnel immediately report any plumbing or steam malfunctions to their supervisors.				
5. All drains are flowing freely.				
6. All exposed water and steam pipes are protected with insulated covering.				
CLEANING AND DISPOSAL				
1. Personnel are trained in proper use of all cleaning supplies and chemicals.				
2. Personnel are trained in proper use of dishwashing equipment.				
3. Wood or metal textured platforms are used in the dishwashing and pot-and-pan-cleaning areas to prevent slips and falls.				
4. Water temperatures are constantly monitored.				
5. There are no obstructions in the traffic lane of the dishwashing and pot-and-pan-cleaning areas.				
6. Adequate scraping space is provided.				
7. Adequate drying space is provided.				
8. Adequate dry dish storage space is provided.				
9. Provision is made for safe disposal of chipped, cracked, or broken dishes and cutlery.				
10. Pot-and-pan-washing areas are provided.				
11. Adequate pot and pan storage space is provided.				
12. Garbage disposals are maintained in safe operating condition.				
13. Trash is disposed in tied plastic bags.				
14. There is a designated, temperature-controlled, trash and garbage storage area.				
15. Garbage and trash disposal areas are free of spills.				

know how to use fire extinguishers and select the appropriate extinguisher for each of the three classes of fire. The three classes of fire are described below:

- Class A fires involve *ordinary combustible items* such as wood, paper, and cloth. Extinguishers for use on class A fires are marked with a triangle and a capital letter A.
- Class B fires involve *flammable liquids* such as fuel oil, gasoline, paint, grease, and solvents. Extinguishers for use in class B fires are marked with a square and a capital letter B.
- Class C fires involve *electrical equipment* such as overheated fuse boxes, conductors, wiring, and motors. Extinguishers for class C fires are marked with a circle and a capital letter C.

Fire extinguishers, which should carry the certification of a nationally recognized testing laboratory such as the Underwriters' Laboratory (UL), must be checked periodically by the fire department to determine whether they are fully charged and whether the fire retardant contained in the cylinder is less than 12 months old. Each extinguisher should have a label attached to indicate the month and year of the last inspection. Extinguishers should be recharged after every use, regardless of the amount of retardant left in the cylinder, and they should be placed away from potential fire hazards and near escape routes. They should be mounted higher than 5 feet if they weigh 40 pounds or less or at least 3½ feet off the floor if they weigh more than 40 pounds.

In addition to an adequate number of correctly located fire extinguishers, at least one automatic sprinkler system with adequate pressure, capacity, and reliability should be in place. Water-flow alarms should be provided on all sprinklers. The system should be periodically inspected and maintained. Shutoff valves in all air ducts located over cooking equipment and heat sources should be provided and inspected at least once a year.

Dry chemical or carbon dioxide firefighting systems should be inspected and tested at least once a year by the fire department and reports of the inspections kept on file. All dry chemical and carbon dioxide systems should benefit from regular maintenance. Food service employees should participate in hospital and department fire drills at least once a year. All fire exits should be well marked and free from obstruction.

First Aid

Most health care institutions have specific policies and procedures for the treatment of injured employees. In many organizations, employee health departments handle minor injuries. However, serious injuries and illnesses are always referred to emergency departments. Emergency telephone numbers (poison control, trauma units) should be posted near each telephone. If deemed appropriate, first aid should be provided immediately.

The Occupational Safety and Health Administration's regulations (29 CFR 1910–151) state that provisions for first aid must be made in the workplace if there is no infirmary, clinic, or hospital near the workplace that can be used for the treatment of injured or sick employees. Health care institutions may offer immediate first aid on the premises; however, OSHA requirements for employee first-aid treatment programs may provide helpful guidelines for food service directors responsible for managing first-aid programs in their departments:

- At least one employee on each shift should be qualified to give first aid, including cardiopulmonary resuscitation (CPR) and the Heimlich maneuver. The employee providing first aid treatment should follow designated procedures to protect him- or herself from communicable diseases.
- First-aid supplies should be readily available and accessible in the work area.

Food service directors can contact their state public health departments for regulations that govern first-aid programs in the workplace. For example, some states have passed laws that require employees in public eating establishments to be trained in performing the Heimlich maneuver.

When feasible, food service directors should encourage workers certified in this technique to train other employees.

☐ Security

Theft is a major problem not only for food service employers but also for employers generally. Employee theft amounts to a loss of more than $20 million annually. It has been estimated that 85 percent of all employees have stolen from their employers. In addition, persons not employed by the operation can take money and property unlawfully. Food service theft can encompass money, food, beverage, supplies, and equipment, so department security should involve implementation of internal and external controls to protect all cash, merchandise, equipment, and supplies.

The most vulnerable areas are purchasing; receiving; storage; inventory control; production; and cafeteria, vending, and catering services. Each of these areas poses unique opportunity for theft and requires specific control procedures (discussed later in the chapter).

Both internal and external security primarily is the responsibility of the food service director, although this responsibility cannot be accomplished without the assistance of departmental staff and the larger facility's security department. Forming a partnership between organizational and departmental security teams is imperative. Employee cooperation in preventing and reporting theft is essential to internal and external security efforts.

Internal Security

Internal security primarily deals with the department's employees. This does not mean, however, that food service directors should overlook the fact that nondepartmental employees (or persons outside the institution) may commit theft. Some causes of employee theft include the following:

- *Poor employee morale:* Anger and resentment may make certain employees feel that the employer "owes them something," or they want to strike back.
- *Leadership deficiency:* Apathetic or poor supervision, management complacency and carelessness, or poor examples set by supervisory and management staff (for example, wastefulness or failure to enforce disciplinary policy) can give the wrong message to employees.
- *Uncompetitive wage structure:* Inadequate wages compromise employees' ability to manage their incomes or meet their expenses and thus may invite temptation to theft.
- *Temptation:* Some people are completely honest, others are incorrigibly dishonest, and still others are only as honest as circumstances permit. Employee access to cash, food, supplies, and equipment should be restricted and closely (but diplomatically) monitored.
- *Rationalization:* People may distance themselves from their actions by viewing their theft not as stealing from a unique entity (their employer) but, rather, as taking from an anonymous large corporation that can "afford the loss."
- *Kleptomania:* Certain persons have a persistent neurotic impulse to steal that is not driven by economic motive.
- *Thrill factor:* Stealing presents a challenge—a titillating taboo—to some people.
- *Personal problems:* Substance abuse, stress, family crisis (divorce, for example), and escalating bills may drive otherwise responsible workers to desperate acts.

To discourage pilferage in the food service department, managers need to deal with the problem immediately, persistently, and consistently. Firm corrective action, enforcement of well-defined policies and procedures that are applied fairly, continuous job-enhancement training, and effective supervisory techniques that boost morale are some deterrents to this problem. Another is a written and sound body of well-publicized internal and external security policies and procedures (within the limits of what reasonably should be disclosed). For example:

- Security begins with the employment process. Check references and, if possible, talk directly to an applicant's previous employer(s). During the screening phase, watch for gaps in job history, references that appear professionally unrelated, questionable addresses or telephone numbers of references, or a social security prefix that does not match an applicant's reported birth state. Another cautionary signal is a space left blank on that portion of an application form that asks whether an applicant has been convicted of a felony or misdemeanor.
- Provide new employees with complete and thorough training and orientation to departmental policy and procedures.
- Occasionally check content of packages taken by employees from the department.
- Routinely check content of trash carts and garbage containers.
- To the extent possible, maintain only one employee entrance and exit that are visible to supervisory staff.
- Lock-and-key procedures should be clear-cut, with key assignment logs maintained and a signout procedure for keys kept in a central lockbox. Duplication of keys should be prohibited. Those locks and combinations to which former employees had access should be changed—especially if the reason for release from employment was security related or if an employee's exit was less than amicable.

As noted earlier, unique security problems can occur in purchasing, receiving, storage, inventory control, production, and services (including cafeteria, vending, and catering). Two security problems in the *purchasing area* that require careful monitoring are potential collusion between purchasing personnel and distributors, and the ordering of excess items that can increase inventory and with it the possibility of theft.

Security problems in *receiving, storage, and inventory control* will affect the quality and quantity of available supplies and therefore the cost of food and supplies. Receiving is vulnerable because it is possible for either delivery or receiving personnel (or both jointly) to short items or substitute lower-quality items and then sell the original items for personal profit. Unless merchandise is immediately accounted for and stored upon receipt, the potential for theft is heightened. In a food service operation, expensive and high-demand items such as alcoholic and carbonated beverages, knives and other small utensils, or candy may have to be placed in locked storage areas. (Procedures discussed in chapter 18 should be implemented to control loss through pilferage, spoilage, and waste.)

A variety of measures can be implemented to prevent pilferage in the *production area*. Close (but nonthreatening) supervision of activities will reduce employee consumption or removal of leftovers or their unauthorized preparation of food items for personal consumption. Meat and cheese are the two most frequent targets of theft from the production storage area. Therefore, cases of meat placed in refrigerated or frozen storage should be opened and inventoried one by one. Again, controlled access to production storage areas is recommended.

Unique security problems in the *service areas*—the cafeteria, vending, and catering operations—are pilferage of food and supplies and control of cash. Commonly, theft in this area ranges from a cashier's charging friends less for meals to not charging for one or more individual items, to "no-sale" transactions or overrings from which the cashier pockets the customer's money. Sometimes a cashier may leave a register unlocked for another employee to take money. Vending machine operations represent another territory susceptible to pilferage, especially if department employees are responsible for filling machines and counting money. Examples that have been observed by managers include:

- Products given away to other employees while machines are being filled.
- Change removed from the change return while the door is open (an area often not secured by vending machine equipment design).
- Money removed directly from the deposit area if the money box is left unlocked. Machines with currency changers are especially vulnerable.

Security measures that can help control service-area pilferage and cash loss are summarized below.

- Monitor portion control and storage of leftovers carefully.
- Purchase cash registers designed with as many safeguards as possible.
- Review all voids, overcharges or overrings, shortages, and "no sales" daily.
- Designate a supervisor to complete or verify cash register currency, coin counts, and reports.
- Monitor cashier's techniques (such as placing extra money into or taking money from the register) to evaluate his or her accuracy and honesty.
- Insist that cash registers remain locked at all times when they are not in use.
- Insist that cashier give a cash register receipt to every customer to prevent possibility of receipt overrings and to permit customers to compare change with the charge.
- Purchase vending machines equipped with electronic counters that reconcile money.
- Promote installation of locks on all vending machine money boxes to eliminate employee access to currency.
- Delegate the duties of filling machines and removing money to different employees to allow for double-checks.
- Make provisions for a security escort during removal of money from vending machines.
- Provide a security escort during deposits from vending and other cash operations.

External Security

External security involves preventing the loss of items once they have left the immediate area. This means securing items from other hospital departments or from customers and protecting the department's property and employees from outsiders.

Food theft may be committed by taking items from patients' or residents' trays or sometimes consuming entire meals. Serviceware is another favored area for theft, one attributed mostly to other staff and represents up to 75 percent of the supply costs for a hospital food service department. Food, trays, bowls, and so on are frequently lost following catered events, when employees may pilfer food or property. The same policy that prohibits food service employees from taking leftover food also should apply to all other employees, including administrative staff.

By no means is theft the province of employees only. Patients, residents, and family members are not exempt from temptation. For example, they may take serviceware as souvenirs, for use at home, or because they feel an item is paid for in the cost of their stay. One hospital implemented a unique approach to this problem: the addition of a serviceware check-off section on the menu, labeled "for food service use only," whereby service personnel listed any serviceware not returned with a patient tray. The operation reduced losses of flatware and serviceware by 55 percent and 50 percent, respectively.

Systems must be in place to prevent unauthorized outsiders from entering the department and to monitor authorized entrants. This should be done for security *and* sanitation purposes. Again, maintaining one entrance and exit is a good measure. All outside doors should be kept locked except for deliveries. Distributors' representatives should have specific times and days allowed for visits and should not be allowed to enter the department from the dock area. Employees' visitors should be limited to the authorized break area and should never be allowed to enter restricted areas (such as production and storage areas).

A formal external security program should be designed in cooperation with the facility's larger security unit. Many of the techniques used in internal security apply to external security measures. (Chapter 21 also discusses some design features that enhance security efforts.) Specific external security strategies may include the following:

- Doors should be checked routinely by supervisors and security personnel to ensure that they are locked.

- The dock area should be electronically monitored to ensure that shipments are taken to their intended destinations in the food service department. Assigning a supervisor in the receiving area when large deliveries are received is recommended.
- Exits should be monitored at shift change to scrutinize employees' packages.
- Boxes on the premises should be broken down before the employee can remove them from the department.
- Supervisors on the evening shift should be rotated occasionally.

Securing and protecting the food service department relies on partnerships between the management staff and the security unit and between employees and management. To prevent loss, all functions of the department must be considered and appropriate policies and procedures established and consistently implemented.

☐ Disaster Planning

For purposes of this discussion, disasters can be classified as either external or internal. *External disasters* take place outside the institution but affect its operation. Examples of external disasters include natural calamities such as damaging snowstorms, hurricanes, earthquakes, and accidents (such as plane crashes, explosions, fires, and mass food poisonings) resulting in large numbers of casualties. External disasters also include national emergencies such as riots, wars, and terrorist attacks. External disasters can overburden an institution owing to the volume of cases the institution may have to handle. They also can affect the institution's ability to provide services, for example, when a flood or a hurricane damages or incapacitates the institution's facilities.

Internal disasters occur within the institution and damage its facilities or threaten the well-being of its patients/residents and employees. Examples of internal disasters include fires, bomb threats, power outages, and radiation accidents. The health care institution's overall disaster plan should include policies and procedures for handling both external and internal disasters.

Design of the Disaster Plan

The Joint Commission on Accreditation of Healthcare Organizations imposes a standard that requires the health care facility to establish a program allowing for continuous care of patients/residents and responding to the needs of others affected by the disaster. Every facility must have clearly defined and understandable guidelines in place as part of an overall disaster plan for the operation during external and internal disasters. The disaster plan must include procedures for treating the injured, providing food and shelter for those seeking refuge, and continuing the care of existing patients.

The institution should appoint a disaster committee whose responsibilities include developing and maintaining the disaster plan and coordinating disaster drills throughout the institution.

The committee also should coordinate with local and state government agencies, the local chapter of the Red Cross, local law enforcement officials, local civil defense authorities, and local fire and rescue departments.

A comprehensive disaster plan should delineate written procedures designed to ensure quick and efficient response to an external or internal disaster. The plan also should include provisions for responding to specific kinds of disasters (such as power outages, plane crashes, and so on). Among factors to be covered in specific disaster plans are the following:

- Allocation of supplies and labor (who is responsible)
- Responsibilities of specific departments and guidelines for interdepartmental cooperation
- Provisions for caring for existing patients/residents as well as for incoming disaster casualties
- Provisions for dealing with victims' families, clergy, and media representatives

351

A system for notifying the institution's employees of an impending disaster is vital to effective disaster planning. Every employee should be able to recognize the public address code or light signal used to announce disaster status in the institution. In addition, the addresses and telephone numbers of all staff and employees should be kept up-to-date so that in the event of an emergency off-duty personnel could be called in. The list should be arranged by department, with the name of the department head at the top. It also might help to arrange employees' names according to their geographic locations throughout the city so that personnel who reside closest to the disaster area could be called first. Supervisors should maintain copies of the call list at home as well as in the office.

Health care institutions should conduct regular disaster drills and disaster training programs for all staff members and employees. These programs should describe types of potential disasters and procedures to be followed during each. The roles and responsibilities of individual employee positions should be explained, and the following questions addressed:

- What identification should the employee wear during a disaster?
- Where should the employee report for work?
- To which department or supervisor should the employee report?
- What duties and responsibilities should the employee perform?
- What should the employee's work priorities be?
- Where will the employee be able to find needed supplies?
- What will be the official communication system?
- What should the employee do once the disaster is over?

The Food Service Department Disaster Plan

The food service department should develop a specific plan to ensure continuous operation and safety while remaining consistent with the plans of the larger health care facility. To ensure this objective, the director (or designee) should confer with the institution's disaster planning team in developing and updating the department plan.

Developing the Food Service Department Disaster Plan

As indicated earlier, the food service department's written disaster plan should support the institution's overall disaster plan. In maintaining and developing the department plan, the director or designee will need to do the following:

- Understand the institution's overall plan for handling internal and external disasters
- Train the food service staff to perform their roles in handling potential disasters
- Know the amount of nonperishable food that must be kept on hand for emergencies according to state law
- Perform regular checks of stores of emergency food and supplies and replace them as necessary
- Reassess the effectiveness of the disaster plan at regular intervals by participating in disaster drills
- Upgrade the department's emergency call list whenever there is staff turnover or there are changes in personnel addresses or telephone numbers

The director may decide to appoint a department disaster planning committee to develop and update the department's plan. Whether disaster planning is handled by the food service director or delegated to a committee, the plan should include provisions for the following items:

- *Menus:* Menus should be planned to use foods that will spoil first—especially when there is no electric power. Menus should be simple so that as few items as possible need to be served. If there has been a refrigeration problem, the freshness of all milk and milk products must be carefully evaluated before being served. Within the first 24 hours of a disaster, meals probably will continue to be served. They should be as simple and nutritious as possible under the circumstances. The type of menu and service depend on the number of people to be fed and what equipment and personnel are available. When possible, consideration should be given to local food preference. Preparation and service procedures for the first 24, 48, and 72 hours after a disaster should be covered in the food service department's disaster plan.

- *Supplies:* The plan should include provisions for maintaining supplies adequate for at least 72 hours at all times. These supplies should include disposable dishes and flatware, cleaning and disinfecting compounds, garbage bags, and sterile water supplies.
- *Sanitation:* The plan should outline procedures for maintaining sanitation at all times during a disaster. Careful attention should be given to checking for spoiled food, sanitizing pots and pans, and cleaning the food production work area.
- *Security:* Security measures should cover food, supply, and employee safety. Provisions against intruders (looting) should be made. Especially during this period employees should wear or carry identification cards at all times.
- *Use of workers from outside the food service department:* The disaster plan should describe the circumstances under which it would be appropriate to use workers from outside the department to perform food service tasks. When staff shortages make it necessary to use unskilled workers, for example, the tasks and roles they are to perform should be clearly designated and their work carefully supervised.
- *Service priorities:* Priorities should be established for providing food service during emergencies. The needs of existing patients/residents and disaster victims should be met first and then staff and employee needs should be served. Of lower priority would be service to members of the press, law enforcement officers, families of victims, and so on.

Planning for Various Disasters

Like the institution's disaster plan, the food service department plan should include specific provisions for a variety of natural disasters common to the facility's geographic area. For example, earthquake planning is especially important in California, Alaska, Washington, and Oregon. Disastrous snow and ice storms should be planned for in the midwestern, northeastern, and mountain states. Floods occur in all areas of the United States, but institutions located in floodplains along waterways should be especially careful to plan for these relatively common disasters. Power shortages and failures often accompany natural disasters and even summer thunderstorms, winter blizzards, and short-term localized power blackouts can put health care institutions on a disaster footing without warning.

Power Failures

The electric power supplied to health care facilities by local utilities can be cut off or decreased as a result of equipment failures, blackouts and brownouts, and natural disasters such as storms, floods, and earthquakes. The problem can last a few minutes or several days. When it is clear that the power may be off for more than a few minutes, the institution's procedures for handling power failures should be followed. The following steps may also be helpful:

- Immediately seal the door frames of all freezers with insulating tape and block the thresholds of walk-in freezers and refrigerators with blankets or other nonporous materials to keep warm air from entering.
- If possible, keep perishable food cold with dry ice.
- Use food stored in refrigerators first because it is the most perishable.
- Ask local vendors or other health care institutions for help.
- Supply consumers with disposable serviceware to make up for limited hot water supplies and incapacitated dishwashers.
- Clean pots, pans, utensils, work surfaces, and other preparation equipment with sanitizing agents.

353

Floods

Facilities located in flood-prone areas should formulate disaster plans that provide for enough food, equipment, and serviceware to serve patients and personnel for five to seven days. Where floods are likely to occur due to seasonal river flooding or hurricanes, the food service department's production and storage areas are best located above ground level to prevent contamination from floodwaters, which contain dirt and sewage. However, most food service storage areas are located at or below ground level, so the storage area for disaster supplies should be well above ground level.

Snow and Ice Storms

In many parts of the United States, travel can become difficult or impossible during heavy snow and ice storms, limiting access to health care facilities. When this happens, employees may be forced to remain at the institution until surface transportation is restored. Therefore, contingency arrangements should be made for delivery of food and supplies by air or mobile snow vehicles.

☐ Summary

The food service director has responsibility for providing a work environment that protects employees from injury and complies with OSHA and other health and safety regulations. The department should have an established safety program that includes designated safety procedures, continuous self-inspection, comprehensive training, and an effective fire-prevention plan. This chapter described working conditions, OSHA regulations, safety policies and procedures, components of safety training, fire safety measures, and first-aid guidelines.

Protecting the food service department against theft requires implementation of internal and external security controls. Theft-prevention techniques were presented for various functional areas. However, no security technique can succeed without a strong partnership between the food service security team and the larger facility's security unit or between management and employees.

A food service department must be prepared to respond to any kind of disaster—earthquake, flood, damaging snowstorms, power outages or reductions, and the like. To do this, the department should establish a disaster plan that complements the institution's plan and meets JCAHO standards. Disaster training should be an ongoing effort, as should participative disaster drills.

☐ Bibliography

All About OSHA. OSHA 2056. Washington, DC: U.S. Department of Labor Occupational Safety and Health Administration, 1985.

All Saints Health Care, Inc. Safety Manual. Ft. Worth, TX: All Saints Health Care, Inc., 1993.

Bureau of National Affairs. *Job Safety and Health: BNA Policy and Practice Service.* Washington, DC: BNA, 1986.

Chaff, L. *Safety Guide for Health Care Institutions.* 4th ed. Chicago: American Hospital Publishing, 1989.

Cherniak, M. J. MSDSs enhance training experience. *Environmental Protection* 3(4):20–21, May 1992.

Hudson, T. Riots in Los Angeles: being prepared—a lesson well-learned for area facilities. *Hospitals* 66(24):9, 15, Dec. 20, 1992.

Joint Commission on Accreditation of Healthcare Organizations. *Accreditation Manual for Hospitals.* Vol. II, *Scoring Guidelines.* Oakbrook Terrace, IL: JCAHO, 1992.

Keiser, J. *Controlling and Analyzing Costs in Foodservice Operations.* 2nd ed. New York City: Macmillan Publishing Co., 1988.

Minor, L. J. *Sanitation, Safety and Environmental Standards.* Vol. 2. L. J. Minor Food Service Standards Series. Westport, CT: AVI, 1983.

National Restaurant Association. *Safety Operations Manual.* Chicago: NRA, 1981.

OSHA Inspection. OSHA 2098. Washington, DC: U.S. Department of Labor Occupational Safety and Health Administration, 1986.

Puckett, R. P. Be prepared: disaster planning. In: J. C. Rose, editor. *Handbook for Health Care Food Service Management.* Rockville, MD: Aspen, 1984.

Somervile, S. R. Safety is no accident. *Restaurant USA* 12(7):14–18, Aug. 1992.

Sabatino, F. Hurricane Andrew: South Florida hospitals shared resources and energy to cope with the storm's devastation. *Hospitals* 66(24):26–28, 30, Dec. 20, 1992.

Stokes, J. F. Control food service theft by beginning security smart. *The Stokes Report* 2(1):1–2, Jan. 1982.

Weinstein, J. The secure restaurant. Part III: external security. *Restaurants and Institutions* 102(27):122–34, Nov. 25, 1992.

Chapter 15

Menu Planning

☐ Introduction

The menu is one of the most important plans a health care food service director develops because the menu serves as a primary control for the operation. It can be viewed as the hub around which all other functions revolve. The menu determines what foods are to be purchased, produced, and served; affects the number and type of personnel hired; and has implications for kitchen design and equipment selection. The menu provides the basis for further departmental planning (for example, service expansion) and serves as a major determinant of purchase scheduling and, ultimately, the financial status of the operation.

Aside from listing the food items offered to target markets, the menu serves other internal and external purposes. Internally, it provides crucial information to food service employees by specifying what items are provided. This enables employees to select which food and supplies to purchase, menu items to prepare, and service arrangements to provide.

The menu also functions externally to communicate the operation's offerings to potential customers. In that the menu facilitates communication between the food service operation and its customers, it also serves as an important marketing tool. It is not too far a reach to say that a food operation's menus can influence customer perceptions about the overall facility's quality of care. Therefore, the menu should be based on information about customers' wants and needs as identified by the facility's marketing information system. The menu should be compatible with the rest of the operation in terms of level and diversity of services offered and marketing mix, for example. It also should be useful in implementing the operation's marketing plan.

According to Robert Reid, a successful menu should:

- Further the goals of the marketing concept
- Contribute to establishing the perceived image of the operation
- Act as a means to influence customer demand for menu items
- Serve as a vehicle to gain a competitive advantage

The menu-planning process must produce a menu designed to satisfy these and other marketing objectives specific to a particular operation.

This chapter will discuss some critical elements of effective menu planning. Some of these are food preferences based on specific sources of information and changing trends; nutrition requirements among different customer markets; budgeted resources; availability and skill levels of the food service labor force; and a number of other factors covered at length.

The chapter then will move to menu specifications. These are driven by considerations such as target markets, meal plans, meal patterns, and types of menus used throughout an operation.

The menu-planning process will be described in detail, so that a menu planner will have a clear picture of what goes into the research, design, implementation, and follow-up evaluation of a good menu. Different types of menus—normal diets, modified diets, and special-service diets (such as gourmet selections)—also are addressed.

The chapter closes with brief summaries of four areas and a number of related methods and techniques of particular import to food service managers and menu planners. These are: (1) menu format, which addresses design of the menu as an effective communication and marketing tool; (2) pricing strategies, which describe several approaches to arriving at what to charge for menu items; (3) menu evaluation, which gives suggestions for pre-and postimplementation review of menu performance; and (4) menu-planning computer applications, which point out some advantages and limitations of computer-assisted menu-planning programs.

☐ Planning Considerations

Because of its impact on the success of the health care food service operation, the menu must be developed with great care. The following factors should be taken into consideration:

- Food preferences of customers
- Nutrition requirements of group(s) being served
- Budget allocations within the department
- Availability and skills of food service workers
- Amount of time required to prepare and serve the food
- Current marketplace conditions and availability of specific food supplies
- Type of production and service system in use
- Amount of space and type of storage, preparation, and service equipment available

Food Preferences

Food preferences are defined by customer wants and are based on personal, cultural, and regional factors. A health care food service operation's marketing information system should provide information about specific food preferences of the operation's target markets. Informal and formal methods can be used to collect data about how patients, employees, staff, visitors, and guests will react to various foods and food combinations.

Sources of Information

Informal observations made in the dining room, the cafeteria, and patients' rooms, for example, can provide valuable insight on preferences. Formal methods—questionnaires, for example—provide information about preferences for menu items already served or new items under consideration. Specifically, patient satisfaction questionnaires may measure reactions to menu items served during a patient's stay. Observations of plate waste for specific entrees, either by visual assessment or by weight, can reveal much for purposes of menu planning. To predict preference or acceptance of specific items, rating forms designed for respondent ranking can be used. This measure generally utilizes a Likert-type scale. With a Likert scale, customers indicate their attitudes by checking how strongly they agree or disagree with a statement, ranging from very positive (extremely high preference) to very negative (extremely low preference). The number of alternatives ranges from three to nine. Preferences for food combinations (for example, cranberry sauce or cranberry relish with turkey, raisin sauce or mustard sauce with ham, dumplings or biscuits with beef stew) also can be determined using this technique.

Food preference and acceptance surveys are particularly important when a limited menu or a nonselective menu is used. Most consumers enjoy frequently being served favorite foods; thus, less-preferred foods should not be repeated too often. Nutrition assessment procedures may also provide essential information about eating behaviors that can be used in planning menus for patients on regular or modified diets.

Trends

In a facility where the population changes frequently, it is important to survey food preferences frequently in order to keep menus current. Even with this information in hand, the task of menu planning is far from easy. Menu planners must keep pace with changing trends to develop new and creative ideas. According to a *Restaurants & Institutions* article written by Brian Quinton, the three most important trends affecting menu planning are changes in tastes, demographics, and habits.

Changing Tastes

Most major food service trade journals track and report the popularity of specific menu items. It is critical that the menu planner keep up with these reports so that the operation's menus can be modified accordingly. For example, according to *Restaurants & Institutions,* chicken fillets were not part of the average menu 20 years ago, but today they are offered on more than 63 percent of all menus. Fried chicken, on the other hand, dropped from 75 percent of menus to 50 percent during the same period.

Trade journals also report that consumers prefer more flavor in their foods, primarily due to the growing popularity of spicier ethnic and regional foods. Of particular popularity are Chinese, Mexican, and Italian menu items, followed by Japanese, Latin American, and European cuisines. Current trends also indicate growing popularity of specialty soups and sandwiches along with increased interest in vegetarian entrees. The menu planner must assess these trends in relation to the preferences indicated by the operation's target markets.

Changing Demographics

The changing demographics presented in chapter 1 have implications for the menu-planning process. Most important among these is the aging of the population. By the year 2000, the older adult segment not only will represent a larger percentage of the general population but also an increased percentage of the patient population in most types of health care operations. The menu planner will need to pay close attention to this market segment not only when developing patient menus but also when planning community ventures such as home-delivered or congregate meals.

Another important segment identified in chapter 1 is the "baby boom" generation, a segment currently at or approaching middle age. Most baby boom households have children whose menu preferences become important when the children become customers either as inpatients or participants in hospital-sponsored child care programs. Most children are accustomed to eating meals away from home and have developed strong preferences. When it comes to satisfying this segment, the four most popular menu items are hamburgers, chicken, french fries, and pizza. To broaden the menu offerings for children, the menu planner should carefully review trade journals to identify changing trends and creative ways to provide food service to children.

As the year 2000 approaches, cultural diversity of the general population will increase. The most rapid growth has been, and will continue to be, in the Hispanic and Asian populations. As nonwhite minorities make up an increasingly larger percentage of the patient and employee segments, menu planners must assess and modify menus to appeal to these markets.

Changing Habits

In addition to monitoring the tastes and demographic makeup of their customers, menu planners must analyze their customers' food attitudes and behaviors. Increased commitment to and concern for health and nutrition has important implications for menu planners. The 1992 Tastes of America Survey indicated that concern with healthful eating continues to grow and has resulted in changes in consumption of specific foods and menu items. A 1989 National Restaurant Association survey categorized consumers in one of three groups—"committed to nutrition," "vacillating," and "unconcerned about nutrition." To meet the wants of committed patrons, the menu planner should incorporate creative, flavorful menu items that conform with dietary guidelines for good health.

Customers continue to eat an increasing number of meals away from the home and at less-regular hours, a life-style change that provides both an opportunity and a challenge for health care food service operators. This is particularly true of breakfast, which has increased in importance as a meal eaten away from home. Because breakfast preferences vary widely among individuals, breakfast menus should offer a range of choices but without wasting food. To enhance breakfast sales, menu planners have incorporated more diverse menus, convenient hours of service, and, in some cases, spirited marketing strategies. To provide menu items that meet customer wants, the menu planner should continue to monitor changing trends.

Nutrition Requirements

Although it is important to focus on customers' wants, the specific nutritional needs or requirements of individual customers and groups of customers also should be considered. The nutrition needs of the general customer segment, which is composed of employees, staff, visitors, and guests, will be discussed first, followed by a brief discussion of the patient market.

General Customer Market

Increased awareness of the importance of nutrition to health, as discussed in the previous section of this chapter, has prompted menu planners to consider the nutritional quality of their menu items offered to general customer markets. Although numerous plans have been developed for the general population, two specific guides are particularly valuable when considering menu planning for this segment: *Nutrition and Your Health: Dietary Guidelines for Americans* and *The Food Guide Pyramid*.

The third edition of *Nutrition and Your Health: Dietary Guidelines for Americans* was released in 1990. These guidelines, shown in figure 15-1, were developed jointly by the U.S. Department of Agriculture (USDA) and the U.S. Department of Health and Human Services (HHS). The seven guidelines are the best, most up-to-date advice from nutrition scientists and make the following recommendations:

1. Eat a variety of foods.
2. Maintain a healthy weight.
3. Choose a diet low in fat, saturated fat, and cholesterol.
4. Choose a diet with plenty of vegetables, fruits, and grain products.
5. Use sugars only in moderation.
6. Use salt and sodium only in moderation.
7. Limit consumption of alcohol.

The Food Guide Pyramid (see figure 15-2) was developed to help healthy individuals implement the dietary guidelines. The pyramid is based on what foods Americans eat, what nutrients are in these foods, and how an individual can make the best food choices. It allows a healthy individual to choose foods that will supply required nutrients without too many calories, fat, saturated fat, cholesterol, sugar, sodium, or alcohol. The three lower sections of the pyramid emphasize foods from the five major food groups. Customers committed to health and nutrition will expect to find choices of menu items that allow them to follow these guidelines.

Figure 15-1. Dietary Guidelines for Americans

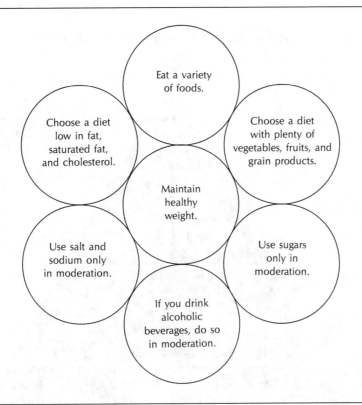

Source: U.S. Department of Agriculture/U.S. Department of Health and Human Services, 1990.

Patient Market

In food service operations that provide three meals a day, as is the case with inpatient service, menus should provide the recommended dietary allowances (RDAs) as defined by the National Research Council in 1989. The RDAs specify nutrition requirements for individuals based on gender and age. Menu planners should evaluate regular patient menus to determine that they indeed satisfy the RDAs. In instances where the patient's medical condition requires modifications to the regular menu, the menu planner should refer to the health care operation's diet manual.

Budget Allocations

The menu is the major factor in establishing and controlling food costs. With some effort and imagination, a skilled menu planner can design a menu that offers variety, interest, and appeal and still remains within most budgets while being planned around up-to-date, tested recipes. Keeping a running total of the cost of items on the menu as it is being planned allows the planner to balance high-cost items with low-cost items so that total daily costs can be kept within the limits of the budget. However, the same cost level should be maintained from day to day rather than balancing overbudget days with days on which the cost is considerably less than the budgeted daily average.

This approach works fairly well for controlling costs with nonselective menus, provided the cost information is current and projected market conditions are considered when menus are planned far in advance. (The different types of menus are discussed later in this chapter.) When a selective menu is offered, a forecast of the demand for each item must be determined before total cost per meal or patient day is computed.

361

Figure 15-2. Food Guide Pyramid

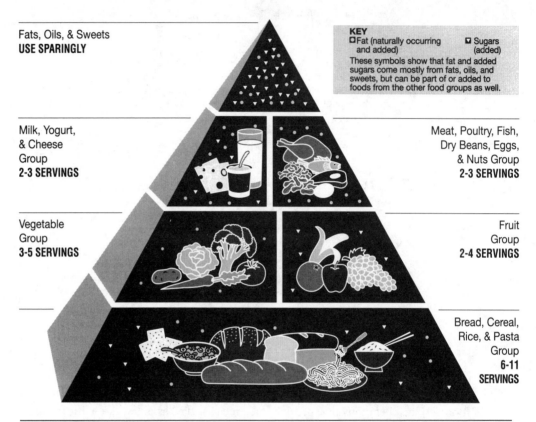

A Guide to Daily Food Choices

Fats, Oils, & Sweets
USE SPARINGLY

KEY
☐ Fat (naturally occurring   ▪ Sugars
and added)   (added)
These symbols show that fat and added
sugars come mostly from fats, oils, and
sweets, but can be part of or added to
foods from the other food groups as well.

Milk, Yogurt,
& Cheese
Group
2-3 SERVINGS

Meat, Poultry, Fish,
Dry Beans, Eggs,
& Nuts Group
2-3 SERVINGS

Vegetable
Group
3-5 SERVINGS

Fruit
Group
2-4 SERVINGS

Bread, Cereal,
Rice, & Pasta
Group
**6-11
SERVINGS**

Source: U.S. Department of Agriculture/U.S. Department of Health and Human Services, 1992.

When menus are planned for employees and guests, cost and selling price must be considered. The selling price should cover ingredients, labor, specified overhead, and profit. (Specific pricing techniques are discussed later in this chapter.) Forecasting demand accurately is difficult because the selling price itself affects the demand for individual items on the menu. Keeping careful histories of the popularity of various food items can sharpen the forecast when the same combination of food items is offered again.

Availability and Skills of Food Service Workers

The availability and skills of production personnel must be considered in menu planning, but they need not limit menu variety and quality. Menu items that require considerable skill and time to prepare can be purchased from commercial manufacturers that supply all or most of the labor involved in preparation. Therefore, menu items that cannot be produced on the premises with available personnel and equipment can still be part of the menu in most operations when the cost of prepared foods fits into the budget.

Employee expectations and satisfaction also should be considered. Plans should be made for the average level of skill and energy but, whenever possible, challenges should be offered to employees who seek to enhance their job skills.

Preparation and Scheduling Requirements

Overloading production schedules by poor menu planning can lead to tired, frustrated employees. Menus that balance the production work load from day to day and leave time for other essential tasks help foster positive employee attitudes.

In the past, managers relied primarily on their intuition and experience in making estimates of the labor involved in preparing individual menu items. Today, however, researchers use industrial engineering methods to determine food service production times. Reliable estimates of the total preparation time for each menu item will help managers plan the menu mix, schedule personnel, forecast labor costs, and develop effective menu pricing systems. Basically, the food for properly planned menus can be produced within the allotted time by employees working at a steady but unhurried pace. Most employees can adjust to occasional miscalculations in the amount of preparation time needed, but they become frustrated and angry when crises become routine. Also, low productivity results when the employees' productivity and skills are underutilized as a result of poorly planned menus or when labor time is not adjusted downward to accommodate the use of more prepared foods.

Marketplace Conditions

Several factors affect the supply and price of foods in the marketplace. Three of these are weather conditions, supply cycles, and geographic location.

Weather conditions may dictate sharp short-term supply and price fluctuations for fresh produce. Favorable weather conditions can result in an unexpected abundance of produce at lower prices, but adverse conditions can bring higher prices and shortages. Fruits and vegetables grown for processing are also affected, with resulting supply problems that may extend over several months.

As for *supply cycles,* improvements in food-processing, distribution, and storage technology have increased the availability of many foods throughout the entire year. However, seasonal fluctuations still occur for some fresh fruits and vegetables that are marketed in unprocessed form.

Geographic location may determine the type and quality of food products available. Improvements in transportation have eliminated this problem for many products. However, other products still may not be available in the ready-to-serve state to hospitals or nursing homes in rural areas.

Production and Service Systems

For production systems in which foods are prepared, held hot or cold, and served on the same day, menus may be limited by the amount of time available for food preparation between meals. The menu planner should try to spread the work load as evenly as possible among employees over the workday and still avoid holding conditions that may damage food quality.

In production systems that incorporate a thermal break, time limits may not be as severe. Once food is produced, it is held in a chilled or frozen state until served. Service deadlines do not limit the production schedules in these two systems, although not all food items are suitable for these holding methods without extensive ingredient or process modification. Menu planners must be completely familiar with the problems associated with certain menu items and revise production procedures accordingly.

The critical relationship between menu items offered and service system selected must be considered. The method of service and the distance that trays or bulk food must be transported can limit the types of menu items that can be served successfully. For example, fried eggs, pancakes, omelets, and ice cream can deteriorate in quality if too much time passes between preparation and service. Or, the number of sauces and casserole dishes may have to be limited in bulk-food distribution because of space limitations in food carts for the extra containers and because of the extra handling required at the point of service.

363

Space and Equipment

Successful menu planning cannot take place without factoring in the amount and type of available storage space for holding foods before, during, and after preparation. Purchasing policies need to take into consideration storage facilities so that deliveries are scheduled in a way that ensures adequate food supplies.

Equipment capability also must be considered during menu planning because a menu item cannot be produced unless the necessary equipment is available when needed. Unfortunately, many small food service operations do not have labor-saving and time-saving equipment such as mechanical slicers, shredders, choppers, and peelers that allow production of more complicated products. Although this equipment is expensive, it can increase productivity and enhance menu variety. In menu planning, demands on equipment must be balanced to avoid overloading ovens, steam equipment, and other production facilities.

☐ Menu Specifications

The food service director must establish basic menu specifications before planning any menus. First, the number of target markets or customer groups for which menus will be developed, along with any special services offered by the department, must be identified. Then, the number of menus that must be developed to meet the needs of different customer groups must be specified. Next, a meal plan and menu pattern appropriate for each customer group must be determined. Finally, such issues as the degree of selection and repetition to offer customers should be specified.

Target Markets

As described in chapter 3, market segmentation can be one of the food service director's most powerful marketing tools for help in determining the markets or customer groups, along with those specified by hospital administration, for which menus will be developed. The most significant distinction is the categorization of potential customers as either patients or nonpatients. Consumer wants and needs with regard to food differ between the two groups, thus influencing the planned menus. The patient customer group can be further segmented based on medical condition, age, and gender, whereas the nonpatient group typically is composed of employees, staff, visitors, and guests. Special services offered by the hospital and/or the food service department may provide the opportunity to serve other markets or groups as well. Examples of special services include child care centers, home-delivered meals for senior citizens, or catering services for off-premises customers. Once the target markets have been selected, the director must determine how many menus to develop. Only then can the menu-planning process proceed to the next step — determining the appropriate meal plans for each customer group.

Meal Plan

The number of meals offered during each 24-hour period varies according to the meal plan. Choosing the patient meal plan appropriate for the facility is an administrative decision that requires input from other patient care departments and the medical staff. For example, the nursing, radiology, and physical therapy departments must schedule patient treatment around mealtimes. Therefore, because meal plans and schedules affect these other departments, their needs should be considered.

The three-meal plan follows the traditional breakfast–lunch–dinner or breakfast–dinner–supper pattern. However, because of changes in American food habits and problems associated with labor scheduling and availability, four-and five-meal plans are being adopted by some health care institutions. The *four-meal plan* consists of a continental breakfast (beverage, cereal, and/or hot roll or quick bread) served early in the morning, a brunch served later in the morning (breakfast and/or lunch items), a main meal served in the late afternoon, and a substantial snack served in the evening. Obviously, this plan must have the full support of nursing and medical services because the entire facility will be affected by it. The *five-meal plan* consists of an early continental breakfast, a midmorning brunch, a light early-afternoon refreshment, a late-afternoon main meal, and an evening snack.

Menus must be planned to balance the day's nutrients among all meals served and to avoid offering an excessive calorie intake, particularly with the four- and five-meal plans. With any meal plan, no more than 15 hours should pass between the last meal of one day and the first meal of the next.

Using the four- or five-meal plan reduces the number of employees needed in the early morning and late evening. For example, items for the continental breakfast can be set up by the afternoon work force, and fewer employees are needed to prepare and serve an evening snack. This leaves the greatest number of employees on duty during one eight-hour period.

The director must determine appropriate meal plans for nonpatient customer groups as well. Again, the customers' wants and needs regarding number and scheduling of meals must be balanced with the resources required to support these plans. Based on this type of analysis, weekend brunches have met with success among health care food service operations. As mentioned earlier, customers' food habits reflect a move away from the traditional three-meal plan to more frequent dining at less-regular hours. This along with the realization that potential customers are available 24 hours a day should be considered when establishing the meal plan for other customer groups. Viewing this situation as an opportunity, the food service director should collect information from these potential customers to develop cost-effective meal plans. Special attention should be given to meal plans that address the needs of the evening and night shift employees of the health care operation.

Menu Pattern

Translating the daily food needs of customers into attractive and appealing meals requires good organization. For inpatients or residents, the *normal diet*—also known as the regular, general, or house diet—is the starting point for planning because it is the basis for all diet modifications. Planning and producing modified diets is easier when the normal diet menu includes several foods that can also be served on modified diets. However, variety in the general menu should not be restricted by this consideration; only slight changes in certain menu items will make them suitable for modified diets.

The menu planner uses the normal diet and the minimum daily requirements for foods from the *Food Guide Pyramid* to develop the patient *menu pattern,* which simply lists the food components to be offered at each meal. For example, the traditional menu pattern for a three-meal plan includes:

- Breakfast
  - Fruit or juice
  - Hot or cold cereal
  - Meat or meat alternative
  - Bread and butter or margarine
  - Beverage
- Lunch
  - Meat or meat alternative, or soup and sandwich
  - Vegetable and/or salad
  - Bread and butter or margarine
  - Dessert or fruit
  - Beverage

- Dinner
  - Appetizer
  - Soup or juice
  - Meat or meat alternative
  - Potato, rice, or pasta
  - Vegetable
  - Fruit or vegetable salad
  - Bread and butter or margarine
  - Dessert
  - Beverage

The traditional menu pattern may offer more food than is necessary because most healthy adults do not consume this many courses at their meals. This pattern should be analyzed to see if the number of courses can be reduced and still meet the customer's nutrition requirements.

With four- and five-meal plans, individual meal components vary from the example and spread total food intake over all meals. The number of items offered at each meal on each day should be about the same to ensure that the recommended number of servings from the food guide pyramid are served and to maintain an even level of food intake from day to day.

Menu patterns for nonpatient customer groups also must be established. The menu patterns established for these groups should balance customers' wants and needs; applicable regulations or requirements, such as with menus for child care facilities; those resources required to support the menu patterns; and the effect of the menu patterns on profitability of nonpatient food service operations. It is helpful to use a form specifically designed for menu planning so that meals for all customer groups conform to the standard set for the facility.

Types of Menus

Once the meal plan and menu pattern for each customer group has been developed, additional menu specifications must be established. These focus primarily on the degree of menu selection and repetition offered to customers.

Selection

Menus can be nonselective, selective, or a combination (for example, a choice of entrees could be offered, but other menu items would be fixed). A nonselective menu gives the patient no choice in what is served. Although many food service directors believe that such a menu saves time, money, and waste, patient dissatisfaction can outweigh such perceived advantages. Even when nonselective menus are carefully planned, some patients may be dissatisfied because they are obliged to eat unwanted foods or leave them as plate waste. However, in many extended care facilities, nonselective menus are used frequently because residents are incapable of making their own choices. In some long-term care and residential facilities that have dining room service, meals are served buffet style. Although there may be no choice of entree, starch, and vegetable, a variety of salads, breads, desserts, and beverages may be offered.

A selective menu offers three obvious advantages: Patients can choose what they want, the amount of plate waste can be lowered, and food costs can be reduced. These advantages are especially attractive when an expensive entree is paired with an inexpensive one, thus allowing the lower-cost item to offset the more expensive one. When patients choose their own food, they are more likely to eat everything served. They may even choose fewer items than would have been served on a nonselective menu. For example, when bread and a starchy vegetable are offered, the patient may select only one.

A selective menu requires that the food service department prepare several different menu items for each meal but in smaller quantities than would be needed for a nonselective menu. Therefore, even a facility with limited equipment and personnel can offer a diverse and interesting menu. Careful item pairing will balance work load, equipment use, and costs.

Carefully planned selective menus also include options that can be used on modified diets. To help ensure that patients select a nutritionally adequate diet, menu items often are grouped in categories from which a specified number of selections can be made, or specific starches and vegetables may accompany each entree. Using selective menus for patients on modified diets also can be an effective aid in teaching patients to manage their own diets. To realize the benefits of this type of menu, selective menus should be reviewed for unnecessary selections and variety. According to an article in the *Hospital Food and Nutrition Focus,* any item that represents less than 10 percent of the regular diet selections probably costs more to produce and serve than it generates in public relations benefits or actual revenue.

Repetition

Menu planning in many institutions is streamlined by using a *cycle menu,* in which a set of carefully planned and tested menus are rotated for a specified number of days or weeks. During a given cycle, no menu is repeated. Depending on the average length of stay, the cycle in an acute care hospital may be 5, 7, 8, or 14 days. Longer cycles are followed in long-term care facilities and for employee cafeterias.

Cycle menus require careful planning and can be either selective or nonselective. When the system is first instituted, the first cycle can be regarded as a test period, after which adjustments are made to increase the attractiveness of meals, to avoid preparation or service difficulties, or to reduce costs. Cycle menus should also be adjusted with the changing seasons, marketplace conditions, and particularly with a change in customer base. As a rule, menus should be reviewed periodically and changed whenever new and appealing food items or food formats are introduced by suppliers. The cycles should be flexible enough to feature holiday foods or to adjust to other social activities, particularly in extended care facilities. A balanced level of item popularity should be maintained throughout the cycle. In addition, the beginning and end of the cycle should be different from one another so that the foods offered show enough variety. Repetition of food items on the same day of every week should be avoided.

Once established, the cycle menu saves time and labor in menu planning, food procurement, and food production. Purchase orders should be filed with the menus to simplify future purchasing and production forecasts. The actual rates of selection for each item should be recorded so that accurate demand forecasts can be made each time the cycle is repeated. The cycle menu is also useful as a training device because it enables employees to become familiar with the production of each item and enhances organizational and time management skills.

Some health care food service operations offer a *static menu* (or set menu) to their customer groups. This menu resembles a restaurant menu in its variety and number of selections and remains the same from day to day, with the possible exception of one or more daily specials. A static menu can simplify purchasing, production, service, and management of the food service operation. However, the characteristics of each customer group, such as patient length of stay, should be analyzed closely to determine if this type of menu is appropriate for any of the operation's customer groups.

The third type of menu based on repetition is the *single-use menu,* which is planned for a specific meal on a specific day, possibly not to be used again in the identical form. The most likely use of this type of menu in a health care operation would be for catered events or as a "monotony breaker" in the employee cafeteria.

☐ Menu-Planning Process

The menu planner should organize the procedure and schedule adequate time and resources for this activity. He or she should gather all reference materials needed for the task, including previous menus, inventory lists, standardized recipes, market reports, results of food preference and acceptability studies, trade publications, other manuals, and the like. Usually, these are available from professional food service and health care associations. A standard menu-planning form (which lists meal patterns, meals served, and days of the week in the period being planned) should be used.

Patient Menus

In a health care operation, the primary customer group is patients. When planning patient menus, the menu planner must weigh the planning considerations described earlier in this chapter, particularly the challenge of balancing patient needs (nutrition requirements) with patient desires (food preferences). To help meet this challenge, a systematic planning process that starts with normal diets should be followed.

Menu Planning for Normal Diets

When planning a normal diet menu, first, select the *meat or meat alternative entrees* for the main meals over the entire menu cycle. Entree choices are made first so that other foods served for each meal can complement and enhance the entree. Given that entree items comprise the biggest cost and because most of the food dollar goes for main dishes, the frequency of their use must be controlled. It is helpful to make a list of possible meat and meat alternative entrees to use in menu planning. A number of menu-planning suggestions are shown in table 15-1. This type of list can save the department time and money, add variety to the menu, and help the menu planner avoid repeating menus on the same day of each week.

Once the entree has been selected, choose the accompanying *vegetables and potatoes, rice, or pasta* on the basis of their color, form, texture, and flavor. A colorful vegetable in whole, sliced, diced, or mashed form makes the meal more attractive. Crisp vegetables complement a soft or creamy main dish.

Next, select *salads* that contrast with the rest of the meal in color, flavor, and texture. For example, chilled salads complement hot entrees. Main-dish salads, chef salads, and cold plates that include salads also are popular entrees.

Vary the type of *bread* served from meal to meal. Include yeast breads, quick breads, sweet breads, and specialty breads.

Select *desserts* that complete and balance the meal in flavor and texture and sometimes in caloric content. Fresh, canned, and frozen fruits are offered as alternatives to desserts in many health care institutions.

Offer the most popular *beverages*. Most institutions provide coffee, tea, and other hot beverages and milk in various forms. Many people prefer low-fat or skim milk to whole milk; chocolate milk may appeal to some patients.

Plan breakfast menus last. Although breakfast menus are simple, they should provide interesting food variations from day to day. Nontraditional items such as breakfast sandwiches might be considered. Trade journals can suggest creative ideas for breakfast menus that are simple yet nutritious, appetizing, and attractive.

Some patients on normal diets may have needs that differ from the general patient population. This is particularly true of children and older adults. For children hospitalized and separated from the familiarity of parents and homes, food takes on added significance. Meals not only should satisfy the nutrition requirements and appetites of hospitalized children, but they also should be fun to eat. Each family should be consulted about its child's food preferences and eating habits. Menu items should suit the child's age and developmental stage, which includes modifying (grinding or pureeing) the physical form of food if necessary. Raw fruits and vegetables that can be eaten as finger foods usually are much more popular than traditional salads. Raw vegetables can be accompanied by nutritious dips for added appeal. Children age 2 to 5 prefer simple foods over mixed dishes; gravies and cream sauces should be avoided in favor of colorful, attractive, and easy-to-handle foods. Midmorning and midafternoon snacks also are options.

Menus should be planned for various age groups, such as 2 to 5, 6 to 12, and 13 to 18. Many pediatric hospitals and institutions use specially designed menu forms with attractive colors and artwork. Nutrition education, particularly for children who may be on modified diets, can be incorporated in an appealing fashion. For example, menus can be designed to teach children about vegetables and fruits by using pictures and personifying each one with a name. Explanations of the body's nutrition needs could be included on the cover of the menu. Coloring books that teach the principles of good nutrition could be distributed at the time each child is admitted.

Table 15-1. Menu-Planning Suggestions

Entrees

Meats

BEEF:
  Corned beef
  Roast beef
  Pot roast
  Broiled steak
    T-bone
    Sirloin
    Filet mignon
    Club steak
  Cubed steak
  Country-fried steak
  Spanish steak
  Swiss steak
  Steak with vegetables
  Steak stroganoff
  Mock drumsticks
  Barbecued kabobs
  Barbecued short ribs
  Braised short ribs
  Beef pot pie
  Beef stew with vegetables
  Beef stew with dumplings
  Beef ragout
  Hungarian goulash
  Chop suey
  Meat loaf
  Swedish meatballs
  Spanish meatballs
  Meatballs with spaghetti
  Tacos
  Enchiladas
VEAL:
  Roast leg of veal
  Roast veal shoulder
  Baked veal chops
  Veal chops in sour cream
  Breaded veal cutlets
  Veal birds
  Veal fricassee with
    poppy-seed noodles
  Veal stew with vegetables
  Veal à la king
  Veal patties with bacon
  Veal paprika with rice
  Curried veal with rice
LAMB:
  Roast leg of lamb
  Roast lamb shoulder
  Broiled lamb chops
  Lamb stew
  Braised lamb riblets
  Barbecued lamb
  Lamb patties with bacon
  Curried lamb with rice
  Lamb fricassee with noodles
PORK (fresh):
  Baked fresh ham
  Roast pork loin
  Roast pork shoulder
  Roast pork with dressing
  Baked pork chops

Breaded pork chops
Deviled pork chops
Barbecued pork chops
Stuffed pork chops
Breaded pork cutlets
Barbecued spareribs
Spareribs with kraut
Spareribs with dressing
Pork birds
PORK (cured):
  Baked ham
  Baked ham slices
  Grilled ham slices
  Baked Canadian bacon
  Ham loaf
  Ham patties
  Glazed ham balls
VARIETY MEATS:
  Braised tongue
  Braised liver
  Liver and bacon
  Liver and onions
  Baked heart
  Braised heart
  Sweetbread cutlets
  Creamed sweetbreads
MISCELLANEOUS:
  Frankfurters with kraut
  Cheese-stuffed wieners
  Egg rolls

Meat Extenders

Baked hash
Corned beef hash
Stuffed peppers
Beef roll
Beef upside-down pie
Spaghetti with meat sauce
Creole spaghetti
Beef and pork casserole
Spanish rice
Creamed beef
Creamed chipped beef
Creamed chipped beef and peas
Chipped beef and noodles
Veal croquettes
Meat turnovers
Veal soufflé
Curried veal with rice
Creamed ham and celery
Ham à la king
Ham croquettes
Ham soufflé
Ham timbales
Ham and egg scallop
Creamed ham on spoon bread
Cold baked ham with potato
  salad
Chef's salad bowl
Russian salad bowl
Baked ham sandwiches
Ham and cheese sandwiches

Ham salad sandwiches
Bacon and tomato sandwiches
Bacon and tomato on
  bun with cheese sauce
Hamburger on bun
Ham biscuit roll
Ham turnover
  with cheese sauce
Ham shortcake
Ham and sweetbread casserole
Sausage and dressing
Sausage and apple dressing
Sausage rolls
Sausage cakes
Fried scrapple
Bacon and potato omelette
Pork and noodle casserole
Baked lima beans
Baked lima beans with sausages
Boiled lima beans with ham
Baked navy beans
Chili con carne
Chili-spaghetti
Ranch-style beans
Baked eggs and bacon rings
Pizza
Cold luncheon meat with
  macaroni salad
Barbecued hamburgers
Wieners with meat
  sauce on bun
Hot luncheon sandwich
Hot roast beef sandwich
Hot roast pork sandwich
Barbecued ham, pork, or
  beef sandwiches
Western sandwich
Toasted chipped beef and cheese
  sandwich

Poultry

TURKEY:
  Roast turkey
  Baked turkey roll
  Hot turkey sandwich
  Sliced turkey sandwich
  Turkey loaf
CHICKEN:
  Baked chicken
  Broiled chicken
  Fried chicken
  Barbecued chicken
  Tahitian chicken
  Breast of chicken with ham
    slice
  Chicken à la Maryland
  Fricassee of chicken
  Chicken with dumplings
  Chicken with noodles
  Chicken pie
  Chicken loaf
  Chicken soufflé

369

continued on next page

Table 15-1. *Continued*

Entrees (continued)

Poultry (continued)

Chicken turnovers
Chicken and rice casserole
Chicken à la king
Singapore curry
Creamed chicken:
  on biscuit
  in patty shell
  on toast cups
  on chow mein noodles
  on spoon bread
Chicken croquettes
Chicken cutlets
Scalloped chicken
Chicken timbales
Chicken chow mein
Chicken biscuit roll
  with mushroom sauce
Chicken salad
Chicken salad in cranberry
  or raspberry mold
Chicken salad sandwich

Fish

FRESH AND FROZEN FISH:
  Fried salmon steaks
  Poached salmon
  Baked halibut steak
  Poached halibut steak
  Fried or baked fillets:
    haddock, perch, sole,
    whitefish, catfish
  Fried whole fish:
    whiting, smelts
  French-fried shrimp
  Creole shrimp with rice
  French-fried scallops
  Fried clams
  Fried oysters
  Scalloped oysters
  Deviled crab

Crab casserole
Broiled lobster
CANNED FISH:
  Salmon loaf
  Salmon croquettes
  Creamed salmon on biscuit
  Salmon biscuit roll
    with creamed peas
  Scalloped salmon
  Salmon and potato
    chip casserole
  Casserole of rice and tuna
  Tuna croquettes
  Creamed tuna:
    on toast
    on biscuit
  Tuna soufflé
  Scalloped tuna
  Tuna biscuit roll with
    cheese sauce
  Tuna-cashew casserole
  Codfish balls
  Tuna and noodles
  Crab salad
  Lobster salad
  Shrimp salad
  Tuna salad
  Salmon salad
  Cold salmon with
    potato salad
  Hot tuna on bun
  Tuna sandwich,
    plain or grilled

Meatless Dishes

Cheese rarebit
Cheese balls on pineapple
  slice
Cheese croquettes
Cheese soufflé
Cheese fondue
Macaroni and cheese
Scalloped macaroni

Baked rice and cheese
Rice croquettes with cheese
  sauce
Chinese omelet
Rice with mushrooms and almond
  sauce
Fried mush
Baked eggs with cheese
Curried eggs
Creamed eggs
Egg cutlets
Egg and noodle casserole
Noodle casserole
Hot stuffed eggs
Eggs à la king
Scalloped eggs and cheese
Scrambled eggs
Omelet
Spanish omelet
Vegetable casserole with pinwheel
  biscuits
Cauliflower casserole
Vegetable timbales
Spinach timbales with poached
  egg
Mushroom puff
Cheese puff
Spoon bread
Corn rarebit
Corn pudding
Scalloped corn
Hot potato salad
Creamed asparagus on toast
French toast
Plain fritters
Corn fritters
Fruit fritters
Grilled cheese sandwich
Egg salad sandwich
Fruit plates
Cottage cheese salad
Deviled eggs
Brown bean salad
Stuffed tomato salad

Vegetables

Green Vegetables

ARTICHOKES:
  With butter or mayonnaise
ASPARAGUS:
  Buttered or creamed
  With cheese or hollandaise
    sauce
BROCCOLI:
  Almond buttered
  With cheese sauce,
    lemon butter, or
    hollandaise sauce

BRUSSELS SPROUTS:
  Buttered
CABBAGE:
  Au gratin
  Buttered or creamed
  Creole
  Hot slaw
CELERY:
  Buttered or creamed
CELERY CABBAGE:
  Buttered
GREEN BEANS:
  Buttered or creamed

Creole
  With almonds or mushrooms
  Southern style
PEAS:
  Buttered or creamed
  With carrots, cauliflower,
    celery, or onions
  With mushrooms or almonds
SPINACH:
  Buttered
  Wilted
  With egg or bacon
  With new beets

Table 15-1. *Continued*

Vegetables (continued)		

Other Vegetables

BEETS:
  Buttered
  Harvard
  Julienne
  In sour cream
  With orange sauce
  Hot spiced
  Pickled
CARROTS:
  Buttered or creamed
  Candied
  Glazed
  Lyonnaise
  Mint glazed
  Savory
  With celery
  With peas
  Parsley buttered
  Sweet and sour
CAULIFLOWER:
  Buttered or creamed
  French fried
  With almond butter
  With cheese sauce
  With peas
CUCUMBERS:
  Scalloped
EGGPLANT:
  Creole
  Fried or French fried
  Scalloped
MUSHROOMS:
  Broiled
  Sauteed
ONIONS:
  Au gratin
  Baked
  Buttered or creamed
  Casserole
  French fried
  Stuffed
  With Spanish sauce
RUTABAGAS:
  Buttered
  Mashed
SQUASH, SUMMER:
  Buttered
  Mashed

TOMATOES:
  Baked
  Breaded
  Broiled sliced
  Creole
  Scalloped
  Stewed
  Stuffed
TURNIPS:
  Buttered
  Creamed
  Mashed
  With new peas

Fruits Served as Vegetables

APPLES:
  Cooked and buttered
  Fried
  Hot baked
BANANAS:
  Baked
  French fried
GRAPEFRUIT:
  Broiled
PEACHES:
  Broiled
PINEAPPLE RING:
  Broiled
  Sauteed

Potatoes, Pasta, and Rice

POTATOES:
  Au gratin
  Baked
  Browned
  Buttered new
  Chips
  Creamed
  Croquettes
  Duchesse
  Fried
  French fried
  Lyonnaise
  Mashed
  O'Brien
  Potato cakes
  Potato pancakes

Potato salad, hot or cold
  Rissole
  Scalloped
  Stuffed baked
POTATOES, SWEET:
  Baked
  Candied or glazed
  Croquettes
  Mashed
  Scalloped
MACARONI AND SPAGHETTI:
  Macaroni and cheese
  Macaroni salad
  Scalloped macaroni
NOODLES:
  Buttered
  Poppy seed
RICE:
  Buttered
  Curried
  Fried rice with almonds
  Green rice
  Croquettes

Other Starchy Vegetables

CORN:
  Buttered or creamed
  On cob
  With tomato
  Pudding
  O'Brien
  Scalloped
  With celery and bacon
  With green pepper rings
  Succotash
LIMA BEANS:
  Buttered or creamed
  With bacon
  With mushrooms
  With almonds
PARSNIPS:
  Buttered
  Browned
  Glazed
SQUASH:
  Baked acorn
  Baked hubbard
  Mashed butternut
  Mashed hubbard

Salads and Relishes		

Fruit Salads

Apple and celery
Apple and carrot

Apple and cabbage
Cranberry relish
Cranberry sauce

Frozen fruit
Mixed fruit
Waldorf

continued on next page

Table 15-1. *Continued*

Salads and Relishes (continued)

Vegetable Salads

Beet pickles
Beet relish
Brown bean
Cabbage relish
Cabbage
Cabbage-carrot
Cabbage-marshmallow
Cabbage-pineapple
Carrot-raisin
Celery cabbage
Coleslaw
Creamy coleslaw
Cucumber-onion in sour cream
Hawaiian tossed
Head lettuce
Potato
Red cabbage
Salad greens with grapefruit
Stuffed tomato
Tossed green
Tomato
Tomato-cucumber
Vegetable-nut

Gelatin Salads

Applesauce mold
Autumn
Beet
Bing cherry

Cabbage parfait
Cranberry ring mold
Frosted cherry
Frosted lime
Grapefruit
Jellied citrus
Jellied vegetable
Jellied waldorf
Molded pear
Perfection
Molded pineapple-cheese
Molded pineapple-cucumber
Molded pineapple-relish
Molded pineapple-rhubarb
Raspberry ring mold
Ribbon mold
Spicy apricot
Sunshine
Swedish green top
Tomato aspic
Under-the-sea

Salad Ices

Apricot
Cherry
Cranberry
Grapefruit
Lemon
Lime
Mint
Orange

Pineapple
Raspberry
Rhubarb
Strawberry
Tomato
Watermelon

Relishes

Burr gherkins
Carrot curls
Carrot sticks
Cauliflowerets
Celery curls
Celery fans
Celery hearts
Celery rings
Cherry tomatoes
Cucumber slices
Cucumber wedges
Green pepper rings
Olives: green, ripe, stuffed
Onion rings
Radish accordions
Radish roses
Spiced crabapples
Spiced peaches
Spiced pears
Stuffed celery
Tomato slices
Tomato wedges
Watermelon pickles

Garnishes

Yellow-Orange

CHEESE:
  Balls, grated, strips
  Rosettes
EGG:
  Hard-cooked or sections
  Deviled halves
  Riced yolk
FRUITS:
  Apricot halves, sections
  Cantaloupe balls
  Lemon sections, slices
  Orange sections, slices
  Peach slices
  Peach halves with jelly
  Spiced peaches
  Persimmons
  Tangerines
SWEETS:
  Apricot preserves
  Orange marmalade
  Peach conserve

Peanut brittle, crushed
Sugar, yellow or orange
VEGETABLES:
  Carrots: rings, shredded, strips
MISCELLANEOUS:
  Butter balls
  Coconut, tinted
  Gelatin cubes
  Mayonnaise

Red

FRUITS:
  Cherries
  Cinnamon apples
  Cranberries
  Plums
  Pomegranate seeds
  Red raspberries
  Maraschino cherries
  Strawberries
  Watermelon cubes, balls

SWEETS:
  Red jelly: apple, cherry, currant,
    loganberry, raspberry
  Cranberry glacé, jelly
  Gelatin cubes
  Red sugar
VEGETABLES:
  Beets, pickled, Julienne
  Beet relish
  Red cabbage
  Red peppers: rings, strips,
    shredded
  Pimento: chopped, strips
  Radishes, red: sliced, roses
  Stuffed olives, sliced
  Tomato, aspic, catsup, chili
    sauce, cups, sections, sliced,
    broiled
MISCELLANEOUS:
  Paprika
  Tinted coconut
  Cinnamon drops (red hots)

Table 15-1. *Continued*

Garnishes (continued)

Green

FRUITS:
Avocado
Cherries
Frosted grapes
Green plums
Honeydew melon
Lime wedges
SWEETS:
Citron
Green sugar
Gelatin cubes
Mint jelly
Mint pineapple
Mints
VEGETABLES:
Endive
Green pepper: strips, chopped, rings
Green onions
Lettuce cups
Lettuce, shredded
Mint leaves
Olives
Parsley: sprig, chopped
Pickles: Burr gherkins, strips, fans, rings
Spinach leaves
MISCELLANEOUS:
Coconut, tinted
Mayonnaise, tinted
Pistachios

White

FRUITS:
Apple rings
Apple balls
Grapefruit sections
Gingered apple
White raisins
Pear balls
Pear sections
VEGETABLES:
Cauliflowerets
Celery cabbage
Celery: curls, hearts, strips
Cucumber: rings, strips, wedges, cups
Mashed potato rosettes
Onion: rings, pickled
Radishes, white
MISCELLANEOUS:
Cream cheese frosting
Sliced hard-cooked egg white
Shredded coconut
Marshmallows
Almonds
Mints
Whipped cream
Powdered sugar

Brown-Tan

BREADS:
Crustades

Croutons
Cheese straws
Fritters, tiny
Noodle rings
Toast: cubes, points, strips, rings
MISCELLANEOUS:
Cinnamon
Dates
French-fried cauliflower
French-fried onions
Mushrooms
Nutmeats
Nut-covered cheese balls
Potato chips
Rosettes
Toasted coconut

Black

Caviar
Chocolate-covered mints
Chocolate sprinkles
Chocolate, shredded
Chocolate sauce
Currants
Olives, ripe
Prunes
Pickled walnuts
Raisins
Spiced prunes
Truffles

Desserts

Cakes and Cookies

CAKES:
Angel food: plain, chocolate, filled
Applesauce
Banana
Boston cream
Burnt sugar
Chiffon
Chocolate and jelly rolls
Coconut
Cupcakes
Fruit upside-down
Fudge
German sweet chocolate
Gingerbread
Lazy daisy
Marble
Pineapple cashew
Poppy seed
Spice
White

COOKIES:
Brownies
Butter tea
Butterscotch
Chocolate chip
Coconut macaroon
Date bars
Oatmeal
Fudge balls
Gingercrisp
Marshmallow squares
Peanut butter
Sandies
Sugar

Pies and Pastries

ONE-CRUST PIES:
Apricot cream
Banana cream
Butterscotch
Chiffon

Coconut cream
Coconut custard
Custard
Date cream
Dutch apple
Frozen ready-to-eat
Fruit-glazed cream
Pecan cream
Pineapple cream
Pumpkin
Rhubarb custard
TWO-CRUST PIES:
Apple
Apricot
Blackberry
Blueberry
Boysenberry
Cherry
Gooseberry
Mincemeat
Peach
Pineapple

continued on next page

373

Table 15-1. *Continued*

Desserts (continued)

Pies and Pastries (continued)

Plum
Prune
Raisin
Rhubarb
Strawberry
COBBLERS, FRUIT:
  Same fruits as for pies

Puddings

Apple crisp
Apple dumplings
Apple brown Betty
Baked custards
Banana cream
Bavarian cream
Bread pudding
Butterscotch pudding
Caramel tapioca
Cherry crisp
Chocolate cream
Coconut cream
Cottage pudding
Cream puffs
Date cream
Date pudding
Date roll
English toffee dessert
Floating island
Fruit gelatin
Fruit whips
Fudge pudding
Icebox dessert
Lemon snow
Meringue shells
Peach crisp
Peach melba
Pineapple cream
Royal rice pudding

Shortcake
Steamed pudding
Tapioca cream
Vanilla cream

Frozen

ICE CREAMS:
  Apricot
  Banana
  Butter brickle
  Caramel
  Chocolate
  Chocolate chip
  Coffee
  Lemon custard
  Macaroon
  Peach
  Peanut brittle
  Pecan
  Peppermint stick
  Pineapple
  Pistachio
  Raspberry
  Strawberry
  Toffee
  Tutti-frutti
PARFAITS, SHERBETS:
  Apricot
  Cherry
  Cranberry
  Greengage plum
  Lemon
  Lime
  Orange
  Mint
  Pineapple
  Plum
  Raspberry
  Rhubarb

Watermelon

Miscellaneous

CHEESE:
  Assorted with crackers and
    fruit
FRUITS:
  Baked or stewed:
    Apples
    Fruit compote
    Rhubarb
  Canned or frozen:
    Apricots
    Berries
    Cherries
    Figs
    Fruit cup
    Peaches
    Pears
    Pineapple
    Plums
    Prunes
    Rhubarb
  Raw:
    Apples
    Apricots
    Bananas
    Berries
    Cherries
    Figs
    Grapefruit
    Grapes
    Melons
    Oranges
    Peaches
    Pears
    Pineapple
    Plums
    Prunes

Leftover Foods

BREADS AND CRACKERS:
  Bread crumbs for crumbing
    cutlets, croquettes, and
    other fried food; for
    thickening steamed and
    other puddings
  Canapes
  Cinnamon toast
  Croutons, as a soup
    accompaniment
  Desserts: bread pudding,
    brown Betty
  French toast
  Hot dishes: cheese fondue,
    scalloped macaroni, soufflé,

    stuffing for meat, poultry, or
    fish
  Melba toast
  Toast points, as garnish
CEREALS:
  Chinese omelet
  Fried or french-fried cornmeal
    mush or hominy grits
  Meatballs with cooked cereal
    as extender
  Rice and tuna
  Rice croquettes
  Rice custard
  Soup with rice, spaghetti,
    or noodles

CAKES AND COOKIES:
  Baked fruit pudding
  Cottage pudding
  Crumbs to coat balls of
    ice cream
  Crumb cookies
  Icebox cake
  Spice crumb cake
EGGS:
  Boiled or poached to add to
    cream sauce, mayonnaise,
    or French dressing, as a
    garnish for vegetables, egg
    cutlets, in salad
  Scrambled for potato salad
    sandwich spread

Table 15-1. *Continued*

Leftover Foods (continued)

EGGS (continued):
  Egg whites, raw, for angel
    food cake, Bavarians, fluffy
    or boiled dressing,
    macaroons, meringue,
    prune whip, white sheet
    or layer cake
  Egg yolks, raw, for cooked
    salad dressing, custard
    sauce, filling, or pudding,
    Duchesse potatoes,
    hollandaise sauce, pancake
    batter, scrambled eggs,
    strawberry Bavarian cream
    pie, yellow angel food cake
FISH:
  Creamed, à la king, or
    scalloped
  Fish cakes or croquettes
  Salad
  Sandwich spread
FRUITS:
  Applesauce cake
  Apricot or berry muffins
  Frozen fruit salad
  Fruit slaw
  Fruit tarts
  Jellied fruit cup or salad
  Jelly or jam
  Mixed fruit salad or fruit cup
  Prune or apricot filling for
    rolls or cookies

Sauce for cottage pudding
MEATS:
  Apple stuffed with sausage
  Bacon in sauce for vegetable
  Baked beef hash
  Boiled lima beans with ham
  Chili con carne
  Chop suey
  Creamed ham or meat
    on toast
  Creamed ham in timbale
    cases
  Creole spaghetti
  Ham or bacon omelet
  Hot tamale pie
  Meat croquettes
  Meat pie or meat roll
  Meat turnovers
  Salad
  Sandwiches
  Scalloped potatoes with ham
  Scrapple
  Stuffed peppers
MILK AND CREAM, SOUR:
  Biscuit brown bread
  Butterscotch cookies
  Fudge cake
  Griddle cakes
  Salad dressing
  Sour cream pie
  Spice coffee cake
  Veal chops in sour cream

POULTRY:
  Chicken and rice casserole
  Chicken timbales
  Creamed chicken in patty
    cases
  Chicken à la king
  Chicken enchiladas
  Croquettes
  Cutlets
  Jellied chicken loaf
  Pot pie
  Salad
  Sandwiches
  Soufflé
  Soup
  Turnovers
VEGETABLES:
  Combinations: carrots and
    peas, corn and beans, corn
    and tomatoes, peas and
    celery
  Fritters
  Potatoes: Duchesse, hashed
    brown, lyonnaise, cakes,
    omelet, salad (hot and cold)
  Salad, in combination
    (when suitable)
  Soup
  Vegetable pie
  Vegetable timbales

Source: Based on S. Fowler, B. West, and G. Shugart. *Food for Fifty*. 5th edition. New York City: John Wiley and Sons, 1971.

Menus for school-age children (including adolescents) need to be adjusted for their nutrition needs and their activity level. Food preferences of this age group, still distinctly different from those of adults, should be carefully considered. A sample pediatric menu for normal diets is shown in figure 15-3.

The second group that may require special attention from the menu planner is older adults whose nutrition needs differ from those of younger adults only in the number of calories required. Fewer calories are needed by older adults because of their decreased physical activity levels and the slowing of their body processes. Frequently, older persons need better nutrition from their meals than they have been receiving, particularly if they live alone or have a physical ailment that limits their food intake or digestion. Lack of motivation to prepare or consume meals on a regular basis may lead to overweight or underweight in this population.

Planning menus for older adults presents many challenges, particularly in long-term care facilities. For one thing, when older persons enter a long-term care facility, the change from a familiar to an unknown environment often produces marked psychological reactions, such as feelings of rejection, insecurity, and despondency. Often new residents express these feelings by complaining about the food, refusing to eat, or insisting on eating only common and familiar foods. For this reason, obtaining a complete profile of the patient's eating habits soon after admission is very important. The resident's family and friends can provide additional information along these lines.

Figure 15-3. Pediatric Menu for Normal Diets

BREAKFAST Please CIRCLE your selections	LUNCH Please CIRCLE your selections	SUPPER Please CIRCLE your selections
Eye Openers	**Savory Beginnings**	**Savory Beginnings**
Orange Juice / Tomato Juice	Vegetable Juice / Cranberry Juice / Soup of the Day	Vegetable Juice / Cranberry Juice / Soup of the Day
Apple Juice / Prune Juice	Apple Juice / Fruit Cup	Apple Juice / Fruit Cup
Cranberry Juice / Banana	Tossed Green Salad / Tangy Cole Slaw / Cottage Cheese	Tossed Green Salad / Tangy Cole Slaw / Cottage Cheese
Fresh Fruit in Season	Potato Salad / Gelatin Salad / Fruit-Flavored Yogurt	Potato Salad / Gelatin Salad / Fruit-Flavored Yogurt
	Lettuce/Tomato Slice	Lettuce/Tomato Slice
Cereals	**Dressings:**	**Dressings:**
Buttered Grits / Raisin Bran	French / Blue Cheese / Thousand Island / Italian	French / Blue Cheese / Thousand Island / Italian
Hot Oatmeal / All Bran	**Main Course Selections (Choose One):**	**Main Course Selections (Choose One):**
Cornflakes / Frosted Flakes	**Hearty Hot Entrees**	**Hearty Hot Entrees**
Rice Krispies / Apple Jacks	*Specialty of the House	*Specialty of the House
Puffed Rice	Roast Beef w/Gravy / Hamburger on Bun	Pizza / Spaghetti w/Meat Sauce
	Fish Sticks w/Ketchup / Vegetarian Manicotti	Baked Ham / Hot Dog on a Bun w/Trimmings
Breakfast Entrees	***Comes with starch and vegetable. Choose salad and dessert.**	***Comes with starch and vegetable. Choose salad and dessert.**
Scrambled Egg / French Toast w/Syrup		
Poached Egg **(OR)** Pancakes w/Syrup	**Deli Delights**	**Deli Delights**
Cheese Omelette	Ham on White Bread / **Meal of a Salad**	Ham on White Bread
Country Sausage Patty	Breast of Turkey Sandwich Platter / Chef's Salad Bowl	Pimento Cheese on Whole Wheat
Crisp Bacon	Peanut Butter and Jelly Sandwich / Tuna Salad Platter	Chicken Salad on Whole Wheat
Grilled Ham Patty	Grilled Cheese Sandwich	Peanut Butter and Jelly Sandwich
	Hot Vegetables of the Day	**Hot Vegetables of the Day**
Breads 'n' Spreads	Whipped Potatoes / Green Beans / Broccoli	Whipped Potatoes / Green Beans / Broccoli
Croissant Roll / Fruit Muffin	Steamed Rice / Whole Baby Carrots / Whole Kernel Corn	Steamed Rice / Whole Baby Carrots / Whole Kernel Corn
Breakfast Roll / Bran Muffin	French-Fried Potatoes	Macaroni and Cheese
Hot Biscuit / Bagel w/Cream Cheese	**Breads 'n' Spreads**	**Breads 'n' Spreads**
Donut / Toasted English Muffin	Hot Roll / Whole Wheat Bread / Crackers	Hot Roll / Whole Wheat Bread / Crackers
Margarine / Jelly / Honey	Cornbread (Mon.-Fri.) / White Bread / Potato Chips	Cornbread (Mon.-Fri.) / White Bread / Potato Chips
	Margarine / Jelly / Honey	Margarine / Jelly / Honey
Beverages	**Sweet Endings**	**Sweet Endings**
Milk / Chocolate Milk	Fruit Pie / Sliced Peaches / Vanilla Ice Cream	Fruit Pie / Sliced Peaches / Vanilla Ice Cream
Low-Fat Milk / Hot Chocolate	Lemon Pie / Flavored Gelatin / Chocolate Ice Cream	Lemon Pie / Flavored Gelatin / Chocolate Ice Cream
Buttermilk	Chocolate Cake / w/Whipped Topping / Sherbet	Chocolate Cake / w/Whipped Topping / Sherbet
	Fresh Fruit in Season / Chocolate Pudding / Chocolate Chip Cookie	Fresh Fruit in Season / Chocolate Pudding / Chocolate Chip Cookie
	Applesauce / Baked Custard (Mon.-Fri.) / Vanilla Wafers	Applesauce / Baked Custard (Mon.-Fri.) / Vanilla Wafers
	Beverages	**Beverages**
	Milk / Chocolate Milk / Iced Tea	Milk / Chocolate Milk / Iced Tea
	Low-Fat Milk / Hot Chocolate / Lemon	Low-Fat Milk / Hot Chocolate / Lemon
	Buttermilk	Buttermilk

The procedures for planning meals for older adults are the same as those followed for planning menus for younger adults on a normal diet, but the quantity and form of foods can be varied to suit the special needs of this group. Note, however, that although the loss of teeth or poor-fitting dentures may make chewing more difficult for some, it should not be assumed that all older adults in this category need very soft or finely ground foods. Offering a variety of food textures and colors in each appetizing meal stimulates interest and appetite. When a selective menu format is feasible, individual preferences can be taken into consideration.

Menu Planning for Modified Diets

After the normal diet menu has been planned, soft and liquid diets and other modified diets can be planned, with substitutions made only as necessary to conform to the prescribed diet as stated in the operation's diet manual. One advantage of this approach is that it keeps the number of modified diet foods at a minimum, thus eliminating the need to prepare many small batches of such foods and reducing labor costs.

Because variety is an important element of satisfying and appealing food service, the menu planner should double-check at the end of the planning process to make sure that repetition has been kept to a minimum. Even liquid diets can be enhanced by offering a variety of flavored seltzer waters, herbal teas, and frozen yogurts. The menu repeat form in figure 15-4 is a useful tool that helps control repetition. The form can identify individual items that appear on the menu too frequently. When this is disclosed, a similar food can be substituted to add variety to the planned menu. For example, mashed potatoes might be replaced with diced potatoes or au gratin potatoes. Or, pudding, canned fruit, or ice cream might be offered in place of gelatin on certain menus.

Figure 15-4. Menu Repeat Form

	Monday B L D	Tuesday B L D	Wednesday B L D	Thursday B L D	Friday B L D	Saturday B L D	Sunday B L D
MENU REPEAT FORM							
DIRECTIONS: List each food item from the menu only once and then check off the meals and days on which each item appears. (B, breakfast; L, lunch; D, dinner.)							
Item Served							
Scrambled eggs	X	X		X	X	X	
Mashed potatoes	X	X		X			X
Carrots	X						X
Gelatin	X	X		X X			X

Source: Adapted from R. P. Puckett, *Dietary Manager's Independent Study Course,* Department of Independent Study by Correspondence, University of Florida, Gainesville, 1985.

Menu Planning for Special Services

Offering options in food service is one way to increase patient satisfaction and improve how the surrounding community views the hospital. Some patients are even willing to pay extra for special services. To satisfy these demands, a number of health care institutions have implemented room service and gourmet meal programs.

A health care room service menu is much like a hotel room service menu in that menus are made available in patients' rooms, and patients or their visitors may call the food service department directly to request service. The order is taken and the price of service is verified over the telephone. After the department checks the patient's diet prescription to verify that the selection is allowable, the order is given to the appropriate production employee for preparation. The food is then delivered to the patient's room by a food service employee who collects cash or credit card payment for the service.

Gourmet meal programs, implemented by some health care food service operations, may include wine with meals, an on-demand meal schedule, and tasty meals presented with flair. Gourmet meal tickets usually are sold in the gift shop and are purchased by friends or family members for patients who are well enough to enjoy the meals. A typical gourmet menu is shown in figure 15-5.

Because gourmet meal service can be costly to start up and maintain, before it is offered the food service director and the institution's administrators must weigh realistically the investment expenses against potential benefits for the institution. Start-up and operating expenses may include the following features:

- Special linens and serving tables
- Fresh flowers for the table setting
- Wine service (possibly a wine steward)
- Design and printing of special menus
- Special food items (such as expensive meat cuts and fresh or out-of-season produce)
- Additional labor for food preparation and individualized service
- A special marketing program for the service

Figure 15-5. Sample Gourmet Dinner Menu

Please circle your selection.

Dinner

Fresh fruit cocktail with honey yogurt dressing	or	Shrimp cocktail
Soup du jour	or	French onion soup
Prime rib of beef au jus	or	Baked stuffed lobster
Hearts of iceberg lettuce and	or	Sliced tomatoes vinaigrette and
Potatoes in butter sauce	or	Rice pilaf
Asparagus spears with hollandaise sauce	or	Vegetable du jour
Fresh-baked rolls with butter	or	Margarine
Marble cheesecake	or	Praline sundae

Coffee *or* Herbal tea *or* Seltzer water

Complimentary Beaujolais

A word of caution: Despite the tight constraints of today's health care environment, some institutions have initiated gourmet meal service programs only to discover, unfortunately, that they are expensive and little used by their patient population. Preliminary market surveys that look closely at patient demographics (especially lifestyle and income levels) will indicate the level of interest in, and affordability of, gourmet meal service. In addition, an informal survey of other health care operations that offer the service would be very informative.

Once gourmet meal service has been instituted, it must be adequately marketed to potential customers. Information about the program should be included in the patients' information directory or notices placed in patients' rooms and in the gift shop. When possible, advertisements in local newspapers and other media can be used.

Nonpatient Menus

In addition to patients, or the primary target market, most health care food service operations provide services to other customer groups. These generally include employees, staff, and visitors. As described earlier, the wants and needs of these groups as identified by the marketing information system should be considered during menu planning.

Employees, Staff, and Visitors

The menu planner should pay special attention to the facility's cafeteria menus that serve employees, staff, and visitors. A well-managed cafeteria can be a showcase for the high-quality food served as well as a profitable operation. When most of the cafeteria items come from the general patient menu, it is recommended that additional items be provided, especially if the menu offered to patients is nonselective. Even when selective menus are the basis of the general patient menu, a cafeteria menu that includes more variety can attract additional customers.

Cafeteria menus should keep customers coming back by offering a variety of foods. Theme or special-event days have been successful in attracting customers, but they usually can be scheduled for only one day each month. To help make customers happy, special health-promoting menus can be offered that include calorie and nutrition information and recipes for favorite items. Other techniques for increasing cafeteria revenues include offering special foods during slow periods, providing takeout services, and selling holiday desserts. Menus that offer a variety of cold and hot sandwiches, salads, main-dish salads, and salad plates also are popular. Variety is needed to keep the operation's employees interested, particularly if the menu is on a relatively short cycle. One or more daily specials can be offered, and some of the items on the general patient menu can be combined for a single-price meal. Consideration should be given to the price mix of cafeteria menu items to ensure affordable alternatives to customers as well as a range of appeal.

Cycle menus can be used in cafeterias as well as for patient service. However, the cycle should be several weeks long when employees use the cafeteria for meals. The many advantages of cycle menus (discussed earlier in this chapter) prevail, with the added advantage of balancing appeal and selling price considerations for the cafeteria.

In acute care hospitals and other short-term care facilities that have relatively large numbers of visitors and outpatients, it may be advantageous to make food available in the cafeteria, in the coffee shop, and from vending machines for most of the day. When there is no coffee shop in the facility, several cold items (sandwiches, rolls, doughnuts, juices, ice-cream products, desserts, and beverages) easily could be provided in a designated area of the cafeteria. Providing microwave ovens that can be operated by customers or employees would allow customers to reheat prepared foods during hours of limited cafeteria service.

Community Residents

Some health care food service operations have implemented services for outside customer groups such as community residents. Depending on the location of the operation and its food service facilities, workers from nearby medical clinics and businesses may be attracted by the facilities' realistic prices and quick service. Serving Sunday brunches, providing delivery service for office parties, and giving weekend and evening discounts to senior citizens are other ways to market the department's services.

Some directors are increasing department revenues by adding off-premises catering services to their business mix. However, this may require nonprofit hospitals to establish a for-profit catering venture. Because of the implications for the hospital's tax status and/or effect on the operation's public image, hospital administration must decide whether to compete with the commercial food service sector by providing nonhospital-related catering services. If off-premises catering is implemented, the food service director may want to expand in-house menus to appeal to a wider variety of catering customers and to develop a reputation for full service.

☐ Menu Format

Because the menu is an important marketing tool, its format must be designed to ensure effective communication. Therefore, the menu planner writes the final menus out in two different formats, one for purchasing, production, and service personnel and the other for patients and other customer groups. The menu used in the kitchen usually provides the names and numbers of the recipes to be followed and the production forecast. Information on portion sizes, special comments about the recipes, and advance preparation requirements can be added. The names of each menu item should be very specific. For example, the kind of fruit juice, the flavor of gelatin, the type of bread item, and so forth should be stated if not already specified in the recipe. This information ensures that the intended balance of flavors, colors, and textures will be produced.

Patient Menus

Selective menus distributed to patients should be informative, accurate, attractive, and easy to understand. Terminology used should be clear, simple, and comprehensible to readers who may be seriously ill or sedated or who may not be fluent in English. Nutrition education information, which can also be included with patient menus, might include general dietary guidelines distributed with all regular menus. Informative notes on modified diet menus could include explanations of the special dietary needs of diabetics and patients with high cholesterol levels. Menus also could contain entertainment features such as crossword puzzles, nutrition trivia questions, or coloring pages for children.

Specially designed forms can be used to make menus more appealing. Forms should be consistent in format and give clear directions for marking choices. The components of the meal should be listed in the expected order of consumption (for example, appetizer, soup, salad, entree, dessert, beverage). Descriptive terms should be accurate; that is, *steamed* vegetables should not be overcooked or pureed. "Truth in menus" is as important as the accurate labeling on commercial food products.

Although foods should be described in appetizing terms, they must be able to live up to the adjectives. *Crisp* salads should be crisp, *hot* rolls should be hot, and *homemade* breads should truly have been baked on the premises. Foods given fanciful names may not be familiar to many patients, who may hesitate to select such items. When colorful names (such as "eye-openers," "savory beginnings," or "sweet endings") are used on the menu, brief descriptions of the items should be included or, alternatively, the choices included in such a category should be clear-cut. An example of a restaurant-style menu used in a hospital is reproduced in figure 15-6.

Figure 15-6. Restaurant-Style Health Care Menu for Normal Diets

BREAKFAST
Please CIRCLE your selections

Eye Openers
Orange Juice — Tomato Juice
Apple Juice — Prune Juice
Cranberry Juice — Banana
Fresh Fruit in Season

Cereals
Buttered Grits — Shredded Wheat
Hot Oatmeal — Puffed Rice
Cornflakes — Raisin Bran
Rice Krispies — All Bran

Breakfast Entrees
Scrambled Egg — French Toast w/Syrup
Poached Egg (OR) Pancakes w/Syrup
Cheese Omelette
Country Sausage Patty
Crisp Bacon
Grilled Ham Patty

Breads 'n' Spreads
Croissant Roll — Fruit Muffin
Breakfast Roll — Bran Muffin
Hot Biscuit — Bagel w/Cream Cheese
Donut — Toasted English Muffin
Margarine — Jelly — Honey

Beverages
Coffee — Milk
Caffeine-Free Coffee — Low-Fat Milk
Hot Tea — Buttermilk
Herb Tea — Chocolate Milk
Hot Chocolate
Lemon
Nondairy Creamer
Artificial Sweetener

LUNCH
Please CIRCLE your selections

Savory Beginnings
Vegetable Juice — Cranberry Juice — Soup of the Day
Apple Juice — Fruit Cup
Tossed Green Salad — Tangy Cole Slaw — Cottage Cheese
Potato Salad — Gelatin Salad — Fruit-Flavored Yogurt
Lettuce/Tomato/Onion Slice

Dressings:
French — Blue Cheese — Thousand Island — Italian

Main Course Selections (Choose One):
Hearty Hot Entrees
Mushroom Burger w/Swiss Cheese
*Specialty of the House
Vegetarian Manicotti
Roast Beef w/Gravy
Baked Fish w/Lemon

*Comes with starch and vegetable. Choose salad and dessert.

Deli Delights — **Meal of a Salad**
Ham on Rye Sandwich — Chef's Salad Bowl
Breast of Turkey Sandwich Platter — Tuna Salad Platter
Grilled Cheese Sandwich — Cottage Cheese and Fruit

Hot Vegetables of the Day
Whipped Potatoes — Green Beans — Broccoli
Steamed Rice — Whole Baby Carrots — Whole Kernel Corn

Breads 'n' Spreads
Hot Roll — Whole Wheat Bread — Melba Toast
Cornbread (Mon.-Fri.) — White Bread — Crackers
Margarine — Jelly — Honey

Sweet Endings
Fruit Pie — Sliced Peaches — Vanilla Ice Cream
Lemon Pie — Flavored Gelatin — Chocolate Ice Cream
Cheesecake — w/Whipped Topping — Sherbet
Chocolate Cake — Chocolate Pudding — Chocolate Chip Cookie
Fresh Fruit in — Baked Custard
Season — (Mon.-Fri.)

Beverages
Coffee — Milk — Lemon
Caffeine-Free Coffee — Low-Fat Milk — Nondairy Creamer
Hot Tea — Buttermilk — Artificial Sweetener
Herb Tea — Chocolate Milk
Iced Tea — Hot Chocolate

SUPPER
Please CIRCLE your selections

Savory Beginnings
Vegetable Juice — Cranberry Juice — Soup of the Day
Apple Juice — Fruit Cup
Tossed Green Salad — Tangy Cole Slaw — Cottage Cheese
Potato Salad — Gelatin Salad — Fruit-Flavored Yogurt

Dressings:
French — Blue Cheese — Thousand Island — Italian

Main Course Selections (Choose One):
Hearty Hot Entrees
Spaghetti w/Meat Sauce
*Specialty of the House
Hot Dog on a Bun w/Trimmings
Roast Beef w/Gravy
Baked Ham

*Comes with starch and vegetable. Choose salad and dessert.

Deli Delights
Ham on Rye Sandwich
Pimento Cheese on Whole Wheat
Chicken Salad Sandwich

Hot Vegetables of the Day
Green Beans — Broccoli
Whole Baby Carrots — Whole Kernel Corn
Whipped Potatoes
Steamed Rice
Macaroni and Cheese

Breads 'n' Spreads
Hot Roll — Whole Wheat Bread — Melba Toast
Cornbread (Mon.-Fri.) — White Bread — Crackers
Margarine — Jelly — Honey

Sweet Endings
Fruit Pie — Sliced Peaches — Vanilla Ice Cream
Lemon Pie — Flavored Gelatin — Chocolate Ice Cream
Cheesecake — w/Whipped Topping — Sherbet
Chocolate Cake — Chocolate Pudding — Chocolate Chip Cookie
Fresh Fruit in — Baked Custard
Season — (Mon.-Fri.)

Beverages
Coffee — Milk — Lemon
Caffeine-Free Coffee — Low-Fat Milk — Nondairy Creamer
Hot Tea — Buttermilk — Artificial Sweetener
Herb Tea — Chocolate Milk
Iced Tea — Hot Chocolate

Nonpatient Menus

If food service is provided to nonpatient customers, appropriate menu formats must be developed to provide adequate communication between the operation and these customers. An appropriate format for the cafeteria would be a menu board. Lettering used on a menu board should be legible and large enough for ease of viewing by customers with differing visual acuity. The board also should be designed to allow changes to be made easily.

In more upscale operations where table service is provided, a printed menu should be developed. The principles of design for printed menus are described in *Marketing by Menu* by Nancy L. Scanlon and *Menu Pricing & Strategy* by Jack E. Miller. Design features include the menu cover, visual format and layout, copy (text), and graphics (pictures). Menu production features deal with typeface style, paper, ink color, and color of graphics. Menu design should reflect current cultural trends, which may mean that customers favor designs that are simple and light (not too crowded or "busy"). In-house desktop publishing can produce menus appropriate for many occasions. However, because of its importance as a marketing tool and the cost of producing this type of menu, the food service director might consider contracting for the services of a menu design consultant.

☐ Pricing Strategies

Pricing the services provided by a food service operation is an extremely important task. The process starts with the cost of producing individual menu items and eventually affects whether the operation achieves its profitability objectives while maintaining quality and cost-effectiveness of service.

Pricing Considerations

To determine what to charge for specific menu items, a number of factors must be considered. Key among these are:

- Customer mix as described by the marketing information system
- Product mix including the type of menu item, the style of service, and the meal occasion or time of dining
- Psychological effects of pricing such as perceived value, price spread between items, and "odd-cents" pricing
- Past prices that customers may have paid for the same menu items
- Competitors and their prices for similar products
- Profit objective as specified in the department marketing plan

Pricing Methods

In his book *Menu Pricing & Strategy,* Jack Miller describes seven menu pricing methods: nonstructured, gross profit, base price, factor, prime cost, actual cost, and forced food cost. Each method has its advantages and disadvantages. Generally, those methods that account for more variables, such as different categories of costs, also require more precise information.

The *nonstructured method* is based on the menu prices established by someone else's food service operation. It does not account for operational differences that exist between any two facilities. The *gross profit method* is designed to determine a specific amount of money that should be made from each customer. The *base price method* prices menu items at a certain level to satisfy the market and then works backward to determine the amount to spend on raw ingredients.

The remaining four methods focus on the costs to produce specific menu items. In the *factor method,* the targeted food cost percentage of the operation is divided into 100 to determine a factor; thus, for a food cost percentage of 35 percent, the factor would be 2.86 (rounded). The menu price is then determined by multiplying the raw food cost by the factor:

$$\text{Raw Food Cost} \times \text{Factor} = \text{Menu Price}$$

In this example, if the raw food cost for a menu item were $1.03, the menu price would be calculated based on the following formula:

$$\$1.03 \times 2.86 = \$2.95$$

The remaining cost-based methods work in a similar fashion but take into consideration other areas of costs such as labor, variable costs, fixed costs, and profit. Although this is an advantage over the factor method, extensive cost records must be maintained and computer-generated data may be necessary to support these systems.

☐ Menu Evaluation

Because of its impact on the food service operation's success, an effective menu evaluation system must be established to provide mechanisms to measure menu performance prior to implementation, with a focus on specific menu features. After implementation, menu performance must be evaluated for customer acceptability and contribution to the financial status of the department. These processes are described below.

Menu Features

Once the menu-planning process is finished, the proposed menus should be evaluated by dietitians to see whether all nutrition objectives have been attained, by food service department managers to determine whether the department's resources have been used effectively, and by customer focus groups to disclose whether the menus will be appealing to customers. The following list, which describes the characteristics of a good menu, can easily be used as an evaluation checklist:

- *Menu pattern:* Each meal is consistent with the established menu pattern (that is, three-, four-, or five-meal plan) and includes all food components and portion sizes specified as necessary to meet the customers' nutrition requirements and, at the same time, minimize plate waste.
- *Color and eye appeal:* The color combinations in each meal are pleasant and blend well, and a variety of colors is used in each meal. Attractive garnishes are included when appropriate.
- *Texture and consistency:* A mix of soft, creamy, crisp, chewy, and firm foods is included in each meal.
- *Flavor combinations:* Food flavors are compatible yet varied. Having two or more strong-flavored foods (such as broccoli, onions, turnips, cabbage, and cauliflower) in the same meal has been avoided. Combinations of foods with similar flavors (such as tomato juice with macaroni–tomato casserole and macaroni and cheese with pineapple–cheese salad) also are avoided.
- *Sizes and shapes:* Meals include a pleasing variety of food sizes and shapes. Having several chopped or mixed items in the same meal (such as cubed meat, diced potatoes, mixed vegetables, and fruit cocktail) has been avoided.
- *Food temperatures:* A balance between hot and cold items is offered for each meal. The climate and/or season of the year also is a consideration in selecting food temperatures. For example, cold vegetable soups are appropriate to summer, whereas hot bean soups are more suited to cold weather.
- *Preparation methods:* Offering more than one food prepared in a particular manner in a meal has been avoided. A balanced distribution of creamed, boiled, fried, baked, and braised foods is offered each day.
- *Popularity:* Popular and less-popular foods are part of the same meal when a selection is offered. Serving all popular foods at one meal and all less-popular foods at another has been avoided.

- *Day-to-day distribution:* The types of food offered for consecutive meals and on consecutive days are varied in ingredients as well as in preparation method. For example, the menus avoid offering meat loaf at lunch and another ground beef entree for dinner or supper. Variations in the foods offered the same day each week are planned. Serving hot dogs every Monday and chicken every Sunday, for example, has been avoided.
- *Customer preferences:* The menus are appropriate for the cultural, ethnic, and personal food preferences of the operation's customers. The menu planner's own food prejudices are not taken into consideration.
- *Availability and cost of food:* Seasonal foods are used frequently. High- and low-cost foods are balanced within each day's menus and throughout the menu cycle so that budget constraints and customer pricing demands are met.
- *Facilities and equipment:* The equipment available is adequate to produce high-quality menu items. Equipment use is balanced throughout the day and the menu cycle. Menu items are compatible with the capacities of transport and service equipment. Enough serving dishes of appropriate sizes and types are available for the attractive presentation of menu items.
- *Personnel and time:* The department's staff is adequate for the preparation and service of items on the menu in terms of the number of workers and their skill levels. The department's work load is balanced from day to day and week to week. Adequate time is available for producing and serving the foods on the menu.
- *Menu form and presentation:* Descriptions of the menu items are specific, appealing, and accurate. The menu follows a consistent and accepted sequence of consumption.

After correcting any problems noted during the preimplementation evaluation, the menu planner should recheck the menus one final time. This procedure should be followed every time menus are planned, but less time is required when cycle menus are used. Whenever a menu is actually produced, any problems encountered should be noted on the master menu form and the appropriate changes made before repeating the menu in another cycle.

Menu Performance

Regardless of how perfect a menu may appear to be, all menu planners must face the periodic elimination and replacement of menu items. Therefore, methods to evaluate menu effectiveness must be employed, ranging from simply counting the number of items selected or sold, to computerized monitoring of consumption practices. Both customer acceptability and menu engineering (using popularity and profitability of menu items as bases for making changes) are key evaluation measures.

Acceptability by Customers

Surveys help determine customer acceptance of various menu items. The form in figure 15-7 asks for customer comments on specific new menu items. Figure 15-8 (p. 386) shows a multipurpose survey asking for suggestions and comments from cafeteria customers on various services and food items. Keeping precise sales histories on menu items helps in demand forecasting and in eliminating unpopular items from the menu. Observing plate waste is another good way to assess the customer acceptance of various menu items. Minimum standards of acceptability based on customer input must be established by the management of the food service department. If the acceptability of a menu item falls below the standard, a change must be considered.

Menu Engineering

Menu engineering is a method used to evaluate the effectiveness of an operation's current menu while providing the basis for future menu-planning decisions. Various theories of menu engineering have been proposed, one of which is to be found in an article by Mohamed Bayou

Figure 15-7. Survey Form for a New Menu Item

CUSTOMER SURVEY

We need your assistance in helping us to meet our goal of serving you high-quality food that tastes good. Please share your comments with us about this new menu item by filling out this questionnaire and dropping it in the suggestion box located in the cafeteria.

1. Menu item _____

2. Menu item served at proper temperature?   Yes _____ No _____

3. Menu item cooked properly?   Yes _____ No _____

4. Did you like the taste of new menu item?

    Enjoyed _____

    Acceptable _____

    Disliked _____

5. Is there anything you can recommend to improve this menu item?

    _____

    _____

---

and Lee Bennett in *The Cornell H.R.A. Quarterly,* giving an excellent review of five menu-engineering methods. The methods described in their article categorize menu items based on both profitability and popularity. One of the methods, developed by Kasavana and Smith, establishes four categories based on contribution margin and volume. The category in which a menu item is placed determines whether the item will be retained, repositioned, or eliminated. These techniques generally require computer support.

☐ Computer Applications

Computer-assisted procedures are used for menu planning in some facilities. To take advantage of the computer's speed, accuracy, and capacity, menu-planning information must be expressed in quantitative terms. Programs can be designed to plan menus that consider labor and raw food costs, nutrient content, color, consistency, frequency, and other factors. However, two variables—nutrient content and raw food cost—are the most widely used in current computer-assisted menu-planning programs.

The greatest obstacle to computer-assisted menu planning has been the absence of sufficient data about each variable. Unless the food service department uses standardized recipes for every item produced, there is little point in planning menus that accurately fulfill nutrient requirements and meet cost limitations. The ingredients used in each recipe must be issued through a controlled procedure, and production workers must follow recipes exactly.

Food composition data must be available for each food item. However, values for some items on the market either are not available or differ from those stated in government handbooks. Nutrient data for many products must be obtained from their manufacturers. In some cases, the data must be developed by the food service director.

Figure 15-8. Survey of Suggestions and Comments from Customers

---

CUSTOMER SURVEY

Several changes are occurring within the Department of Food and Nutrition Services to better meet the needs of our customers. We have changed our menu, and we are providing additional services such as Healthful Food for Life. These changes are for you! Therefore, we want your ideas and opinions on how the new menu and additional services can best meet your needs. Please share your comments and suggestions with us so that we can meet our primary goal–pleasing you!

1. Age _____ Sex _____

   Years employed at hospital _____

2. Have you read any of the "Good News" handouts?

   Yes _____ No _____

   If so, did you find them interesting and informative?

   Yes _____ No _____

   Would you like us to provide them on a regular basis?

   Yes _____ No _____

3. Have you tried the Healthful Foods for Life menu?

   Yes _____ No _____

4. Did you find the Healthful Foods for Life menu worthwhile?

   Yes _____ No _____

5. Which one of the following types of foods do you prefer?

   Mexican _____   Seafood _____

   Italian _____   Vegetarian _____

   Southern _____   Other _____

6. Do you find that the new menu meets your food preferences?

   Yes _____ No _____

7. Please share any additional comments or recommendations.

   _____

   _____

   _____

8. If you would like to be interviewed, please leave your name and phone number during the day. We will contact you to arrange an appointment.

   Name _____ Telephone _____

The menu planner must specify such variables as the frequency with which menu items may be served and the food combinations allowed on one menu. This process involves coding for ingredients, color, flavor, shape, and other factors in such a way that the computer can identify these considerations and deal with them. Menu cost is a combination of raw food cost and labor cost. Yet, because accurate production time data are not available for most food items and are difficult to obtain, precise labor cost planning may be impossible. Flexibility in adjusting to the special needs of customers or incorporating new items is severely limited as well. These are a few of the problems involved in computer-assisted menu planning that have led many operations to continue using manual procedures. Applications in which the computer is utilized to support the menu-planning process, such as with menu engineering, have experienced more success.

☐ Summary

In many respects, successful operation of the food service department depends on the effectiveness and appropriateness of the department's menus, which can affect perceptions of the facility's overall quality of care. In today's competitive environment, the revenue brought in by various food service department ventures can make a valuable contribution to the hospital's profits—or losses. Menu planning involves designing meals that meet the nutrition needs of a variety of customer groups, both patient and nonpatient. At the same time, menus must fulfill the customers' appetite for good-tasting and attractive food.

☐ Bibliography

Axler, B. H. *Foodservice: A Managerial Approach.* Lexington, MA: D. C. Heath, 1979.

Bayou, M. E., and Bennett, L. B. Profitability analysis for table-service restaurants. *Cornell Hotel and Restaurant Administration Quarterly* 33(2):49–55, Apr. 1992.

Carmen, J., and Norkus, G. Pricing strategies for menus: magic or myth? *Cornell Hotel and Restaurant Administration Quarterly* 31(3):44–50, Nov. 1990.

Eckstein, E. F. *Menu Planning.* 2nd ed. Westport, CT: AVI, 1978.

Foltz, M. B., and Stephens, G. Marketing food and nutrition services. *Hospital Administration Currents* 29(2), 1985.

Food Guide Pyramid. Washington, DC: U.S. Department of Agriculture, Human Nutrition Information Service, Home and Garden Bulletin no. 249, 1992.

Gisslen, W. *Professional Cooking.* 2nd ed. New York City: John Wiley and Sons, 1989.

Hoover, L. W., Waller, A. L., Rastkan, A., and Johnson, V. A. Development of on-line real-time menu management system. *Journal of The American Dietetic Association* 80(2):46, Jan. 1982.

Kochilas, D. Making a menu. *Restaurant Business* 90(17):92–102, Nov. 1991.

Konz, S. *Work Design: Industrial Ergonomics.* 2nd ed. Columbus, OH: Grid, 1983.

Kotschevar, L. H. *Management by Menu.* Chicago: National Institute of the Foodservice Industry, 1975.

McCarthy, B., and Straus, K. Tastes of America 1992. *Restaurants & Institutions* 102(29):24–44, Dec. 1992.

Menu planning to control costs. *Hospital Food & Nutrition Focus* 7(4):1–3, Dec. 1990.

Miller, J. E. *Menu Pricing & Strategy.* 3rd ed. New York City: Van Nostrand Reinhold, 1992.

Nutrition and Your Health: Dietary Guidelines for Americans. 3rd ed. Washington, DC: U.S. Departments of Agriculture and Health and Human Services, Home and Garden Bulletin no. 232, 1990.

Peterson, L. C. Top of the morning. *Food Management* 27(5):168–80, May 1992.

Puckett, R. P. *Dietary Manager's Independent Study Course.* Gainesville, FL: Department of Independent Study by Correspondence, University of Florida, 1985.

Quinton, B. Menus & markets. *Restaurants & Institutions* 101(8):12–32, Mar. 1991.

Reid, R. D. *Hospitality Marketing Management.* 2nd ed. New York City: Van Nostrand Reinhold, 1989.

Sanson, M. Live long & prosper. *Restaurant Hospitality* 70(2):112–26, Feb. 1990.

Scanlon, N. L. *Marketing by Menu.* 2nd ed. New York City: Van Nostrand Reinhold, 1990.

Sherer, M. Responding to the age of maturity. *Food Management* 27(12):88–100, Dec. 1992.

Shugart, G. S., Molz, M., and Wilson, M. *Food for Fifty.* 9th ed. New York City: John Wiley and Sons, 1992.

Solomon, J. A guide to good menu writing. *Restaurants USA* 12(5):27–30, May 1992.

Spears, M. C. *Foodservice Organizations: A Managerial and Systems Approach.* 2nd ed. New York City: Macmillan Publishing Company, 1991.

Stephenson, S. Hospital catering: for profit or not for profit? *Restaurants & Institutions* 101(27)83–88, Oct. 1991.

Stokes, J. W. Planning the menu, in *How to Manage a Restaurant.* Chapter 4. Dubuque, IA: William C. Brown, 1982.

Townsend, R. Young diners. *Restaurants & Institutions* 101(24):22–42, Sept. 1991.

West, B. B., and Wood, L. In: V. F. Harger, G. S. Shugart, and J. Payne-Palacio, editors. *Foodservice in Institutions.* 6th ed. New York City: Macmillan Publishing Company, 1988.

Woodard-Polster, T. Taking your menu on the road. *Restaurants USA* 11(1):29–31, Jan. 1991.

Chapter 16

Product Selection

☐ Introduction

Product selection (food, serviceware, and preparation equipment) is a critical factor in meeting customer expectations, adhering to nutrition guidelines, and containing expenses for a health care food service operation. The purchasing agent for the department must be knowledgeable about food and ingredients, menu patterns, and production and service systems before he or she can select food supplies with any degree of accuracy and cost-effectiveness.

This chapter will present basic information on all the food groups (meats and seafood, eggs and egg products, milk and other dairy products, fruits and vegetables, grains and cereals, and beverages). Specifically, topics on meat inspection, meat grades, meat specifications, and processed meats will be presented. The same will be done for most of the other food groups, so that a purchaser can make informed and economic choices that will complement rather than hamper operation controls.

Food substitutes and equivalents will be addressed, as will national and local regulations regarding interstate and intrastate purchasing decisions. Food nutrients, federal standards of quality, and methods of food processing also will be described. For example, the fat content of dairy products, moisture content of dehydrated foods, and hydrogenation features of various oils will be examined.

Finally, the chapter will discuss considerations pertinent to purchasing equipment (utensils, serviceware, dinnerware, hollowware, for example). Upon completing this chapter, food service directors and purchasing agents will be able to communicate freely and collaborate on purchasing decisions that will facilitate departmental and organizational goals, profitability, and service delivery.

☐ Meat and Meat Products

Meat is the most costly component of the daily menu, but it also is one of the most important sources of protein in the diet and must be selected carefully for use in the food service department. Both wholesomeness and quality of meat products must be considered, keeping in mind that various cuts are marketed in different quality grades. The cut and grade of meat selection should be based on the meat's intended use. Purchasers must be familiar with meat inspection parameters, grades of meat, market forms of meat, meat specifications, and processed meats.

Meat Inspection

Meat products sold in interstate commerce must be inspected for wholesomeness and stamped for approval. Figure 16-1 illustrates the federal stamp that is affixed to the carcass of meat, on the label of processed meat, or on the meat product if the product has met specific standards. Each label designates that the product has been examined for disease and that any unwholesome part has been removed and destroyed; that the meat has been handled and prepared in a sanitary manner in a processing plant that meets federal sanitation standards; and that no harmful substances have been added to the meat. The combined letter and numeric designation in certain inspection stamps identifies the plant at which the meat was processed and inspected. (See figure 16-1.)

Products purchased from processing plants within a certain state must meet minimum state sanitation criteria. The criteria and inspection program vary significantly from state to state and may not always be reliable. With the increased concern regarding the safety of meat, the purchasing agent should carefully consider the risk and liability implications of purchasing meat that has not met federal standards. For purchases made locally, it is advisable to tour the plant and obtain a copy of the standards.

The stamp or seal *kosher* ("fit to eat") refers to the ritualistic manner in which meat was slaughtered and butchered by a *sochet* (a religious slaughterer) according to Orthodox Jewish dietary law. The symbol does not guarantee the wholesomeness or quality of the meat, but indicates approval by the Union of Orthodox Jewish Congregations that the meat has met the standards of kosher and *kashrut* ("*kosher*-ness").

Meat Grades

The U.S. Department of Agriculture (USDA) has an established voluntary system for grading the quality of products. There are two types of grade: yield grade and quality grade. All operations utilize quality grade when selecting meat because it is a measure of the palatability, that is, the eating quality of the product. Operations that purchase wholesale or primal cuts will need to know the desired quality and yield grades. Quality grades are based on the following criteria:

- Shape or conformation of the carcass
- Class (kinds) of animal
- Sex of animal
- Amount of exterior fat (finish)
- Amount of intermuscular fat (marbling)
- Firmness of lean and fat

The yield or cutability grade indicates the amount of lean that can be obtained from the carcass. Whether to continue yield grading is currently being debated.

Each general type of meat (described in the following subsections), as well as poultry and eggs, is graded according to a specific set of requirements. After the grading process, the external surface of the meat carcass is marked with a shield indicating the federal grade (figure 16-1). Because grading is not required by law, the food buyer must specify on the purchase order the USDA grade of meat desired when graded meat is to be purchased.

Beef

Beef is graded for quality according to seven USDA grades: Prime, Choice, Select, Commercial, Utility, Cutter, and Canner. Beef also is graded according to a system of yield grades, which are guides to the amount or cutability of usable meat in a carcass. High-cutability carcasses combine a minimum of fat covering with very thick muscling and yield a high proportion of lean meat. The USDA yield grades are numbered 1 to 5, with 1 having the highest cutability. All beef that is quality graded is also yield graded.

Figure 16-1. Grade Stamps and Inspection Marks Used for Meat, Poultry, Eggs, and Seafood

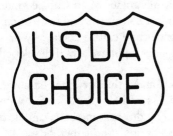

Federal Grade Stamp for Meat

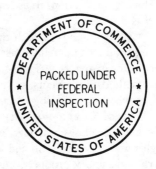

Federal Inspection Stamp for Seafood

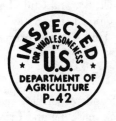

USDA Poultry Inspection Mark

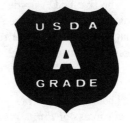

USDA Poultry Grade Mark

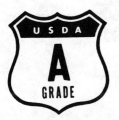

USDA Shell Egg Grade Mark

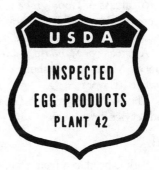

USDA Egg Products Inspection Mark

Prime grade is the most tender, juicy, and flavorful beef available on the market because of its abundant marbling and thick external fat cover. However, the external fat cover and marbling give Prime beef a high fat content, which is unacceptable in many health care institutions. In addition, the price per pound for all USDA Prime cuts usually is too high for most health care institutions to use except for special occasions, and the supply of this high-quality beef is limited.

Choice grade is of high quality but has less fat than Prime grade. More Choice-grade beef is produced than any other grade, and it is preferred by most consumers and institutions because of its tenderness and flavor. Rib and loin cuts are tender and can be cooked by dry-heat methods. Other cuts, such as round or chuck, also are tender and have a well-developed flavor when prepared by moist-heat methods.

Cuts of *Select grade* have less marbling within the muscle and a thinner outer fat cover. The meat is relatively tender, but it lacks much of the juiciness and flavor associated with higher grades of beef. Rib and loin roasts and steaks prepared by dry-heat methods can yield fairly satisfactory products, but other cuts are best prepared by moist-heat methods.

Commercial grade is produced from mature animals and lacks the tenderness of the higher grades. Institutions find it economical to use this grade for ground beef and stew meat, which becomes tender and full-flavored when cooked slowly with moist heat.

The three other USDA grades for beef—*Utility, Cutter,* and *Canner*—usually are not sold as fresh beef. Instead, they are used in processed meat products.

Lamb

The five USDA grades for lamb are Prime, Choice, Good, Utility, and Cull. The standards for these grades are similar to those for beef. *Choice* or *Good* is the grade selection usually specified for institutional use. *Utility-* and *Cull-grade* lamb is used primarily in processed meat products.

Veal

The six USDA grades for veal are Prime, Choice, Good, Standard, Utility, and Cull. A veal carcass of *Prime grade* is superior in quality and has thick muscling and firm, fine-textured flesh. The cut surface of the flesh looks and feels velvety. The bones are small in relation to the size and weight of the carcass.

The carcass of *Choice grade* is moderately blocky and compact, with fairly thick fleshing. The flesh is firm and fine-textured and may look and feel moist. The bones are moderately small in proportion to the size and weight of the carcass.

A carcass of *Good grade* is blocky and compact, with thin fleshing and no evidence of plumpness. The flesh is moderately soft and on a cut surface looks and feels moist. The bones are large in proportion to the size of the carcass.

A carcass of *Standard grade* is not thickly fleshed and has a higher proportion of bone to meat. Moist-heat methods of cooking are needed to produce a juicy meat with a well-developed flavor.

The two other grades of veal are *Utility* and *Cull*. They are rarely used in institutional food service operations.

Pork

Pork is produced from young animals and is less variable in quality than beef. The USDA rates pork according to two quality levels: acceptable and unacceptable. The USDA grades for pork are numbered from 1 to 4 for animals of acceptable quality. Grade differences are related to the ratio of lean to fat and the yield of the loin, the ham, the picnic, and the Boston Butt. Pork that is not acceptable for use as fresh meat and pork that is watery and soft is graded *Utility*. The yield grades for pork are similar to those for beef, but the grades for pork reflect the differences in carcass yield for the four major cuts rather than the differences in eating quality. Most pork marketed today is grade 1 or 2. If a food service operation purchases carcass or packer-style (split-carcass) hogs, the following guidelines should be used to assess quality:

- *Cuts:* Muscles should not have more than a moderate amount of interior fat.
- *Bones:* Bones should be porous with cartilage present. Avoid brittle or flinty bones.
- *Lean:* Color should range from light pink to bright red and be smooth and fine-textured, similar to calf.
- *Fat:* Fat should be firm, creamy white, and evenly distributed.
- *Skin:* The skin should be smooth, thin, and pliable.

Market Forms of Meat

Meat can be purchased in several market styles: by the half- or quarter-carcass, in wholesale or primal cuts, or in oven-ready or portion-control cuts. Carcasses and primal cuts seldom are used in most food service departments today because of the amount of chilled storage space, cutting equipment, and skilled labor needed to prepare them for use. In addition, disposing of bones and other waste is a problem. Also, it is difficult to use all the different meat cuts effectively within a menu cycle. Carcasses and primal cuts are not even available from many institutional meat purveyors because suppliers purchase only the wholesale cuts they use most frequently and break them down into the oven-ready and portion-control cuts used by their food service customers.

The advantages of using oven-ready and portion-controlled meats are many. Roasts can be purchased in uniform sizes, weights, and trims. This gives the food service director greater control over portion yields and cost per serving. Specification of serving size for individual portion cuts offers maximum control of production quantity and quality, with little or no waste. Greater customer satisfaction can be achieved because each person receives the same-size portion.

Meat Specifications

All meat products should be purchased according to specifications based on a sound knowledge of the factors that influence preparation needs. A *specification* is a clear, concise, yet complete description of the exact item desired so that all vendors have a common basis for price quotations and bids. As such, it is an essential communication tool between buyer and seller. Specifications should be realistic and should not include details that cannot be verified or tested or that would make the product too costly. Without up-to-date product information, specifications will be useless. The specific information varies with each type of food, but all specifications should include at least the following information: name of product, grade or quality designation, size of container or package on which the price will be based, and the number of units to be purchased. A purchaser's ability to recognize various meat cuts and identify quality is essential. The Institutional Meat Purchase Specifications (IMPS) represent the USDA's official requirements for inspecting, packaging, packing, and delivering specific meats and meat products. For a detailed description of each of these requirements, refer to *SPECS: The Comprehensive Foodservice Purchasing and Specification Manual* by Reed. The IMPS are the most widely known and accepted specifications for meats used in the United States.

The *Meat Buyer's Guide* contains the meat specifications agreed on by the National Association of Meat Purveyors (NAMP). The *Meat Buyer's Guide to Standardized Meat Cuts* and the *Meat Buyer's Guide to Portion Control Meat Cuts* (also by NAMP) were written to simplify the IMPS and to provide graphic descriptions of the most commonly used cuts of meat. The meat buyer's guides (MBGs) illustrate the proper dimensions of meat cuts and should be used when writing specifications. Meat purveyors know the specifications in these publications and have no problem providing the meat cuts specified. These guides were last revised in 1984. The specification numbers from the *Meat Buyer's Guide to Standardized Cuts* are as follows:

- Fresh beef (No. 100)
- Fresh lamb and mutton (No. 200)
- Fresh veal and calf (No. 300)
- Fresh pork (No. 400)
- Cured, cured and smoked, and fully cooked pork products (No. 500)
- Cured, dried, and smoked beef products (No. 600)
- Edible by-products (No. 700)
- Sausage products (No. 800)

The specifications in the *Meat Buyer's Guide to Portion Control Meat Cuts* were developed by members of the meat-purveying industry who worked closely with food service customers and representatives of the USDA. These specifications use the following numbering system:

- Beef (Series 1100)
- Lamb (Series 1200)
- Veal (Series 1300)
- Pork (Series 1400)

When writing food service product specifications, both the IMPS numbers and the MBG numbers should be used. In many cases, the numbers are the same; for example, IMPS No. 110 for rib roast/ready (boneless and tied) is the same as MBG No. 110. The boneless and tied roast/ready rib is that portion of the roast/ready rib (item 109) that remains after the ribs, feather bones, and intercostal meat (rib fingers) have been removed. Boning procedures must be accomplished by scalping, which produces a smooth inner surface on the rib. The boneless roast/ready rib must be tied to produce a firm, compact roast. It must be held together by individual loops of strong twine uniformly spaced girthwise and lengthwise around the outside of the roast.

Food service departments that buy relatively small quantities of meat may not find it practical either to follow the lengthy specifications found in the IMPS or to make use of the Meat Acceptance Service, which is based on the IMPS, offered by the USDA. When a purchaser uses this service, the supplier has a USDA meat grader examine the product concerned to certify that the meat and meat products comply with the IMPS. This method of meat purchasing assures the buyer of a wholesome product as well as the grade, trim, weight, and other options specified. The service is provided on a fee-per-hour basis.

For best quality, meat items that will not be used within three to five days after delivery (within one day for ground beef) should be purchased frozen. The blast-freezing processes used by meat purveyors provide the best conditions for quality retention. The common practice of freezing fresh meat in the food service department usually results in quality deterioration because most food service departments have freezers capable of holding meat in the frozen state but not of freezing meat rapidly.

Regardless of how much meat is purchased at any one time, the written specifications to be given the vendor should include the following information:

1. Name of the cut
2. Requirements for boning, rolling, and tying (if applicable)
3. USDA grade or other quality designation
4. Weight of cut or individual portion (state tolerances allowed)
5. IMPS or MBG number (if applicable)
6. Chilled or frozen delivery
7. Packaging or number of units per shipping container

Following are some examples of specifications that adhere to these rules:

- Beef, inside round roast, USDA Choice, 8 to 10 pounds, IMPS No. 168, chilled, 32- to 40-pound polylined boxes preferred

- Beef, ground (special) bulk, USDA Commercial or Utility, 18 to 22 percent maximum fat content, IMPS No. 137, frozen, 10-pound bag
- Beef liver, portion cut, Selection No. 1, 4-ounce portion, IMPS No. 703, frozen, 10- to 15-pound polylined boxes preferred
- Bacon, sliced, layout pack, skinless, cured and smoked, Selection No. 1, 8- to 12-pound bellies, 18 to 22 slices per pound, IMPS No. 593, chilled, 10- to 15-pound polylined boxes preferred

Processed Meat

Processed meat is a term used to identify meat that has been changed by cooking, curing, canning, drying, or freezing or by a combination of these processes. Meats commonly described as processed include sausages, cold cuts, hams, bacon, and frankfurters. Some are fully cooked and can be served as purchased, whereas others require heating. Table 16-1 lists the characteristics of common processed meats.

☐ Seafood

More than 200 kinds of seafood are on the market today, including fresh and saltwater fish and various kinds of shellfish. *SPECS: The Comprehensive Foodservice Purchasing and Specification Manual* provides descriptions of many of these varieties. The kinds and prices of fresh fish and shellfish products available vary with the geographic location of the facility and the season of the year. Because frozen fish and shellfish products are widely available and easy to use, most food service departments use frozen rather than fresh seafood. Most kinds of frozen seafood are available throughout the year. The increasing popularity of fish has taxed the supply and resulted in increased prices for many of the most popular species. Consequently, many less-familiar fish are being marketed in fresh and frozen forms. Because many of these fish are satisfactory and economical, they deserve consideration.

Fish may be sold by different names in different parts of the country. For example, bass has many names: The Pacific bass may be called rockfish, sea bass, or striped bass; the Atlantic variety may be called striped bass, sea white bass, or common bass.

Some fish may be common to a particular area but are frozen and shipped to other areas of the country for consumption. Some of these include:

- Redfish, common to the South Atlantic and the Gulf of Mexico
- Halibut, common to both the Pacific and the Atlantic
- Mullett, common to the South Atlantic and the Gulf of Mexico
- Northern pike, common to Canadian lakes
- Pompano, common to the South Atlantic and the Gulf of Mexico
- Salmon, common to the North Pacific
- Scrod, common to the North Atlantic
- Whitefish, common to the Great Lakes

Inspection for sanitary conditions and wholesomeness—which is required for meat, poultry, and egg products—is not as widely applied to seafood. The Seafood Quality and Inspection Division of the National Marine Fisheries Service, U.S. Department of Commerce (USDC), conducts a voluntary seafood inspection program on a fee-for-service basis for processors and other interested parties. Contract plant inspection means that the processing plant, equipment, and food handlers have met all required sanitation standards. In addition, a federal inspector has examined samples of the product and found it to be safe, wholesome, and properly labeled.

Seafood packed under federal inspection will bear a statement of inspection on the label or the "Packed under Federal Inspection" (PUFI) mark. (See figure 16-1.) Product grading, which is voluntary, is an additional guarantee to the consumer that the product meets a certain level

Table 16-1. Descriptions of Common Processed Meats

Meat	Description
Bacon	The cured and smoked belly of the hog. Available sliced shingle style or on parchment paper ready to grill.
Beef, dried	Also known as chipped beef. A slow-cured product made from beef round; cured, smoked, dehydrated, and thinly sliced. Available in cans, jars, and vacuum packages.
Bologna	Made of cured beef and pork; finely ground with seasonings similar to those in frankfurters. Available in rings, rolls, or slices of various diameters; fully cooked and ready to serve. • Beef bologna: made exclusively of beef and has a definite garlic flavor. • Meat bologna: a mixture of beef and pork. • Poultry bologna: made of chicken or turkey or a combination of chicken and turkey.
Bratwurst	Pork or a pork and veal mixture, highly seasoned, made in links slightly larger than frankfurters. Available both fresh and fully cooked.
Braunschweiger	Liver sausage that has been smoked after cooking or includes smoked meats as ingredients.
Chorizos	Dry pork sausage of Spanish origin; meat coarsely cut, smoked, highly spiced and hot to the palate; size similar to large frankfurters or bulk style.
Ham	Cured pork leg available with bone in or boneless; sold in a variety of forms, dry cured or with water added for economy, tenderness, and a juicy flavor. Generally supplied fully cooked and ready to heat and serve.
Knockwurst (or knackwurst)	Similar in ingredients to frankfurters and bologna, with garlic added for stronger flavor; made in wide natural casings or in skinless style; fully cooked but usually served hot; also known as knoblauch or garlic sausage.
Liverwurst, liver sausage	Finely ground selected pork and livers; seasoned with onions and spices; may also be smoked after cooking or may include smoked meat such as bacon.
Luncheon meat	Chopped pork, ham and/or beef, seasoned and ready to serve. Available in loaves, in cans, and in vacuum packages, sliced.
Mettwurst	Cured beef and pork ground and lightly seasoned with allspice, ginger, mustard, and coriander; smooth, spreadable consistency; cooked before serving.
Pastrami	Flat pieces of lean beef, dry cured, rubbed with a paste of spices, and smoked.
Polish sausage	Coarsely ground lean pork with beef added, highly seasoned with garlic; frequently referred to as kielbasa, once a Polish word for all sausage.
Pork sausage, fresh	Made only from selected fresh pork; seasoned with black pepper, nutmeg, and rubbed sage; sold in links, packaged patties, or bulk; thorough cooking required.
Pork sausage, fresh country style	Made of selected fresh pork; ground more coarsely than other fresh pork sausage; generally sold in casings, but also in bulk and links; thorough cooking required.
Pork sausage, smoked country style	Fresh pork sausage, mildly cured and smoked; thorough cooking required.
Salami	General classification for highly seasoned dry sausage with characteristic fermented flavor; usually made of beef and pork; seasoned with garlic, salt, pepper, and sugar; most air dried and not smoked or cooked (cooked salamis are not dry sausage).
Salami, cooked	Made from fresh meats; cured, stuffed, then cooked in a smokehouse at high temperatures; may be air dried for a short time; softer texture than dry and semidry sausages (cooked salamis are not dry sausage); refrigeration required.
Salami, Cotto	Cooked salami; contains whole peppercorns; may be smoked as well as cooked.
Salami, Genoa	A dry sausage of Italian origin; usually made from all pork but may contain a small amount of beef; moistened with wine or grape juice; seasoned with garlic; cord wrapped lengthwise and around the sausage at regular intervals.
Salami, Italian	Includes many varieties named for towns and localities (for example, Genoa, Milano, Sicilian); principally cured lean pork, coarsely chopped and some finely chopped lean beef added; frequently moistened with red wine or grape juice; usually highly seasoned with garlic and various spices; air dried; chewy texture.
Salami, kosher	All beef; meat and processing under rabbinical supervision; mustard, coriander, and nutmeg added to regular seasonings.
Smoky links	Coarsely ground beef and pork; seasoned with black pepper; stuffed and linked like frankfurters.
Sausage, thuringer style	Made principally of ground pork; may also include veal and beef; seasoning similar to that in pork sausage, except no sage is used; may be smoked or unsmoked.

of quality. Graded products may bear the appropriate grade mark: USDC Grade A, B, or C. The grade stamp signifies that the product meets the following criteria:

- The product is clean, safe, and wholesome.
- Specified quality standard as indicated by grade designation has been achieved.
- Condition of the establishment in which the fish was processed was acceptable as required by food-control authorities.
- The product was processed under supervision of federal food inspectors and was packed under sanitary conditions.
- Common or usual name is accurately reflected on label.

The grading service is used primarily by large processors and only rarely by small ones. However, fresh and frozen products of excellent quality can be obtained from uninspected sources when the vendors are reputable and are known to follow adequate sanitary standards.

Fresh Fish

High-quality fresh fish has firm, elastic flesh with a smooth, slippery slime and shiny surface. The eyes should be bulging and clear, the gills should be pink to bright red, and there should be no strong "fishy" odor. As fish deteriorates, the slime becomes more viscous (sticky) and grainy, the odor changes from smelling like seaweed to smelling like ammonia, and the flesh softens. Because fresh fish deteriorates quite rapidly, great care must be taken in handling it during harvest and processing. This task becomes more difficult when markets are far from the source. For this reason, a large percentage of fish on the market is sold frozen.

Frozen Fish

Frozen fish, if properly processed, packaged, and stored, shows no sign of freezer burn. Packages are free from dripping and ice. Individually quick-frozen (IQF) fillets and steaks are best to purchase (except for breaded fish products). The fish should have little or no odor. If handled properly, frozen fish will remain in good condition for relatively long periods. If the fish is purchased as a ready-to-cook breaded product, the ratio of fish to breading should be checked to ensure that the department is getting its money's worth of fish.

Shellfish

Shellfish are marketed live or cooked whole in the shell, headless, or shucked. The meat can be purchased fresh or frozen, cooked or raw, plain or breaded, and canned. Shellfish purchased live in the shell must be kept alive until cooked. Buyers of fresh shellfish should be well acquainted with their source of supply and should check to make sure that the products have been harvested from uncontaminated waters. A high proportion of shellfish is marketed frozen, and the quality characteristics of frozen shellfish are the same as those described for other frozen fish.

Market Forms of Fish and Shellfish

Fresh and frozen fish are available in several forms. Some are:

- *Whole and drawn:* Only the scales and entrails are removed.
- *Whole and dressed:* Scales, entrails, and usually the head, tail, and fins are removed.
- *Headed and gutted:* Head, tails, fins, and entrails removed.
- *Steaks:* Cross-sectional slices are cut from large dressed fish with the skin off, usually ⅝ to ¾ inch thick.
- *Fillets:* The sides of fish are cut lengthwise, away from the bone. Fillets are practically boneless and come with or without skin.

- *Portions and sticks:* Large, solid, frozen blocks of boneless fish are machine cut. Pieces are dipped in batter or breading and may or may not be partially cooked. The designation *precooked* means that only the batter or breading is cooked and that the fish is raw. Fillets are available in many shapes and sizes and are ready to cook as purchased.

Currently, many other seafood products are processed and sold in convenience form, either frozen or in a freeze-dried state. Frozen fish fillets or portions may be filled with stuffing, sauce, or nuts. Shrimp and crab are available freeze-dried, which helps reduce the amount of labor involved in preparation. Both products can be stored for long periods because they are cooked and cleaned before being frozen, freeze-dried, or canned. Reconstitution in water takes little time, the flavor and color are good, and the cost may be less than that of the fresh product at certain times of the year.

Specifications for Fish and Shellfish

When developing specifications for fresh or frozen fish and shellfish, the following information should be included:

- Species (kind) of fish or shellfish
- The PUFI seal or grading stamp, if applicable
- Market form or portion shape and size
- Raw or precooked, plain or breaded
- Chilled or frozen
- Pounds per package
- Packages per case

Some sample specifications include the following:

- Cod, breaded, 4-ounce portions, U.S. Grade A, ten 6-pound boxes per case
- Cod fillets, skinless, 6-ounce portions, individually quick-frozen, U.S. Grade A, ten 5-pound boxes per case
- Pollock, breaded, 2-ounce precooked portions, minced white meat, PUFI, USDC, six 5-pound boxes per case
- Shrimp, round, breaded, 30/35 count, U.S. Grade A, six 4-pound boxes per case

Canned Fish

Many kinds of canned fish products are available including salmon, tuna, mackerel, crab, shrimp, sardines, clams, herring, anchovies, and caviar. Of these, only salmon and tuna are available in several species and styles.

On the Pacific Coast, salmon usually is sold by species name because of the differences in color, texture, and flavor among species. Chinook (or king) salmon, for example, which ranges in color from white to deep-salmon color, is the highest-quality salmon and therefore the highest priced. Very little of this salmon is canned because most is sold fresh or smoked. Sockeye is the reddest of all varieties, is of high quality, and also is high in price. Silver, medium-red, or coho salmon, usually a rich orange color slightly touched with red, is widely used for canning. Pink or humpback salmon is lighter in color but has excellent flavor and is good for use in many combination recipes. Chum or keta salmon is light colored and bland in flavor.

Tuna canned in the United States is produced from four species of the mackerel family: albacore, yellowfin, bluefin, and skipjack. Albacore has the lightest meat and is the only tuna that may be labeled white meat. The other species are labeled light meat.

Canned salmon and tuna are available packed in oil, water, and brine. Four styles of pack are available: fancy or solid pack, which must contain 82 percent solid pieces; chunk style, in which 50 percent of the weight must be pieces ½ inch or larger in diameter; flakes, in which 50 percent or more of the pieces are less than ½ inch in diameter; and grated. Specifications for canned fish should state the species and variety, packing medium, style of pack, size of can, and number of cans per case. Some sample specifications include the following:

- Tuna, solid pack, light meat, oil pack, six 64-ounce cans per case
- Tuna, solid pack, light meat, water pack, twenty-four 6½-ounce cans per case
- Salmon, pink, PUFI, six 64-ounce cans per case

☐ Poultry

Poultry products are used extensively in food service menus because of their great versatility in both general and modified diets. Availability of poultry is rarely a problem because the production and processing techniques used today provide a consistent supply of the desired kind, quality, and quantity of poultry in almost any season. Prices fluctuate according to market conditions and the prices of red meats, but in general most poultry products are less expensive than other meat items.

Market Forms of Poultry

Many of the different market forms of poultry are popular because they save time in preparation and eliminate waste. For example, turkey rolls come in many styles: all white meat, all dark meat, mixed light and dark meat, and in specified proportions by weight. Light and dark meat can come mixed together throughout the roll or separately in distinct sections of it. Turkey rolls usually are cooked and ready to heat and serve, but sometimes they are available raw.

Turkey roasts of boneless white, dark, or mixed light and dark meat are available in a range of weights. They are marketed raw, usually seasoned, and ready to cook from the frozen state. Frozen, cooked, diced white or dark meat of chicken or turkey, separate or mixed, is an ideal product for use in many food service recipes. Cooked fried chicken products, breaded or battered, are available in a wide range of portion sizes and styles.

All poultry products should be handled carefully after delivery, and they should be refrigerated or frozen under the conditions appropriate and recommended for specific items. Of course, all precooked or uncooked frozen products should be thawed under refrigeration or reheated without thawing.

Poultry Specifications

Because of the wide variety of poultry products and market forms, the food buyer must keep abreast of the marketplace and use well-written specifications for all poultry items. Adequate descriptions of poultry items include the following information:

1. *Kind* refers to the species, such as chicken, turkey, duck, capon, goose, and quail.
2. *Class* refers to physical characteristics related to age and sex, as follows:
   - Broiler-fryer chicken—a young chicken of either sex, 9 to 12 weeks old, weighing 1½ to 4 pounds, ready to cook
   - Roaster chicken—young chicken of either sex, 3 to 5 months old, weighing 4 to 6 pounds or more, ready to cook
   - Hen or stewing chicken—female chicken, more than 10 months old, weighing more than 4 pounds, ready to cook
   - Rock Cornish game hen—female chicken, 5 to 7 weeks old, weighing less than 2 pounds, ready to cook
   - Fryer-roaster turkey—less than 16 weeks old, weighing 3 to 7 pounds, ready to cook
   - Young hen or young tom turkey (or young turkey)—16 to 24 weeks old, weighing 8 to 16 pounds (hens) or 16 pounds or more (toms), ready to cook
   - Yearling or mature turkeys—older than 12 months and of heavy weight

3. *Grade* refers to the quality of the product and is determined by factors such as conformity, fleshing, fat covering, and freedom from various types of defects such as cuts, tears, broken bones, and discoloration. The USDA grades for ready-to-cook poultry are A, B, and C. Almost all chicken or turkey marketed fresh-chilled or frozen is Grade A; Grades B and C are used for processed forms. All poultry must be inspected for wholesomeness. Inspection and grade marks for poultry are shown in figure 16-1. Birds that have a wing, tail, or drumstick missing because of damage during processing but whose eating quality has not been affected are labeled "Parts Missing."

4. *Style* indicates whether the bird is to be cut up or left whole. When ready-to-cook poultry is purchased, the buyer's preference for parts, quarters, eight-piece cut, nine-piece cut, breasts, legs, thighs, boneless, and so forth should be indicated.

5. *State of delivery* indicates whether the poultry should be delivered fresh-chilled, frozen, or cooked and frozen.

6. *Weight or size* indicates weight range allowable for individual birds and/or ounces per portion for convenience forms.

7. *Delivery unit* refers to weight or number per delivery box or package.

Some sample specifications for poultry are as follows:

- Chicken, U.S. Grade A, 2½- to 3-pound broiler, quartered, fresh, chilled, or frozen as specified
- Chicken, boned, cooked, ready to use, minimum 91 percent meat, maximum 6 percent broth and 3 percent fat, natural proportion of light and dark meat, seasoned with salt only, six 30-ounce rolls per case, prepared under continuous USDA inspection
- Chicken, diced, ½-inch cubes, white, dark, or mixed meat, cooked, frozen, three 10-pound polybags per case
- Chicken, fryer, cooked in batter, frozen, nine-piece cut, quartered or individual parts, 9 pounds per case
- Turkey, young hen, U.S. Grade A, whole, fresh or frozen, 12 to 14 pounds
- Turkey, young tom, U.S. Grade A, whole, fresh or frozen, 20 to 26 pounds
- Turkey breast, U.S. Grade A, boneless, frozen, uncooked, natural skin cover, four 8- to 10-pound polybags per case
- Turkey roll, natural proportions white and dark meat, cooked, frozen, 4½ to 5 inches in diameter, four 10-pound rolls per case
- Turkey, diced, ½-inch cubes, white, dark, or mixed meat, cooked, frozen, three 10-pound polybags per case
- Turkey ham, cooked, frozen, two 7- to 8-pound polybags per case
- Turkey franks, chilled, 10 per pound, 10 pounds per case

☐ Eggs and Egg Products

Egg production is a highly automated business that yields superior fresh eggs for the food service and retail markets. Modern technology and the federal regulations covering shell eggs, as stated in the Egg Products Inspection Act of 1972, prevent the distribution or use of eggs that have not been graded.

Grades of Shell Eggs

The USDA provides a voluntary grading service for producers of shell eggs. Eggs that have been graded under this program can be identified by the official USDA shell egg grade symbol on the package (see figure 16-1). The symbol indicates that the eggs have been graded for quality under both federal and state supervision.

Grades refer to the interior quality and condition of the egg, as well as to the appearance of the shell. Official consumer grades are U.S. Grade AA, U.S. Grade A, and U.S. Grade B.

The higher-quality eggs—AA and A—have a firm and thick white, a well-rounded yolk, and a delicate flavor. They are ideal for any purpose, but are particularly good for frying and poaching when appearance is important. Grade A eggs are less expensive than Grade AA and are entirely satisfactory for the same purposes as the higher grade. Grade B eggs have thinner whites and somewhat flatter yolks that may break easily. They are less expensive and are suitable for general cooking and baking.

Weight and Size of Shell Eggs

Shell eggs also are classified according to size, although size has no relation to quality. Large eggs can be of any quality, just as eggs of any quality can be of any size. Official size categories are based on the minimum weight per dozen. Eggs for institutional use are sold in cases of 30 dozen and half-cases of 15 dozen. The official size categories and weights per dozen and the minimum weights per case, excluding the weight of the container, are listed in table 16-2. The most common sizes are extra large, large, and medium.

The weight of cases of eggs received from various suppliers should be checked periodically. An empty carton that contains the filler flats should be weighed to get an approximate weight of the carton. Then a full case should be weighed and the results, minus the weight of the carton, checked against the weights given in table 16-2.

Price Considerations in Purchasing Shell Eggs

The size and grade of eggs purchased should depend on the price per ounce and the intended use of the eggs. In some areas, shell color can affect the egg's price even though color does not affect its grade, nutritional value, flavor, or cooking performance. Egg prices vary by size for the same grade, but the degree of price variation depends on the supply of the various sizes. To determine which size is the most economical, the price per ounce of various sizes should be compared by dividing the price per dozen by the weight in ounces for a dozen eggs of a particular size. For example, if large eggs are 80 cents per dozen, with a minimum weight of 24 ounces for a dozen eggs of that size, the price per ounce would be 3.3 cents. Medium eggs at 70 cents per dozen, weighing 21 ounces per dozen, also would cost 3.3 cents per ounce. In this case, either size would be an equally good buy. However, medium eggs at any price per dozen over 70 cents would cost more per ounce than large eggs at 80 cents per dozen and would not be a good buy.

Egg Products

Egg products are a convenience item for food service operations and commercial food manufacturers. Whole eggs, yolks, whites, and various blends can be obtained in liquid, frozen, and dried forms.

Table 16-2. Official USDA Size Categories for Shell Eggs

U.S. Weights or Classes, Size	Minimum Weight per Dozen, Ounces	Minimum Weight per 30-Dozen Case, Pounds
Jumbo	30	56
Extra large	27	50½
Large	24	45
Medium	21	39½
Small	18	34
Peewee	15	28

The Egg Products Inspection Act of 1970 requires that liquid, frozen, and dried egg products be inspected under the USDA's continuous mandatory inspection program. This requirement applies to products shipped between states, within a state, and in foreign commerce. The official USDA egg products inspection mark (see figure 16-1) means that the products were processed under continuous supervision of a USDA-licensed inspector, that the products were processed in an approved plant that had adequate facilities, and that the products were pasteurized in accordance with USDA requirements and were truthfully and informatively labeled.

Institutional packs of liquid, frozen, and powdered eggs are available in various sizes. Containers for frozen packs range in size from 3 to 45 pounds. Many food service operations find the smaller containers, which resemble half-gallon milk cartons, to be the most convenient to use within a short time after thawing. The containers should be stored at 0°F (−18°C) or below and thawed under refrigeration. Dried egg products also are available in many pack sizes, and the 5-pound container is the easiest to use. Because dried egg products can be contaminated easily and deteriorate in quality rapidly, they should be stored in the refrigerator in a tightly covered container.

The food service buyer should become familiar with the product variety provided by local vendors and develop specifications in accordance with need and market availability. Table 16-3 summarizes the manufacturing and inspection specifications for several egg products.

Specifications for Eggs and Egg Products

Specifications for fresh eggs should include the form, quality designation, size, and unit of purchase. No quality designation (such as grade) is used for egg products because they are not graded; the words *USDA inspected* are used in place of a grade. Some sample specifications for eggs and egg products follow:

1. Eggs, fresh, Grade AA, large, 45-pound net per 30-dozen case
2. Eggs, frozen, whole, pasteurized, homogenized, USDA inspected, six 4-pound cartons per case
3. Eggs, dried, whole, six 3-pound cans per case

□ Milk and Other Dairy Products

Effective sanitation in production, transport, and processing is the key to high-quality milk and other dairy products. For this reason, the regulations concerning sanitary production of dairy products are very strict. The U.S. Public Health Service's Milk Ordinance and Code is the basis for state and local milk regulations. The Grade A classification for milk and milk products is a designation based on compliance with sanitation requirements of applicable laws. Only Grade A pasteurized milk can be shipped interstate, and in most states it is the only grade available for purchase and use as a fluid product. A food service buyer should be familiar with all state and local regulatory standards that apply to the suppliers with whom he or she deals.

Grades of Milk

Grades are related to the conditions under which milk is produced and handled and the bacterial count in the final product. Pasteurization destroys pathogenic (disease-causing) organisms and most other bacteria commonly found in milk. Most fluid milk is *homogenized,* a process that divides the fat globules into tiny particles that remain in permanent suspension in the milk. Food and Drug Administration (FDA) standards for the composition of milk specify the minimum amounts of milk solids and milk fat contained in milk or cream products.

Table 16-3. Manufacturing and Inspection Specifications for Selected Egg Products

| Specification | Liquid or Frozen | | | Solids | | | | | | |
| | | | | Whites | | Whole | | Yolk | | |
	White	Yolk[a]	Whole	Spray Dried	Pan Dried	Plain	Free Flowing[b]	Plain	Free Flowing[b]	Scrambled Egg
Moisture (%)	–	–	–	8.0	14.0	5.0	3.0	5.0	3.0	2.5
Total solids (%)	11.0	43.0	24.7	–	–	–	–	–	–	–
Crude protein (%)	10.0	14.0	12.0	80.0	74.0	45.0	45.0	30.0	30.0	34.3
Total lipids (%)	Nil	28.0	10.5	± 0.02	Nil	40.0	40.0	56.0	56.0	36.5
pH	8.9 ± 0.3	6.2 ± 0.1	7.3 ± 0.3	7.0 ± 0.5	5.5 ± 0.5	8.3 ± 0.3	8.3 ± 0.3	6.4 ± 0.3	6.4 ± 0.3	–
Carbohydrates[c] (%)	–	–	–	Glucose free	Glucose free	SOP	SOP	SOP	SOP	17
Total microbial count (grams)	<5,000	<5,000	<5,000	<10,000	<10,000	<10,000	<10,000	<10,000	<10,000	<10,000
Yeast (grams)	10 max.	10 max.	10 max.	10 max.	10 max.	10 max.	10 max.	10 max.	10 max.	–
Mold (grams)	10 max.	10 max.	10 max.	10 max.	10 max.	10 max.	10 max.	10 max.	10 max.	–
Coliform (grams)	10 max.	10 max.	10 max.	10 max.	10 max.	10 max.	10 max.	10 max.	10 max.	–
Salmonellae (grams)	Negative[d]	Negative	Negative	Negative 100%[e]	Negative SOP	Negative 100%	Negative 100%	Negative 100%	Negative 100%	Negative
Granulation	–	–	–	USBS 60	–	USBS 16	USBS 16	USBS 16	USBS 16	–
Others[f]	–	–	–	–	–	–	–	–	–	–

Source: American Egg Board.

[a]Egg yolk contains 17 percent egg white; natural egg yolk contains about 52 percent solids.

[b]Free-flowing products contain less than 2 percent sodium silicoaluminate.

[c]Most egg white solids are desugared. Whole egg and yolk products are desugared if specified on purchase (SOP).

[d]Negative by approved testing procedures.

[e]U.S. Bureau of Standards (USBS) Screen No. 80.

[f]Additives and performance specifications may be specified on purchase.

403

Forms of Milk and Dairy Products

Milk and dairy products are available in a wide variety of forms. The most familiar are whole milk, skim milk, low-fat milk, cultured buttermilk, cream, evaporated milk, sweetened condensed milk, and a number of other forms as described in the following subsections.

Whole Milk

According to FDA standards, whole milk must contain at least 3.25 percent fat and 8.25 percent milk solids. This applies to plain or flavored milk.

Skim Milk

To meet FDA standards skim milk, plain or flavored, contains less than 0.5 percent fat and at least 8.25 percent milk solids. Total solids can range from 8.0 to 9.25 percent depending on state standards.

Low-Fat Milk

Low-fat milk must be fortified with vitamin A at levels specified by FDA regulations. Fortification with vitamin D is optional. Standards for milk products in certain states may vary from federal standards, which require that low-fat milk in plain or flavored form contain at least 0.5 to 2 percent fat and 8.25 percent milk solids.

Cultured Buttermilk

Cultured buttermilk, which has a characteristic flavor that is produced by bacterial fermentation, is processed from pasteurized skim milk to which lactic acid and bacteria have been added. Partial fermentation produces some coagulation of the milk protein. Small butter granules may be added. Buttermilk is a by-product of butter production. No federal standards have been established for buttermilk.

Cream

Several forms of cream are commonly available on the market. Half-and-half, by federal standards, contains 10.5 to 18 percent fat, and light cream 18 to 30 percent fat. Light whipping cream contains 30 to 36 percent fat and heavy whipping cream 36 percent or more.

Evaporated Milk

Evaporated milk is prepared by removing about half the water from fresh whole milk. The milk fat content is no less than 7.5 percent, and the milk solid content is no less than 25.5 percent. Evaporated milk must contain 25 international units (IUS) of vitamin D per ounce; the addition of vitamin A is optional. Evaporated low-fat and skim milks also are available, which are useful in reducing the amount of fat in the diet.

Sweetened Condensed Milk

Another type of milk used occasionally is sweetened condensed milk. This product is made from whole milk by removing about half the water and adding 40 percent sugar in the form of sucrose, dextrose, or corn syrup before evaporation takes place.

Yogurt

Yogurt is a cultured product that can be made from whole milk, low-fat milk with added milk solids, and skim milk with added milk solids. It is available plain or in flavors and with various levels of fat content. Because of the variation in yogurt composition, the buyer should check local sources for product information and nutrient composition.

Sour Cream and Sour Half-and-Half

Sour cream and sour half-and-half are cultured milk products that can be used in food service operations. Cultured sour cream contains about 20 percent milk fat and cultured half-

and-half about 12 percent milk fat. Sour half-and-half can be substituted for the richer product in most recipes and is less expensive.

Nonfat Dry Milk

Nonfat dry milk is economical for institutional use in cooked and baked products. Standards in the United States for grades of nonfat dry milk are U.S. Extra Grade and U.S. Standard Grade. Nonfat dry milk contains no more than 5 percent moisture and no more than 1.5 percent milk fat unless otherwise specified. Instant nonfat dry milk, made by a special process that gives it improved solubility, is the most popular form. However, noninstant nonfat dry milk also is available and can be used satisfactorily in baked products when mixed with the dry ingredients. Fortification of nonfat dry milk with vitamins A and D is optional and, if desired, should be stated in the specification.

Dry Buttermilk

Dry buttermilk is another useful product for baking purposes. The grades for this product are the same as for nonfat dry milk. All dry milk products are made from pasteurized milk. Dry buttermilk is more stable than fresh, fluid buttermilk.

Ice Cream

Federal standards for ice cream specify a minimum content of 10 percent milk fat and 20 percent milk solids. The quality of ice cream is related to its composition, the quality of its ingredients, the weight per gallon, and the quality and quantity of flavoring materials. Differences in these components influence the price of the various products and brands. Ice cream is available in a wide variety of forms suited to food service use, including such time-savers as individually wrapped slices and individual cups. Novelty items add variety to the menu.

Ice Milk and Sherbet

Ice milk, hardened or soft, is available in a wide variety of flavors. Ice milk contains at least 2 percent milk fat and 11 percent milk solids. Fruit sherbets contain a minimum of 1 percent milk fat and 2 percent milk solids. Because compositional requirements vary from state to state, food buyers must be familiar with state regulations.

Specifications for Milk and Milk Products

Written specifications for milk and other dairy products are just as important as specifications for other foods. Additions or deletions from the following sample specifications may be needed to suit particular situations:

1. Milk, whole, homogenized, pasteurized, fortified, minimum 3.25 percent milk fat, half-pint carton
2. Milk, low-fat, homogenized, pasteurized, fortified, minimum 2 percent milk fat, half-gallon carton
3. Buttermilk, cultured, homogenized, pasteurized, minimum 8.25 percent milk solids, quart carton
4. Cream, half-and-half, pasteurized, 10.5 to 18 percent milk fat, pint carton
5. Milk, nonfat, dry, instant, U.S. Extra Grade, 5-pound bag
6. Yogurt, low-fat, minimum 8.5 percent nonfat solids, plain-flavored, 8-ounce carton

☐ Nondairy Substitutes for Milk and Cream

Cream substitutes, dessert toppings, and imitation milk are among a group of products developed as substitutes for dairy products. There are no compositional standards for these products, so food buyers must check the ingredient lists provided by the manufacturer. Some nondairy products, including many coffee whiteners, contain no milk or other dairy products and are available fresh or frozen in liquid or powdered form. Dessert toppings are marketed in pressurized containers and in powdered or frozen form. The stability of nondairy toppings and their low cost compared to dairy products have made them extremely popular for food service use.

Imitation milk, available in some states, can have utilitarian value for some modified diets. These products combine fats or oils other than milk fat with food solids but exclude milk solids. Sodium caseinate is frequently used as the protein source.

Cultured nondairy sour cream is another imitation dairy product. Lauric acid oils—including coconut oil, hydrogenated coconut oil, and palm kernel oil—are frequently used in this product. The manufacturer should be consulted for specific content information.

☐ Natural, Processed, and Imitation Cheeses

The many varieties of cheese available have tremendous potential for use in interesting menus and are a challenge to the food buyer. Making good cheese purchases requires knowledge of the quality and flavor characteristics of each cheese and of the ways it can be used.

Natural cheeses are made from whole, partially defatted, or skim milk, depending on the variety of cheese. Federal standards of identity specifying the processing methods and setting minimum fat and maximum moisture contents have been established for the primary cheese varieties.

Varieties of Natural Cheese

Natural cheeses are classified into several groups by degree of hardness: soft, such as cottage cheese, ricotta, and cream cheese; semisoft, such as brick, Muenster, and mozzarella; hard, such as cheddar and Swiss; and very hard, such as Parmesan and Romano. Further distinctions are made on the basis of the organism (bacteria or mold) involved in the ripening process and the length of ripening or aging.

Cheddar Cheese

Cheddar is a whole-milk cheese that is perhaps the most popular of all the natural cheeses in the United States. Also known as American cheddar, it can be identified by its shape or style, classified as longhorn or daisy. In addition, it is often identified by the locale where it was produced, such as Wisconsin or New York. Standards for cheddar cheese specify a minimum of 50 percent milk fat content and a maximum of 39 percent moisture by weight. The USDA grades for cheddar cheese—AA, A, B, and C—are based on the cheese's flavor, body, texture, color, and appearance. Some states also have their own grades.

Flavor terminology also is used to specify age of the cheese. As cheddar cheese ages, its flavor becomes sharper. The market flavors available are fresh or current, medium or mellow, aged or sharp, and very sharp. Aged cheddar melts faster and produces a smoother product than cheese less than three months old.

When purchasing cheddar cheese, the desired form and size should be specified: 20-, 40-, or 60-pound blocks; 12-pound cylindrical longhorns; 20-pound cylindrical daisies; 5- to 20-pound loaves; or any other size or form available from vendors. Sliced forms also are available. In addition, the desired degree of aging and USDA or state grade should be specified.

Swiss Cheese

Swiss cheese, produced from pasteurized whole and skim milk, has a lower fat content than cheddar cheese. Standards require a minimum of 43 percent milk fat and no more than 41 percent moisture. The characteristic holes, or "eyes," are formed when bacteria produce gas bubbles during the aging process. The activity of bacteria also creates the sweet, nutty flavor characteristic of Swiss cheese. USDA-graded Swiss cheese is available. Aging for three to nine months is typical, although the desired aging should be specified.

Cottage Cheese

Cottage cheese is the soft, uncured curd from pasteurized skim milk. Cream is added to the dry cheese curd to make creamed cottage cheese. The milk fat content and moisture should not be less than 4 percent and 80 percent by weight, respectively, in the finished product. Creamed or dry cottage cheese comes in small curd, with particles about ⅛ to ¼ inch in diameter, and in large curd, with particles up to ⅜ inch in size. Specifications for this product should state the curd size to be ordered. Cottage cheese is available in many container sizes, from 1 to 30 pounds. Because cottage cheese, particularly large-curd cottage cheese, has a limited shelf life once the container has been opened, the quantities served and how long a container lasts should be considered when purchasing the product.

Other Natural Cheeses

Because the variety of natural cheeses is so extensive, other specific types are not described here in detail, but the reader can refer to *SPECS: The Comprehensive Foodservice Purchasing and Specification Manual* for additional information about the various varieties. Table 16-4 gives examples of cheese classifications and describes the characteristics of commonly used cheeses. Except for mozzarella, federal grades and standards have not been established for most of the varieties listed. However, familiarity with the quality standards of various manufacturers and careful product evaluation will help the food buyer select high-quality cheeses.

Processed Cheese

Pasteurized processed cheese is a blend of two or more varieties of the same cheese or two or more varieties of different cheeses, fresh and aged, that are heated to stop further ripening. The varieties are noted on the product's label. Emulsifying agents are added to yield a smooth texture and prevent separation. Because of the heating process, the texture and flavor of the cheese remain constant after processing.

Pasteurized processed cheese is similar to natural cheese, except that the former has a lower fat content, a higher moisture content, and added whey or milk solids. Other ingredients, such as sausage, vegetables, and nuts, are sometimes added. Processed cheese usually has a less-pronounced cheese flavor than natural cheese but melts more readily during cooking.

Pasteurized processed cheese spread has less fat and more moisture than the other products already described. It is soft and can be spread with a knife. A stabilizer is usually added to prevent separation of the ingredients. None of the processed cheese products are federally graded.

Imitation Cheese

The Filled Cheese Act of June 6, 1896, imposed a tax on cheese and licensed its manufacture and sale under special labeling and packaging procedures. Various states also imposed other restrictions that inhibited or discouraged development of filled-cheese products. The Filled Cheese Act was repealed in October 1974. As a result, filled-cheese foods are now subject solely to the provisions of the Federal Food, Drug, and Cosmetic Act and the Fair Packaging and Labeling Act. Today, they move freely in interstate commerce as nonstandardized foods, but their sale is prohibited in some states.

At present, two types of imitation cheese are available to consumers: those made with skim milk plus vegetable fat and those made with calcium caseinate or sodium caseinate plus vegetable fat. Most of these products have the body, texture, and appearance of regular cheese, although some consumers find the flavor to be different. Cheese substitutes also are functionally equivalent to their natural cheese counterparts. Various convenient package sizes are available for food service use.

Table 16-4. Descriptions of Common Cheeses

Cheese	Description
American (pasteurized process)	Semisoft to soft; light yellow to orange; mild. Made of cow's milk (whole), cheddar, and/or colby cheese.
Blue	Semisoft; white with blue-green mold; flavor similar to Roquefort. Made of cow's milk (whole).
Brick	Semisoft; smooth; light yellow to orange; flavor mild but pungent and sweet. Made of cow's milk (whole).
Brie	Soft; edible white crust; flavor resembles Camembert. Made of cow's milk (whole, low-fat, or skim).
Camembert	Soft; almost fluid; mild to pungent flavor. Made of cow's milk (whole).
Cheddar	Hard; smooth; light yellow to orange; mild to sharp. Made of cow's milk (whole).
Cottage	Soft; moist, delicate, large or small curd. Mildly acid flavor. Unripened; usually made of cow's milk (skim). Cream dressing may be added to cottage dry curd.
Cream	Soft; smooth; buttery; mild, slightly acid flavor. Unripened; made of cream and cow's milk (whole).
Edam	Semisoft to hard; rubbery; mild, sometimes salty flavor; cannonball shape. Made of cow's milk (low-fat).
Gorgonzola	Semisoft, less moist than blue; marbled with blue-green mold; spicy flavor. Made of cow's milk (whole) or goat's milk or mixture of these.
Gouda	Hard; flavor like Edam. Made of cow's milk (low-fat).
Gruyere	Hard with tiny gas holes; mild sweet flavor. Made of cow's milk (whole).
Monterey Jack	Semisoft (whole milk), hard (low-fat or skim milk); smooth; mild to mellow. Made of cow's milk (whole, low-fat, or skim).
Limburger	Soft; strong, robust flavor, highly aromatic. Made of cow's milk (whole or low-fat).
Muenster	Semisoft; flavor between brick and Limburger. Made of cow's milk (whole).
Neufchatel	Soft; creamy; white; mild flavor. Unripened or ripened 3 to 4 weeks. Made of cow's milk (whole or skim) or a mixture of milk and cream.
Parmesan	Very hard (grating) granular texture. Made of cow's milk (low-fat).
Provolone	Hard, stringy texture; bland acid to sharp, usually smoked flavor; pear, sausage, or salami shaped. Made of cow's milk (whole).
Roquefort	Semisoft; white with blue-green mold; sharp, piquant flavor. Made of sheep's milk.
Stilton	Semisoft; white with blue-green mold; spicy but milder than Roquefort flavor. Made of cow's milk (whole with added cream).
Swiss	Hard with gas holes; mild, nutlike, sweet flavor. Made of cow's milk (low-fat).

Cheese Specifications

Sample specifications for cheese include the following:

- Cheese, American, processed, medium blend, pasteurized, six 5-pound blocks
- Cheese, cheddar, natural, U.S. Grade A, medium aged, six 5-pound blocks
- Cheese, mozzarella, part skim, low moisture, six 5-pound blocks
- Cheese, cottage, creamed, minimum 4 percent milk fat by weight, maximum 80 percent moisture, small curd, 5-pound container

☐ Fruits and Vegetables

A significant amount of information is needed to purchase fresh or processed fruits and vegetables. As with other food products, it is important to select the form (fresh, canned, or frozen), style, and quality best suited to the planned use. The *Blue Goose Purchasing Guide to Fresh*

Fruits and Vegetables and *Produce 101* are excellent references for use in purchasing fresh produce.

Grades of Fruits and Vegetables

The USDA's Agricultural Marketing Service has developed quality grade standards for fruit and vegetable products. The grading of fresh, frozen, and canned fruits and vegetables is voluntary. Any grower, processor, or buyer who wants the product graded requests and pays for the grading service. After the products have been graded by a USDA inspector, they can be labeled with the U.S. grade name. When a product is labeled with one of the official grade names, such as Fancy, but without the prefix U.S., that product still must meet the USDA's standard for the grade, whether or not it has actually been inspected.

Although most fresh fruits and vegetables are sold wholesale on the basis of U.S. grades, not many are marked with the grade when they are resold. The typical range of grades for fresh fruits and vegetables includes U.S. Fancy, U.S. No. 1, and U.S. No. 2. For some products, there are grades above and below this range.

Grades for canned and frozen fruits and vegetables are U.S. Grade A (Fancy), U.S. Grade B (Choice for fruits and Extra Standard for vegetables), and U.S. Grade C (Standard). *Grade A* fruits and vegetables are the most tender, succulent, and uniform in size, shape, and color. *Grade B* is very good quality, but grade B fruits and vegetables may be slightly less uniform in size and color, and the products may have a few blemishes. Grade B fruits usually are packed in heavy syrup. *Grade C* products are of fairly good quality, just as wholesome and nutritious as the higher grades, and they may be the best buy for use in combination recipes when appearance is not important. Grade C fruits are more mature and usually are packed in light syrup. Grade C fruits also are used in most water-packed and low-calorie fruit products.

Most processors and distributors have their own quality control programs and quality designations, whether or not they use USDA's grading service, and most pack more than one grade of product. Food buyers should be aware of the various quality designations used by the processors and distributors in their areas.

Net Weights of Canned Fruits and Vegetables

Various federal and state laws require that a statement of net quantity appear on the label of canned fruits and vegetables. However, none of these laws specifies what the labeled weight or volume should be for these products. The fill, which affects the net weight or volume, varies with each product, but cans must be as full as practical, usually about 90 percent.

Considerations in Buying Fruits and Vegetables

The intended use of fruits and vegetables and the size of container to select should be considered before fruits and vegetables are ordered for use in the food service department. These two considerations are discussed below.

Intended Use

The intended use of a product determines which product style to buy, and in turn the product style affects the cost of fruits and vegetables. Canned whole fruits and vegetables usually cost more than cut styles but should be used when appearance is important. Short cuts, dices, and vegetable pieces are the least expensive and are good for use in soups and stews. Less-perfect fruits can be chosen for cooked desserts and mixed salads when appearance is not as important.

In purchasing fresh fruits and vegetables, the quality, variety, and size of the produce needed should be considered. For some fresh items, the labor and waste involved in trimming and preparation should be considered. For example, fresh broccoli requires some preparation time, and some net loss occurs from trimming stems and cutting bunches into uniform serving sizes. Apples purchased for eating raw are different in variety and size from those purchased for cooking.

Container Size

The container size selected can affect cost, quality of food, and ease of handling. Using large containers can involve a lower cost per serving if the quantity of food they contain can be used while it is at peak quality. If purchased in too large a unit, some food may have to be discarded due to staleness or spoilage, thus increasing food costs.

The No. 10 can, packed 6 per case, is the most common packing container for canned fruits and vegetables. However, for items used in smaller quantities, No. 303 cans, packed 24 per case, may be a better purchase size.

Frozen vegetables are most commonly found in 2- or 2½-pound packages and are packed 12 per case. However, some are available in 20-, 30-, and 50-pound packages.

As stated earlier, the acronym IQF used in relation to frozen fruits and vegetables means individually quick-frozen. Pieces of the product are frozen separately and then packed loosely so that the right amount of product can be measured without having to thaw the whole package. Generally, IQF fruits and vegetables are available in 2½-pound packages and in 20-pound polybags; sometimes they are available in larger quantities.

Fresh fruits and vegetables are usually purchased by weight, but in some cases the count per shipping container also should be specified. Many different sizes of cartons, boxes, and other shipping containers are used for fresh produce, depending on the type of product and where the product is produced. A list of common container sizes for fresh fruits and vegetables is available from the United Fresh Fruit and Vegetable Association (see the bibliography).

To retain their color and flavor, many fruits are packed in sugar syrup. Because fruit-to-sugar ratios vary, suppliers should be consulted for specific information.

Fruit and Vegetable Specifications

Specifications for fresh, frozen, and canned fruits and vegetables should include the following information:

- Name of product
- Style or type of product (whole, cut, trimmed, and so forth)
- USDA grade, brand, or other quality designation
- Size of container
- Quantity or weight per shipping unit
- Other pertinent factors, depending on the product (packing medium, syrup density, variety, stage of maturity, drained weight, and so forth)

Specifications for fruit and vegetable products should be based on the quality and type of product needed in a particular operation. Some sample specifications for fruit and vegetable products follow:

1. Bananas, fresh, No. 1, green tip, six 8-inch, 40-pound carton
2. Fruit cocktail, canned, U.S. Grade A (Fancy), heavy syrup, minimum drained weight 72 ounces, six No. 10 cans per case
3. Blueberries, frozen, whole, U.S. Grade A, IQF, 20-pound box
4. Cabbage, fresh, green, U.S. No. 1, 1½- to 2-pound heads, 50-pound mesh sack
5. Corn, canned, yellow, whole kernel, U.S. Grade A (Fancy), liquid pack, minimum drained weight 70 ounces, six No. 10 cans per case
6. Broccoli, frozen cuts, U.S. Grade A, twelve 2-pound packages per case

Dehydrated Fruits and Vegetables

Dehydrated fruits and vegetables have been available to American consumers for many years. Today, more and more dehydrated products, particularly potatoes, are used in food service operations. Two basic types of dehydrated products are available: regular moisture and low moisture. Regular-moisture products contain 18 to 20 percent of the food's original moisture. Apples, apricots, raisins, dates, peaches, and prunes are available in this form. Low-moisture dehydrated products contain only 2.5 to 5 percent moisture; these foods are less perishable. Onions, parsley, green peppers, potatoes, garlic, and many other vegetables are sold in this form.

Two processing methods for drying foods are used. In warm, dry areas of the country, fruits are dried in the sun. In colder climates, foods are dried by *vacuum dehydration,* a process that involves vacuum chambers and exposure to dry, warm inert gas.

Federal standards of quality exist for nearly all dried and low-moisture fruits. These standards are U.S. Grade A, U.S. Grade B, and U.S. Grade C. No standards are available for low-moisture vegetables except for dried legumes (beans, peas, and lentils). Nearly all peas and lentils and about a third of all beans are officially inspected before or after processing, even though retail packages seldom carry the federal or state grade stamp.

The USDA grades for dried legumes are generally based on the food's shape, size, and color and on the presence or absence of foreign material. State grades are based on quality factors similar to those for federal grades. The low grades usually contain more foreign material and more kernels of uneven size and nonstandard color. The high grades are U.S. No. 1 for dry, whole, or split peas, lentils, and black-eyed peas. USDA No. 1 Choice Handpicked or simply Handpicked are the high grades for great northern, pinto, and pea beans. U.S. Extra No. 1 is the high grade for lima beans, large and small.

The specifications for dehydrated fruits and vegetables should call for a clean product that has been prepared and packed under sanitary conditions. The product should have a bright color and good aroma.

Specifications for dehydrated potatoes should include the style required: flaked, granulated, sliced, or diced. In addition, it should be specified when instant mashed-potato products are to include dry milk and/or vitamin C. Other important considerations are the quality and yield of instant dehydrated potatoes. The actual number of pounds the product yields in the reconstituted state should be checked against the yield given on the label. Cooking samples of dehydrated potato products is the best way to check their quality.

Some sample specifications for dehydrated foods follow:

1. Potatoes, sliced (cross-sliced ⅛ inch thick), dehydrated, maximum 7 percent moisture, four 5-pound bags per case
2. Potatoes, instant, granules, without milk, Fancy, six 10-pound bags per case
3. Beans, dry, navy, U.S. Grade No. 1, 25-pound bag
4. Peas, dry, split, green, U.S. Grade No. 1, 25-pound bag
5. Raisins, processed, Thompson seedless, natural, U.S. Grade A, small, 30-pound box

☐ Fats and Oils

Food service operations use several kinds of shortening and oil products. Manufacturers offer specific products for baking, frying, and general cooking purposes.

Lard

Lard is fat rendered from hogs. Its quality varies according to its color, texture, and flavor. The shortening ability and texture of lard are well suited for use in pastry. However, ordinary leaf lard is not satisfactory for frying because its smoking point is lower than that of vegetable oils. Hydrogenated lard is of higher quality and has a higher smoking point than leaf lard. Blends of lard and tallow (rendered from cattle and sheep) are marketed, as well as blends of meat fat and vegetable shortenings. These products are suitable for most general cooking purposes. Also available are hydrogenated meat-fat shortenings that are designed for stability in deep-fat frying.

Hydrogenated Vegetable Shortenings

Hydrogenated vegetable shortenings can be used for many food production purposes. The process of hydrogenation changes vegetable oils from liquid form to a solid form that is creamy and plastic at room temperature. Fully hydrogenated vegetable shortening is used in baking, grilling, and other cooking operations. Commercial shortenings, for the most part, are mixtures of unsaturated and saturated fatty acids combined with glycerol.

Vegetable Oils

Vegetable oils for general and specialized uses include those from a single source and blends of several different vegetable oils. The most widely used vegetable oils include corn oil, cottonseed oil, soybean oil, olive oil, and peanut oil. Safflower, sunflower, and sesame seed oils are more unsaturated than the other common oils and therefore are being incorporated into many new products. Most vegetable oils are deodorized, bleached, and clarified for use in foods, but any of these processes may be omitted in the processing of specialized oils. The quality of vegetable oils can deteriorate from exposure to air, light, and moisture. Oils also can become cloudy under cold conditions if they have not been *winterized,* a process that keeps them clear at refrigerator temperatures. Cooking oils not processed in this way become solids at low temperatures.

Oils and Shortenings for Deep-Fat Frying

Shortenings and oils that were specifically designed for good performance in deep-fat frying are best for food service use. Oils with high smoking points are needed to help prevent fat breakdown. A minimum smoke point of not less than 426°F should be specified.

Fat and Oil Specifications

Before products for deep-fat frying, baking, and general-purpose cooking are purchased, detailed information about their ingredients and performance should be obtained from their manufacturers. Specifications for these products may be similar to the following:

1. Oil, mixed (cottonseed, soybean, and corn), 5-gallon container
2. Shortening, all vegetable, high ratio, hydrogenated, 50-pound container
3. Shortening, all vegetable, all purpose (smoking point 435°F [223°C]), hydrogenated, 50-pound container
4. Shortening, liquid, all vegetable with stabilizer (smoking point 440°F [227°C]), three 10-quart, six 5-quart, or six 1-gallon containers per case

Butter

By law, butter must contain no less than 80 percent milk fat. It may or may not contain salt and coloring. The U.S. grades for butter are based on flavor, body or texture, salt, and color. The grades, based on a numerical point system, are U.S. Grade AA (score of 93), U.S. Grade A (score of 92), and U.S. Grade B (score of 90). Many states also have established grades for butter. Purchase units for butter include pound prints, chips, patties, and cubes. Local suppliers can offer information about the availability of various forms that meet specific needs. The quality desired, style (prints, chips, and so forth), number of chips per pound, and total weight of the container should be included in a specification for butter.

Margarine

Margarine is manufactured under federal standards of identity and must contain 80 percent fat, which may be of approved animal or vegetable origin. The kinds of fat used in the manufacture of margarine must be listed on the label. If animal fat is used, the margarine must be manufactured under government inspection. Other ingredients include milk, salt, flavoring, color, emulsifiers, and preservatives. Fortification of margarine with 15,000 IUs of vitamin A per pound is mandatory; vitamin D fortification is optional. Margarine for cooking can be purchased in 1-pound packages. For table use, chips and patties are available in different sizes. Many states have laws requiring food service operators to inform customers when margarine is used as a table spread. The information needed in written specifications is similar to that needed for butter.

☐ Grains and Cereals

Food service operations, especially those that prepare bakery products from scratch, may select several kinds of flours. Pasta and rice products are basic elements of the menu in health care institutions, as are breakfast cereals.

Types of Flour

Several types of flour made from different kinds of wheat are available for specific uses. Flours are classified by their density (hard, semihard, or soft), color, protein strength, and use. Hard or bread flours have a higher protein content than other types of flour. These proteins help form gluten, the strong, elastic structure needed in yeast-leavened doughs.

All-Purpose Flours

All-purpose flours can be blends of hard wheat flours, soft wheat flours, or both hard and soft wheat flours. Although all-purpose flours are suitable for many purposes, they are not as satisfactory as bread flour for baking high-rising breads. However, all-purpose flour can be used for almost any other baked product with excellent results. All-purpose flour is available bleached or unbleached. Self-rising, all-purpose flour also is available; this flour contains baking powder, baking soda, and salt.

Pastry and Cake Flours

Pastry and cake flours usually are milled from soft wheats and are used mainly in pies, cakes, and other desserts. These flours have a lower protein content and a higher starch content than other flours. In purchasing white flour products, the buyer should specify that the flour be enriched with thiamin, riboflavin, niacin, and iron. Fifty and 100-pound bags are the most convenient sizes for food service use.

Whole Wheat or Graham Flour

Whole wheat or graham flour is made from the entire wheat kernel with only the outer bran layer removed. Because the wheat germ, which is high in fat, is left in whole wheat flour, it becomes stale or rancid when not stored properly.

Rye Flour

Rye flour, made from rye grain, contains the proteins needed for gluten formation in bread baking, but not in the same proportion as in wheat flour. For this reason, some wheat flour is used in rye bread recipes.

Soy Flour

Soy flour, with varying amounts of fat removed, is high in protein. Incorporation of some soy flour into bakery products improves their protein content, moistness, and tenderness.

Flour Specifications

Specifications for flours commonly include the percentage of protein required and the ash content. The following examples illustrate suggested specifications for some wheat flours:

1. Flour, wheat, white, all-purpose enriched, 0.46 percent maximum ash, 9 percent minimum protein on 14 percent moisture basis, 50-pound bag
2. Flour, wheat, bread, enriched, 0.46 percent maximum ash, 9 percent minimum protein on 14 percent moisture basis, 50-pound bag
3. Flour, whole wheat or graham, 1.9 percent maximum ash, 11 percent minimum protein on 14 percent moisture basis, 25-pound bag

Types of Pasta

Enriched macaroni products are made from wheat. High-quality macaroni products are made from a hard, amber durum wheat, which yields a glutinous flour. The wheat is milled into a golden-toned, coarse product called semolina, into granules that contain more flour, or into flour itself. Water is added to a mixture of durum meals or flour, semolina, and farina to make a dough that is forced through dies to make tubular macaroni products and cordlike spaghetti. Because enrichment of these products with thiamin, riboflavin, niacin, and iron is not mandatory, the buyer must specify that the product be enriched. Macaroni products can be made with other kinds of wheat flours, so durum wheat pasta products should be specified for high quality.

Noodle products are similar in composition to macaroni except that they contain liquid eggs, frozen eggs, dried eggs, egg yolks, dried yolks, or any combination of these at a minimum level of 5.5 percent. As for macaroni products, enrichment is optional and, if desired, should be stated in the specification.

Pasta Specifications

Examples of pasta specifications include the following:

1. Macaroni, shell, durum, enriched, small, 10-pound box
2. Egg noodles, durum, enriched, broad, 10-pound box
3. Spaghetti, durum, enriched, long, 10-pound box

Cornmeal

Cornmeal, made from white or yellow corn, is available in either coarse or fine grinds. Enrichment with B vitamins and iron is common but not mandatory; calcium is another optional enrichment ingredient. Regular cornmeal, which contains most of the corn kernel, contains more than 3.5 percent fat. Degermed cornmeal has a fat content of less than 2.25 percent. Self-rising cornmeal, with added baking soda, baking powder, and salt, also can be purchased. Common purchase units are 5- or 25-pound bags. The size that best suits an institution's needs should be selected. If only small amounts are used at any one time, smaller bags are easier to handle. A sample specification for cornmeal would include the following information: yellow, enriched, coarse, 25-pound bag.

Types of Rice

Rice can be classified as short, medium, or long grain. Each type has different cooking characteristics. For example, short-grain rice tends to be stickier after cooking and is suitable for use in recipes in which it is used as an extender and binder. Both medium- and long-grain rice remain separate and more distinct in form after cooking. Varieties of rice include Pearl (American and California), Short Grain (Calora, Magnolia, Zenith), and Medium Grain (Blue Rose, Early Prolific). Rice is available in several forms: regular milled white, parboiled or converted white, precooked white, and brown or husked.

Regular White Rice

Regular milled white rice has the outer hull removed and is polished. Because this processing removes significant amounts of B vitamins and some of the minerals, enrichment is desirable and should be specified in the purchase order. A sample specification for white rice would include the following information: milled, long grain, enriched, U.S. Grade No. 1, 25-pound bag.

Converted Rice

Parboiled or converted rice is regular white rice treated to retain its B vitamins by either parboiling or subjecting the rice to steam pressure before hulling. After cooking, the grains tend to be more separate and plump and have better holding qualities than regular white rice.

Precooked Rice

Precooked rice is milled, cooked, and dehydrated. It usually is enriched.

Brown Rice

Brown rice has only the rough outer husk removed and thus has a higher calorie, protein, and mineral content than enriched white rice. The firmer texture and characteristic nutty flavor have helped increase the popularity of brown rice. It is well suited to many kinds of recipes and is a staple for vegetarian fare. The specification information needed is similar to that for other kinds of rice.

Wild Rice

Wild rice is not actually a rice but, rather, the seed of a grasslike plant. Because it is more expensive, it usually is purchased as part of a mixture that includes white or brown rice and that often is preseasoned. Relatively small quantities of wild rice produce large cooked yields because wild rice continues to absorb water throughout the cooking process.

Breakfast Cereals

Many kinds of hot cooked cereals can be found on menus in health care facilities. These include oatmeal (rolled oats), farina, grits, cream of wheat, cream of rice, and rolled wheat. Regular, quick-cooking, and instant forms are available for many of these products. Except for the whole wheat products, enrichment should be specified.

Ready-to-eat breakfast cereals add great variety to breakfast selections. Individual boxes and ready-to-serve individual bowl packs are available for the most popular varieties. If patients are unable to handle individual boxes, bulk retail packages should be considered. These are less expensive but require more labor to serve. Sweetened cereals cost more per ounce than unsweetened cereals.

Following are sample specifications for two types of breakfast cereal:

1. Farina, enriched, regular, six 5-pound packages per case
2. Cereal, whole wheat meal, malted, six 5-pound packages per case

☐ Other Staples

Many other food items are staples in food service operations, but purchasing decisions for these are easier to make than for the products covered thus far. For example, many kinds of prepared bread and bakery products are available. Developing specifications requires a knowledge of local market offerings and terminology. For breads, specifications should include size or weight of loaf, number of slices, and enrichment. Although federal laws require enrichment of some bread products sold interstate, some states do not require enrichment of breads produced and sold within their boundaries. Frozen bread and roll dough have become very popular because they provide the desirable fresh-baked characteristics with greatly reduced labor and equipment requirements. The quality of products from various vendors as well as cost should be evaluated before purchasing decisions are made.

Their consistent quality and labor-saving advantages make baking mixes an important staple in many food service operations. Cake mixes, pudding mixes, quick bread mixes, and other dessert mixes are just a few examples of the products available that can add variety to the menu at a low labor cost. When purchasing such products, the food buyer should compare the product quality and yield from various brands and calculate the cost per serving.

☐ Beverages

Popular beverages include coffee, tea, cocoa, and carbonated potables. Customer preferences, food cost, and available equipment are factors to consider when selecting these products. Chapter 21 describes beverage-dispensing services.

Coffee

Different blends of coffee beans result in the unique flavor characteristic of various brands. Some varieties and origins of coffee beans include:

- *Armenia*—full bodied (Colombia)
- *Blue Mountain*—full bodied (Jamaica)
- *Cooptepec*—full bodied (Mexico)
- *Java*—mild, good quality (Indonesia)
- *Marciabo*—light, rich (Venezuela)
- *Santo*—somewhat acid, high quality (Brazil)

Other varieties are described in *SPECS: The Comprehensive Foodservice Purchasing and Specification Manual.*

Selection should be based on consumers' preference and the amount they are willing to pay. Specifications for coffee should include: roast, grind, percentage of types desired in the blend, and packaging. In that the volume of coffee purchased by most food service operations is significant, the food buyer should order several brands "in the bean" and send to the Coffee Brewing Center for quality evaluation. Results should be used in writing coffee specifications.

Tea

Tea quality depends on the altitude, soil, and climate at which it is grown and the processing technique used. There are three types of tea, with varying classes for each type: green, oolong, and black. Teas are marketed based on their geographic area of origin.

Cocoa

Cocoa is processed by roasting, grinding, and defatting the niles of cocoa beans. Cocoa must have at least 22 percent but not more than 35 percent cocoa butter. The higher the cocoa butter content, the richer the product. Cocoa that has been treated with an alkali during processing is darker in color, has a less acidic flavor, and is more soluble.

Specifications for Other Staples

When writing specifications for other miscellaneous items, such as spices, condiments, sweeteners, and specialty beverages, the various brands available should be considered and the quality of each evaluated. Prices for various package sizes should be compared, and the food buyer should keep up-to-date on price trends. Package sizes, particularly for spices, should be considered. Some may be used in much larger quantities than others and should be purchased in 1-pound or larger units; those used only occasionally should be purchased in the smaller retail market packages so that they retain their quality until used. If available, federal standards and grades should be used. Federal grades have been defined for honey, maple syrup, nuts, olives, pickles, and catsup. Federal standards of identity also are available for many products.

The following specifications for some food staples may be useful in developing others:

1. Walnuts, U.S. No. 1, small pieces, latest season crop, six 5-pound boxes per case
2. Olives, green, giant, U.S. Grade A or Fancy, six No. 10 cans per case
3. Pickles, dill, thin, cross-cut, fresh pack, U.S. Grade A or Fancy, six No. 10 cans per case
4. Honey, light amber, U.S. Grade A, extracted, six 5-pound containers per case

☐ Small Equipment and Utensils

Adequate and appropriate equipment and utensils are required for maintaining control in preparation and service. These items are not classified as equipment, and there is no depreciation account for their replacement. This class of equipment includes measuring devices, pans, knives, cutting boards, scales, thermometers, and portioning utensils. Careful selection of utensils can influence work efficiency, product quality, portion control, and initial cost.

General selection factors include appearance, durability, cost, and satisfaction for specific use. Most utensils are made according to standard manufacturer's specifications. Thus, the purchasing agent usually selects the items from a manufacturer's or equipment supplier's catalog rather than by writing a detailed specification.

Measuring Devices

Liquid and dry measuring devices range in size from a cup to a gallon. Liquid measures should have a pouring lip, and dry measures should have a level top. Measures should be made of durable materials, because accuracy can be affected by dents and bends in lightweight metals. Both measures and measuring spoons are available in either stainless steel or heavy-duty aluminum. Although aluminum may be satisfactory, the extra cost of stainless steel may be balanced by its longer life. There is also some current concern over the relationship between the use of aluminum utensils and Alzheimer's disease. For safety reasons, glass measures should not be used in institutional food service departments.

Pans

Preparation equipment should be standardized as much as possible. Perhaps the most important application of that principle is in the selection of pans. Most standardized recipes are based on the standard pan that measures about 12 by 20 inches—the size that fits the openings in the hot-food serving table or cart. Standard pans, used for many purposes such as cooking, holding, and storing foods under refrigeration, are available in 2½-, 4-, 6-, and 8-inch depths. Smaller pans of several sizes are based on the 12-by-20-inch serving table opening: half-sizes measuring 12 by 6⅔ inches (three to fill an opening) and other smaller sizes.

Considerations other than size that apply to pan selection are type and weight of the metal and design. Both stainless steel and aluminum pans are available. For stainless steel pans, 18- to 22-gauge metal usually is used. Standard pans have either solid or perforated bottoms.

Pan design is important for storage reasons. Pans that taper slightly from top to bottom nest well and can be stacked without becoming wedged together. Covers come in several designs: flat, hinged, and domed.

Besides the serving table pans, sheet pans (bun pans) also are needed. Sheet pans are 18 by 26 inches or 20 by 24 inches, with a depth of ¾ inch to about 2 inches. Sheet pans are usually made of 16-gauge aluminum.

If pots, kettles, saucepans, and stockpots are needed for food preparation, heavy-gauge metal pans are more durable and will help prevent scorching and sticking. Saucepans and stockpots are available in various thicknesses of aluminum and stainless steel as well as other metals. Although the bright appearance and durability of stainless steel are desirable, this material does not conduct heat as evenly as heavyweight aluminum when used in surface cooking. Handles should be sturdy, and large saucepans should have an additional bracket handle on the side opposite the long handle to make lifting easier and safer.

Pan sizes should be selected keeping in mind the kind of cooking to be done and matching burner sizes on ranges with circular heating units. Four-quart saucepans are useful for many purposes; however, the capacity of small pans should be based on portion sizes and the total quantity needed of any product. Lids should be purchased for pans to be used in surface cooking because they help to reduce the cooking time needed for some products and thus save energy.

Knives

The quality of a knife is determined by the material of the blade and handle and its shape and construction. Most knife blades are made of carbon steel. A high-carbon steel blade has the finest cutting edge when it is properly cared for and sharpened. When chrome is added to the alloy, the result is stainless steel. When vanadium is added, the blade is stronger and tends to hold its cutting edge longer.

Knife handles can be made of wood, plastic, wood and plastic combinations, even bone. Possibly more important than the material used in the handle is how the handle is attached to the blade. High-quality knives have a continuous piece of metal extending from the knife tip through the handle. In such knives, the handle is usually made of two pieces that are attached to the blade with heavy rivets. The blade must be well fastened into the handle, or it will loosen with use. Several types of knives are needed including French cooks' knives that have a 10-inch blade for chopping, paring knives, utility or boning knives with slim 5- or 6-inch blades for trimming, and carving knives for slicing.

Cutting Boards

Cutting boards must provide sanitary cutting surfaces that are thoroughly cleanable and that will not absorb juices from foods or allow food particles to collect. Hard-composition rubber or plastic cutting boards are superior to the wooden variety and are frequently required by local or state health departments. Small 10-by-12-inch boards are convenient for employees to use in cutting small amounts of food. In the cooking or salad preparation areas, 18-by-24-inch boards are adequate.

Scales

Scales are needed for checking deliveries, weighing ingredients in food preparation, and controlling serving portions. Scales must be accurate, easy to use and read, durable, and easy to clean. Types used in food service facilities include floor scales; suspended platforms; overhead tracks (in large facilities); built-ins; and portion, counter, and table scales. Some of the new models can generate a printout with the date, time, and weight of the product.

The capacity of bakers' scales ranges from 5 to 20 pounds. For all-purpose use in preparation areas, a 25- to 50-pound capacity scale that will weigh in fractions of an ounce is ideal. For controlling portion sizes, a scale with quarter-ounce gradations and a capacity of up to 2 pounds should be available.

Thermometers

Thermometers are essential in the control of food quality. Oven thermometers should have a temperature range of 200° to 600°F (93° to 315°C). Several bimetallic thermometers with a tubular metal stem equipped with a dial or digital temperature indicator should be available to monitor temperature of food products.

Thermometers for refrigerators, freezers, and dry storage areas also are needed. In newer models of cold storage equipment, they can be built in. Periodic checks using a freestanding shelf thermometer will validate their accuracy. Deep-fat thermometers are essential for frying equipment that is not thermostatically controlled.

Portioning Utensils

Portioning equipment such as scoops, ladles, and spoons should be available in both the production and service areas. Scoops are numbered from 6 to 60, the number referring to the number of scoops it takes to equal 1 quart. Equivalent measures of scoops in cups, tablespoons, and teaspoons are printed in most quantity food cookbooks and manufacturers' catalogs.

Portioning ladles, usually made of 18-gauge stainless steel, are available in sizes of 1, 2, 4, 6, 8 ounces and larger. Most are labeled with the number of ounces they hold. Large ladles, which hold 1 to 4 quarts, may be needed to transfer foods from steam-jacketed kettles or stockpots to serving pans.

In addition to scoops and ladles, stainless steel and heavy-duty plastic spoons are needed. The spoons are made with varied handle lengths and with solid, slotted, or perforated bowls.

☐ Service Supplies

The selection of appropriate service supplies (trays, dinnerware, tableware, hollowware, glassware, and disposables) is important for presenting meals attractively. The initial investment; the replacement cost; labor, water, and energy costs; and waste-disposal costs are essential factors to consider. The kind and size of trays required for patient and resident service depends on the delivery system used (these are described in chapter 20). Whatever system is used, preserving food quality is of prime importance. Trays should be made of durable materials that will not bend, dent, warp, or lose their shape over continuous use. Trays of hard rubber, plastic, and molded fiberglass in a variety of shapes and sizes are designed to withstand repeated washing. Attractively colored trays that are plain or have designs molded under a protective surface layer eliminate the need for place mats at all meals.

The type of dinnerware chosen may be reusable, single-service disposable, or a combination of these. *Reusable ware* should be durable, easy to clean, stain resistant, and attractive. Its colors and designs should be compatible with the trays and the food items served. If reusable dinnerware is purchased, vitrified china is recommended. Three weights are available: thick, hotel, and medium. However, weight does not necessarily indicate strength; only the quality of materials and the manufacturing methods determine durability.

Food service directors who prefer china because of its appearance but also want to minimize breakage have found that dinnerware made from glass components and modified to resist breakage, crazing, chipping, and staining is very satisfactory. A number of sizes and shapes, plain white or with designs, are available. Food service departments that use microwave ovens for heating foods prior to service find these dishes very useful.

Another type of dinnerware, light in weight and easy to handle, is made of melamine plastic. Melamine costs less than conventional dinnerware and is more resistant to breakage. However, melamine dishes lose their finish with use, thus are susceptible to stains and scratches and are difficult to sanitize.

The tableware (flatware and hollowware) chosen for institutional use should be designed for durability and attractiveness. Eating utensils made of stainless steel meet both these criteria because they have the added advantages of being tarnishproof and easy to clean. The size of flatware selected for tray service should be based on ease of handling and size of the tray. Choosing the same size and pattern for both patient and nonpatient service reduces sorting and washing time and replacement cost.

The types and sizes of beverage serviceware needed vary among food service departments. The type of material selected (glass, plastic, or single-service) is influenced by service requirements and available labor and warewashing equipment. Whichever type of serviceware selected should be durable, easy to clean, and suitable for the portion sizes served.

Single-service disposable dinnerware and tableware are used in part or exclusively by some food service departments. Customer acceptance; local regulations; temperature retention capability; and supply, labor, storage, and disposal costs should be analyzed before selection. Disposables, available in a variety of materials, colors, and designs, should be selected for their strength and rigidity on the basis of service needs. Attractive geometric, floral, or modern patterns can enhance tray or cafeteria service. Plates used for entrees should resist cutting, sagging, and soaking. Beverage containers should be appropriate for maintaining the temperature of either cold and hot liquids. Eating utensils must be sturdy enough not to break.

☐ Summary

The role of a health care food service purchasing agent is not simply to approve purchase requisitions submitted by the food service director. Purchasers must be familiar with current quality standards established by the USDA, national and local legislation as it pertains to wholesomeness, and quality of all categories of food and ingredients (especially meats and meat products, given that they comprise the biggest cost outlay).

Purchasers must work cooperatively with food service department managers to ensure proper production scheduling, storage times, and shelf life of products—without overstocking or understocking inventory. This balancing act must be done in keeping with meeting customer expectations while staying within a prescribed budget. A key component of this effort is writing up purchase specifications, which depend on USDA mandates as well as IMPS, NAMP, and MBG standards (for meat and meat product purchases). The chapter described the federal grade stamps and inspection marks used for meat, poultry, and eggs, as well as the USDC standards and PUFI inspection mark for seafood.

Even the most nutritionally sound and carefully prepared foods will not meet customer expectations in the presentation area without tastefully selected service supplies. Making appropriate tray, dinnerware, tableware, hollowware, glassware, and disposable ware purchases also is a key purchasing responsibility. Therefore, texture, color, and durability of service equipment must be synchronized as closely as possible with the aesthetic features of menu offerings.

☐ Bibliography

The Almanac of the Canning, Freezing, Preserving Industry. 71st ed. Westminster, MD: Judge and Sons, 1986.

American Egg Board. *A Scientist Speaks about Egg Products.* Park Ridge, IL: American Egg Board, 1981.

American Meat Institute. *Answers to Predictable Questions Consumers Ask about Meat.* Washington, DC: American Meat Institute, 1982.

Blue Goose Purchasing Guide to Fresh Fruits and Vegetables. Fullerton, CA: Blue Goose, Inc., 1980.

Folsom, L. A., editor. *The Professional Chef: Foodservice Buying and Specifying Guide and Product Delivery.* Boston: Cahners, 1979.

Food and Nutrition Service. *Food Service Purchasing Pointers for School Food Service.* Washington, DC: U.S. Department of Agriculture, 1977.

Food Purchasing Specifications for Foodservices. Madison, WI: Wisconsin Department of Agriculture, Trade, and Consumer Protection, 1978.

Kotschevar, L. H., and Terrell, M. *Foodservice Planning: Layout and Equipment.* 3rd ed. New York City: Macmillan, 1986.

National Association of Meat Purveyors. *Meat Buyer's Guide.* McLean, VA: NAMP, 1984.

National Association of Meat Purveyors. *Meat Buyer's Guide to Portion Control Meat Cuts.* McLean, VA: NAMP, 1984.

National Association of Meat Purveyors. *Meat Buyer's Guide to Standardized Meat Cuts.* McLean, VA: NAMP, 1984.

National Restaurant Association. *Current Issue Report: A Review of U.S. Food Grading and Inspection Programs.* Chicago: NRA, 1989.

O'Neill, W., editor. *The Packer's 1986 Fresh Produce Foodservice Directory.* Shawnee Mission, KS: Vance, 1986.

Pedderson, R. B. *Foodservice and Hotel Purchasing.* Boston: Cahners, 1981.

Pedderson, R. B. *SPECS: The Comprehensive Foodservice Purchasing and Specification Manual.* Boston: Cahners, 1977.

Peterkin, B., and Evans, B. *Food Purchasing Guide for Group Feeding.* Agriculture Handbook 284. Washington, DC: Government Printing Office, Superintendent of Documents, 1985.

Produce Marketing Association. *Produce 101.* Newark, DE: Produce Marketing Association, Foodservice Division, 1992.

Reed, L. *SPECS: The Comprehensive Foodservice Purchasing and Specification Manual.* 2nd ed. New York City: Van Nostrand Reinhold, 1992.

Spears, M. C., and Vaden, A. G. *Foodservice Organizations: A Managerial and Systems Approach.* Chapter 7. New York City: John Wiley and Sons, 1985.

United Fresh Fruit and Vegetable Association. *Fruits and Vegetables: Facts and Pointers.* Washington, DC: UFFVA, 1985.

Warfel, M. C., and Frank, H. W. *The Professional Food Buyer: Standards, Principles and Procedures.* Berkeley, CA: McCutchan, 1979.

Chapter 17

Purchasing

☐ Introduction

Food purchasing plays an essential role in meeting customer needs and ensuring the success of the health care food service operation. Aside from being well versed in product selection and food quality standards as discussed in the preceding chapter, the purchasing agent (or buyer) should be knowledgeable about product availability, trends directing customer expectations, the purchasing process, market conditions, production demand, and purchasing methods. The buyer/purchasing agent provides leadership in establishing partnerships with distributors and serves on the product evaluation team. Knowledge of the food distribution system, the structure of wholesale markets in which purchasing occurs, and ethical issues that arise in purchasing also is important to the buyer role.

This chapter will discuss trends that influence purchasing decisions and the purchasing process. Specific trends explored are continuous quality improvement, technology, distributors' changing product line, and the changing role of distributors' sales representatives.

Food marketing and wholesaling will be examined within the context of a larger food distribution system that tracks the flow food from its place as a raw product grown by a farmer to an item for consumer consumption in the health care environment. The intermediary points—food assembly, grading, storing, processing, transport, and the like—are translated to the food service area and expedited to buyer and distributor.

A 10-step procurement model will be broken down into its component parts and examined, starting with assessing needs for a new product, service, or piece of equipment, and ending with receipt and distribution of items throughout the production area in a food service operation. Buyers and department directors will be able to adapt the model to suit their individual needs. The buyer's responsibilities and optimum qualifications needed to perform the functions of procurement will be delineated.

Methods of "power-purchasing" strategies will be described. Some of these are group purchasing organizations, just-in-time purchasing, one-stop purchasing, and prime vendor agreements. Their advantages and disadvantages are explored, along with other distinctions— such as centralized versus noncentralized and contract versus noncontract purchasing.

The chapter will give an in-depth look at how vendors are selected, the buyer–vendor relationship, and ethics issues that can arise in the purchasing process. Finally, a brief "how-to" list of computer-assisted procurement will be given. (The term *buyer* will be used throughout this chapter to describe the individual primarily responsible for acquiring food products, equipment, and services for the health care food service department.)

☐ Trends Influencing Purchasing Decisions

Like all other functions of the food service department, purchasing is influenced by, and must respond to, changes in the internal and external environments. Trends that will affect the purchasing function include:

- Continuous quality improvement
- Technology
- Distributors' changing product lines
- Changing role of distributor's sales representatives

An overview of some these trends was presented in chapter 1. Specific impact of these trends on the purchasing function is discussed below.

Continuous Quality Improvement

Purchasing is an area that should be integrated with continuous quality improvement (CQI). Because CQI is designed to be customer driven, it has a direct link with product selection. If food service is to provide products and services to meet the demands of different customers, it is imperative that feedback be obtained from the patients, employees, administrators, and guests. Unfortunately, data collected on what customers really want too often are ignored by food service staff who think they know better what customers desire. Instead of using information collected to identify new products and develop or modify specifications, the information is ignored.

Continuous quality improvement can be used to enhance the relationship between the food service department and brokers and distributors. This is particularly critical in a prime vendor arrangement. Open communication, sharing of information, and being customer focused are essential elements in the CQI process. Benefits include faster introduction of new products, provision of product information that will meet a specific operation's needs, and enhanced training on product use and marketing. (A more detailed discussion of vendor relations is presented later in this chapter.)

In addition to selecting and evaluating products, a product evaluation team should be empowered to identify the need for new products, select them, evaluate their acceptability, and recommend purchases The team may be composed of food production employees, the production manager, the buyer, tray line and cafeteria employees, and customers.

Group purchasing organizations can implement CQI in providing services to their members. The process should help overcome some of the barriers described later in this chapter.

Technology

The most rapidly changing trend that affects food service distributors and health care operations is to be observed in technological developments, which will influence distributors' interactions with customers, order placement, and inventory control. Predictions are that by the year 2000, electronic data interchange (EDI) will replace face-to-face meetings and other modes of communication such as the telephone, facsimile (fax) machine, and written message. Described as a totally automated process whereby data are transmitted, received, and processed by computers without direct interaction between sender and receiver, EDI already is processing orders. By the year 2000, 80 percent of all ordering will be done directly by the buyer using personal computers with software distributed by a specific distributor or generic direct-order-entry software application that processes purchase orders. Electronic data interchange will be used to monitor customers' buying habits and provide nutritional breakdown of all products in the distributor's line, as well as assess market outlook and menu suggestions.

Advantages to using EDI systems for food service order placement include immediate order confirmation; notification of out-of-stock items, with a list of suggested substitutions; automatic price updates; menu analysis; inventory control; and portion control. The expansion of cost-effective radio frequency (RF) communication systems will provide at least three benefits: immediate customer access to the distributor's computer while decreasing telephone expenses; the transfer of inventory data to a personal computer within the food service operation; and bar-code scanning that can facilitate deliveries and receiving. In the future, any member of the management team can use electronic data bases from the distributor to obtain product information including a color photo of the product, unit cost, and other data needed in planning menus and analyzing cost implications of different menu items and menu mixes. The use of electronic mail (e-mail) also is predicted to increase.

Distributors' Changing Product Line

Distribution will continue to be a people business in which service is the name of the game for distinguishing one distributor from another. The move toward "full-line" food service distribution is predicted to continue, with distributors' product mix expanding and the number of items available greater than ever before. Food distributors will become the primary source for supplies and equipment to food service operations. Specialty distributors in meat, poultry, paper products, and so on will be forced to expand their product line to compete with full-line distributors for national accounts. The specialty distributor of the 1980s will become the broad-line distributor of the 1990s. Distributors will place more emphasis on packaging relative to its impact on the environment and the "green movement." They will work in partnership with food service organizations and the packaging industry to develop packages that are less dense and contain recycled materials.

To become more competitive, distributors are offering *value-added services,* those services that go beyond simply completing the delivery accurately and on time. Value-added services to providers include:

- Computerized services that incorporate EDI and advanced technology
- Advice on new products, nutrition information, food cost, and so on
- Continuing education seminars
- Menu development, merchandising, and marketing services
- Floral service
- Consulting services on design, layout, and equipment
- Coordination of a food service operation's recycling efforts

Today's competitive environment requires distributors and their sales representatives to continue to provide and expand value-added services to retain customers and acquire new ones.

Changing Role of Distributors' Sales Representatives

Distributors' sales representatives (DSRs) will become consultants and problem solvers rather than mere order takers. Because purchase orders will be processed using EDI, DSRs will be trained to be more customer oriented and to provide information on products, packaging, economics, environmental issues, commodities, market trends, inventory control, conditions influencing costs, availability of products and supplies, and promotional and recipe ideas. Each DSR will need to have thorough knowledge of their accounts and of their company's product lines. In effect, they will provide value-added services as a strategy to increase customer loyalty.

☐ Food Marketing and Wholesaling

The food distribution and marketing system is part of the food and fiber system, the largest industrial system in the United States. Using inputs of technology, capital, machinery, fertilizers, chemicals, petroleum, and labor, farmers produce the nation's supply of raw food and fiber products. They then wholesale these basic raw products to the marketing sector of the food and fiber system.

Marketing System

The American food marketing system serves the country's population by supplying farm products in the desired forms and at the appropriate times. The system assembles, grades, stores, processes, packages, transports, wholesales, retails, prices, takes risks on, controls the quality of, merchandises, exchanges ownership of, brands, regulates, develops, and tests most of the food products—old and new—consumed in the United States.

Food processors and manufacturers are a direct-market outlet for vast quantities of raw farm products as well as the source of supplies for hundreds of thousands of distributors. This large, complex system must mesh smoothly to overcome problems of food perishability, seasonal availability, volume, and logistics. To remain dynamic and responsive, the system must provide not only a means for product flow from producer to consumer, but also a communication system for the flow of information about consumer preferences and demands from consumer to producer.

The food marketing system includes more than half a million businesses that employ the equivalent of more than 5 million full-time employees. Persons employed by restaurants and other food service facilities make up almost half of that total. The output of farms in the United States combined with food products from other countries around the world are gathered by wholesalers and distributors within the marketing system and processed to various degrees by the nation's food manufacturers and processors.

Wholesaling

Wholesaling is the link in the marketing system responsible for distributing food from the producer or processor to the retailer. The principal wholesaling activities involve gathering foods from many sources and distributing them to retailers, hotel and restaurant operators, and other institutions.

Because of the extensive number of products available and the variety of items stocked in relatively small amounts in food service operations, food service managers could not possibly search out and deal with the producers and processors of all the food products needed. Conversely, processors could not (in many instances) profitably provide the limited quantities needed by individual food service units. The job of the food wholesaler is to set up an efficient system for gathering the various products in sizable quantities from various producers and processors and then to sell them in smaller quantities to direct users of the materials.

As shown in figure 17-1, the structure of a typical food distribution system, the food wholesaler (who buys and assembles the needed products) is the central figure in the distribution process. Some processors can perform the function of wholesaling through their sales offices and branch warehouses. The fact that processors' sales agents specialize in a limited product line means that they can concentrate their expertise and sales effort on fewer products. These agents do not take title, submit bills, or set prices for the goods sold. Some processors distribute a limited product line or a limited volume of products through food brokers and commissioned agents who act as their sales representatives. This group of intermediaries in the distribution system helps the processors by keeping them informed of current trade conditions and requirements of the market. In turn, the broker's sales staff provides goods and services for the retail and food service trade without taking actual possession of the products for sale. Brokers and commissioned agents are paid by the food processors for their services.

Figure 17-1. The Food Distribution System

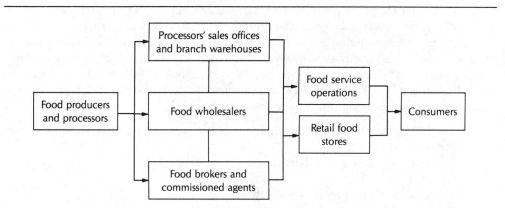

Food wholesalers are classified on the basis of their position and their activities in the marketing system. One category includes full-function wholesalers. *Full-function* wholesalers perform all the marketing functions in varying degrees. Their knowledge of the market, buying methods, and techniques for merchandising items to the best advantage is their strongest asset. Because wholesalers must be able to supply their customers with relatively small quantities at frequent intervals, they purchase large quantities of food and store the food and other goods in the form of stock in inventory. *Full-service* wholesalers extend credit to the customer and deliver goods when ordered. This type of wholesaler is the one most commonly used by food service operations.

In contrast, *limited-function* wholesalers carry a limited product line, may or may not extend credit, and establish order-size requirements for delivery. Processors' sales forces usually fall into this category.

Wholesalers also can be classified according to the types of products they handle. For example, wholesalers that stock a wide variety of goods so that the buyer can obtain a significant percentage of the items needed from one source are known as *general-line* wholesalers. There has been a trend toward expansion of the types and lines of products and services handled by institutional wholesalers so that volume feeding establishments can purchase virtually all their supplies from one wholesaler. This strategy is sometimes called *one-stop shopping.* (More information about this trend is provided later in this chapter.)

In contrast to general-line wholesalers, *specialty wholesalers* handle only one line or a few closely related lines of products. For example, some specialize in perishable products, such as fresh produce; they may handle some frozen fruits and vegetables and other related products as well. The number and economic importance of specialty wholesalers is declining in the American food distribution system.

☐ The Procurement Process

Procuring products and services for the food service department is a complex process involving much more than the buyer simply acquiring products and services from reputable distributors and organizations. The term *procurement* involves a broad range of product selection and purchasing activities required to meet the needs of the food service department.

The process depends on a complex decision-making process that includes determining quality and quantity standards for the facility; specifying and ordering foods that meet those standards; and receiving, storing, and controlling the food supply inventory. (Inventory control, receiving, and storage are discussed in detail in chapter 18.) Effective procurement requires that buyers have immediate access to a great deal of current and accurate information so as to make the best decision given the resources at their disposal.

Buyer's Responsibilities

Responsibility for the procurement process varies depending on the size and philosophy of the health care institution and on available expertise in the food service department. In smaller facilities, the food service director or manager often performs and/or coordinates procurement activities. Large organizations may employ an individual with special training or expertise in procurement. The buyer may be a food service employee if decentralized purchasing is used, or an employee of the purchasing department if the facility has centralized its purchasing activities. Responsibilities of the food buyer include:

- Determining food service department needs in terms of product, equipment, and services
- Selecting the method(s) of purchasing
- Selecting vendor(s)
- Soliciting and awarding bids or contracts
- Placing and following up on orders
- Training and supervising employees in receiving, storage, and issuance of food and supplies
- Establishing and maintaining an inventory control system
- Conducting research, including evaluating new products and conducting value analyses and make–buy studies
- Participating on the product evaluation team
- Maintaining effective vendor relations
- Assessing cost–benefit of value-added services provided by the distributor
- Providing product information such as cost data and nutrition information to others in the food service department
- Tracking changes in market and economic conditions through open communication with DSRs, attending trade and food shows, and keeping abreast of trends by reading trade and professional publications
- Utilizing current technology to facilitate the procurement process
- Maintaining open communication lines throughout the food service department and the larger institution

Buyer's Qualifications

Ideally, a buyer's educational and experiential qualifications should encompass the following areas: food quality; product specifications; computer skills, especially in spreadsheet applications and marketing and distribution channels in the food distribution system (see figure 17-1); and accounting and other business activities associated with purchasing such as soliciting and awarding bids and contracts and performing make–buy analyses. Experience in food production and service also is beneficial. In addition, the buyer should possess certain managerial, interpersonal, and personal attributes. Some of these are organizational skills and a penchant for detail and accuracy; a team mind-set; initiative; good human relations and communication skills; and high ethical standards. Due to the complexity of activities performed, the buyer must be organized and follow through on tasks. Good human relations and communication skills are essential because he or she must meet the needs of several individuals in the food service department and communicate these needs to DSRs, members of group purchasing organizations (GPOs), and all other parties with whom the buyer interacts. Not only must the buyer demonstrate initiative in continuously assessing opportunities to increase or maintain food quality, but he or she must do so while decreasing cost whenever feasible. Attention to detail is critical because accuracy in purchase orders and inventory affects operating costs and service delivery. The buyer must maintain high ethical standards at all times, avoiding conflict of interest and kickbacks, for example. (More will be said on ethics in purchasing later in this chapter.)

No matter who has ultimate authority for the procurement function, a procurement specialist or the food service manager, the individual must maintain high standards in product quality. The buyer must continuously assess how to obtain products, equipment, and services to meet the needs of various components of the food service department while remaining within the financial constraints imposed on the operation.

Steps in the Food Service Procurement Process

As illustrated in figure 17-2, the procurement process in a food service department is a 10-step sequence of activities. This process may be adjusted as needed to accommodate a particular facility or organizational structure. The following sections discuss the procurement-process steps, and more information on receiving and storing is provided in chapter 18.

Figure 17-2. The Procurement Process

1. Complete needs assessment
   - Evaluate menu
   - Standardize recipe
   - Gather input from product evaluation team
   - Gather input from management staff
   - Forecast production demand

2. Select purchasing method(s)
   - Consider size and philosophy of operation
   - Determine purchase volume
   - Determine frequency of delivery
   - Consider distributor location
   - Evaluate department storage facilities
   - Determine available personnel

3. Develop approved vendor/distributor list
   - Decide whether to use a prime vendor

4. Establish and maintain inventory system
   - Just-in-time purchasing?
   - Perpetual inventory?
   - Physical inventory?
   - Consider value of inventory
   - Determine frequency of delivery

5. Determine order quantity
   - Forecast menu portions
   - Determine standard portions
   - Determine serving supplies
   - Assess food on hand

6. Obtain bid/price quotes
   - Develop specifications for each item
   - Obtain best prices/terms

7. Place order
   - Specify price
   - Specify quantity
   - Specify payment method
   - Distribute copies of order

8. Receive order
   - Request minimum number of shipments

9. Store Order
   - Consider type of food

10. Issue items

Needs Assessment

The purpose of a needs assessment is to determine the operation's requirement for food, supplies, equipment, and services including quality, quantity, and required time frame. Information sources the buyer should rely on in completing the needs assessment include menu(s), standardized recipes, production demand forecasts, input from the product evaluation team and management staff, and the image the operation wants to project. Current and projected needs should be determined. Maintaining a master calendar of catered functions and other special activities that would influence the procurement process is strongly recommended.

Selection of Purchasing Method

The next step in the process is selection of the procurement method(s) most appropriate for a particular facility. Factors influencing the decision may include size and philosophy of the food service operation, purchase volume, frequency of delivery desired, distributors' location, department storage facilities, available personnel and their skill levels, and type of purchasing system—centralized or decentralized, for example. Purchasing methods most frequently used by health care food service providers are discussed later in this chapter.

Approved Vendor/Distributor List

Identification of the vendor/distributor/suppliers with whom the organization will conduct business is a critical step of the procurement process. Specific factors to consider, which are discussed more fully later in this chapter, also may influence the selected method(s) of purchasing. These factors also may determine whether a distributor would meet a particular organization's needs or even conduct business with the facility.

Inventory System

The inventory system established will help determine whether to implement just-in-time purchasing, a perpetual inventory, or a physical inventory (among other choices). It also will determine quantity of supplies maintained on hand, value of the inventory (in other words, how much money is tied up in inventory and unavailable for other uses), and frequency of delivery.

Order Quantity

The planned menu tells the buyer what kinds of food are needed, but only careful planning can ensure a supply of food sufficient for producing the anticipated number of meals with a minimum amount of leftovers. The quantities of food needed can be calculated by following four steps:

1. Forecast as accurately as possible the number of serving portions required for each item on the menu. When a selective menu is used, the forecast can be based on records of the number of selections previously made when the same combinations were served.
2. Determine a standard portion size for each food item. The standard portion size should correspond to the portion size stated on the standardized recipes to be used. Standardized recipes also should state the amount of each ingredient to be purchased for the stated yield.
3. Determine the quantities of food supplies required for the number of serving portions needed.
4. Check the amount of food on hand in refrigerated, frozen, and dry storage areas and subtract that amount from the quantity needed for the planned menus. Prepare a list of supplies that must be purchased and a list of those to be requisitioned from the storeroom.

Regardless of the purchasing method used, order quantities should be large enough to make transactions economically worthwhile for vendors. The advantages of price comparison and product choice are lost if small orders are split among several vendors because of price.

Bid/Price Quotes, Order Placement, and Record Keeping

If purchasing is centralized, the food service department usually completes a purchase requisition form like the one shown in figure 17-3 to inform the purchasing agent of the quantity and quality of specific foods to be ordered. The purchase requisition should contain complete specifications for each item, the unit of purchase (dozen or case, for example), the total quantity of each item, and the requested delivery date. In addition, a vendor and a price may be suggested; however, the purchasing agent is responsible for obtaining bids and awarding the purchase to the supplier quoting the best prices and terms. This approach works best when the director of the food service department and the purchasing agent can pool their knowledge and communicate freely.

Administrative policy usually requires that purchase requisitions be approved by a designated person in the food service department before being sent to the purchasing department. The purchase requisition should be prepared in multiple copies, the number depending on the organization's record-keeping system. At least one copy should be kept on file in the food service department.

Whether purchasing is done by a purchasing department or by the food service department, a purchase order should always be used to inform the vendor of specific requirements. A purchase order is a legal document authorizing a supplier to deliver merchandise in accordance with the terms stated on the form. Purchase order forms, such as the example shown in figure 17-4, are standardized by the institution and used by all departments.

The information contained in these forms includes the name and address of the supplier; a complete specification for each item, unless the vendor already has the specification on file (in which case the specification number can be used along with a brief description); the total quantity of each item ordered; the price per unit quoted by the vendor; the total price for the amount ordered; the terms of delivery; and the method of payment. The number of copies of the purchase order to be made varies among institutions, but because it is the record of merchandise ordered and the form used to check the receipt of deliveries, all departments dealing with supplies or with payments need copies.

Order Receipt, Storage, Issuance of Items

Delivery schedule requests should be considered carefully. Increased transportation costs will affect food costs if deliveries are requested more often than necessary. The delivery schedule required depends on the size of the institution, its geographic location, its storage facilities, and the size of the food service staff. In general, however, economy of food delivery and storage can be achieved as follows:

- Meat, poultry, and fish delivered once a week or less frequently, depending on whether the products are chilled or frozen
- Fresh produce delivered once or twice a week, depending on the storage space available and the quantities needed
- Canned goods and staples delivered weekly, semimonthly, monthly, or quarterly, depending on the storage space available, quantities needed, and price quotes for specific volume
- Milk, milk products, bread, and baked goods delivered daily or every other day, although suppliers should be consulted because many dairies and bakeries have reduced delivery frequency
- Butter, eggs, and cheese delivered weekly
- Frozen foods delivered weekly or semimonthly, depending on the storage space available, usage rate, and price quotes for the quantities needed

Upon delivery, acceptance, and storage, items can be dispensed as needed to production areas.

Figure 17-3. Example of a Purchase Requisition

PURCHASE REQUISITION					

To: Purchasing Office   Requisition No.: _____

Date: _____   Purchase Order No.: _____

From: _____   Date Required: _____

Unit	Total Quantity	Description	Suggested Vendor	Unit Cost	Total Cost

Requested by: _____   Approved by: _____   Date Ordered: _____

Figure 17-4. Example of a Purchase Order Form

		PURCHASE ORDER		

To: _____

_____

Purchase Order No.: _____
(Please refer to the above number on all invoices)

Date: _____

Requisition No.: _____

Department: _____

Date Required: _____

Ship to: _____ F.O.B. _____ Via: _____ Terms: _____

Unit	Total Quantity	Description	Price per Unit	Total Cost

Approved by: _____

□ Purchasing Methods

The purchasing method used by the buyer varies depending on the organization's size, philosophy and policies, purchasing volume, and financial stability, as well as the distributor's location and current environmental trends. The most common methods of purchasing used by health care food service facilities include group purchasing, consortium purchasing, prime vendor, one-stop purchasing, just-in-time purchasing, and formal (competitive) and informal (off-the-street) purchasing.

Group Purchasing Organizations

Some institutions are combining their buying power by forming purchasing cooperatives, or group purchasing organizations (GPOs), to effect cost savings. These units are also known as co-ops, buying groups, and purchasing support groups. Generally, the term *cooperative* is used to describe nonprofit organizations, whereas the term *group purchasing* describes the relationship among for-profit organizations that pool their purchasing power. Regardless of which term is used, approximately 90 percent of all health care organizations belong to one or more of these groups. Compared with other health care departments, purchases by food service departments account for less than 10 percent of purchases made by the largest national and regional GPO.

The concept of group purchasing is based on the premise that several organizations have more purchasing power when negotiating collectively than any *one* entity alone. The organization of purchasing groups can occur on a local, state, regional, or national level. The requirements for membership and services provided vary. In most instances, members of the GPO pay a membership fee that is often based on bed count, dollar value of operating budget, or some other scale based on volume of purchases. These fees provide capital for operating the central office, employing procurement personnel, and legal services attendant to negotiating contracts. Some GPOs require members to purchase a specified volume of products, whereas others expect members to use their contractual agreements to their fullest potential.

Most GPOs have several characteristics in common. These include:

- At least one full-time procurement person who works with members to identify their needs and to negotiate contracts.
- Members usually meet formally to establish or update policies and operating procedures, establish specifications, evaluate products, share information, and assess the GPO's function.
- Group purchasing organizations frequently function as agents for the members, acting on members' behalf when negotiating contracts.
- A membership fee is required.
- Many GPOs are currently establishing prime vendor programs requiring committed volume contracts. Members are required to purchase a minimum of 80 percent of their purchases from prime vendors with whom the GPO has contracts. In some instances, members are prohibited from joining other GPOs with prime vendor arrangements.
- Competitive bidding is the primary procedure used for determining pricing, terms, and contract conditions between the GPO and the supplier.
- Value-added services such as product quality testing, value analysis, computer systems and software, employee development seminars, recipe ideas, and menu planning may be provided to GPO members.

Savings in excess of 20 percent is the primary reason food service directors use group purchasing. Other benefits include product standardization, increased quality, decreased administrative cost for processing multiple purchase orders, and less time spent in purchasing products and supplies. Members also cite improved knowledge of new and existing products and enhanced networking as a result of participation in GPO meetings. Membership commitment and support of the GPO's philosophy are essential for success of the group.

Some barriers that influence the effectiveness and cost savings of participating in a GPO include difficulty in obtaining consensus on product specifications; loss of control over supplier selection, product variety, quality, and contract awards; and unwillingness of representatives of competing health care organizations to work as team members. Group members who join multiple GPOs decrease the negotiating power of the group because the volume of purchases is diminished. The group's purchasing power is increased only when volume is significantly more than it would be for each individual food service department.

When selecting a GPO, the buyer and food service director should adhere to certain guidelines. Among them:

- Select a group composed of members from organizations sharing similar characteristics.
- Interview current members and the GPO's employees to assess potential savings in excess of required fees.
- Answer the following questions:
  - What are membership requirements? Is a guarantee to purchase a specified quantity (%) or dollar volume through the GPO required?
  - How does the GPO operate?
  - What value-added services are provided to members?
  - Is a prime vendor contract used? If so, what product lines are available?
  - What is the GPO doing to obtain data on current market prices, new products, and trends?
- Discuss findings with food service management staff and members of the quality product evaluation team.
- Consult with the financial officer when evaluating the cost–benefit ratio of membership.
- Present a proposal for joining a GPO to the administration.

One-Stop Purchasing or Single Sourcing

One-stop purchasing or *single sourcing* is defined as the strategy of selecting and using a single supply source. This purchasing method is used by large and small health care facilities (including long-term care facilities). The method is based on a cooperative relationship between the food service department and the vendor.

One vendor (a full-line distributor) supplies the buyer with most of the food and supplies needed. The efficiency of food purchasing is improved by eliminating the time-consuming processes of placing bids and getting quotations. A substantial reduction in warehousing costs is possible if deliveries are made frequently. Lower net costs of products can result because the supplier knows relatively far in advance that certain food services will be needing specific products; thus the vendor can buy from wholesalers in larger quantities.

Certain disadvantages can arise with relying on one vendor exclusively. For one thing, backup suppliers might be difficult to find should the single-source vendor fail to deliver the supplies ordered. For another, the quality of available foods might be inferior or inconsistent. For larger food service departments, the number of distributors able to supply one-stop services may be limited; nonetheless, the supplier pool for this service provision is definitely growing. The effectiveness of one-stop purchasing is directly related to the efficiency and credibility of the supplier. Most food service departments generally have found this method to work very satisfactorily.

Prime Vendor Agreements

The *prime vendor* method involves a formal agreement between the food service department (buyer) and one vendor (supplier), whereby the buyer contracts with the vendor to supply a specified percentage of a given category (or categories) of product. The percentage ranges from 60 to 80, with 80 percent being more common today. The prime vendor contract, also referred to as a *systems contract,* includes an agreement to purchase certain items for a specified time period and frequently specifies a minimum quantity of any or all items to be ordered during the contract period.

The steps involved in establishing a prime vendor relationship are outlined below. The bidding system is similar to contract purchasing, which is discussed later in this section.

1. Buyer completes an ABC analysis of purchases to determine which items make up the majority of purchases. (See chapter 18.)
2. Food service solicits bid proposals from several distributors for an estimated, committed volume (annual or monthly usage), product specification and designated delivery, services, and inventory.
3. Food service director (or other buyer) reviews the bid and determines lowest bidder that meets all criteria.
4. Buyer negotiates and awards contract.
5. Food service department (via the director or other channel) provides feedback to the vendor on quality of service, delivery, and products. The food service representative can require the vendor to "open the books" and provide information on the structure of its cost and pricing data if this privilege is a condition of the contract. It is imperative that the purchasing agent continue to track prices and market conditions.
6. Buyer develops secondary sources for products and supplies.

Benefits of a prime vendor agreement are increased competition and lower price; reduced cost of inventory, space, and order processing; and availability of value-added services. One value-added service that many health care food services utilize is computer systems provided by the prime vendor that allow the operations to place orders; obtain current price information and availability of products and supplies and product information (including nutrient analysis); and implement menu-planning and merchandising ideas. Some prime vendors provide a variety of software programs to their customers.

Disadvantages include potential gradual price increases, a decrease in competition, and a limited number of vendors with whom the operation conducts business. A reduction in service level can occur, especially in areas where only a limited number of vendors are available to conduct business. For the concept to be effective, continued enhancement of the vendor–buyer relationship is essential. The buyer must treat the DSRs and individuals delivering the product as partners rather than adversaries.

Just-in-Time Purchasing

Just-in-time (JIT) purchasing is a production planning strategy adopted by many manufacturing firms. The process involves purchasing products and supplies in the exact quantity required for a production run or limited time period and only as they are needed ("just in time"). Distributors deliver small quantities of supplies more frequently, and deliveries are timed more precisely based on production demand. Thus, just-in-time has an impact on both purchasing and inventory. Three goals are achieved with the JIT process: Inventory is decreased significantly as are related costs; space management is simplified; and problems must be resolved immediately as they occur. Unlike the manufacturing industry, each day food service operations produce a large number of perishable products in smaller quantities. The effectiveness of JIT warrants investigation because of potential cost reductions.

The ability to implement this method depends on several factors. These include complete support and cooperation of suppliers, commitment of all employees (including top administrators), accurate production demand forecasts, and changes in most aspects of the operation from menu planning through final service.

Locating food service distributors willing to provide frequent deliveries may be a challenge to some buyers, given that most distributors are requesting that customers accept fewer deliveries so as to decrease costs. Like the prime vendor concept, JIT requires building partnerships with distributors, and adoption of the JIT philosophy could require a change in attitude regarding quantity of supplies to maintain in inventory. Just-in-time purchasing practices emphasize ordering smaller quantities rather than storing large quantities just in case additional product is needed.

Centralized Purchasing

With centralized purchasing, the most common method of purchasing used in health care institutions, a separate department in the institution specializes in purchasing the materials and supplies needed by the institution's various services and departments. In this system, the food service director (like all other department heads) requisitions supplies from the purchasing department. Only representatives from the purchasing department deal directly with outside vendors and suppliers. Vendors have direct contact with end users of the supplies only if new products or services are being brought into the purchasing system. In many institutions that use centralized purchasing, receiving and storage are also handled by the purchasing department rather than by the individual departments that use the supplies.

Contract and Noncontract Purchasing

Two other general methods of buying are contract purchasing and noncontract purchasing. *Contract purchasing* (sometimes called formal buying) involves a binding agreement between vendor and purchaser. With this process, food service directors develop written specifications for each product and an estimate of the quantity needed for the designated bid period. A written notice of requirements, or a bid request (see figure 17-5), is made available to vendors, who are invited to submit price bids based on the quality and quantity needed. The bid request includes instructions about the method of bidding, delivery schedule required, and frequency of payment; the date bids are due; the basis for awarding contracts; and any other information needed by buyer and seller. This process may be formal, with notices of intent to bid published under "Legal notices" in the local newspaper. Alternatively, it may be informal with copies of the bid distributed widely through the mail or by other means.

In addition to specifications for each item to be purchased, the bid request may include general provisions. For example:

- A performance bond by the seller
- Errors in the bid
- Alternate or partial bids
- A discount schedule
- Definition of the term of the contract
- Time frame for performance
- Requirements for the submission of samples
- Requirements for delivery points
- Inspection provisions
- Provisions for certification of quality
- Packing requirements
- Billing instructions
- Payment methods
- Requirements for standard package size
- Cancellation clause

Obtaining firm, fixed prices for the specified bid period is desirable. However, when product prices fluctuate frequently or rise steadily, vendors may be unable (or unwilling) to quote firm prices for an extended period. Bid requests that state a maximum amount required, as well as a minimum quantity to be purchased from the successful bidder, allow some flexibility for both

Figure 17-5. Example of a Bid Request

BID REQUEST	

Bids will be received until _____ for __[indicate type of]__ delivery on the date indicated.

Issued by: _____ Address: _____

_____

Date Issued: _____ Date to Be Delivered: __[5-10 days after bid is awarded]__

Increases in quantity up to 20 percent will be binding at the discretion of the buyer. All items are to be officially certified by the U.S. Department of Agriculture for acceptance no earlier than two days before delivery; costs of such service to be borne by the supplier.

Item No.	Description	Quantity	Unit	Unit Price	Amount
1	Chickens, fresh-chilled fryers, 2½ to 3 lb., ready-to-cook, U.S. Grade A	500	Pound		
2	Chickens, fresh-chilled hens, 4 to 5 lb., ready-to-cook, U.S. Grade A	100	Pound		
3	Turkeys, frozen young toms, 20 to 22 lb., ready-to-cook, U.S. Grade A	100	Pound		
4	Eggs, fresh, large, U.S. Grade A, 30 dozen cases	150	Dozen		
5	Eggs, frozen, whole, inspected, six 4-pound cartons per case	60	Pound		

Vendor: _____

buyer and vendor when prices of the product needed are likely to fluctuate considerably. Although price is a major consideration in awarding the contract, the buyer should carefully consider quality of the product and ability of the vendor to meet the delivery schedules specified in the contract. In addition, the vendor's reputation, previous performance, and compliance with specifications and government regulations are important considerations. All bidders, including those not awarded the contract, should be informed when the contract has been awarded.

Noncontract purchasing (sometimes called informal buying) is done through verbal and written communications between buyer and vendor via telephone sales representatives. However, it may be handled without direct contact with the sales representative through the open market. Price quotations are obtained from two or more suppliers. Quotation sheets, or call sheets, such as those shown in figure 17-6, are useful. A quotation sheet provides spaces for the name and description of food items, amount of food needed, and prices quoted by various suppliers. After the price quotes have been received, the service and quality record of the supplier that gave the lowest quotation is checked. If the supplier has a history of providing good-quality products on schedule, the order usually is placed there. Although small institutions may use this method to purchase most of their foods, larger ones may use it only for perishable fresh products or foods needed in limited quantities. One disadvantage of noncontract purchasing is the amount of time required to check and compare prices, interview sales representatives, and place orders. Problems also can result from verbal commitments to buy. Some of these problems, however, can be avoided by providing vendors with a list of accurate product specifications as a communication aid.

☐ Vendor Selection and Relations

All distributor/vendors cannot meet the needs and expectations of all food service operations. Thus, it is imperative to select those compatible with a specific operation and with which the buyer can work cooperatively to obtain products that meet established standards and the operation's financial constraints. Quality, price, dependability, and service are factors that must dictate supplier selection. The buyer should strive to achieve the following objectives when evaluating potential vendors:

- Negotiate a fair price.
- Receive consistent quality and quantity as specified.
- Receive order on time.
- Develop relationships with vendors based on trust.
- Avoid internal conflicts over vendor relations.
- Build relationship with local vendors to develop goodwill within the community.

Achievement of these objectives is essential to the overall success of the procurement process.

Selection

Supplier selection involves a four-stage process, which is best remembered by the mnemonic SINE:

1. *Survey:* Explore all possible sources of supply.
2. *Inquiry:* Compare and evaluate prospective vendors to identify qualifications, advantages, and disadvantages.
3. *Negotiation and selection:* Enter into effective and clear dialogue with candidates to secure the best price, quality, and delivery commitment.
4. *Experience:* Monitor vendor service and product quality to ensure that what is promised is delivered.

Figure 17-6. Examples of Quotation Sheets

QUOTATION SHEET

Type of Product: __Fresh produce__   Day: __Monday__   Date: __2/10/88__   Approved by: _____DL_____

Amount on Hand	Quantity	Unit	Description and Specifications	Supplier and Quotations per Unit			
				Smith	Brown		
21	23	50# bag	Carrots	11.40	13.85		
0	1	40# bag	Bananas, #4	12.00	13.40		

QUOTATION SHEET

Type of Product: __Canned goods__   Day: __Wednesday__   Date: __4/6/88__   Approved by: _____DL_____

Amount on Hand	Quantity	Unit	Description and Specifications	Supplier and Quotations per Unit			
				Smith	Brown		
3	6	Case	Applesauce, regular #10 can	10.09	10.83		
4	6	Case	Peas, early June, #10 can	11.39	13.46		

The *survey stage* is devoted to identification of the need for new products, the need to investigate new suppliers, or the need to reevaluate current suppliers. Questions in this regard include:

- What is available on the market?
- Who can supply the product(s) or service(s)?
- Who can supply it (them) most (or more) economically within the required time period?
- Who are the distributors that service this area?

This stage results in a list of potential suppliers. The goal is to use the management information system (MIS) described in chapter 10 to identify as many sources as possible. A buyer who is new to an area must also network with other food service directors or buyers to assemble the list. Additional sources of information include past experience, interviews with DSRs, trade journals and shows, yellow pages, and buyer's guides.

In the *inquiry stage,* after identifying all potential sources the buyer must compare and analyze sources that appear capable of meeting the needs of the food service department. Criteria for evaluation include, but are not limited to, price, quality, service, delivery schedule, and available quantity. Also during this phase, the buyer should contact other buyers or managers for their feedback and experience with the suppliers from which they purchase. Sample questions that could be asked include:

- Is the firm reliable?
- Is quality consistently excellent?
- Are deliveries accurate and on time?
- How would you rate DSRs and other vendor employees with whom you have interacted?
- What additional value-added services do you use?
- How would you evaluate these services?
- What do you like most about this distributor?
- What problems, if any, have you experienced in conducting business with this vendor?

Another factor that must be evaluated is whether to use local or national vendors, each of which offers advantages and limitations. Additional criteria for comparing distributors are financial stability of the firm, technical expertise of the distributors' staff, and compatibility of business practices with regard to ethics standards. Business practices include strict adherence to delivery schedule, credit terms, minimum order requirement, lead time, return policy, and product line variety. If possible, a visit to the vendor's facility is recommended, especially if there has been no prior business relationship. After comparing all the potential distributors based on these criteria, the buyer narrows the options and prepares a second list called a qualified supplier list (QSL).

During the *negotiation and selection stage,* the buyer uses information obtained during the inquiry stage to issue an initial purchase order. Before doing so, however, he or she should meet with the suppliers to discuss payment, delivery, and contract terms, if applicable.

During the *experience stage,* the buyer follows up to ensure that the chosen vendor is providing the type of service and quality of products previously agreed on. If problems occur, the buyer should document them and provide immediate feedback to the distributor so that corrective action can be taken. Any problems (and their resolution) should be documented for future reference and evaluation.

The goal of the supplier selection process is to establish several product, supply, and equipment sources that can consistently provide the quantity and quality of products required at the right price and the right time. Communication and feedback are critical ingredients for a long-term and effective buyer–vendor relationship.

Buyer–Vendor Relations

Sound business practices and well-stated purchasing policies are the bases for good purchasing decisions. Careful planning and an accurate statement of food needs are the starting points in building good buyer–vendor relations. As always, fairness and honesty are essential. Product requirements should be specified and complete information as to availability and prices should be obtained. The buyer should establish an appointment schedule with sales representatives and adhere to it. At no time should one vendor's price information be discussed with another vendor. Accepting gifts, favors, coupons, and other promotional offers can create a potentially unhealthy obligation to a vendor that can adversely affect the buyer's freedom to make objective vendor selections. Buyers should be familiar with and follow the fair business policies of their institutions. Special services that ordinarily would not be available from vendors should not be requested.

☐ Basic Purchasing Guidelines

As a quick-reference tool, the following purchasing guidelines are summarized. They provide the fundamental "how-to's" of purchasing:

- Develop a specification for each food item. Government and industry specifications can provide a starting point to help food service managers and buyers develop their own. For some products, specifications can be quite brief, whereas others will require substantial detail.
- Make sure that a copy of specifications developed by the food service department is available to and used by the buyer. Many departments find it convenient to provide a complete set of their specifications (classified by commodity group and number) to vendors with which they routinely do business. This decreases the time required to get a price quotation.
- Compare food quality and yield in relation to price. A food of higher quality and a higher unit price may yield more serving portions of better quality and at a lower cost per serving than the same food of lower quality and price. Frequent studies of the net yield in serving portions and of the cost per serving of various brands make it possible to base buying decisions on cost per serving rather than on unit purchase price.
- Use bid requests or quotation sheets to get price quotations.
- Purchase only the types, quality, and quantities required for the planned menu and/or production forecasts. However, if a special buy becomes available and the quality is acceptable, a surplus of the product may be purchased if adequate storage space and conditions permit. For example, prices on the previous year's pack of canned or frozen fruit or vegetable items may be quite reasonable just before the new pack reaches the market.
- Purchase foods only from vendors known to maintain approved levels of sanitation and quality control in accordance with government regulations and recommended practices of food handling and storage.
- Purchase foods by weight, size, or count per container. The minimum weights acceptable for purchase units should be stated in the specifications.
- Establish a purchase and delivery schedule based on the storage life of various foods, the location of vendor in relation to the buying facility, delivery costs, storage space, inventory policies, and the food needs specified in the menu(s).
- Ensure that all purchases are inspected upon delivery. Rejection of an item should be done at the time of delivery unless there is a prior agreement that the vendor will give credit for any defective products or gross errors. Delivery sheets or invoices should not be initiated or signed until the quality and quantity of foods delivered have been checked against the purchase order.
- Maintain written purchase and receiving records for all foods and supplies ordered and received.

☐ Standards of Ethics

Several ethics issues should be addressed when establishing purchasing policies. Along with responsibility for spending large quantities of money on behalf of an operation comes certain temptations that involve making ethics-based decisions. Implicit in the buyer role is the basic requirement to remain loyal to the employer and to the ethics standards established by the organization. This means avoiding conflicts of interest, whereby personal gain could be derived from conducting business with a specific vendor. Most organizations' policies proscribe against accepting gifts or services from vendors with which the facility conducts business if such gifts or services are for personal use. Accepting bribes, kickbacks, and gifts in exchange for special ordering consideration, then, is not only unethical but illegal.

Many dilemmas will occur for which there is no one "right" or "wrong" action. When this happens, a buyer's personal ethics imperative and organizational policies must provide a framework for action. For example, sensitive issues that have occurred in food service and interfered with fair and honest business practice include the following:

- Gaining confidential information about a competitor from suppliers
- Accepting free trips, entertainment, and gifts beyond the dollar amount set by the organization
- Purchasing from suppliers favored by the administration
- Disclosing one vendor's quote to another vendor
- Using the organization's economic clout to force a vendor to lower prices

The best way to avoid these situations is to adhere to defined policies and procedures for conducting good and ethical business practices with vendors. The food service director may consider adopting the National Association of Purchasing Management's Principles and Standards of Purchasing Practices as a guide for everyone involved in the procurement process (available from the NAPM, P.O. Box 22160, Tempe, AZ 85285-2160).

☐ Computer-Assisted Procurement

Technology's impact on food service distributors and health care food service operations has already been discussed. Predictions of the role electronic data interchange will have on the procurement process also has been described.

This section provides a brief footnote to the earlier section so that buyers understand the fine points of computer-assisted procurement from actual practice. The steps enumerated below are intended as another quick-reference tool explaining computerized purchasing by buyers whose computer terminals are connected to a central processing unit (CPU).

1. The buyer calls up from the computer's files a listing for the product to be purchased. The computer record shows the specification for the product, its unit price, and a list of vendors who can supply the product.
2. The buyer selects the vendor, the quantities needed, and the desired delivery date and time.
3. After the products have been delivered and accepted, delivery confirmation is entered into the computer record and conveyed (or telecommunicated) to the vendor's computer.
4. The vendor's computer sends an invoice directly to the institution or to the institution's bank for payment for the products delivered. The invoice may be communicated by computer or with hard copy of the invoice printed out from the computer's record.
5. For an invoice communicated directly to the bank, the institution's bank automatically credits the vendor's account and debits the institution's account for the purchase.

In addition to the system described above, a number of spreadsheet applications might facilitate record keeping and provide current cost information. Examples include vendor evaluation, bid analysis, usage reports, and inventory analysis and valuation. Point-of-sale systems can be directly linked to a perpetual inventory (additional applications were discussed in chapter 10).

☐ Summary

Whether a health care facility hires a procurement specialist or charges the task of purchasing to the food service director or a centralized purchasing department, procurement activities ultimately have one objective. That objective is to ensure that everything needed to produce menu items is in place, on time, and within budget boundaries.

To accomplish this massive objective, buyers must survey supplier sources, inquire about prospective vendors, negotiate for the best selection at the most favorable price, and monitor selected vendor/suppliers to make sure they deliver what they promised when they promised it. Buyers must do this while minimizing leftovers, plate waste, and rampant overstocking.

Certain trends affect these efforts significantly. For example, distributors no longer can rely on the traditional "sales call." Their service representatives—DSRs—now must promote value-added services to retain a buyer–client base they once could take for granted. Thus, technology such as direct computer linkups between buyers and distributors' product or service line can expedite the buyer's order process and inventory control methods. Such services provided by distributors create distributor–buyer alliances whose common goal is customer retention. What's more, this interaction can be accomplished without either party leaving his or her office.

☐ Bibliography

Anasari, A., and Modarress, B. *Just-in-Time Purchasing.* New York City: Free Press, 1990.

Birkman, I. Food service needs controls to contain cost. *Hospitals* 54:79, Mar. 16, 1980.

Casper, C. A new way to manage inventory. *Institutional Distribution* 28(40):44–45, 48–49, Sept. 1, 1992.

Casper, C. Information 2000—computer wizardry will radically alter how distributors and their customers communicate. *Institution Distribution* 27(12):45–50, Dec. 1991.

Casson, J. The economic importance of the hospitality industry. In: A. Pizam, R. C. Lewis, and P. Manning, editors. *The Practice of Hospitality Management.* Westport, CT: AVI, 1982.

Coltman, M. M. *Hospitality Industry Purchasing.* New York City: Van Nostrand Reinhold, 1990.

Dion, P. A., Banting, P. M., Picard, S., and Blenkhorn, D. L. JIT implementation: a growth opportunity for purchasing. *Journal of Purchasing and Materials Management* 28(4):32–36, Fall 1992.

Hamann, T., Scott, W. G., and Conner, P. E. *Managing the Modern Organization.* 4th ed. Boston: Houghton Mifflin, 1982.

Heinritz, S., Farrel, P. V., Giuniperro, L., and Kolchin, M. Institutional purchasing. In: *Purchasing Principles and Application.* 8th ed. New York City: Prentice Hall, 1991.

Hoffman, M. DSRs in basic training. *The Food Service Distribution* 5(9):26–27, Aug. 1991.

King, P. In central Pennsylvania colleges. *Food Management* 28(4):98, Apr. 1993.

King, P. In nursing homes in New Hampshire. *Food Management* 28(4):102, Apr. 1993.

Lambert, H. R. Partnerships needed to create customer value. *Institutional Distribution* 28(1):16, Jan. 1992.

Murai, S. State of the industry: purchasing cooperatives. In: *Impact of Food Procurement on the Implementation of the Dietary Guidelines for Americans in Child Nutrition Programs Conference Proceedings.* University, MS: Food Service Management Institute, 1992.

National Association of Meat Purveyors. *The Meat Buyer's Guide.* McLean, VA: NAMP, 1984.

Newman, R. G. Single sourcing: short-term saving versus long-term problems. *Journal of Purchasing and Materials Management* 25(2):20–25, Summer 1989.

Ninemeir, J. D. *Purchasing, Receiving, and Storage: A Systems Manual for Restaurants, Hotels, and Clubs.* Boston: CBI Publishers, 1983.

Ouellette, R. P., Lord, N. W., and Cheremisinoff, P. N. *Food Industry Energy Alternatives.* Westport, CT: Food and Nutrition Press, 1980.

Reid, R. D., and Riegel, C. D. *Purchasing Practices of Large Food Service Firms.* Tempe, AZ: Center for Advanced Purchasing Studies/National Association of Purchasing Management, Inc., 1989.

Salkin, S. The growing clout of healthcare purchasing groups. *Institution Distribution* 28(2):101–5, Feb. 1992.

Salkin, S. Value added services add value, but you provide the service. *Institutional Distribution* 27(12):18, Dec. 1991.

Salkin, S. Why GPOs are booming. *Food Service Director* 59(3):60, Mar. 15, 1992.

Schechter, M., and Boss, D. Putting quality management to work. *Food Management* 57(11):102–4, 106, 110–13, Nov. 1992.

Schuster, K. In hospitals in California. *Food Management* 28(4):100, Apr. 1993.

Sneed, J., and Kresse, K. H. *Understanding Food Service Financial Management.* Gaithersburg, MD: Aspen, 1989.

Spears, M. C. *Foodservice Organizations: A Managerial and Systems Approach.* 2nd ed. New York City: Macmillan, 1991.

Stefanelli, J. M. *Purchasing: Selection and Procurement for the Hospitality Industry.* 2nd ed. New York City: John Wiley & Sons, 1985.

Trace, T. L., Lynch, J. F., Fischer, J. W., and Hummrich, R. C. Ethics and vendor relationships. In: S. J. Hall, editor. *Ethics in Hospitality Management: A Book of Readings.* East Lansing, MI: Educational Institute, 1992.

Weisburg, K. Why more hospitals eye group purchasing options. *Food Service Director* 65(3):65, Mar. 15, 1991.

Wetrich, J. G. Group purchasing: an overview. *American Journal of Hospital Pharmacy* 44(7):1581–92, July 1992.

Wolkenhauer, S. Selling something other than product at a price. *Institutional Distribution* 28(10):23, 90, Oct. 1992.

Receiving, Storage, and Inventory Control

☐ Introduction

The processes of receiving, storing, issuing, and inventory control not only influence a health care food service's costs, but also the quality of the food served to its customers. Critical steps in each process should be monitored as part of the department's continuous quality improvement (CQI) efforts.

This chapter will examine these processes and how they are related to and influence the health care food service operation. How to receive goods, inspect them for correlation between the quality and quantity specified in the purchase order and those of the materials delivered, and maintain receipt documentation will be discussed.

Once shipments are accepted (and rejections returned immediately), they must be stored properly. Procedures and conditions for dry storage items and low-temperature storage items will be delineated. Conditions for proper storage area upkeep (cleaning and sanitizing) will be outlined. For example, floor, window (if applicable), wall, and ceiling maintenance recommendations will be provided, along with shelf height, shelf–wall clearance, lighting and light fixture, and ventilation suggestions. Ideal storage temperatures and humidity levels for specific foods also will be detailed. Ancillary storage equipment—refrigerators and freezers, thermometers, and mobile equipment, for example—will be described.

Because food service inventory represents the bulk of the department's financial investment, inventory control, cost containment, and continuous quality initiatives are critical factors that department directors and buyers must always keep in mind. Therefore, the chapter will give significant attention to how foods and supplies are issued throughout the production and service areas. Specific inventory control tools will be provided; these include perpetual inventory calculations and physical inventory taking. Other techniques (all oriented to the accounting concept of FIFO, that is, first in, first out) will be described as well.

☐ Receiving Procedures

An effective procurement system requires adequate receiving procedures to ensure that the food and supplies delivered match the quality and quantity of the items ordered. The economic advantage gained from competitive bidding based on well-written specifications easily can be lost as a consequence of poor receiving practices. Acceptance of poor-quality products or incorrect amounts can mean financial loss to the food service department. This risk can be eliminated or minimized if sound receiving procedures and properly trained personnel are in place.

Receiving procedures vary among institutions, but some basic rules apply to all facilities. Responsibility for checking quantities should be assigned to receiving or storeroom personnel. In very small organizations, this may be one of several tasks assigned to production personnel. Inspection for quality should be the responsibility of someone who knows the specifications or at least is qualified to judge the quality of the goods being delivered. Whoever is charged with inspecting shipment deliveries should prepare ahead of time for each one. This means knowing the delivery dates and approximate times so that space and equipment can be made available. Because most deliveries are made on a regular schedule, this should be relatively easy.

Receiving staff immediately should check the merchandise; perishable items first, preferably while the delivery person is still present. The count, weight, quality, and condition of the merchandise should be compared to the purchase order or quotation sheet before delivery is accepted. Scales should be available for checking items ordered by weight. Any cases or cartons that appear damaged should be opened right away. The quality of fresh produce should be inspected at the top *and the bottom* of each container. Internal temperature of all frozen foods should be 0°F (−18°C). If the temperature exceeds 0°F, the foods should be rejected. If such a detailed check is not possible, the receiving staff should inspect packages for signs indicating that the product may have been subjected to undesirably high temperatures. Wet or dripping packages should never be accepted.

Next, the staff should date or tag all chilled, frozen, and nonperishable foods as they are received to ensure their use on a FIFO basis. Such foods should be stored immediately. (The price per unit can be recorded on frozen and nonperishable items at this point.)

Only after foods have been inspected, dated, tagged, and approved should the staff sign the delivery slip from the vendor and fill out the required receiving report. Unordered or rejected merchandise should be returned immediately. Nonperishable foods and supplies should be transferred to appropriate storage areas as soon as possible (nonfood items should always be stored separately from food supplies).

Institutions with a centralized receiving department usually require a written report for all merchandise received. The food service director and the buyer should have copies for their files.

Two receiving methods are used most often in food service operations. These methods are invoice receiving and blind receiving.

Invoice Receiving

Invoice receiving involves having a receiving clerk check the items delivered against the original purchase order or telephone order (documented in writing) and note any discrepancies. This method makes it easy for the clerk to check the quantity and quality of the materials delivered against the specifications. Invoice receiving is quick and economical, although it loses its advantage if the clerk fails to compare items delivered with the specifications and simply uses the delivery invoice as a reference.

Blind Receiving

With *blind receiving,* the clerk uses an invoice or a purchase order that has the "quantity ordered" column blacked out. The clerk records the quantity actually received for each item on the invoice or purchase order—not on the supplier's invoice. This method takes more time than invoice receiving because it requires that the clerk prepare a complete record of all merchandise delivered. Even so, blind receiving is the more reliable method of the two.

Record Keeping

Maintaining records of all merchandise delivered is as important as inspecting deliveries for quality and quantity. The methods and forms used for this purpose may be simple or complex, depending on the level of documentation required. A receiving record must be kept so that all personnel involved in purchasing, using, and paying for supplies are informed of what was received. Depending on whether receiving is centralized or takes place in the food service department, one or more of the following records may be used.

Merchandise Receipt

A merchandise receipt like the one shown in figure 18-1 may be required for each shipment received. This type of form is completed by a receiving clerk in the central stores area, who sends copies to appropriate department staff members in purchasing, food service, accounting, and so forth to inform them that the goods have been received. Notations of items ordered but not delivered or items returned may be included on this form or on a separate form (called a credit memo) used for this purpose. The merchandise receipt and the credit memo should be signed by the person taking delivery and either attached to the invoice or sent separately, depending on the department's policy. (The procedure for routing receipts and credit memos should be clearly stated in the department's policy and procedures manual.)

Receiving Record

A daily receiving record similar to the one shown in figure 18-2 may be required, in addition to the merchandise receipt. Alternatively, it may be the only form used to record incoming goods. Either or both records can be used to verify receipt of merchandise. The forms also are a source of information for processing payments in the accounting department or for updating inventory records.

☐ Storage Procedures

Dry storage and low-temperature storage facilities should be accessible to both the receiving and food preparation areas so that transport time and corresponding labor costs can be kept to a minimum. Ideally, these facilities should be on the same floor as the production area, but if this is not possible, space should be allocated in the production area for one or more days' supply of foods. (Recommended storage temperatures and times are listed in table 18-1.)

Dry Storage Maintenance

The amount of space required for dry storage depends on the types and amounts of foods needed, the frequency of deliveries, the facility's policies on inventory size, and the amount of money invested in inventory. These factors vary from one institution to another.

Storage areas should be dry and easy to keep free of rodents and insects. Walls and ceilings should be constructed of nonporous materials, and ceilings should be free from water and heating pipes. Any windows should be screened and equipped with an opaque security sash to protect supplies from direct sunlight. Floors, preferably made of quarry tile, terrazzo, or sealed concrete, should be slip resistant. All components—walls, ceilings, and floors—should be easy to clean.

All parts of a storage room should be well lighted so that supplies and labeling are visible and so that housekeeping can be achieved properly. Light fixtures covered with wire mesh help protect against breakage and shield employees from falling glass should breakage occur. About two or three watts of light per square foot of floor area is recommended, with fixtures centered over the aisles.

Ventilation and temperature control are critical to dry storage rooms for retarding deterioration of food supplies. A temperature range of 50° to 70°F (10° to 21°C) is recommended. A thermometer placed in a highly visible location (for example, at the entrance) is essential. Ventilation should be provided by fans or other specially designed systems.

Figure 18-1.   Merchandise Receipt

MERCHANDISE RECEIPT		
Date: _____		
No: _____		
Received from: _____		
Purchase Order No.: _____		
Quantity	**Description**	**Distribution**
Merchandise Received and Inspected by: _____		

Figure 18-2. Daily Receiving Record

							Distribution	
Quantity	Unit	Description of Item	Name of Vendor	Quantity Verified by	Unit Price	Total Cost	To Kitchen	To Storeroom

RECEIVING RECORD

Merchandise Received and Inspected by: _____ Date: _____

Table 18-1. Recommended Storage Temperatures and Times

Food	Refrigerator Storage (32°F-40°F [0°C-4°C])	Freezer Storage (0°F [−18°C] or Below)	Dry Storage (50°F-70°F [10°C-21°C])
Roasts, steaks, chops	3-5 days	Beef and lamb: 6 months Pork: 4 months Veal: 4 months Sausage, ham, slab bacon: 2 months Beef liver: 3 months Pork liver: 1-2 months	Never
Ground meat, stew meat	1-2 days	3-4 months	Never
Ham, baked whole	1-3 weeks	4-6 months	Never
Hams, canned	12 months	Not recommended	Never
Chicken and turkey	2-3 days	Chicken: 6-12 months Turkey: 3-6 months Giblets: 2-3 months	Never
Fish or shellfish	30°F-32°F (−1°C-0°C) on ice, 2-3 days	3-6 months	Never
Shell eggs	1-2 weeks	Not recommended	Never
Frozen eggs	1-2 days after thawing	9 months	Never
Dried eggs	6 months	Not recommended	Never
Fresh fruits and vegetables	5-7 days	Not recommended	Never
Frozen fruits and vegetables	—	Variable, depends on kind	Never
Canned fruits and vegetables	—	Not recommended	12 months
Dried fruits and vegetables	Preferred	Not recommended	2 weeks
Canned fruit and vegetable juice	—	—	Satisfactory
Regular cornmeal	Required over 60 days	Not recommended	2 months
Whole wheat flour	Required over 60 days	Not recommended	2 months
Degermed cornmeal	Preferred	Not recommended	Satisfactory
All-purpose and bread flour	Preferred	Not recommended	Satisfactory
Rice	Preferred	Not recommended	Satisfactory

To promote security, it is preferable to have only one entrance to the storage area so that deliveries and supplies can be monitored. Access should be limited to those employees responsible for inventory control and receiving. Secure locks should be installed on all doors, and keys should be carefully safeguarded (for example, by a key signout system). A door width of at least 42 inches allows easy movement of supplies into and out of the area.

Miscellaneous supplies and broken (open) case lots can be stored on adjustable metal shelves installed at least 2 inches from the walls. Specific guidelines for shelving and spacing between shelves are discussed in chapter 21. The aisles between shelves and platforms should be wide enough to accommodate mobile equipment.

Metal or plastic containers with tight-fitting covers should be used for storing dry foods such as cereals, cereal products, flour, sugar, and broken lots of bulk foods. Containers, which should be legibly and accurately labeled, can be placed on dollies for ease of movement from one place to another.

Toxic materials used for cleaning and sanitation should be clearly labeled and kept in a locked storage area away from food supplies. *Empty food containers must never be used for storing broken lots of toxic materials, nor must empty cleaning and sanitation containers be used to store food.* Food should be stored only in food-grade containers.

A worktable should be provided near the entrance of the storeroom for unpacking supplies, putting up small orders of bulk products, and assembling orders. Large and small scoops should be on hand for each food container in use, such as bins for flour, sugar, cereal, and so forth. Scales need to be accessible for weighing small and large quantities of food. Several types of mobile equipment, such as platform dollies and shelf trucks, may be needed for delivering supplies to the various work areas. Hand-washing facilities are essential and should be located near the storeroom entrance.

A regular cleaning schedule should be developed and a staff member or crew assigned to the tasks of cleaning the floor, walls, ceiling, light fixtures, shelves, and equipment in the storeroom. Routinely, the food service director or a supervisor should inspect the area. Any violations of sanitation standards and facility policies should be corrected immediately.

Fireproof refuse containers that are located in conformance with local public health laws should be emptied at least daily. Leaking or bulging cans of food and spoiled foods must be disposed of promptly. The storeroom should be treated regularly for the control of rodents and insects. Further information on safe and sanitary preservation of food and supplies in dry storage areas is available from local and state public health departments (see also chapter 13).

Stock should be systematically arranged and inventory records should follow the same system to save time when stock is issued or inventoried. New stock should be placed behind like items so that the older stock will be issued first, again using the FIFO method. As mentioned, each item should be marked or stamped with its date of delivery and unit cost as it is placed on the shelf. The cost can thus be noted on the inventory sheets as the actual count is taken in the physical inventory. This method permits rapid computation of the cash value of inventory on hand. Price marking also is an effective way of familiarizing production personnel with the cost of foods.

Quantity lots of bagged items, such as flour and sugar, should be cross-stacked on slatted platforms or racks raised high enough above the floor to permit air circulation. Bulk cereals, dried vegetables, and dry milk should be refrigerated if the storeroom temperature cannot be maintained below 70°F. When cases of canned foods are stacked, their labels should be exposed for easy identification. Cartons of foods packed in glass jars should be kept closed because light tends to change the color and flavor of some foods. Dried fruits can be stored satisfactorily for a limited time in their original boxes if the storeroom temperature can be kept below 70°F and the humidity below 55 percent. If refrigerated space is available, storing dried fruits at lower temperatures will retard mold growth.

Bananas should be kept in the dry storage area or at a temperature of 60° to 65°F (15° to 18°C). To prevent bruising, they should be left in the delivery boxes. Because a temperature of 58°F (14°C) or below darkens the flesh of bananas, they should not be refrigerated. Unripened fruits and vegetables should be placed in dry storage until they become edible (unripe melons, peaches, pears, pineapples, plums, avocados, and tomatoes ripen at 65° to 70°F [18° to 21°C]; colder temperatures, however, can damage these products so that they will not ripen).

Potatoes should be stored away from light, if possible, in a dry, well-ventilated room at a temperature of 40° to 55°F (4° to 14°C). If peeled potatoes are purchased, they should be refrigerated and held no longer than the number of days suggested by the processor. Sweet potatoes and winter squash keep best in a well-ventilated room at a temperature of 50° to 60°F (10° to 15°C). Sweet potatoes spoil more quickly under refrigeration than in dry storage. Onions keep best in dry storage at a temperature of 40° to 60°F (4° to 15°C). It is important to avoid indiscriminate overbuying because food quality can deteriorate even under the most ideal storage conditions.

Low-Temperature Storage Maintenance

To preserve their nutritional value and appeal, perishable foods should be placed in refrigerated or frozen storage immediately after delivery and kept there until they are to be used. The type and amount of low-temperature storage space required varies with the facility's menu and purchasing policies. Some food service operations are fortunate to have separate refrigerated units for meats and poultry, fish and shellfish, dairy products, and vegetables and fruits, with separate freezers for ice cream and other frozen foods. Separate facilities are desirable because each kind of food has its own ideal storage temperature. However, satisfactory storage conditions can be maintained with fewer units following these temperature guidelines:

- Fruits and vegetables (except those requiring dry storage): 40° to 45°F (4° to 7°C)
- Dairy products, eggs, meats, poultry, fish and shellfish: 32° to 40°F (0° to 4°C)
- Frozen foods: −10° to 0°F (−23° to −18°C)

If separate refrigerators and freezers are available, foods should be stored at the following temperatures:

- Fruits: 45° to 50°F (7° to 10°C)
- Vegetables, eggs, processed foods, and pastry: 40° to 45°F (4° to 7°C)
- Dairy: 38° to 40°F (3° to 4°C)
- Fresh meats: 34° to 38°F (1° to 3°C)
- Fresh poultry: 32° to 36°F (0° to 2°C)
- Frozen foods: −10° to 0°F (−23° to −10°C)

In large institutions, walk-in refrigerators and freezers are common. In smaller operations, the trend is away from walk-ins and toward reach-ins because available storage space is used more efficiently, less floor space is required, and cleaning is much easier. Regardless of the type of refrigeration available, location is the key for saving labor and avoiding nonproductive work. Walk-in refrigerator doors should be flush with the floor so that movable racks or shelves can be wheeled in and out with ease. Employees should be trained to obtain all supplies needed at one time to eliminate the constant opening of doors, which increases energy usage.

Refrigerators and freezers should be provided with one or more thermometers, such as a remote-reading thermometer, a recording thermometer, and a bulb thermometer. The *remote-reading thermometer,* placed outside the refrigerator, shows the temperature inside. The *recording thermometer,* also mounted outside the refrigerator, has the added feature of continuously recording the temperature in walk-in, low-temperature storage. One can see at a glance any fluctuations in temperature. The *bulb thermometer* probably is the most common one used for refrigerators and freezers that do not have a thermometer built into the door. The warmest area of the unit should be determined and the thermometer placed there. Whichever type of thermometer is used, a staff member should be assigned to check the temperatures in all units at least once a day and to record them on a chart.

Humidity also is important for maintaining food quality because perishable foods contain a great deal of moisture and evaporation will be greater when the air in the refrigerator is dry. Evaporation causes foods to wilt, discolor, and lose moisture. Food held at low humidity shrinks considerably and requires extra trimming. Although a humidity level as low as 65 percent is suggested for some products, a range between 80 and 95 percent is recommended for most foods.

Good air circulation should be provided throughout the refrigerators and freezers at all times, with foods arranged so that air can circulate to all sides of the pan, box, or crate. For sanitary reasons, foods should not be stored on the floor. All foods are to be covered and labeled with the receiving date. Most foods should be left in their original containers—a requirement mandatory for frozen foods—to reduce the possibility of freezer burn and drying. Fresh produce should be examined for ripeness and spoilage before it is stored and may be transferred to specially designed plastic containers if it passes inspection. The paper wrappings on fruit should be left on to help keep them clean and to prevent spoilage, moisture loss, and bruising.

□ Inventory Control Procedures

Inventory represents money in the form of food, supplies, and small equipment. Efficient inventory control keeps the size of inventory at a level appropriate for the facility and ensures the security of goods on hand. Food service inventory management starts with the menu-planning process. The quantities of food supplies needed to produce the menu items are projected on the basis of how frequently individual items appear on the menu and on the probable demand for each item as determined from records of its past popularity. Once appropriate inventory levels have been established for various food supplies, they should be monitored continuously and adjusted periodically to correct for any shortages and overstocks.

Issuing of Food and Supplies

Issuing is the process of providing food and nonfood supplies to other areas within the food service department, including the production and service units. Products such as milk, bread and other bakery items, and fresh produce may be issued directly from the receiving area to the appropriate production units without the products ever going into storage. Referred to as *direct issuing,* this method bases the quantities of items issued on records of past usage. The majority of food and supplies, however, are issued from dry, refrigerated, or frozen storage. Issuing is essential to control the quantity of food removed from storage and to provide cost-accounting information to the accounting department and to the storeroom clerk if the food service operation uses a perpetual inventory system. In addition, usage data are required for budgeting.

All food and issues that are not direct issues should be requisitioned from the designated storage area. However, many operations only issue goods from the dry storage area.

Many facilities have two or more types of storage areas for dry goods: one for bulk supplies and the other for supplies used daily. The main storage area for bulk supplies is kept locked, and goods are issued by a stock clerk after the clerk receives a stores requisition like the one shown in figure 18-3. With this system, someone in the department determines the amount of supplies that will be needed over the next day or week and then fills out a requisition. The supplies are delivered and stored in the production area. A locked storeroom is recommended because it affords better control.

To increase control of the issues, requisitions should be prenumbered to permit tracking of lost or duplicate forms. The type of information to include on the form is determined by whether the cost-accounting system is manual or computerized. For a manual system, information should include the unit requesting supplies, date, product description, quantity, supply unit, unit price, and total cost. For a computerized system, the above information (excluding unit price and total cost) and an inventory number for the item should be included. Some computerized systems generate requisitions. Requisition forms should provide for the initials or signatures of the person completing the requisition and the storeroom clerk (or other employee) responsible for filling the request.

In operations too small to justify a full-time clerk to issue foods and keep records, other systems can be considered. For example, one staff member can be designated to issue food and keep records during a specified time of day. Alternatively, a signout sheet can be placed in the storeroom so that staff members responsible for food production can prepare a list of the kinds and amounts of foods they use. At the end of each day, the lists are given to a manager,

Figure 18-3.   Stores Requisition

STORES REQUISITION						

_____ Hospital

Day to Be Used: _____   Day Issued: _____

Order by: _____   Issued by: _____

Stock Number	Total Quantity	Order Unit	Item Description	Issued to	Price per Unit	Total Cost

who records on the inventory record the supplies used each day. The last two methods, however, can create security and control problems in the department.

Some larger food service operations issue ingredients from an ingredient control room. If this system is used, the personnel in this unit requisition supplies from the different storage areas. Ingredients are weighed and measured prior to being issued to the production area at specified time periods. Some ingredient control rooms maintain a limited inventory of frequently used nonperishable products and supplies such as flour, sugar, and shortening.

Record Keeping

In addition to effective receiving and issuing procedures, good inventory records are essential for providing management with the information needed to calculate and monitor food and supply expenses. Four reasons have been cited for maintaining accurate inventory records:

1. To provide data for cost control
2. To assist in identifying purchasing needs
3. To provide accurate information on type and quantity of food and supplies on hand
4. To monitor usage of products and prevent theft and pilferage

The actual quantity of each item in inventory is another important aspect of an inventory control system. There are two basic methods used to determine the quantity of goods on hand: a perpetual inventory system and a physical inventory system.

Perpetual Inventory

The process of recording all purchases and food issues is known as *perpetual inventory*. Under this system, a continuous record of the quantities of supplies on hand at any given time, as well as their value, is created. Perpetual inventory records provide the food service director with up-to-date information on product usage and the need for further purchases.

A perpetual inventory record alone is not sufficient for an accurate accounting of all food and supplies in the inventory. The inventory should be verified monthly by taking a physical inventory of goods on hand (discussed in the next section) and adjusting the inventory accordingly.

Perishable foods delivered directly to the production area are not usually kept on the perpetual inventory because they are usually consumed shortly after they come in. Perishable supplies may require only a monthly consumption record compiled from purchases.

Maintaining a perpetual inventory system is time-consuming. Therefore, small institutions may not have the staff or the need for such detailed records. For them, a physical inventory and a record of purchases are sufficient, especially when limited amounts of supplies are kept on hand.

To estimate the amount of time required to maintain a perpetual inventory system, the following formula can be used:

Number of items purchased per week × 4 weeks per month = number of purchases per month

Number of items issued per day × 30 days per month = number of issues per month

Number of items counted to verify perpetual system = number of items counted per month

(Purchases per month + issues per month + number of items counted per month) ÷ time required to enter each item

For example, if a food service purchased 500 items per week and issued 1,000 items per day and it took the storeroom clerk 30 seconds to enter each item, a total of 270.83 labor hours per month would be required to maintain a perpetual inventory system in this operation.

500 items per week × 4 weeks per month = 2,000 items

1,000 items issued daily × 30 days per month = 30,000 items issued per month

500 items counted × 1 time per month = 500   32,500 ÷ 0.5 minutes = 270.83 labor hours per month   **457**

Labor cost required to maintain a perpetual inventory must be justified. Before an operation can justify using a perpetual inventory system, data calculated and maintained must be used frequently by management and be essential to cost control.

Physical Inventory

Periodic physical counts of all stock are necessary even when a perpetual inventory is maintained. Regardless of how well systems and personnel perform, errors can be made in recording transactions, foods can spoil, and pilferage can occur. In small operations in which the labor involved makes keeping a perpetual inventory impractical, physical inventories can be taken monthly to determine the cost of foods used during the preceding month.

Taking a physical inventory is simplified when the storeroom is organized by food categories and the foods in each category are stored alphabetically. A form for recording goods on hand should be developed to correspond to the storeroom's organization. Each item on the inventory form should be listed on a separate line. If more than one package size of an item is stocked, it still should be listed separately. The form should include space for the product description, the unit size, the quantity on hand, the unit cost, and the total value of the amount on hand.

After a physical inventory has been conducted, the cost of the food used can be calculated in the following manner. The value of the beginning inventory plus the cost of the foods purchased equals the value of the food on hand. When the value of the final inventory is subtracted from the value of the food on hand, the result is the cost of the food used between inventories. In other words:

$$\text{Beginning inventory} + \text{purchases} = \text{food on hand}$$
$$\text{Food on hand} - \text{final inventory} = \text{food used}$$

An example of a physical inventory record is given in figure 18-4. Inventory records are essential not only for calculating costs but also for managing purchases and making the best use of available funds. With continued emphasis on cost containment in today's health care industry, food service directors must stay on top of inventory distribution and cost control in their departments.

Inventory Control Tools

Several types of inventory records are maintained in an effort to monitor food cost, determine purchase quantity, and identify inventory levels to maintain. Six of them are outlined in the following subsections: valuing inventory, ABC method, fixed-item inventory, par stock system, mini-max system, and economic order quantity.

Valuing Inventory

One of the most common records food service departments keep is the dollar value of the assets in inventory. The first step in calculating inventory value is to count the number of each type of item on hand. This value is computed by multiplying the quantity of the item by a predetermined cost. The following three methods are used most frequently to determine cost:

- *Last in, first out (LIFO):* All products counted are valued at first price paid during the accounting period.
- *First in, first out (FIFO):* Products are valued at the last price paid during the accounting period. This method is used by operations that attempt to ensure that the oldest items in inventory are used first.
- *Weighted average:* Actual price paid for an item is multiplied by number of units on hand for a specific order. The sum of the total actual dollar value is divided by the number of units on hand to compute the average cost per item.

Figure 18-4. Example of a Physical Inventory Record

PHYSICAL INVENTORY

Date: _____ Taken by: _____ Beginning Inventory: $ _____

Quantity on Hand	Order Unit	Article	Description	Unit Cost	Total
	#10	Apples	Sliced, 6 #10/case		
	#10	Apples	Dehydrated, low moisture, 6 #10/case		
	#10	Apple rings	6 #10/case		
	#10	Applesauce	6 #10/case		
	#10	Apricots	Unpeeled halves, 6 #10/case		
	#10	Blueberries	Water pack, 6 #10/case		
	#10	Cherries	RSP, water pack, 6 #10/case		
	1 gallon	Cherries	Maraschino halves, 4 gallons/case		
	#10	Cranberry sauce	6 #10/case		
	1 pound	Dates	Pieces, 25-pound box		
	#10	Fruit cocktail	6 #10/case		
	#10	Fruit for salads	6 #10/case		
	#3	Grapefruit sections	Whole, 12 #3		
	#3	Grapefruit-orange sections	Whole, 12 #3 cylinder; 46 ounces/case		
	#10	Mincemeat	Solid pack, 6 #10/case		
	#10	Mandarin oranges	6 #10/case		
	#10	Peaches	Halves, 6 #10/case		
	#10	Peaches	Sliced, 6 #10/case		
	#10	Pears	Halves, 6 #10/case		
	#10	Pineapple	Crushed, 6 #10/case		
	#10	Pineapple	Sliced, 6 #10/case		
	#10	Pineapple	Tidbits, 6 #10/case		
	#10	Plums	Purple, 6 #10/case		
	#10	Prunes	6 #10/case		
	1 pound	Raisins	Dried, seedless, 24 16-ounce/case		
	#10	Rhubarb	6 #10/case		

The method selected for valuing the inventory will influence the calculation of cost of goods sold in the operation's financial statement. This value in turn influences the profit or loss status of the food service department. (Chapter 11 provides more information regarding financial controls.)

ABC Method

The concept of the ABC method is based on the premise that a small number (15 to 20 percent) of the items purchased accounts for the majority of the inventory value. Items in the inventory that constitute the greatest value are the ones on which management should spend most of its tracking effort. These items are often referred to as the A items and represent approximately 20 percent of all inventory items but account for about 80 percent of inventory value. Only the minimum quantity required to meet current demand should be maintained in inventory. The B items represent 10 to 15 percent of the inventory items and 20 to 25 percent of total inventory value. The low value items, the C items, contribute only 5 to 10 percent of inventory value and consist of 60 to 65 percent of the total number of items in inventory. Examples of each class of items are listed below.

- A items—Meat, frozen convenience entrees, seafood
- B items—Dairy products, china
- C items—Staples (for example, beans, flour, and sugar), breakfast cereals, paper products

Fixed-Item Inventory

The fixed-item technique for monitoring inventory is similar to the ABC method except that the food service director selects only a limited number of items to track the usage. Order quantity and flow of these products are carefully monitored. Steaks would be an example of one meat item that might be included on an operation's fixed-item inventory list.

Par Stock System

The par stock system requires that a certain quantity level be established for each item that must be kept on hand to meet the needs of the planned menu and any unusual circumstances that might occur. Orders are placed at regular fixed intervals over a specified period. Each time the ordering date comes around, enough stock is purchased to replenish the supply to the predetermined level. The usage rate of each item must be carefully planned between order dates.

Mini-Max System

The mini-max system involves establishing both a minimum and a maximum amount of stock to have on hand. Goods are ordered whenever the minimum is reached and only in the quantity needed to attain the maximum level. With this system, the amount of each food ordered will be the same each time, but the time at which it is purchased will vary. Again, the usage rate of each item must be carefully scrutinized so that the determined minimum and maximum levels remain appropriate.

Figure 18-5 compares the par stock and mini-max systems. Both approaches work to help prevent overstocks and avoid shortages of frequently used foods.

Economic Order Quantity

Economic order quantity (EOQ) is a method to calculate reorder points to ensure that the best price is obtained after taking into consideration the carrying cost or the cost of maintaining the item in inventory for an extended period of time. The EOQ method is not used frequently by food service directors but may be a helpful tool in operations that order very large quantities at one time or for group purchasing organizations (GPOs). Unless the inventory system is computerized, the calculation of EOQ is time-consuming and cumbersome. A detailed discussion of the method is provided by Spears in *Foodservice Organizations*.

☐ Summary

Receiving, storage, and inventory control are critical aspects of the food service department's procurement system that are directly affected by menu planning. Inventory control is vital to department survival because it represents money in the form of food, supplies, and small equipment. Enough food should be kept on hand to ensure that the menu can be prepared and that emergency situations can be handled. On the other hand, food spoilage, theft, and pilferage as a result of overstocking must be avoided. A periodic count of items on hand determines whether the proper controls are in place.

Figure 18-5. Comparison of Par Stock and Mini-Max Inventory Systems

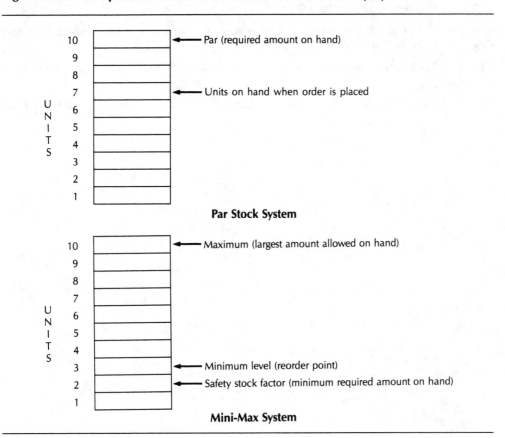

Receiving procedures must ensure that the quantity and quality of food and supplies ordered match those of the materials received. Upon receipt, inspection, and approval, goods should be date-stamped, costed, and stored in the proper area. Invoices of goods received should be checked for accuracy.

Items should be stored appropriately, always with the FIFO method in mind. Storage areas should be clean, have proper temperature controls and adequate maintenance, and be monitored by efficient security systems. Toxic chemicals used for cleaning and sanitizing should be stored away from food products.

☐ Bibliography

American Dietetic Association. *Standards of Professional Responsibility*. Chicago: ADA, 1985.

Axler, B. H. *Foodservice: A Managerial Approach*. Lexington, MA: D. C. Heath, in cooperation with the National Institute for Foodservice Industry, 1979.

Back to basics: inventory control. *Hospital Food & Nutrition Focus* 6(11):1, 3–5, July 1990.

Determining and controlling costs. *Hospital Food & Nutrition Focus* 8(5):1, 3–6, Jan. 1992.

Determining and controlling production and service costs. *Hospital Food & Nutrition Focus* 8(7):1, 3–4, Feb. 1992.

Ninemeier, J. D. *Purchasing, Receiving, Storage: A System Manual for Restaurants, Hotels and Clubs*. Boston: CBI, 1983.

Produce 101. Newark, DE: Bill Communication, Inc., and Fresh Produce Marketing Association, 1992.

Reed, L. *SPECS: The Comprehensive Foodservice Purchasing and Specification Manual.* 2nd ed. New York City: Van Nostrand Reinhold, 1993.

Spears, M. C. *Foodservice Organizations: A Managerial and Systems Approach.* 2nd ed. New York City: John Wiley & Sons, 1991.

Virts, W. B. *Purchasing for Hospitality Operations.* East Lansing, MI: American Hotel and Motel Association, 1987.

Zenz, G. J. *Purchasing and the Management of Materials.* 5th ed. New York City: John Wiley and Sons, 1981.

Chapter 19

Food Production

☐ Introduction

Food production plays a critical role in meeting the objectives of the health care food service department and satisfying the expectations of its customers. This system is responsible for translating the menu into food of the highest caliber possible in the required quantities. Nutritious, carefully prepared, flavorful, and attractive foods are vital tools for restoring and/or maintaining the health of patients or residents and in satisfying the wants of the nonpatient market.

Two of the most important management decisions that affect the system's success are which food production system to use and which production forecasting method to apply. Several alternatives have evolved for both these functions. A health care operation considering a change or evaluating the effectiveness of these functions should study closely the factors described in this chapter as they affect food quality, microbiological safety, customers' expectations and needs, and the operation's financial status.

The food service director is responsible for developing food quality standards (as described in chapter 4), implementing those standards, and following procedures to control the quality and quantity of food provided. Production controls vital to this process include standardized recipes, ingredient and portion standards, and production schedules. Well-trained production workers should strive to maintain the nutritional value and the natural flavor, color, and appeal of the foods they prepare.

The operation's food production processes should be based on proper cooking procedures and the controls listed above. The section of this chapter that discusses food production processes focuses on methods of food preparation. For issues regarding quality standards, ingredient characteristics, safety and sanitation, and food storage, refer to the appropriate chapters.

This chapter will describe and compare four food production systems: cook–serve, cook–chill, cook–freeze, and assembly–serve. Next, production forecasting techniques—that is, determining what menu items need to be prepared, in what quantities, and over what time frame—will be outlined.

Because a food service department manager must balance the production schedule with work load, food quality standards, and employee skills (among other demands), the elements that make up a workable production schedule will be delineated. Methods and devices for portion control, recipe standardization (including techniques for testing recipes), ingredient control, and the benefits of a centralized ingredient room or area will be detailed.

The chapter will give an in-depth breakdown of food production processes for the key food groups. For example, optimal cooking procedures for various meats and meat products (dry heat, roasting, broiling and grilling, and so forth) will be suggested. The same will be done for poultry, fish and shellfish, eggs and egg products, and the dairy group (including milk and milk products). Storage guidelines for these food groups will be provided as well. Similar selection, preparation, and storage pointers will be presented for fresh and frozen fruits and vegetables; for starches (potatoes, pasta, rice, and cereals); breads (yeast and quick varieties specifically); and beverages.

☐ Food Production Systems

The food production systems used most commonly today are classified as cook–serve (conventional), cook–chill, cook–freeze, and assembly–serve (convenience). The systems differ in several areas: in the market form in which foods are purchased, in the amount and type of labor required, in the timing of production relative to service, in the holding methods used prior to service, and in the types of equipment required. Although each system has certain strong and weak points that have been identified by researchers and acknowledged by users, all the systems have successfully provided food of acceptable quality in operational situations. The key to their success lies in adequate managerial control of the critical control points in each production system (as described in chapter 13) and in thorough employee training.

Cook–Serve System

In a cook–serve system, most menu items are prepared primarily from basic ingredients on the day they are to be served. Most cook–serve systems incorporate ingredients with some degree of processing. The prepared items used most frequently are bakery goods, canned and frozen vegetables and fruits, and ice cream. Portion-cut chilled or frozen meats have replaced the traditional meat-cutting operation. Bread products and dessert items are still baked on-site in some cook–serve systems. Baked items are made by starting from scratch with basic ingredients or by using standard production methods along with some mixes and frozen pies, bread doughs, and desserts. Vegetables are purchased in many forms: canned, frozen, fresh, prewashed or prepeeled, and dehydrated.

The number of different food supply items kept in inventory for cook–serve systems is relatively high. The availability and cost of labor, the equipment available, and the facility's supply sources affect purchasing decisions, but rising labor costs have accelerated the trend toward purchasing more extensively processed foods.

The cook–serve system can be further categorized based on the amount of holding required between production and service of food items to customers. These subcategories include limited holding and extended holding of finished food products.

Cook–Serve with Limited Holding

Cook–serve with limited holding systems, often referred to as *à la carte cooking,* is utilized extensively by full-service and quick-service restaurants. Because customers dine at varying times and usually select items from a written menu, individual food items are cooked "to order" rather than cooked ahead. This type of system, as opposed to the other types of food production systems, minimizes the holding time between food preparation and service to customers. On the other hand, this system requires rather extensive pre-preparation of ingredients so that food preparation can be expedited once the customers have placed their orders. This type of system is appropriate if the health care organization operates a full-service or quick-service restaurant.

Cook–Serve with Extended Holding

Cook–serve with extended holding is the traditional system of food production for health care operations. It differs from the previous system in that most menu items are held hot or cold until they are served. Production may take place in a kitchen located in the facility or in a separate kitchen or commissary that supplies several sites. Food service directors who use a cook–serve with extended holding system believe that they have better control over menus, recipes, and overall quality. Menus can reflect changes in seasonal supply and marketplace conditions as well as the food preferences of patient and nonpatient markets. Also, menus can be tailored to the specific standards of the facility. In some cases, however, menu variety may be more limited than in other systems because of the amount of production time allowable, the skill levels of employees, or the availability and capacity of equipment.

A 12- to 15-hour production and service day is common for facilities using cook–serve with extended holding because foods are produced just before assembly and service. Periods of increased activity are necessary because the quality and nutritional value of some foods are adversely affected by extended holding. However, it is difficult to produce all the foods on the menu within the ideal period, and the holding that becomes necessary often results in having to serve lower-quality food.

Both skilled and semiskilled employees are needed in a cook–serve with extended holding system, and the need for skilled employees often leads to higher labor costs than is the case with other production systems. In addition, the availability of skilled employees may be limited because of the location of the facility or because of the undesirable working hours characteristic of the cook–serve with extended holding system.

Production is scheduled on a seven-day workweek. The level of productivity in cook–serve with extended holding systems may not be as high as in other systems because it is difficult to schedule a balanced daily work load that covers service time peaks and yet minimizes the number of employees on duty during slow periods. As a result, skilled employees are frequently assigned routine cleaning jobs to equalize the work load even though these tasks could be performed by less-skilled employees.

Many types and sizes of equipment are needed in a cook–serve with extended holding system. More total capacity may be needed for certain pieces of equipment because of the volume demand and same-day service that characterize the system. Poor utilization of equipment can occur, depending on the menu item mix, because both hot-holding and cold-holding equipment are needed. However, a cook–serve with extended holding system can require less energy than other systems because chilling and freezing hot foods are not necessary. Another shortcoming of the system is evident when foods must be prepared well in advance of service time, because it is difficult to maintain proper temperatures during extended holding. Food perishability increases with overcooking, and foods held at a high temperature for a long period lose their palatability and some of their nutritional value.

Cook–Chill and Cook–Freeze Systems

Cook–chill and cook–freeze systems do not have the labor, productivity, and cost problems associated with the cook–serve system or the problem of diminished food quality associated with extended holding. In a cook–chill system, prepared menu items are chilled, ready for assembly and reheating one or more days after production. Foods can be purchased at any stage of processing as basic ingredients for recipe preparation, as partially prepared recipe components, or as fully prepared items. After initial preparation, menu items may be individually portioned or stored in bulk. These food production systems require two stages of heat processing: initial cooking and reheating before serving.

The quality of food can and should be high in cook–chill and cook–freeze systems because chilled or frozen food is less perishable and retains its nutrients longer than food cooked and held in the cook–serve system. Menu selections can be more varied, particularly when menu items are individually portioned before chilling or freezing. It is possible to offer a restaurant-style menu when production does not take place on the same day as service. These foods smell, look, and taste good because they are not overcooked during holding, as in the cook–serve system. This is because the cooking process is finished during reheating. However, an internal temperature of at least 140°F (60°C) must be reached during the initial partial cooking process to ensure that foods are not contaminated by bacterial growth. (See chapter 13.)

Recipe quantities may need to be increased for large-volume production runs for frozen items. In such cases, the traditional steps in preparation are often changed to accommodate the expanded volume and to save time.

Not all foods can be held successfully in cook–chill or cook–freeze systems without extensive modification of the ingredients and/or recipes. Special ingredients, such as thickening agents, are needed for some recipes. Foam and sponge products, gels, coatings, and emulsions pose other problems. When foods are frozen, structural and textural changes occur because of cell damage and protein coagulation. As a result, odd flavors can develop in some vegetables and meats.

The extended period between initial preparation and consumption of the food in cook–chill systems creates many opportunities for the mishandling of food. Food service directors are responsible for controlling potential microbiological hazards at critical control points. This process involves monitoring equipment sanitation and time–temperature conditions at all stages from food procurement through service. During the production stage, quick-chilling procedures are essential to bring the temperatures of cooked foods to 45°F (7°C) or lower in less than four hours after initial cooking. Factors that influence the cooling rate of foods include the initial internal temperature of the food, size or depth of the batch, dimensions of the food mass, density of the food, and temperature and load of the refrigerator.

Similar quick freezing is necessary in a cook–freeze system in order to optimize the taste and smell of the frozen food as well as to ensure a product free of contamination. It is recommended that a temperature of 0°F (–18°C) or lower be reached within 90 minutes after initial cooking. Frozen food should be stored at 0°F or lower and must be properly packaged to prevent dehydration. Entrees should be thawed in a refrigerator and used within 24 hours after thawing. In all cook–chill and cook–freeze systems, the temperature of the entrees should be kept at 45°F (7°C) or lower during portioning, assembly, and distribution.

As in cook–serve systems (and all food production activities), good personal hygiene for food handlers is a critical control point at all stages of processing food in cook–chill and cook–freeze systems: initial preparation, portioning, assembly, and service. Employees can directly and indirectly contribute to microbiological contamination through poor personal hygiene and work habits. (See chapter 13.)

In both cook–chill and cook–freeze systems, production usually can be scheduled into a 40-hour workweek with regular 8-hour shifts. For this reason, these systems (because they incorporate production tasks that require high skill levels) usually require fewer skilled employees. In cook–chill systems, the plating of food can be spread over a longer period because all items are held cold during plating and tray assembly. This system can reduce the number of employees needed and possibly increase their productivity and satisfaction.

More balanced and efficient use of equipment is possible in cook–chill and cook–freeze systems because production can be distributed over the entire work shift rather than being done in the limited time just before service. Total equipment requirements may be lower than in a cook–serve system, but the types of equipment and capacities needed depend on whether a cook–chill or a cook–freeze system is being followed. For example, specialized quick-chill refrigerators are needed for both systems, but blast or cryogenic freezers also are needed for a cook–freeze system.

Adequate refrigerated space must be available for storing foods and holding them during the assembly process. Also, the amount of refrigeration space needed for preplated items is greater than for bulk storage items. The acquisition of needed equipment adds to capital investment costs. Research also indicates that more energy is used in the cook–chill and cook–freeze systems than in the cook–serve system because of the significant amount of energy required to chill or freeze, thaw, and reheat foods.

Cook–chill and cook–freeze systems may operate in an on-premises kitchen, or they may be located in a commissary separate from the service area. Many commissaries use these systems because the scheduling and control of production and service are easier for chilled and frozen foods than they are for hot foods.

Assembly–Serve System

With an assembly–serve food production system (sometimes called a convenience system), most or all foods are obtained from a commercial source in a ready-to-serve form. This includes entree items that are purchased frozen, canned, or dehydrated; ready-to-serve dessert and bakery products that are purchased fresh, frozen, or canned; salads and salad ingredients that are purchased ready to assemble; canned, frozen, or dehydrated sauces and soups; frozen concentrated, portion-packed, canned, or dehydrated fruit juices and beverages; and individual portion packets of condiments such as sugar, jelly, syrup, salad dressing, and cream.

Menu variety can be wider in assembly–serve systems than in cook–serve systems, but it depends on the facility's access to suppliers who can provide a wide range of products. However, the variety of preplated items is not as large as that offered in bulk-packaged products. Inconsistent quality among different products and among different lots of the same products has been observed. Because of this inconsistency, it is desirable to try several potential vendors before implementing an assembly–serve system. Also, the geographic location of the food service operation and small purchase volumes may intensify problems in obtaining products of the same quality from one purchase period to another.

An assembly–serve system requires minimal use of skilled labor. Labor costs should decrease if the foods used in the system are at a maximum convenience level. However, labor savings must compensate for the higher food costs characteristic of an assembly–serve system.

The system should eliminate the need for most standard production equipment, but in many cases it does not. Many operations are reluctant to abandon the option of on-premises production in case the quality, availability, or cost of the prepared items fails to meet expected standards. Thus, a primary economic advantage is lost.

Questions related to the feasibility of implementing an assembly–serve system include the following:

- Do available products meet the operation's nutrition standards for normal and modified diets?
- Are enough products available to provide variety throughout the menu cycle?
- Do products meet the quality standards of the operation and its customers?
- Is the cost per serving within an acceptable range?
- Is the operation's storage space sufficient for handling disposable ware?
- Will changes be required in the type and amount of equipment needed for reheating foods?
- Is the facility's refrigerator and freezer space adequate?
- How many labor hours can be eliminated with this system?
- How will tray assembly and delivery be performed?
- Will additional packaging materials create waste disposal problems?

In an assembly–serve system, attention must be paid to prevention of microbiological contamination at critical control points. Some of the hazards present in other systems are eliminated because there is little or no on-premises food preparation. The amount of freezer and refrigeration space needed for storing and thawing frozen foods before final heating exceeds that needed in cook–serve systems. Thawing or tempering frozen products must be carried out under refrigeration, and storage times for purchased chilled foods should be kept to a minimum. Perishable foods must be maintained at 45°F (7°C) or lower during portioning, assembly, and distribution. In the reheating stage, foods must reach temperatures of at least 140°F (60°C) as rapidly as possible. For maximum safety and palatability, an end-point temperature of 165°F (74°C) is recommended for most hot foods. Food temperatures should be routinely checked before service. As in other systems, personnel and equipment sanitation are essential to control microbiological hazards.

☐ Production Forecasting

In addition to determining the type of food production system (or combination of systems) to be implemented, the food service director must decide which forecasting technique is appropriate for the food service operation. *Forecasting* is the process of estimating a future event based on past data. Because most food production systems require extensive advanced preparation of menu items, *production demand forecasting* is critical to satisfying customer expectations.

Forecasting Techniques

Forecasting techniques can be divided into three categories: qualitative, time series, and causal models. *Qualitative* techniques are less analytical and are more appropriately used for such activities as strategic planning of marketing decisions. The *quantitative* models, both time series and causal, can be used for production forecasting.

Time Series Forecasting Techniques

Time series forecasting techniques rely solely on historical data about demand for menu items. These techniques, which assume that demand for menu items follows a pattern over time, are appropriate for short-term forecasting, such as demand for menu items. They are the forecasting techniques most frequently used by health care food service operations.

Examples of time series techniques include simple moving average and weighted moving average. Both combine data about demand for menu items over several periods or menu cycles. They result in an average, or the forecast, for the number of servings to prepare during the next menu cycle. Exponential smoothing is another time series technique that is available in computerized software packages. It differs from the averaging techniques in that it does not weigh data from the past menu cycles equally.

Causal Forecasting Techniques

In addition to historical data, causal techniques use additional types of data as well. These techniques might relate demand for menu items to other variables believed to influence demand, such as patient census or the number of patients on normal and modified diets. Causal techniques generally are more costly to implement than time series techniques. For short-term forecasting, these techniques do not result in increased accuracy over the time series techniques.

Regression analysis is the causal technique used most commonly. It draws on past data to establish a relationship between two variables, such as the number of patients on a normal diet and the number of servings of a particular entree, to forecast the number of servings to prepare.

Designing a Forecasting System

An effective forecasting system is key to health care food service operations. A number of factors must be considered when designing or redesigning a forecasting system. Ann Messersmith and Judy Miller, in their book *Forecasting in Foodservice,* indicate that the nature of the information to be forecast and the availability of data essential to generate the forecast are key concerns. Prior to selection of a specific forecasting technique, each technique should be evaluated on the basis of the accuracy of the forecast and the cost of implementing and operating the technique. Implementation issues include personnel training, modification of operational procedures, and consideration of computer-assisted applications. In addition, a strategy should be developed to evaluate the technique after it has been implemented.

☐ Production Schedules

Daily schedules for food production can be valuable management tools for controlling the use of labor while ensuring food quality. A daily production schedule assigns specific tasks to each employee. The work load is distributed according to the assigned duties and the specific skills of individual employees, and a time sequence for all production activities is established by management. In a cook–serve food production system, efficient production timing is perhaps the greatest benefit of following a daily production schedule. It can ensure that foods will not be cooked too far in advance of service and yet can allow adequate time for preparation.

For each item to be prepared, daily food production schedules should state the name of the item; the name of the employee assigned to prepare the item; preparation start and completion times; and specific details regarding ingredients, portion control, assembly, and so forth. In smaller operations, one production schedule for the entire kitchen staff may be sufficient. Larger operations with several employees in each specialized unit may require separate schedules for each work group. When work assignments are not highly specialized, production schedules can eliminate confusion about which tasks are to be performed by each employee.

Daily food production schedules should be developed concurrently with menu planning. This prevents a work load imbalance from day to day and allows adequate time for preparation of foods for later service. During scheduling, the equipment to be used for preparing each food item should be considered so that all necessary equipment will be available when needed.

☐ Portion Control

Individual food service departments should determine the appropriate portion size their facilities can accommodate for each category of food served. In setting portion sizes, the type of customers and their nutrition needs, the type of menu served, and the food budget should be considered. In most situations, evaluations solicited from patients, residents, or nonpatient customers are very helpful in judging their acceptance of portion sizes and the overall quality of the food produced.

Many measures can be taken to ensure that equal portions of food are served. For example, purchased supplies should meet well-defined specifications, recipes should be standardized, and the right utensils should be used for portioning and serving. Slicing machines can ensure that equal portions of meat, cold cuts, and cheese are cut. Gram scales can also be used for accurate portioning of meats and other entree items. Dough cutters and pie/cake scorers can be used to portion breads, rolls, biscuits, and desserts. Portion control of other items is done by count, such as number of slices of bread, packages of crackers or cookies, pats of margarine, and so forth.

☐ Standardized Recipes

Standardized recipes are followed in the ingredient control area (discussed later in the chapter) well as in the production area to control the quality, quantity, and cost of the menu items prepared. A *standardized recipe* is one in which the amounts and proportions of ingredients, as well as the method of combining them, have been developed and tested for a particular food service operation. The ingredients needed and the preparation procedures to be followed must be stated accurately so that a high-quality product and an exact number of portions can be produced every time the recipe is used. Substitutions for specified ingredients and changes in procedures must be avoided.

When standardized recipes are used, changes in personnel should not affect food quality because each ingredient and preparation detail is precisely stated in the recipe. Purchasing is simplified because the exact quantities and forms of food needed for each food item were established when the recipe was tested. Job satisfaction is increased because employees know they will produce a successful product when they follow directions carefully. In addition, new employees can be trained much more rapidly when they have standardized recipes to follow.

Although recipes are available from many sources, each food service department should reevaluate and test all new recipes used to ensure that the quantities produced, the portion

469

sizes stated, and the overall quality meet customer needs and are suited to the equipment available. When reviewing new recipes, the director should compare the stated portion size with the portion size established for the operation.

Elements of Recipe Standardization

Before a recipe can be standardized, a number of factors should be analyzed. These are discussed in the following sections.

Proportion of Ingredients

Each recipe should be read carefully, particularly if it has not yet been tried, because it may prove to be inappropriate or the number of ingredients used or the complexity of the procedures may make it impractical to use. The proportions of ingredients should be analyzed in relation to one another. For example, in a cake recipe, the sugar, flour, and shortening ratios should be appropriate for the product. Finally, the new recipe should be compared with other tested recipes for similar products.

Quantity of Ingredients

The quantities of ingredients should be listed in the recipe in both weight and volume measures. Because weighing ingredients is more accurate than measuring them by volume, volume measurements should be converted to weights. Small amounts of spices and seasonings can be measured by volume rather than weighed.

Form of Ingredients

The form of ingredients should be described in the recipe. Descriptive terms placed before the name of the ingredient designate the kind and form of food as purchased or the cooking or heating required before the food is used, such as *canned* tomatoes, *fresh* chopped spinach, *cooked* chicken, and *hard-cooked* eggs. Descriptive terms are placed after the ingredient name to indicate the preparation necessary to make the form of the ingredient different from the form as purchased or cooked: for example, onions, *chopped;* canned diced carrots, *drained;* and apples, *pared and sliced.* If waste is likely to occur in the initial preparation steps for some ingredients, the quantity should be listed as edible portion (EP) rather than as purchased (AP). The purchase amount should be recorded in a separate section on the recipe card.

Order of Ingredients

Ingredients should be listed in the order in which they will be combined. Ingredients requiring pretreatment before they are combined should be listed first or specially marked to indicate that advance preparation is needed.

Procedures

If possible, preparation procedures should be simplified or some steps eliminated to save time, equipment, and ware washing. For example, in a kitchen equipped with steam-jacketed kettles, the easiest way to prepare a cooked pudding is to place measured cold milk in the kettle, combine all dry ingredients, blend them into the milk with a wire whip, and then heat the entire mixture. The procedure for combining ingredients should be stated clearly. Specific terms—such as *blend, whip, cream,* and *fold*—tell the cook exactly what to do. Mixing speeds and times, as well as the type of beater to be used, should be stated in recipes to be prepared in the mixer. When batch size is increased or decreased, mixing times may need to be adjusted accordingly. If chilling is required before the entire recipe can be completed, the chill time should be stated.

Recipe Format

Standardized recipes may be written in a variety of ways. A standard format for all recipes should be developed for ease of use. (A sample format is shown in figure 19-1.) Spaces for

Figure 19-1. Example of a Standardized Recipe Format

RECIPE: PIZZA CASSEROLE		

Portions: 96   Cooking Temperature: 350°F (177°C)   Total Recipe Cost: _____

Pans: 3   Cooking Time: 20-25 minutes   Cost per Portion: _____

Pan Size: 12 × 20 × 2½ inches   Portion Size: 8 × 4 inches   Date Calculated: _____

Portion Utensil: Spatula

Ingredients	Amount	Procedure
Ground beef Pork sausage, bulk	3 pounds 3 pounds	1. Sauté ground beef and sausage until cooked. 2. Drain excess fat.
Spaghetti, thin Salt Cooking oil	4 pounds, 8 ounces 4 tablespoons 2 tablespoons	3. Cook spaghetti in boiling salted water in steam-jacketed kettle. Add 2 tablespoons oil to water to prevent boiling over. 4. Drain. 5. Put in pans.
Canned tomato sauce	1 #10 can	6. Pour equal amounts of sauce over spaghetti. 7. Sprinkle cooked meat over sauce.
Oregano, crushed Sweet basil, crushed Mozzarella cheese, grated Onions, chopped Green peppers, chopped Mushrooms, drained Ripe olives, sliced	3 tablespoons 3 tablespoons 9 pounds 1½ cups 1½ cups 3 1-pound cans 3 cups	8. Sprinkle oregano and basil over meat. 9. Sprinkle cheese over oregano and basil. 10. Top with chopped onions, green peppers, mushrooms, and ripe olives. 11. Bake.

recording calculations of portion cost and for other batch sizes also can be included. Recipes can be filed according to types of items in a standard recipe box, a file drawer, a notebook, or on a computer system. Transparent plastic envelopes or laminated cards can be used to protect recipes in the kitchen.

Batch Size Adjustment

The batch sizes for tested recipes often need to be altered to make handling easier or to suit the capacity of the facility's equipment. To adjust the total recipe yield, the number of servings needed is determined first. That number then is divided by the number of servings stated in the original recipe to arrive at a factor for adjusting the ingredient quantities. To increase batch size, the amount of each ingredient is multiplied by the factor and rounded off to the nearest convenient weight or measure. To decrease batch size, the amount of each ingredient in the original recipe is divided by the factor to arrive at the appropriate quantity for the reduced recipe. It is important that ingredient proportions never be changed when recipes are increased or decreased, although mixing and cooking times should be adjusted as necessary. Decimal equivalents and rules for rounding weights and volume measures of ingredients in recipes are listed in tables 19-1, 19-2, and 19-3.

Other Details

The recipe should specify pan type, size, and method of pretreatment. To get an accurate yield of uniform portions, the weight or volume of the mixture to be placed in each pan must be stated in the recipe and followed. It is helpful to note the total weight or volume of the batch as well. Cooking times and temperatures should be double-checked, because those in the original recipe may not be suitable for the type of equipment available. For example, baking

Table 19-1. Decimal Equivalents for Different Units (in Parts of 1 Pound, 1 Cup, or 1 Gallon)

Number of Units (ounces, tablespoons, or cups)	Decimal Equivalent of 1 Pound, 1 Cup, or 1 Gallon					
	+0 Unit	+¼ Unit	+⅓ Unit	+½ Unit	+⅔ Unit	+¾ Unit
0	–	0.016	0.021	0.031	0.042	0.047
1	0.062	0.078	0.083	0.094	0.104	0.109
2	0.125	0.141	0.146	0.156	0.167	0.172
3	0.188	0.203	0.208	0.219	0.229	0.234
4	0.250	0.266	0.271	0.281	0.292	0.297
5	0.312	0.328	0.333	0.344	0.354	0.359
6	0.375	0.391	0.396	0.406	0.417	0.422
7	0.438	0.453	0.458	0.469	0.479	0.484
8	0.500	0.516	0.521	0.531	0.542	0.547
9	0.562	0.578	0.583	0.594	0.604	0.609
10	0.625	0.641	0.646	0.656	0.667	0.672
11	0.688	0.703	0.708	0.719	0.729	0.734
12	0.750	0.766	0.771	0.781	0.792	0.797
13	0.812	0.828	0.833	0.844	0.854	0.859
14	0.875	0.891	0.896	0.906	0.917	0.922
15	0.938	0.953	0.958	0.969	0.979	0.984

Note: The units are read at the side and top of the table as follows: If the units are ounces, the decimal equivalents given in the body of the table are parts of 1 pound; if the units are tablespoons, the decimal equivalents are parts of 1 cup; if the units are cups, the decimal equivalents are parts of 1 gallon.

Example 1: To convert 10½ ounces to the corresponding decimal equivalent of a pound, find 10 in the first column and follow this line across to the column headed ½, which shows that 0.646 pound corresponds to 10½ ounces.

Example 2: To convert the decimal 0.531 pound to ounces, find 0.531 in the body of the table. Then in the first column find the number that is on the same horizontal line, which is 8. Next, add the number from the heading of the column in which 0.531 was found, which is ⅔. Thus, 0.531 pound corresponds to 8⅔ ounces.

Source: USDA Guides for Writing and Evaluating Quantity Recipes for Type A School Lunches, September 1969.

temperatures and times for standard ovens may have to be reduced for convection ovens. Portioning instructions should be stated, as well as any instructions for cooling or holding prior to portioning. The portioning tools to be used may be stated in certain recipes. Suggested garnishes also may be listed.

New recipes should be prepared exactly as the procedures state. It often is tempting to begin modifying ingredients, quantities of ingredients, or preparation steps before discovering what kind of product would have been produced by the original recipe. Measurements should be checked for accuracy. If the original recipe does not list weight as well as volume measures, quantities should be weighed as the recipe is prepared and the actual yield carefully noted to determine whether it is the same as the stated yield. The finished product should be evaluated for eye appeal, quality, and acceptability. Because products fully acceptable to food service department personnel may be less appealing to customers, in most operations, seeking evaluations from customers is very helpful in determining the level of acceptance.

If careful evaluation indicates that changes are needed in the recipe, they should be made and carefully noted on the recipe. It is very important to have the cooks' cooperation because they may find it hard to resist asserting their individuality by changing the ingredients or procedures without authorization.

☐ Ingredient Control

The preparation of high-quality food is the most important task of the food service department. Ingredient control is a vital component of the total system, as illustrated in figure 19-2.

Traditionally, each person responsible for food preparation performed all the tasks, from collecting and weighing the ingredients to portioning the final product. Because of the need for greater control over quality and costs, some food service operations have centralized the preparation of recipe ingredients in ingredient areas or a single ingredient room. Centralized ingredient control frees skilled cooks from performing repetitive tasks that do not require their level of skill. Food quality can be controlled by eliminating the possibility that production workers might alter the ingredients or batch size. In some operations, only dry ingredients are weighed or measured. In others, all the steps necessary to weigh recipe ingredients accurately are performed in a central location. The latter system achieves the greatest degree of control but requires more labor and equipment.

In the ingredient area, the quantities of ingredients stated in the standardized recipe are weighed, measured, and collected for each menu item. The worker weighing the ingredients uses a production forecast that indicates the batch size needed for each recipe. Premeasured ingredients that bear labels listing the recipe name, ingredient name, and quantity are delivered to the cooks in the kitchen at the appropriate point in the production schedule.

The physical layout of the ingredient room can take many forms. When enough space is available, an area within the storeroom itself can be equipped to handle this function.

Table 19-2. Rules for Rounding Weights and Volume Measures of Ingredients in Recipes

If the Total Amount of an Ingredient Is	Adjust as Follows[a]	Example
Weights[b]		
Less than 2 ounces	Volume measure only unless weight is ¼, ½, ¾ ounce, and so forth	⅞ ounce of salt would be shown only as 2 tablespoons
From 2 to 10 ounces	Nearest ¼ ounce	Round 2⅓ ounces to 2¼ ounces
More than 10 ounces but less than 2 pounds 8 ounces	Nearest ½ ounce	Round 1 pound 5⅜ ounces to 1 pound 5½ ounces
2 pounds 8 ounces to 5 pounds	Nearest full ounce	Round 3 pounds 6⅝ ounces to 3 pounds 7 ounces
More than 5 pounds	Nearest ¼ pound	Round 5 pounds 9½ ounces to 5 pounds 8 ounces
Volume Measures[b]		
Less than 2 tablespoons	Nearest ¼ teaspoon	Round 1⅔ teaspoons to 1¾ teaspoons
2 tablespoons to ½ cup	Nearest teaspoon	Round 3 tablespoons ⅓ teaspoon to 3 tablespoons
More than ½ cup but less than ¾ cup	Nearest tablespoon	Round ½ cup 1⅓ tablespoons to ½ cup 1 tablespoon
More than ¾ cup but less than 2 cups	Nearest 2 tablespoons	Round 1 cup 2¾ tablespoons to 1 cup 2 tablespoons
2 cups to 2 quarts	Nearest ¼ cup	Round 1 quart 3 cups 11⅓ tablespoons to 1 quart 3¾ cups
More than 2 quarts but less than 4 quarts	Nearest ½ cup	Round 3 quarts 9 tablespoons to 3 quarts ½ cup
1 gallon to 2 gallons	Nearest full cup	Round 1 gallon 1 quart 3¼ cups to 1 gallon 1¾ quarts
More than 2 gallons	Nearest full quart	Round 2 gallons 1 quart ½ cup to 2¼ gallons

Source: USDA Guides for Writing and Evaluating Quantity Recipes for Type A School Lunches, September 1969.

[a]When a weight or volume measure is at the midpoint, round up.

[b]The weights and volume measures have been grouped so that the percentage error in rounding does not exceed the error normally introduced in handling food ingredients.

Table 19-3. Rules for Rounding Amounts to Purchase for a Marketing Guide

If the Total Amount of an Ingredient Is	Adjust as Follows[a]	Example
Weights[b]		
Between 2 and 10 ounces	Up to next ¼ ounce	Round 6⅛ ounces to 6¼ ounces
More than 10 ounces but less than 2 pounds 8 ounces	Up to next ½ ounce	Round 1 pound 3¾ ounces to 1 pound 4 ounces
Between 2 pounds 8 ounces and 5 pounds	Up to next 1 ounce	Round 4 pounds 7¼ ounces to 4 pounds 8 ounces
More than 5 pounds	Up to next even 2 ounces (use only amounts of 2, 4, 6, 8, 10, 12, or 14 ounces, or full pounds)	Round 8 pounds 8¾ ounces to 8 pounds 10 ounces
Cans, Packages, Loaves[b]		
No. 10 can	Up to next ⅛, ¼, ⅓, ½, ⅔, ¾, or 1 can	Round 0.60 can to ⅔ can
No. 3 cylinder	Up to next ¼, ⅓, ½, ⅔, ¾, or 1 can	Round 0.40 can to ½ can
Package	Up to next ¼, ½, ¾, or 1 package	Round 0.80 package to 1 package
Loaf of bread	Up to next ¼, ½, ¾, or 1 loaf	Round 0.57 loaf to ¾ loaf

Source: USDA Guides for Writing and Evaluating Quantity Recipes for Type A School Lunches, September 1969.

[a]When a weight or volume measure is at the midpoint, round up.

[b]The weights and volume measures have been grouped so that the percentage error in rounding does not exceed the error normally introduced in handling food ingredients.

Figure 19-2. Production System Based on Ingredient Control

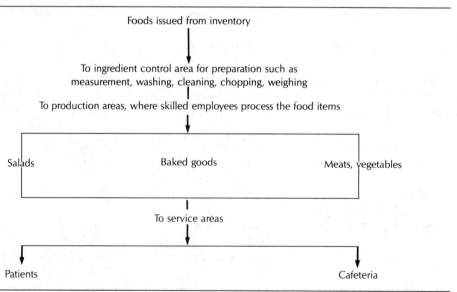

Source: Adapted from R. P. Puckett, *Dietary Manager's Independent Study Course.* Gainesville, FL: Department of Independent Study by Correspondence, University of Florida, 1985.

Otherwise, a location close to the storeroom and refrigerators can be used. Regardless of the physical layout, the equipment needed includes large and small scales, measures, a sink, storage bins, large and small containers for measured ingredients, trays or baskets, and carts. Even without a separate ingredient area, some of the advantages of this system can still be realized. During slow periods in the workday, employees can be assigned to weigh ingredients for the next day's production.

Accurate measurement is important for consistent results with standardized recipes. Measuring tools and scales must be easily accessible in all work areas when centralized ingredient control is not used. It is quicker and more accurate to weigh ingredients when the right kinds of scales are provided. Standard measuring spoons and measuring cups for both dry and liquid ingredients are needed. The purchase of heavy-grade metal measures is well worth their extra cost because they are not as likely to be dented and distorted as are cheaper measures. In each work center, measuring equipment should be stored in an easily accessible place.

☐ Food Production Processes

Selection of appropriate food production processes affects the quality of the finished menu item. This is especially true when heat is used to cook the product. Following proper cooking procedures enhances the flavor, appearance, color, digestibility, and palatability of meat. Proper cooking also conserves the nutrients in food. The food service director must be familiar with the recommended methods for cooking and/or preparing each category of food.

Meat

The flavor, tenderness, juiciness, and color of cooked meat are the primary measures of quality in meat products. In addition to maintaining these sensory qualities of meat, the food production director must know the total quantity and number of servings obtainable after the meat has been cooked. Cooking methods that produce the highest yield of palatable, edible meat must be selected to control the cost of each serving. Cooked yields are reduced by shrinkage caused by excessive evaporation of water from the surface of meat and through drip loss of fat, water, and natural flavoring substances from the tissue.

The control of cooking temperatures and times is critical in minimizing shrinkage of meat during preparation. Research has shown that low temperatures consistently produce higher meat yields that are more evenly cooked. The other basic factor that affects shrinkage is length of cooking time. As cooking time increases, losses from evaporation increase, with undesirable changes in meat texture, flavor, and carvability.

Several factors affect cooking time. Among these are size of the cut and uniformity of its shape. Usually, the larger the roast, the longer the cooking time required. If the cut is not uniform in shape, one end of the cut can become overcooked before the rest is done. A large flat roast cooks faster than one of similar weight that has been rolled and tied.

Cooking time also is affected by the composition of the meat itself. The more plentiful the fat covering and marbling, the less cooking time is required, because fat is a better heat conductor than muscle. For roast meats, cooking times are also increased by multiple oven loads and by the degree of doneness desired. Overcooking is a particularly wasteful practice because it not only causes higher losses in yield, but it also diminishes tenderness and palatability.

Cooking methods for meat usually are designated as dry-heat or moist-heat methods, depending on the atmosphere surrounding the meat. The differences are in the rate of heat transfer to the meat and in the temperatures to which the meat surface is exposed. Water vapor, used in moist-heat cooking, is a more efficient heat conductor than air, so it helps supply heat energy more rapidly to the meat. The temperature to which meat is subjected in moist-heat cooking should be no higher than the boiling point of water. In dry-heat cooking, the heat transfer is slower, but the meat surfaces are subjected to much higher temperatures.

Dry-Heat Methods

Dry-heat methods cause the caramelization, or browning, of meat surfaces, which makes meat more palatable but does not provide additional moisture to soften the collagen in the meat. For that reason, the dry-heat methods of roasting, panfrying, grilling, and deep-fat frying usually are recommended only for naturally tender meat cuts. Muscles that received relatively little exercise during the meat animal's life, such as rib and loin cuts of beef and pork and cuts that come from higher-grade animals, usually are suitable for dry-heat cooking. Meat from young animals, such as veal and lamb, also is tender but often is cooked by moist-heat methods to develop its flavor.

Because of changes in methods of beef production as well as in consumer preferences over the past decade, other exceptions apply to these general recommendations. Less-tender chuck and round roasts may be cooked by dry heat to the rare and medium-rare states and then thinly sliced to yield a flavorful, tender finished product. Other methods are used by food service operations to tenderize less-tender cuts enough to allow dry-heat cooking. Some of these treatments also are used by meat processors. To physically break down muscle fibers and connective tissue, mechanical means—such as cubing, dicing, grinding, and chopping— often are used. Marinating less-tender cuts in oil and acid mixtures can break down muscle fibers as well. Tomato juice, vinegar, lemon juice, wine, and sour cream commonly are used in marinades. Enzymatic tenderizers, which often contain papain (a protein from papaya), can be applied to meat surfaces, used as a marinade, or injected into the muscle. Surface applications of such tenderizers are most effective on thinner cuts of meat.

Roasting

Meats can be roasted in several different types of ovens (conventional, convection, deck, among others), but the cooking procedure is similar in each. The meat is placed on a rack in an open pan with no moisture added. The heat in a regular oven or the heated moving air in a convection oven helps produce surface browning. It was once common to sear roasts in a very hot oven for 20 to 30 minutes and then reduce the temperature to about 300°F (149°C) for the remainder of the cooking time. Searing, or coagulating the surface proteins, was supposed to prevent loss of juices and nutrients. However, studies have shown not only that this is not the case, but that searing can increase total cooking losses from the surface. Without searing, there is no hard outer crust and slicing is easier. Repeated studies have shown that roasting at low, constant temperatures ranging from 225° to 250°F (107° to 121°C) decreases the amount of shrinkage and produces meat that is juicier, more uniformly cooked, and more tender. The lower temperature is recommended for convection ovens.

A meat thermometer should be used to determine the interior temperature and doneness of meat. The thermometer should be inserted so that the tip is in the center of the largest muscle and is not touching bone or embedded in fat. Because the internal temperature of meat continues to rise after it has been removed from the oven, the meat should be taken out of the oven slightly before the desired temperature has been reached. If a roast is allowed to stand in a warm place for 10 to 15 minutes, its texture will become more firm and it will slice more easily.

Tables that list roasting times in minutes per pound at best provide only a guide to help estimate total cooking time. It is essential to use meat thermometers to determine doneness and to keep careful records of the actual cooking times needed to reach that state of doneness for each quality, style, and size of roast prepared.

Table 19-4 lists standard end-point temperatures for roasted meats. It should be noted that the internal temperature for well-done pork (170°F [77°C]) is lower than earlier recommendations. Research has shown that 170°F is ideal for flavor, tenderness, and palatability; is well above the safety point for destruction of possible trichinae (140°F [60°C]); and produces a greater yield of sliceable meat.

Table 19-4. Standard End-Point Temperatures for Roasted Meat

Meat	Internal Temperature
Beef	
Rare	130°F (54°C)
Medium-rare	140°F (60°C)
Medium	150°F (65°C)
Medium-well	155°F (68°C)
Well-done	160°F (71°C)
Veal	170°F (77°C)
Lamb	160°F (71°C) to 180°F (82°C)
Pork, fresh	
Well-done	170°F (77°C)
Pork, cured	
Ham, ready-to-eat	140°F (60°C)
Ham, uncooked	160°F (71°C)
Shoulder	170°F (77°C)
Turkey	180°F (82°C) to 185°F (85°C)

Broiling and Grilling

Broiling and grilling are dry-heat cooking methods in which direct or radiant heat from gas flames, electric coils, or charcoal briquettes provides the heat source. This method is most successful for relatively tender cuts between one and two inches thick. Thinner cuts tend to dry out and thicker cuts are difficult to broil to the more well-done stages. Cuts should be turned only once during broiling and should not be seasoned until cooking is complete. Adding salt tends to draw moisture from the meat surfaces and delays browning.

Many kinds of equipment can be used for broiling and grilling, so cooking times vary from one unit to another. Timetables for broiling and grilling are not particularly useful because thickness of the cut, distance of the meat from the heat source, and degree of doneness affect total cooking time. Frozen cuts can be broiled with consistent results, but they should be placed farther from the heat or cooked at a lower temperature to reach uniform doneness. Broiling time is almost doubled for most frozen steaks. Cuts over 1½ inches thick should be thawed before broiling.

Panfrying

In panfrying, heat is conducted from the surface of a grill, braising pan, or skillet to the meat surface. The metal surface should be oiled before very lean cuts are placed on it, but most meats generate enough melted fat to prevent sticking. Moderate temperatures should be used to avoid overbrowning and crusting the meat surfaces. Excess fat can be removed as it accumulates, and care should be taken to avoid temperatures high enough to cause smoking, which make the meat taste off flavor. Many meat cuts (such as hamburger, steak, liver, cube steak, ground lamb, lamb chop, ham steak, Canadian bacon, and other similar thinner cuts) can be completely cooked by this method. Many recipes combine an initial sautéing or grilling with moist-heat finishing.

Panfrying large quantities of the cuts mentioned is often too time-consuming to be practical. For this reason, oven frying is substituted. With this method, meat is placed in well-greased, shallow pans with or without additional fat dribbled over it. Meats may be dredged in seasoned flour or crumbs and cooked at temperatures ranging from 375° to 400°F (190° to 204°C). The pan is left uncovered and no liquid is added.

Deep-Fat Frying

Deep-fat frying is not a primary method for cooking meats but, rather, usually is the initial step for browning meats that will be finished by another method. For example, round steaks or pork chops may be browned in deep fat and then finished in the oven. Meats should be coated or breaded before deep-fat frying; the fat temperature should be kept at 350°F (177°C), high enough to avoid overabsorption of fat and yet low enough to produce a tender product and avoid breakdown of the fat. Meat that is to be deep-fat fried should be free of excessive moisture and loose particles of breading. Moisture will cause the fat to spatter or bubble and will speed fat breakdown.

When meat is deep-fat fried, uniformly sized pieces should be loaded into the fryer basket and lowered slowly into the hot fat. The fryer should not be overloaded because this will reduce the fat temperature and increase the amount of fat absorbed into the meat (particularly important when frying frozen meat). The meat should be cooked until the outside is properly browned or until the cut is completely done. The degree of doneness should be checked by cutting into a sample piece from the batch. When the meat is removed from the fat, the fryer basket should be lifted and allowed to drain over the fryer kettle and care taken to avoid shaking excess crumbs from the coating into the fat. Because salt hastens the deterioration of fat, the meat should be salted after its removal from the fryer basket. Additional fat should be added during the cooking process to maintain the correct frying level and extend the life of the fat. The fat should be brought up to proper cooking temperature before more meat is fried. Frying fat should be filtered at least once daily—more often if the fryer is used extensively or if breaded foods are cooked in it.

Moist-Heat Methods

Meats cooked by moist heat are surrounded by steam or hot liquid. The external surface of the meat is exposed to temperatures no higher than that of boiling water, except when the meat is cooked under pressure. Moist-heat methods are used to tenderize tougher muscles and cuts that contain larger amounts of collagen. In general, the cooking times for moist-heat methods are considerably longer because the temperatures are lower than in dry-heat cooking. Many cuts that could be cooked by dry heat are cooked in moist heat to add greater variety and appeal to entree selections. For example, certain tender cuts such as pork or veal steaks, chops and cutlets, and beef and pork liver are cooked this way. Slow cooking develops flavor, tenderizes meat, and reduces handling time.

Braising

Braising (also called *pot roasting, Swissing,* and *fricasseeing*) is one of the most frequently used moist-heat cooking methods. Meat cuts are cooked slowly in a covered utensil in a small amount of liquid. The meat may be browned first in a small amount of fat, in which case the cut can be dredged first in seasoned flour to enhance browning.

In food service facilities, several different pieces of equipment can be used to braise meat. Steam-jacketed kettles or tilting braising pans are ideal because they speed the cooking process, create uniform cooking temperatures, and make handling the cooked meat easier. Covered shallow, heavy-duty pans also can be used for braising on the range top or in an oven at 300° to 325°F (149° to 163°C).

Stewing

Stewing meat involves cooking in a large amount of liquid at temperatures just below the boiling point. Although the method is sometimes described as boiling, temperatures between 185° and 200°F (85° and 93°C) are better than boiling temperatures (212°F [100°C]) because they produce a more flavorful and tender product. Boiling makes meat stringy and difficult to slice, and it causes more shrinkage.

Stewing is suitable for less-tender cuts of meat, such as fresh or corned beef brisket; beef, lamb, or veal cubes for stews or casseroles; and any meats, such as shank and neck, being used to make soup stock. For additional flavor and color, some meats may be dredged in seasoned flour and browned before stewing. Although stewing can be done in many different types of equipment, it is important to select pots, kettles, and pans that are large enough to accommodate efficient handling of batches.

Steaming

Meat can be steamed by using pressure steamers or by wrapping it in heavy foil. This moist-heat method tenderizes less-tender cuts, but shrinkage and drip loss may be greater than with other cooking methods. Many food service operations use compartment steamers to reduce the cooking time required for meat that will be used in salads, creamed dishes, and sandwiches. However, the flavor and color of steamed meats usually are less attractive than the flavor and color of meats cooked by other methods. Experiments with the heavy foil wrapping of beef roasts have shown that cooking time is increased, cooking losses are higher, and the meat is less tender.

Preparing Frozen Meat

More and more food service operations are moving toward purchasing more types of frozen meat items. Most frozen meats can be cooked with essentially the same yield and quality as fully or partially thawed meats. The same cooking procedures and temperatures apply, but additional cooking time and energy are needed to reach the desired degree of doneness. In roasting meat from the frozen state, the cooking time should be increased about one and a half times. This additional time and the cost of fuel for the extra roasting must be considered in production scheduling. A meat thermometer should be inserted midway in the cooking process so that accurate end-point temperatures can be determined.

Some cuts of meat, such as fabricated veal and pork cutlets, should not be thawed before cooking. Thawed cuts of these kinds are difficult to handle, and when they are breaded, there is a tendency for the breading to fall off when the cuts are thawed before cooking. Also, browning may be more uneven when these cuts are thawed before cooking. When cooked frozen meats are used, the manufacturer's instructions for thawing and reheating should be followed exactly to obtain optimum quality and avoid food safety hazards.

Portioning Meat

Standard portion sizes for each type of meat served must be determined to ensure adequate cost control and consumer satisfaction. A chart giving individual portion sizes can be developed in the department and made available to the workers responsible for portioning. For roasts and other large cuts, electric slicing is the most efficient way to produce uniform portions. The sliced meat should be weighed for the desired individual portion size, and equal numbers of portions should be placed in each pan (covered to prevent moisture loss). For fully cooked meats, such as hams, turkey rolls, and beef roasts, the meat should be sliced and put in a pan before heating. The manufacturer's instructions for handling should be followed.

Electric slicers must be carefully cleaned immediately after each use and maintained in a sanitary condition. In operations that do not have an electric slicer, sharp knives and properly sanitized cutting boards will be needed. The work area used for portioning cooked meats also should be kept in a sanitary condition. Knives and boards used in preparing raw meat or poultry products must always be sanitized before they are used with cooked products.

Holding Cooked Meat

Cooked meats must be held at temperatures of 140°F (60°C) or higher. Prior to holding, the meat should be brought to a safe temperature of at least 140°F or higher as needed for palatability and safety. Most holding equipment is designed to maintain these temperatures and not to reheat cold foods. Ideally, meat and menu items containing meat should be held for as short a time as possible and never for more than two hours. In many situations, however, holding for transport or an extended service period is necessary. Meats cooked by moist heat are more suitable for extended holding, but medium-rare beef roasts can be held for a short time without becoming overdone. Pork should be brought to a temperature of 170°F (77°C) prior to holding.

In many food service operations, staggered production schedules reduce the necessity for extended holding and decrease the probability of quality loss, shrinkage, and lower acceptability.

479

Batch production is almost always necessary for fried and breaded items because they do not hold well on the steam table.

Storing Cooked Meat

Regardless of how accurately the department forecasts production, unused cooked meat items occasionally may remain at the end of the service period, as well as meat items that were cooked in advance of the service time. Despite care in preparation and holding, the risk that these foods have been exposed to microbiological contamination is always present. For that reason, cooked meats must be stored very carefully to prevent the possibility of causing food-borne illness in consumers.

Cooked meat and foods containing meat must be quickly chilled to temperatures below 45°F (7°C) within two hours. For some items, cooling will be more rapid if the hot food is placed in a shallow layer in shallow pans and refrigerated immediately. The food should be covered after it has cooled. For dense foods, such as lasagna, quick cooling can be accomplished by placing the pan of food on ice or in a sink containing ice and water. Stews, soups, and other semiliquid foods should be treated similarly and be stirred frequently during the initial cooling period. Hot foods should not be placed in deep pots, jars, or pans because doing so slows the cooling rate. Hot stock, gravy, and other liquid products should not be added to a pan that contains leftovers. The risks in doing so are twofold: The entire batch may be warmed to temperatures that can support bacterial growth, and the safe storage life of the newly cooked food will be shortened.

In a cook–chill production system, a specially designed quick-chilling refrigerator should be used to bring hot foods containing meat down to 45°F within four hours. After chilling, the foods should be stored at 32° to 38°F (0° to 3°C) and used within 48 hours to avoid safety risks and loss of palatability.

Using Leftover Meat

Leftovers should always be stored separately, dated, and kept for no longer than 48 hours. If it is known that the products will not be used within that period, they should be frozen immediately after service in a freezer that has adequate air circulation. Pans of food should not be stacked and refrigerator shelves should not be covered with foil or trays because this can block the flow of cold air around the foods.

Leftovers should not be combined with fresh products; for example, leftover beef stew should not be added to a fresh batch of beef stew. However, many kinds of leftover meat can be used in casseroles, salads, sandwich fillings, and soups. When devising ways to use leftovers, department managers must consider the cost of additional labor needed to make the items usable. If considerable labor will be expended in reworking the item, it may be more economical to serve it with fewer changes or to freeze it until it appears again in the menu cycle.

Leftover meats to be frozen should be packaged in moistureproof and vaporproof materials such as freezer wrap, freezer bags, and heavy-duty foil. Plastic or foil containers are suitable for casseroles, stews, and other semiliquid products that can be thawed in the refrigerator before reheating. These products should be reheated to at least 165° to 170°F (74° to 77°C). After one reheating, leftovers should be discarded.

Poultry

Most poultry purchased today is ready to cook either fresh chilled or frozen. Many forms of cooked poultry are also available to food service facilities. The most widely marketed poultry—broiler-fryer chickens, turkeys, Cornish game hens, ducks, and geese—are all young, tender birds. For that reason, broiling, frying, and roasting are the preferred preparation methods. Moist-heat cooking methods offer wide menu variety and appeal, and today's poultry does not need long cooking in moisture to yield a tender product.

Poultry must be properly handled during preparation, cooking, holding, and cooling to prevent contamination that might cause food poisoning. Chilled fresh poultry should be stored at 28° to 32°F (−2° to 0°C) for not more than two or three days. If poultry must be purchased more than two or three days prior to service, it should be purchased frozen.

Poultry should always be thawed in the refrigerator. For large birds, this can mean up to four days. Frozen whole turkeys, ducks, and geese can be thawed more rapidly by placing them, in their original wrappers, in cold water. Defrosting at kitchen temperature or in warm water is hazardous because this can promote growth of bacteria on the surface of the poultry. The body cavity is especially rich in Salmonella bacteria, which are capable of causing food poisoning. Thawed poultry should be washed inside and out in cold water, drained, refrigerated, and cooked within 24 hours. Breaded or battered chicken pieces, either cooked or uncooked, should not be thawed prior to cooking or reheating. Fully cooked frozen turkey rolls, frozen diced turkey and chicken, and other similar forms may be thawed in the refrigerator before use. Knives and cutting boards used to prepare uncooked poultry should be sanitized before they are used to prepare other food products.

Dry-Heat Methods for Cooking Poultry

There are also dry-heat methods for cooking poultry. These are discussed in the following subsections.

Roasting

One of the most common methods of preparing poultry uses the dry-heat method of oven roasting. Turkey can be roasted whole, cut in half, or cut in pieces. The results are similar in all cases, but the decreased oven space and roasting time required may make the cut forms more efficient to use. Overcooking white meat can be avoided by roasting the white pieces in a separate pan and allowing a shorter cooking time. A turkey to be roasted whole should not be stuffed, and roasting should be done in one continuous period. Raw turkeys can be cooked from the frozen state or partially thawed and then cooked.

Whole turkeys and chickens should be placed on a rack in a shallow pan and roasted at 300° to 325°F (149° to 163°C). Low oven temperatures ensure higher yields of edible meat, with better flavor and succulence. The skin can be brushed with margarine, oil, or shortening. If desired, the body cavity of whole birds may be seasoned with salt, pepper, and herbs. A meat thermometer can be used to determine the degree of doneness. For turkeys, the thermometer should be inserted in the thigh muscle adjoining the body cavity or in the thickest portion of the breast. Doneness is indicated when the thermometer registers 180°F (82°C). Doneness also is indicated when the thigh or breast meat feels soft or when the leg moves readily at the thigh joint and the juice is clear, with no pink color.

A tent of aluminum foil placed loosely over the breast of a whole turkey will delay browning and excessive drying of the breast meat, but it should be removed for the last 30 minutes of roasting. (Wrapping the whole bird in foil or cooking it in a covered pan results in steam cooking, and the rich browning and true flavor of roasted poultry does not develop.) Basting should be done as needed during cooking.

In roasting ducks or geese, no basting is needed. Fat should be poured off as it accumulates in the roasting pan. A small amount of water may be added to each pan to reduce spattering, but the birds should be roasted uncovered, following the same procedures as described for turkey and chicken.

For easier slicing, roasted poultry should be allowed to stand for 15 to 20 minutes after removal from the oven. This permits the hot juices to be absorbed into the meat so that they flow less freely during slicing. Also, the flesh will be firm and therefore will slice with less tearing and crumbling.

Oven Frying

Fried chicken has long been a favorite entree, and an easy way to prepare it in quantity is to oven-fry it. Chicken pieces are washed and dried, dredged in seasoned flour, and placed in a single layer on a well-greased sheet pan or in a 12-by-20-inch pan. The chicken is then cooked in a 400°F (204°C) oven for 45 to 50 minutes. Variations on the basic oven-fried chicken recipe are almost unlimited. The chicken may be dipped in milk, buttermilk, undiluted cream soup, or margarine before coating. Coatings include bread crumbs, cornflake crumbs, and cracker crumbs seasoned with herbs, paprika, and Parmesan cheese. Instant potato flakes make a crunchy coating, and commercial coatings can provide further variety for this popular menu item.

Deep-Fat Frying

Deep-fat frying produces chicken pieces with a uniform golden color. This method, however, requires more attention than oven frying. To ensure that the chicken is thoroughly cooked, many food service operations fry it until it is golden and then place it in a 325°F (163°C) oven to complete the cooking. The temperature of the fat should be 350° to 365°F (177° to 185°C), and the same procedures described for frying meat apply. Deep-fat frying can be used for reheating the breaded or battered chicken pieces that are used in many food service operations, although oven frying yields a product lower in fat. The poultry processor's instructions for cooking time and temperature should be followed.

Broiling and Grilling

Tender young chickens can be broiled or grilled if the food service operation's equipment capacity is sufficient for the quantity needed. Halves or parts may be brushed with melted fat, seasoned, and placed skin side down on the broiler rack about six inches away from the heat source or directly on the grill. The chicken parts should be turned after 10 or 15 minutes and brushed with fat. Total broiling time will be 35 to 50 minutes, depending on the size of the pieces. For calorie-restricted or fat-restricted diets, brushing the chicken with fat should be eliminated. Also popular for both modified and normal diets are recipes for boneless, skinless chicken breasts, which can be marinated for flavor enhancement and then broiled or grilled to the proper degree of doneness.

In extended care facilities, an outdoor chicken barbecue can provide a welcome change from the regular summer meal routine. Several times during cooking, chicken quarters, halves, or pieces may be brushed with oil, a mixture of equal parts of oil and vinegar, or a seasoned barbecue sauce. Seasoned barbecue sauces should not be added until the last 15 or 20 minutes. The chicken pieces should be turned every 10 or 15 minutes during the 45 to 60 minutes required for doneness. To shorten the cooking time, the pieces can be partially cooked in a steamer or oven just before barbecuing.

Moist-Heat Methods for Cooking Poultry

Several moist-heat methods may be used for cooking older, less-tender poultry or for menu variety. These methods include braising, stewing, simmering, and steaming and may be used for cooking whole or split poultry to be sliced, creamed, or made into soups and stews. The flavor that develops depends on the concentration of the broth. In braising, only enough liquid is used to cover the bottom of the pan; in stewing and simmering, the meat is fully covered with liquid. In all moist-heat methods, the pan or kettle is covered tightly, and the temperature is kept at about 185°F (85°C). Cooking time depends on the age and size of the bird, as well as the quantity in the pan. The poultry should be cooked until fork tender. Poultry parts also may be steamed in low- or high-pressure steamers according to the manufacturer's instructions.

If moist-heat methods are used to produce cooked boneless meat to be used in other recipes, the poultry should be removed from the cooking liquid as soon as it is done. The pieces should be placed in a single layer on a flat pan and allowed to cool only enough to ensure safe handling. The meat should be quickly boned by using a fork, tongs, and plastic disposable gloves. The boneless meat should be placed in a shallow layer on a flat pan, refrigerated immediately, and kept refrigerated until used. The broth should be cooled separately by adding ice, if the broth is concentrated, or by placing the hot broth in a pan in a sink filled with ice water and stirring until cold. Cooked poultry meat should be stored in the same manner as other meat products.

Fish and Shellfish

Good-quality fish that is well prepared can compete with the finest meat or poultry. Fish flesh is delicate and contains some connective tissue and variable amounts of fat. Fat content is one of the characteristics that determine the best cooking method for a particular species of fish, although almost any cooking method will produce a tender product. Most finfish and all shellfish are lean, with less than 5 percent fat. This means that they are susceptible to drying, by exposure to either air or heat. Other considerations are the size, texture, form, and strength of the fish's flavor.

Well-done (the point at which the flesh becomes opaque, flakes easily, and is moist) is always the stopping point when cooking fish. High cooking temperatures or overcooking yield a hard, dry, pulpy fish that breaks up easily. Table 19-5 lists recommendations for cooking methods for several common species of freshwater and saltwater fish. Fish should be served as soon as possible after cooking because holding makes unbreaded products dry and breaded products mushy.

Handling and Storage of Fish and Shellfish

Proper handling and storage are necessary to protect the quality of fresh and frozen fish. Ease of handling, product quality, and microbiological safety are all primary concerns. Fresh fish and shellfish should be stored in the refrigerator at about 35° to 40°F (2° to 4°C) for no longer than two days.

Frozen unbreaded fish products should be thawed in the refrigerator; 24 to 36 hours should be allowed for thawing one-pound packages and 48 to 72 hours for five-pound, solid-pack packages and one-gallon cans. If faster thawing is necessary, sealed containers can be thawed under cold running water. This is not a recommended practice, however, because soluble flavors will leach out into the water if the fish pieces become waterlogged. Breaded products should not be thawed before cooking.

Methods for Cooking Fish and Shellfish

No matter what recipe is used, certain basic principles and procedures should be followed when cooking fish and shellfish. Some of these are discussed in the following subsections.

Baking

One of the easiest ways to prepare fish in quantity is to bake fillets, steaks, or unbreaded pieces. Pieces of uniform size should be placed on a well-oiled pan and baked in a 350° to 400°F (177° to 204°C) oven for the shortest time that will produce a cooked product. Herbs, lemon juice, paprika, chopped parsley, chives, or seasoned salts can add flavor and appeal to baked fish. In baking already breaded and cooked pieces of fish, the manufacturer's instructions should be followed.

Broiling

Broiling requires careful watching and thus increases labor time. However, broiled fish adds variety to menus and, if prepared properly, is well accepted by many people. It is best to thaw frozen fish to reduce cooking time. Lean fish should be brushed with melted margarine; fish containing more fat may not need the added fat. The fish should be placed on an oiled broiler pan, with skin (if any) away from the heat source, and broiled two to four inches away from the heat for 5 to 15 minutes, depending on the thickness of the fillet. The fillets may be brushed with melted margarine as needed to keep them moist.

Table 19-5. Recommended Cooking Methods for Fish

Species of Fish	Fat or Lean	Broil	Bake	Simmer, Steam, Poach	Fry, Panfry
Alewife	Fat		Best	Good	
Barracuda	Fat	Good	Best		Fair
Black bass	Lean	Good	Good		Good
Bloater	Fat				Best
Bluefish	Fat	Good	Best		Fair
Bonito	Fat	Good	Best		Fair
Buffalo fish	Lean	Good	Best		Fair
Bullhead	Lean		Fair	Good	Best
Butterfish	Fat	Good	Fair		Best
Carp	Lean	Good	Best		Fair
Catfish	Lean			Good	Best
Cod	Lean	Best	Good	Fair	
Croaker (hardhead)	Lean	Good	Fair		Best
Drum (redfish)	Lean		Best	Good	
Eel	Fat		Good	Fair	Best
Flounder	Lean	Good	Fair		Best
Fluke	Lean	Good	Fair		Best
Grouper	Lean		Best		
Haddock	Lean	Best	Good	Fair	
Hake	Lean	Fair	Best	Good	
Halibut	Fat	Best	Good	Fair	
Herring (lake)	Lean	Good	Fair		Best
Herring (sea)	Fat	Best	Fair		Good
Hog snapper (grunt)	Lean	Good			Best
Jawfish	Lean		Best		
Kingfish	Lean	Best	Good	Fair	
King mackerel	Fat	Best	Good		
Lake trout	Fat	Fair	Best		Good
Ling cod	Lean	Best	Good	Fair	
Mackerel	Fat	Best	Good	Fair	
Mango snapper	Lean	Good			Best
Mullet	Fat	Best	Good		Fair
Muskellounge	Lean	Best	Good		Fair
Perch	Lean	Good	Fair		Best
Pickerel	Lean	Fair	Good		Best
Pike	Lean	Fair	Good		Best
Pollock	Lean	Fair	Good	Best	
Pompano	Fat	Best	Good		Fair
Porgy (scup)	Fat	Good	Fair		Best
Redfish (channel bass)	Lean	Good	Best		
Red snapper	Lean	Good	Best	Good	
Robalo (snook)	Lean	Good	Best		
Rockfish	Lean		Good	Best	
Rosefish	Lean		Good		Best
Salmon	Fat	Good	Best	Fair	
Sablefish (black cod)	Fat			Good	
Sardines	Fat		Best		
Sea bass	Fat	Best	Fair		Good
Sea trout	Fat	Best	Good		Fair
Shad	Fat	Good	Best		Fair
Shark (grayfish)	Fat		Best	Good	
Sheepshead (freshwater)	Lean		Good	Best	
Sheepshead (saltwater)	Lean	Best	Good		Fair
Smelts	Lean	Good	Fair		Best
Snapper	Lean	Good	Best	Fair	
Sole	Lean	Good	Fair		Best
Spanish mackerel	Fat	Best	Good		Fair

Table 19-5. *Continued*

Species of Fish	Fat or Lean	Broil	Bake	Simmer, Steam, Poach	Fry, Panfry
Spot	Lean				
Striped bass (rockfish)	Fat		Good	Best	
Sturgeon	Fat	Good	Best	Fair	
Sucker	Lean	Good	Fair		Best
Sunfish (pumpkin seed)	Lean	Good			Best
Swordfish	Fat	Best	Good	Fair	
Tautog (blackfish)	Lean	Best	Good		Fair
Trout	Lean	Good	Fair		Best
Tuna	Fat	Fair	Best	Good	
Walleye (pike, perch)	Lean			Best	
Weakfish (sea trout)	Lean	Best	Good		Fair
Whiting (silver hake)	Lean			Best	
Whitefish	Fat	Good	Best		Fair
Yellowtail	Fat		Good	Best	

Panfrying

If small quantities of fish are prepared, panfrying, or sautéing, may be a suitable method. Thawed, dried fish should be dusted with seasoned flour or coated with breading and fried in ⅛ inch of hot oil over moderate heat, first on one side and then the other, until each side is browned. Breaded frozen fish should not be thawed before panfrying.

Oven Frying

A simple procedure that requires little direct labor time is oven frying. A standard oven should be heated to 500°F (260°C) or a convection oven to 450°F (232°C). Thawed fish fillets may be dipped in beaten egg or milk and then in flour or breading. Frozen breaded portions or sticks should not be thawed. The fish should be placed on a well-greased baking pan, and some added fat may be poured over the fish. Fat should not be added to cooked breaded portions. Precooked items will reheat rapidly, so the cooking time should be watched carefully.

Deep-Fat Frying

If properly prepared, fried fish and shellfish have good visual appeal, flavor, and texture. To obtain an attractive brown, crispy crust, the oil for deep-fat frying should be heated to a temperature of 350° to 365°F (177° to 185°C). Fish or shellfish should be dipped in batter, milk, or egg and breading; excess breading should be shaken off. The pieces should be placed carefully in the fryer without overloading and fried about four or five minutes, depending on thickness, until the coating is golden brown and done. The fish should then be drained and served as soon as possible. If necessary, fish can be held for a short period uncovered in proper hot-holding equipment or in open pans under infrared food warmers. For breaded products, the manufacturer's instructions should be followed.

Batter ingredients are a critical factor in producing a good deep-fried product that is crisp, not greasy, and maintains the characteristic flavor of the specific fish. Common batter ingredients are flour, egg, baking powder, salt or other seasoning, and a liquid. Although baking powder helps produce a fluffier, lighter batter, it increases fat absorption. Many batter recipes use a carbonated beverage instead of baking powder to avoid this problem. Egg also increases the tendency for fat absorption but helps the batter adhere to the product. Some experimentation may be needed to develop and standardize a suitable batter recipe or to find an acceptable commercial batter mix.

The frying oil should be kept in good condition by periodically filtering it, adding more oil as needed, and controlling the temperature. Oil that has begun to break down will cause the food to overbrown, absorb more fat, and take on strong off flavors. Too high a temperature, as well as the presence of food particles, moisture, and salt in the oil, will hasten fat breakdown. When the fryer is not in use, the thermostat should be set at 200°F (93°C) or the fryer turned off.

Steaming, Poaching, and Simmering

Steaming and poaching are good ways to prepare fish or shellfish without adding fat or calories. In steaming, the fish is placed on a rack in a shallow pan with liquid on the bottom, covered tightly, and cooked in the oven or on the range top until the fish is done. A low- or high-pressure steamer also may be used following the manufacturer's instructions.

In poaching, the fish is placed in a shallow pan containing a small amount of seasoned hot liquid such as water, water and lemon juice, or milk. The pan is covered, and the fish is simmered gently at about 185°F (85°C) until it flakes easily. Portions should retain their shape.

For chowders and stews, the fish is cooked at simmering temperatures in a larger amount of liquid used as stock. Shellfish such as shrimp, lobster, and crab also should be cooked in large amounts of seasoned water at temperatures between 185° and 200°F (85° and 93°C) only long enough to cook through. However, for most operations, it is more economical and efficient to purchase such fish in a partially prepared form to eliminate the labor involved in shelling and handling.

Eggs and Egg Products

An egg is one of the most versatile and valuable foods available. Served at breakfast, lunch, or dinner, in appetizers, soups, entrees, salads, or desserts, eggs are a good source of many nutrients. In addition to regular shell eggs, a number of processed egg products are available and appropriate for use in health care food service operations.

Using Processed Egg Products

The term *egg products* refers to liquid, frozen, dehydrated, and freeze-dried eggs produced by breaking and processing shell eggs. These products include separated whites and yolks, mixed whole eggs, and blends of the whole egg and yolk. Using egg products can save labor time, effort, and storage costs; furthermore, there is less waste than with shell eggs.

Chilled or Frozen Egg Products

Chilled or frozen egg products are available in four- or five-pound paper cartons and in 30-pound containers. The products are suitable for use in almost any menu item. Handled properly, they are even safer to use than fresh shell eggs because they are pasteurized at temperatures high enough to destroy bacteria. Additional ingredients and special production processes improve and preserve the performance characteristics of many egg products.

Chilled egg products should be stored at 38°F (3°C) or lower. These products have a longer shelf life than thawed frozen eggs and usually can be held at least five days. Manufacturers usually list recommended storage conditions and times on the product labels.

Frozen egg products should be stored at 0°F (−18°C) or lower. They should be thawed in the refrigerator for two or three days or placed under cold running water for quicker thawing. Once thawed, they should be refrigerated and used within four days.

Other available convenient frozen egg products include omelets, scrambled eggs, and hard-cooked eggs. These products should always be handled according to the manufacturer's instructions.

Dehydrated Egg Products

New processes that remove the small amount of glucose in eggs have permitted development of improved dried egg products. Glucose removal is necessary for longer shelf life. The products are treated at temperatures high enough to destroy pathogenic organisms.

Dried egg solids are available in several forms: egg white, whole egg, egg yolk, and fortified products. For quick breads, yeast breads, cookies, and cakes, the dry egg solids can be blended with the other ingredients, and the water required for reconstituting is added to other liquids in the recipe. For other recipes, dried eggs are reconstituted before they are combined with the other ingredients. Table 19-6 lists the conversion factors to use in substituting one form of egg for another.

Most quantity recipe files and manufacturer's labels provide information on reconstituting dried whole eggs. However, as a general rule, equal measures of dried egg and water are used. If products are weighed, one part dried whole egg to three parts water should be used.

Egg Substitutes

Cholesterol-free egg substitutes are useful in some modified diets. Individual manufacturers use different formulas, but in general the natural egg white is retained and a substitute for the yolk is added. Yolk substitutes contain vegetable or other oils, carotenoids as coloring, and nutritional additives. Although manufacturers suggest various uses, egg substitutes do not have all the functional properties of eggs, their satisfactory performance being limited to scrambled eggs, omelets, and binders in other recipes. The manufacturer's directions should be followed for storage and preparation of egg substitutes.

Methods for Cooking Eggs and Egg Products

Eggs may be cooked either in or out of the shell. Typical breakfast fare includes hard-cooked, poached, fried, scrambled, and baked eggs. For variety, they can be served as omelets or soufflés, or they can be incorporated in other meal components. Whatever the method of preparation, prolonged cooking and high heat are to be avoided.

Some general suggestions that apply to cooking eggs follow:
- Only eggs that are free from dirt and cracks should be purchased or used.
- Eggs should be kept refrigerated (45°F or less) until preparation time unless they are being prepared for egg foam. In that case, they should be allowed to stand at room temperature for 30 minutes before use.
- Eggs and egg combinations should be cooked at moderate to low temperatures. High temperatures and prolonged cooking should be avoided.
- According to a recent interpretation of the Food and Drug Administration (FDA) model for food service sanitation codes, shell eggs should be cooked to an internal temperature of at least 140°F and held at that temperature if not served immediately. At this temperature, the white is firmly set and the yolk is beginning to thicken. Commercially pasteurized eggs or egg products can be substituted for raw eggs in such items as Caesar salad.
- Appropriate techniques should be used when beating eggs. For a binding or coating mixture, whole eggs should be beaten lightly with a fork or wire whip. For lightness and volume, they should be beaten thoroughly with an electric mixer until they are

Table 19-6. Conversion Factors for Substituting Egg Products

	Frozen	Shell Egg Equivalent	Dried Egg Solids
Whole	1 pound	9 eggs	4½ ounces + 11½ ounces water
Yolk	1 pound	23 yolks	7¼ ounces + 8¾ ounces water
White	1 pound	15 whites	2¼ ounces + 13¾ ounces water

thick and light yellow. For stiffness, they should be beaten until peaks form that fold over slightly as the beater is withdrawn.

- Egg whites should be combined carefully with other ingredients by folding (rather than stirring) with a wire whip or an electric mixer at low speed.
- Hot liquids should be added to eggs slowly and beaten constantly.

Medium and Hard Cooking

Eggs can be cooked in the shell to various degrees of doneness by using any one of several different pieces of equipment. However, regardless of the equipment used, time and temperature are the critical factors. Medium- and hard-cooked eggs can be prepared in a compartment steamer, a steam-jacketed kettle, or a pan on the range top. Eggs at refrigerator temperature are more likely to crack when placed in hot water if the pan method is used. This can be prevented by placing them in warm water for a few minutes before cooking.

Medium-cooked eggs require cooking for five to seven minutes in water brought to a boil (212°F [100°C]) and then reduced to a simmer. Small-batch cooking is necessary when serving medium-cooked eggs. Holding for even a short time will cause them to overcook. Hard-cooked eggs need 15 to 20 minutes when cooked by this method. Excessive temperatures and prolonged cooking cause hard-cooked eggs to toughen, and a greenish black ring forms around the yolk, the result of hydrogen sulfide in the white combining with iron in the yolk to form ferrous sulfide.

Hard-cooked eggs placed in cold water immediately after cooking will be easier to peel. Quick cooling also helps prevent formation of the ring around the yolk. Hard-cooked eggs should be thoroughly cooled before being mixed with other ingredients, particularly in salads.

A timesaving method for making hard-cooked eggs that are to be chopped is to cook them out of the shell in a shallow, greased pan. The pan is placed either uncovered in a steamer for 20 minutes or covered in an oven at medium temperature for 30 to 40 minutes. After cooling, the eggs can be removed from the pan with a spatula and chopped with a French knife or food chopper. With this method, however, timing is critical because overcooking results in a product of inferior quality.

Poaching

In poaching eggs, the addition of 1 tablespoon of salt or 2 tablespoons of vinegar to 1 gallon of water will help reduce spreading of the egg whites. Fresh Grade AA or A eggs and simmering water should be used to retain the eggs' shape. A four-inch-deep, full-size pan filled with about two inches of water should be used. The eggs should be gently slipped into the water and cooked for three to five minutes, until whites are coagulated and yolks are still soft. In a cafeteria, eggs can be poached in a counter insert pan in the hot-holding counter. Whichever method is used, small-batch cooking is recommended.

Frying

Fried eggs lend variety to the menu, particularly for residents in long-term care facilities. However, more labor time may be needed to produce good-quality fried eggs than eggs prepared by other methods. Careful handling during the preparation and holding processes is necessary. Small-batch or continuous preparation during the service period is suggested. A grill, griddle, tilting braising pan, or large skillet can be used to fry the eggs, depending on the number of servings needed and equipment available. Fresh Grade AA or A eggs should be fried in ample fat heated to about 275°F (135°C). The fried egg should have a firm white that is free from browning or crispness, and the yolk should be set but not hard or dry, unless that is the consumer's preference.

Scrambling

Scrambling is one of the easiest ways to prepare eggs. Large quantities can be cooked in a short time by using a griddle, tilting braising pan, oven, steamer, or large skillet. Eggs lower than Grade A quality result in a high-quality product when scrambled. High cooking temperatures and long cooking and holding times in a heated serving unit will cause scrambled eggs to curdle. An undesirable flavor and greenish color also may result.

If scrambled eggs must be held at serving temperature for an extended period, a buffer such as powdered citric acid should be added at the ratio of 0.1 percent (3 grams per gallon of egg). Cream of tartar also may be used at 0.5 percent (5 grams or ½ teaspoon per gallon of eggs). Today, many food service operations purchase frozen blended egg products to use in scrambling. The buffers in these products enable them to hold well for extended periods. Frozen egg mixtures require less preparation time and provide a consistent product. If mixtures are prepared on the premises, milk, cream, or medium white sauce can be used to make the egg mixture; the ratio is ½ cup (4 ounces) liquid to 1 pound of whole eggs.

For best appearance, eggs for scrambling should be beaten just enough to blend the yolk, white, and liquid. They should then be cooked over low heat or in the oven, with occasional stirring, to form a tender, moist food.

Baking

Eggs for baking are broken into individual greased baking dishes or greased muffin tins. An attractive way to serve baked eggs is to remove the crusts from a bread slice, butter it, press it into a greased muffin tin, and drop a shelled egg in the center. It should then be baked in a slow oven (325°F [163°C]) for 12 to 20 minutes, depending on the firmness desired.

Making Omelets

Omelets require greater skill and time in preparation than many other egg products. For this reason, it is not feasible to serve them to large numbers of patients or residents. However, frozen prepared omelets are currently available from several food processors. If menu variety is desired and the facility's resources of time, personnel, and equipment are limited, omelets should be considered.

Making Soufflés

Soufflés add interest and consumer appeal to menus. They are similar to fluffy omelets but have a thickening agent (such as thick white sauce or tapioca) added to the beaten egg yolks before the whites are folded in. The soufflé mixture is placed in a well-oiled pan that is set in water and baked at 375°F (190°C). A lower temperature (300°F [149°C]) can be used if the pan is not set in water, although more cooking time is required. Soufflés should be light, fluffy, tender, and delicately browned.

Cheese

Flavorful and rich in nutrients, cheese is a good source of complete protein that can substitute for meat and add variety to menus. Like other protein-rich foods, cheese must be cooked at a low temperature. A high temperature or prolonged heating causes stringiness and fat separation, which give a curdled appearance to the product. Cheese blends into most recipes more smoothly if it is first grated or chopped.

Some recipes use several varieties of cheese, each with its own distinctive flavor and characteristics. Processed cheese and cheese foods often blend into recipes more smoothly because they have already been heated during processing and contain an emulsifier. However, processed cheeses lack the distinctive flavor of natural aged cheese. If a strong cheese flavor is desired, a combination of the two can be used. Dried cheeses also are used to heighten the cheese flavor in some products.

Milk

Milk, an important component of many prepared foods, requires careful preparation procedures to prevent curdling and scorching. High temperatures and prolonged cooking coagulate

489

and toughen milk protein, change milk flavors, and cause caramelization of the lactose in milk. But the curdling and coagulation of the milk protein can be caused by other factors as well. For example, table salt and curing salt such as that used in ham and bacon can cause milk to curdle, as can tannins, found in many vegetables such as potatoes and in chocolate and brown sugar. Strong food acids can cause almost immediate curdling. Because milk scorches easily, it should be heated over water or in a steam-jacketed kettle with low steam. Prolonged heating at low temperatures may darken milk (by caramelization of the lactose) or cause it to lose some of its flavor.

Several techniques can be used in preparing foods that contain milk to decrease the risk of curdling. For example, the milk can be thickened with flour or cornstarch, as in white sauce and puddings, to stabilize the milk protein during the cooking process. Salt should not be added early in the cooking process. Acid ingredients, which should be at the same temperature as the milk, should be added in small amounts toward the end of the cooking time.

Evaporated milk is whole milk with 50 percent of the water removed. Diluted with an equal quantity of water, it can be substituted for fresh whole milk in most recipes with very good results because it is more heat stable and resistant to curdling. It produces smooth, even-textured puddings and white sauces.

For reasons of economy and convenience, nonfat dry milk can be used for many cooking purposes. Fourteen ounces of nonfat dry milk and 1 gallon of water produce the equivalent of 1 gallon of fresh skim milk. Adding 5 ounces of margarine or other fat to this recipe makes the equivalent of 1 gallon of fresh, whole milk in fat and calorie content. In many recipes, ½ to ¾ cup of nonfat dry milk can be added for each cup of liquid to supplement the nutritional value and protein content of the food.

Dry milk can be combined into food products by several methods. In cakes, cookies, quick breads, and instant mashed potatoes, milk solids can be added to the other dry ingredients, and the water needed to reconstitute the dry milk is added with the other liquid ingredients. For custards, puddings, and similar dishes, dry milk solids should be combined with the sugar. The water required for reconstitution is added separately. If the milk is to be reconstituted and used in liquid form, the amount of dry milk specified by the manufacturer's instructions should be weighed and the water carefully measured. Once reconstituted, the milk should be refrigerated immediately and protected from contamination.

Dried cultured buttermilk also is available and convenient to use in many recipes. It is combined with recipe ingredients in the same manner as nonfat dry milk. Dried cultured buttermilk should be refrigerated after the container has been opened.

Many desserts use dairy product foams. When air is beaten into cream or evaporated milk, a semistable foam is produced. Cream that contains less than 30 percent milk fat will not whip without the use of special methods or ingredients. Whipping cream foams to about twice the original volume and evaporated milk to about three times the original volume. The cream or milk must be cooler than 40°F (4°C), and bowl and beaters should be thoroughly chilled. One tablespoon of lemon juice per cup of evaporated milk will help stabilize the foam produced. The lemon juice should be added after whipping.

In substituting nondairy whipped toppings for whipping cream in recipes, it is important to remember that the nondairy products whip to larger volumes. Therefore, substitutions should be made according to the quantity of whipped material required by the recipe, rather than by equal volumes of unwhipped liquid.

Vegetables

With the abundant variety of vegetables in every season and every region, good vegetables that are well prepared should have an almost universal appeal. *Well prepared* means that the texture, flavor, and appearance are up to standard, the serving temperature is right, and the vegetable harmonizes with the rest of the meal. The nutritional value and quality of vegetables depend on the nutrient content of the fresh vegetables, storage and preparation methods, and the length of time between preparation and service.

Preparation of Vegetables

Because many nutrients are concentrated under the skin of raw vegetables, care must be taken in their preparation to minimize nutrient loss. Ideally, vegetables should be prepared just before cooking or service. However, this is not always possible because of limited personnel and time. Vegetables that are cleaned, peeled, chopped, or sliced in advance must be refrigerated in covered containers or tightly sealed plastic bags until needed. Vegetables that darken when peeled and are exposed to air must be treated with an antioxidant before storage. To avoid severe losses of vitamins and minerals, peeled or cut vegetables should not be stored in water.

Vegetables should be washed thoroughly in cool water before further processing. Leafy green vegetables should be rinsed several times. Long soaking periods in salted water are no longer necessary to remove insects from broccoli, cabbage, brussels sprouts, and cauliflower because commercial vegetable growers now wash produce before it is shipped. However, these vegetables still need a thorough washing in plain water.

Many kinds of equipment can be used to reduce the labor required to prepare raw vegetables. Shredders and mixers with grater and slicer attachments are frequently used. More sophisticated food cutters, choppers, slicers, and vertical cutter-mixers have been designed to uniformly process large quantities of vegetables in a short time. If machine peeling is used for vegetables, the time should be carefully controlled to reduce loss and control cost.

The overall purpose of preparing vegetables is to make them more digestible and to give them a more desirable flavor. Cooking may be needed to soften cellulose or to make the starch more digestible. Cooking methods for various vegetables differ in some respects, but several general principles apply. A cooking method that best preserves nutrients by a short cooking time and use of a limited amount of water should be chosen. It is not always possible to achieve optimum nutrient retention. For example, steaming under pressure reduces nutrient losses that occur when vegetables are cooked in water, but the higher cooking temperature may increase loss of heat-sensitive vitamins. However, shorter cooking times in low- or high-pressure steam equipment reduce this kind of loss. Flavor enhancement also should be a guide in selecting a cooking method. In most instances, the best method for nutrient retention also produces the most desirable flavor. To preserve nutrients as much as possible and make them aesthetically pleasing, vegetables should be cooked only until they are fork tender or slightly crisp.

Although general charts listing cooking times for various types of equipment are available, each facility should use the information provided by equipment manufacturers. The times given should be tested and posted on a chart beside pieces of equipment used for vegetable preparation. Cooking times vary according to steam pressure and design of equipment. A timer should be used no matter what equipment is used. It is very difficult to obtain the desired quality of vegetables in large-batch cooking either in a steam-jacketed kettle or on the range. Production workers may need to be retrained to use the batch method and to time batches to match the demands of the serving period.

Methods for Cooking Vegetables

Cooking methods for vegetables vary depending on a number of factors. Some of these—color, flavor, canned versus fresh vegetables, and the like—are discussed in the following subsections.

Color

The vibrant colors of properly cooked vegetables add greatly to their appeal, but an unattractive color can cause a vegetable to be rejected even before it has been tasted. For that reason, color preservation and enhancement are primary objectives in vegetable cooking. The pigments that create vegetable colors are affected in different ways during cooking—by heat, acid, alkali, and cooking time.

Chlorophyll, the pigment in green vegetables, is slightly soluble in water and is changed to olive green by acids and heat when the vegetables are cooked in a covered pan or are overcooked. Although alkalis such as baking soda intensify the bright green color, they should not be used because they destroy some vitamins and alter the texture of the vegetable. Steam cooking is ideal for green vegetables because the continuous flow of steam around the vegetable carries off the mild acids that cause undesirable color changes, and vitamin losses into water are eliminated. When steam equipment is not available, green vegetables should be cooked uncovered in a small amount of rapidly boiling water for as short a time as possible.

Yellow and orange vegetables, tomatoes, and red peppers contain the *carotenoid pigment,* which is insoluble in water and unaffected by acid and alkali. Overcooking affects the texture of yellow and orange vegetables and can dull the color. Because corn and carrots contain relatively large amounts of sugar, overcooking or extended holding can cause the sugar to caramelize, giving the vegetables a brownish color. Yellow vegetables may be cooked in a steamer or in a covered or uncovered pan with a small amount of boiling water.

Anthocyanin pigments color beets, red cabbage, and eggplant. Anthocyanins are extremely soluble in water; they turn blue in alkaline solution but become brighter red in acid solutions. Adding a small amount of mild acid is an acceptable way to maintain the color of red cabbage. However, it usually is unnecessary to add acid to beets while cooking. Cooking times for these red vegetables should be short. With long cooking, anthocyanin pigments turn greenish and eventually lose most of their color.

Light-colored vegetables contain pigments that are colorless, slightly colored, pale yellow, or brown. This group of *flavonoid pigments* is adversely affected by heat and alkali. In mild acid solutions, they remain white. In the presence of alkali, as in hard water, they become yellow or gray. Although the color change to yellow may not detract from the appearance of cooked onions, the graying that can occur in cauliflower and turnips is unattractive. Adding a small amount of cream of tartar to the cooking water or cooking in a steamer can prevent this color change.

Strong-Flavored Vegetables

Onions, cabbage, cauliflower, broccoli, brussels sprouts, rutabagas, and turnips all have strong flavors. Members of the onion family contain *sinigrin,* which is driven off when onions are cooked to leave a sweet flavor. The cabbage family develops sulfide compounds during cooking and becomes sulfur flavored if cooked too long. Cooking methods for these vegetables differ. Onions should be sautéed in fat or cooked in relatively large amounts of water for the best flavor. Members of the cabbage family are best cooked in a steamer for short periods. However, when a steamer is not available, they can be cooked in a small amount of water on top of the range, in shallow pans, uncovered or loosely covered. Rutabagas and turnips should be cooked in a moderate amount of water, uncovered, and only until tender to keep the flavor as sweet as possible.

Canned Vegetables

Canned vegetables offer several real advantages in food service operations: moderate cost, year-round availability, consistent quality, reduced energy use, and good variety. However, poor handling can yield cooked products that have lost much of their appeal and nutrient content. Canned vegetables are fully cooked and should be reheated only enough to meet immediate needs, with batch heating throughout the serving period. They can be reheated in a steamer, steam-jacketed kettle, or a kettle on the range top. The vegetable should be cooked only long enough to heat through, with very little stirring. A No. 10 can of any vegetable reheats to 150°F (65°C) in about five minutes. However, the vegetable should not be reheated on a steam table because reheating will take too long and spoil the quality. If cooked vegetables will not be used for extended lengths of time, they should be refrigerated and reheated before use to keep the product in good condition. Imaginative seasoning can greatly enhance the appeal of canned vegetables. Herbs, small amounts of meat, nuts, mushrooms, lemon juice, sauces, and cheese can be used for variety.

Frozen Vegetables

In many instances, frozen vegetables are fresher than fresh vegetables, having been blanched and flash frozen within an hour or two of harvesting. High-quality frozen vegetables provide freshness, beautiful color, and portion control and save labor time and waste. Small-batch cooking is essential for top-quality cooked products.

Many products are available in individually quick-frozen (IQF) forms that make it very convenient to cook only the amount needed immediately. Most frozen vegetables should be cooked from the frozen state. Only a few, such as spinach, need tempering in the refrigerator before cooking to allow more uniform heat transfer. Frozen vegetables should be cooked in shallow layers in half- or full-size steam-table pans to eliminate handling time and damage in transferring from cooking to serving container. A full-size (12-by-20-by-2½-inch) pan will hold three 2- to 4-pound packages of vegetables. As with any other form of vegetable, frozen vegetables should be undercooked if they are to be held hot for more than 15 or 20 minutes.

Steam is the best method for cooking frozen vegetables. The manufacturer's directions for the type of steamer to use should be followed. Range-top cooking time should be carefully watched to avoid overcooking, and serving pans should be used rather than large kettles.

Frozen vegetable combinations add excitement to vegetable offerings. In such combinations, blanching times are adjusted to produce a uniform cooking time for the mixture. Package directions indicate cooking time.

Starches

Foods that are composed primarily of starch serve an important role in meals from both an aesthetic and nutrition perspective. High-carbohydrate foods, or starches, appear at almost all meals. The most popular starches are potatoes, pasta, rice, and cereals.

Potatoes

Potatoes can be cooked in many ways (in water or in sauce, steamed, fried, or baked) and are one of the most versatile and well-liked vegetables. The sugar, starch, and moisture content varies with the variety of potato and method of preparation. New potatoes and red-skinned potatoes, which often have a higher moisture content, are suitable for boiling and steaming.

All-purpose potatoes are especially useful for mashing, although a number of highly acceptable dehydrated products also are available. In addition, this type of potato can be used in a number of recipes that require baking in a pan or casserole, such as potatoes au gratin.

Russet or Idaho potatoes produce a more desirable baked product, with a fluffy, mealy texture. Baked potatoes should not be wrapped in foil because foil slows down the cooking process, adds to the cost, and produces a steamed product. The potato skin should be oiled or perforated with a fork before baking to allow steam to escape. Specially designed racks for baking potatoes are used in many food service operations. The metal pins on the racks allow potatoes to be placed vertically in the oven and promote faster cooking.

French fried potatoes are popular among certain customer groups. Although most french fries served are made from frozen products, some are made from fresh potatoes. The steps for deep-fat frying presented earlier in this chapter should be followed for this menu item. Frozen french fries that can be oven-cooked also are available.

Pasta

Macaroni, noodles, and spaghetti form the basis of many combination entrees. Pastas enriched with B vitamins and iron should be used. Those made from durum wheat remain firmer and do not stick together as much after cooking. Pastas are cooked in a large volume of rapidly boiling salted water in a kettle or steam-jacketed kettle until they are tender and yet firm. A compartment steamer also could be used. Adding oil to the cooking water keeps the pasta from sticking together and helps keep the water from boiling over. If the pasta is to be combined with other ingredients for further cooking, it should be slightly undercooked. Durum wheat pastas usually do not need rinsing after cooking. However, any pasta can be rinsed in a colander under either hot or cold water to remove excess starch. If pasta is to be served hot, it should be rinsed with hot water; cold water should be used if the pasta is to be included in a combination salad. Pasta served from a steam table should be tossed with a small amount of fat (such as olive oil) prior to placing it in the pan.

Rice

Rice is available in brown, milled, parboiled, and partially cooked forms. Rice combinations with seasonings also are available but are more expensive. The amount of water and cooking time vary according to the type of rice, so it is necessary to follow the preparation methods recommended for the specific form used. Rice can be cooked in a tightly covered pan on the range, in the oven, in a compartment steamer, or in a steam-jacketed kettle. Rice held for later service should be kept in shallow pans to prevent packing. To avoid losing the vitamin B content, enriched rice should not be rinsed either before or after cooking. Long-grain rice should be used when the rice is to be served plain or in combination with entrees. When cooked, the grains remain firm, fluffy, and separate. Leftover rice can be refrigerated or frozen. Half a cup of water is added for each quart of rice when it is reheated for service.

Cereals

When dry cereal is added to water, the starch granules absorb moisture, become greatly enlarged, and thicken after heating. Instant and quick-cooking cereals have been further processed by various methods that allow them to cook within a few minutes. The manufacturer's directions should be followed in preparing cooked cereals. The amount of liquid needed and cooking times vary according to the type of cereal being prepared. The cereal should be kept covered until served to prevent drying.

Sandwiches

Sandwiches are popular in any season and with nearly everyone. Sandwiches add variety and interest to menus and provide the needed nutrients alone or in combination with other foods.

Sandwich Ingredients

Sandwiches can be made from any number of ingredients. They can be open or closed faced, cold or hot, and served in a variety of shapes and forms. The essential things to remember are that they should have good flavor, texture, and appearance and that they should be served fresh at the appropriate temperature.

So many varieties of specialty breads, rolls, and buns are available from commercial sources today that the problem is which one to choose. Using bread with a close-grained, firm texture is desirable to prevent the sogginess caused by moist fillings. Spreads such as salad dressing, mayonnaise, and combinations of these with other ingredients can be used for flavor. Sandwich fillings should contain a combination of ingredients with some contrast in flavor, color, and texture. Mixed fillings, especially those that contain meat, fish, poultry, or eggs, must be handled in accordance with safe food preparation practices. Cheese and meats for sandwiches can be purchased already sliced for uniformity. Some meats—ham, roast beef, corned beef, and turkey—can be machine sliced paper thin and stacked high for appeal and easy eating.

Food service magazines are helpful for new ideas that can appeal to patients and staff. Attractive sandwiches can be convenient and profitable items in employee and visitor cafeterias and can add interest to traditional menu patterns.

Sandwich Assembly

Assembly lines should be used to streamline sandwich making. After the steps for sandwich assembly have been determined, the ingredients should be arranged in the proper order.

To save steps, time, and motion and to be efficient enough to meet production schedules during sandwich assembly, employees should do the following:

- Wear disposable gloves, use both hands, and arrange the slices of bread in two or four rows on a cutting board.
- Distribute the spread on the bread with a spatula and cover each slice with a circular motion.
- Use both hands to place slices of meat, cheese, poultry, or tomato on the bread slices in alternate rows.
- Scoop mixture portions onto the center of bread slices and spread with a spatula, using one stroke moving in and one stroke moving out.
- Use both hands to place lettuce on top of the filling.
- Close sandwiches by turning a slice of bread over the filling-covered slices.
- Stack sandwiches two or three high and cut through the entire stack.
- Transfer unwrapped sandwiches to trays or pans; cover with foil, plastic film, or the pan lid; and store in the refrigerator.
- Wrap sandwiches individually in plastic bags or film before storing.

If a large volume of sandwiches is to be made, these steps can be divided between two or more employees.

Salads

Well-prepared salads add appeal and flavor variety to any menu. They are an excellent means of serving nutrient-rich vegetables and fruits and provide good sources of fiber. Careful handling and imagination in combining flavors and colors make the difference between appealing and mediocre salads. Using well-designed recipes and careful preparation methods, anyone trained in food preparation can achieve attractive results.

The colors, flavors, and textures of salad ingredients should be balanced. Salad underliners of lettuce, endive, or other greens can complement and enhance the appearance of almost any salad. Garnishes and dressings accent salad flavors and add color and eye appeal. There are several basic types of salads, such as mixed-green and combination salads, main-dish salads, and molded salads, but almost endless variations are possible.

Combination Salads

The simplest salad is lettuce torn into bite-size pieces tossed with a savory dressing; a combination of greens can be used for variety in color, texture, and flavor. Salad recipes that specify weights of ingredients are useful when substituting one green for another as availability or cost changes. The wide variety of salad greens available allows plenty of latitude for varying basic combination salads. Iceberg lettuce, leaf lettuce, bibb lettuce, Boston lettuce, endive (chicory), escarole, romaine, spinach, watercress, and Chinese cabbage can be used in various combinations. Other ingredients such as radishes, tomatoes, cauliflower, red cabbage, fresh mushrooms, green onions, red onion rings, sprouts, cucumber, broccoli, croutons, and hard-cooked eggs can be added with appealing results.

All salad ingredients should be clean, crisp, and mixed lightly to avoid breaking or crushing. To keep the greens from wilting, dressings should be added just before service or they can be added by the customer. Whenever possible, a choice of dressings, either prepared on the premises or selected from the wide variety of commercial dressings, should be offered.

Main-Dish Salads

A salad served as the main course of a meal should contain some protein-rich food, such as chicken, seafood, eggs, cheese, ham, turkey, or other meat, usually combined with raw or cooked vegetables. For added flavor, meat and vegetable pieces may be marinated in a tart French dressing, drained, and combined with mayonnaise or a cooked dressing before serving.

Such mixtures can be used to stuff tomatoes or can be served with tomato wedges as garnish. Care in handling the meat or other protein food is essential to maintain safety. Marination in the acid salad dressing provides some protection from bacterial growth, but clean utensils and refrigeration are still required.

Julienne strips of poultry, meat, and cheese can be used to top combination green salads for main-dish entrees. Salad plates offering a salad mixture accompanied by cold cuts, cheese slices, and fresh fruits are attractive and appealing year-round. In cold seasons, a cup of hot soup or consommé provides a good accompaniment.

In arranging main-dish salads, different shapes should be used to make an interesting pattern. The food shapes can be varied for contrast and accented with contrasting and complementary colors. Visual appeal is just as important as substantial character and a pleasing blend of flavors and textures. Salads should be kept thoroughly chilled at all times.

Molded Gelatin Salads

Molded salads usually are sweetened mixtures made with flavored gelatin mixes or plain gelatin. Water, fruit juice, and vegetable juice can be used as the liquid. For fast congealing, only enough hot water to dissolve the gelatin should be used before adding cold water or other liquid for the remaining quantity. In very hot weather or when unrefrigerated holding is necessary, the amount of liquid used should be reduced slightly. Before other ingredients (such as chopped vegetables, fruit pieces, and cottage cheese) are added, the mixture should be cooled until it has the consistency of unbeaten egg whites. This step will keep the added ingredients from sinking to the bottom of the pan.

For quantity service, standard 12-by-20-inch pans should be used so that the gelatin can be cut for serving. Individual molds are attractive, but they are more time-consuming to prepare. Molded salads should be made the day before service.

Preparation of Salad Ingredients

Efficient salad preparation and assembly calls for good tools, equipment, and work procedures. Some basic rules should be followed in preparing all salad ingredients. All ingredients should be of top quality and should be kept in the refrigerator except during actual preparation. Salad greens should be thoroughly washed, dried, and stored in vaporproof containers until used. Trays of finished salads should be refrigerated until they are served. All salads can be attractively arranged and garnished by using the natural color and shape of each ingredient to advantage. For example, a salad composed of salad greens can be enhanced by the contrasting colors and shapes supplied by purple onion slices, tomato wedges, and ripe olives. Maximum sanitation control in work methods and equipment should be observed. Automated equipment should be used whenever possible to reduce labor time and to produce uniform results.

Assembly of Salad Ingredients

Most individual salads can be assembled in advance, put on trays, and refrigerated until they are needed. To save time and steps in assembly, all equipment and ingredients should be arranged within easy reach of the employee. Mobile carts can be used to extend work space and to store salad trays. Trays should be stacked on the work counter, and each tray should be stacked with all the plates or bowls it will hold. Both hands should be used during assembly and appropriate portion utensils or disposable plastic gloves should be used to handle ingredients.

Fruits

Fresh, canned, dried, and frozen fruits, either plain or in combination, are often served as a salad, dessert, or snack as well as with breakfast foods. Fresh fruits in season, carefully selected for quality, can be a regular and popular menu item. When selective menus are used, fresh fruit should be offered daily. Bowls of whole fresh fruit can be used on cafeteria lines as an attractive merchandising tool and as a simple serving method.

Whole fresh fruits should be thoroughly washed before they are served. Cutting clusters of grapes makes them easier to serve, but many fresh fruits need almost no preparation before service. Cut-up fresh fruits can be combined in a virtually infinite number of variations or combined with canned fruits. Peeled and cut fresh fruits should be stored in fruit juices to maintain their juiciness and flavor. Varied shapes and sizes of fruits and complementary flavors and colors should be used.

Breads

Whole-grain and enriched breads, cereals, and cereal products are a significant part of the daily diet because they supply carbohydrates, protein, B vitamins, and iron. The wide range of bread and cereal foods offers many opportunities for menu variety.

Yeast Breads

To save time and labor, most institutions purchase commercially baked bread and rolls, supplementing them with mixes for quick breads or frozen dough products for yeast breads. Quick-bread mixes also can be prepared on-site and kept on hand for many uses. Facilities that have adequate equipment and labor time can prepare yeast bread products on-site. The use of standardized recipes and procedures makes it possible for any experienced person to produce high-quality yeast breads.

Two basic methods are used for mixing yeast breads: the sponge method and the straight-dough method. The *sponge method* includes two mixing processes and two fermentation processes in alternating sequence. Part of the flour, water, yeast, sugar, and shortening is mixed and allowed to ferment. This mixture is then combined with the remaining ingredients, mixed again, and allowed to ferment a second time. In the *straight-dough* method, all ingredients are mixed at one time before any fermentation takes place. This latter method is the most practical and saves time.

Bread structure depends on developing the gluten by mixing and kneading. If bread flour is used, more kneading is needed to develop the gluten than when all-purpose flour is used. Overkneading is preferable to underkneading.

During fermentation (rising), a humid atmosphere prevents dehydration or crusting of the dough surface. A temperature of around 85°F (29°C) is ideal to ensure adequate yeast growth. After the first rising, the dough should be punched down, scaled, shaped, and put in pans. The second rising will be more rapid, because more yeast cells are present in the dough. The bread is ready for baking when the dough has doubled in size. A relatively high baking temperature is used to allow the gas in the dough to expand further, to firm the bread's structure, and to develop a golden brown color.

After baking, the loaves should be removed from the pans and placed on racks to allow steam and alcohol to escape. Bread can be held for long periods if frozen in moistureproof and vaporproof material. For freezing, it is recommended that baked bread be wrapped while it is still warm to reduce moisture loss in the freezer.

Unbaked dough also can be refrigerated for at least 12 hours or overnight. The first rising will occur during refrigeration. By refrigerating dough in this manner, the traditional early morning baking schedule can be avoided. Dough will be ready to shape and bake when employees arrive at standard starting times, and yet the products will be ready for main meals of the day. Although dough can be frozen immediately after mixing and before fermentation, recipes for frozen bread dough must contain enough yeast to perform effectively after thawing.

Quick Breads

Quick breads leavened with baking powder, baking soda, or steam can add appeal to any meal with a minimum of labor. Prepared mixes for muffins, biscuits, pancakes, popovers, and other items require only the addition of liquid and/or eggs to produce high-quality products. Mixes, purchased or made on the premises, minimize the skill and time needed for preparation.

Two basic methods are used in mixing quick breads: the muffin method and the biscuit method. In the *muffin method,* dry ingredients are mixed together. Then liquids, including oil or melted shortening, are added. The ingredients are mixed only enough to be thoroughly combined. Extended mixing will overdevelop the gluten and cause toughness, tunnels, and holes in the finished product. The muffin mixture should be portioned with a scoop for uniformity.

The *biscuit method,* which is used for soft doughs, also involves a minimum of mixing. Solid fat is cut into the combined dry ingredients. Liquid is then added and mixed just enough to moisten the ingredients. Then the dough is rolled out on a floured board and cut or rolled directly on the baking pan. The labor-saving method of rolling directly on the baking pan may make it possible to serve freshly made biscuits more often. The dough can be cut into squares or triangles before or after baking. All the dough can be used without the reworking involved in traditional methods of cutting.

Desserts

Imaginative dessert planning and thoughtful preparation can complement the rest of the menu, balance cost, and add nutritional value to the entire meal. Dessert choices balance the satiety level of a menu, for example, a fruit or light dessert with a hearty meal and a cool, delicately flavored dessert after a spicy main dish or salad.

Food service operations with limited resources can increase the variety of desserts they offer by using mixes and other convenience dessert products. Cake mixes in particular yield consistent, uniform results when directions are followed carefully. Manufacturers provide recipes for variations on the basic cakes, which can be substituted for many cakes requiring on-site skilled labor for preparation. Frozen dessert products such as cakes, cheesecakes, pies, and other pastries also have been widely accepted. When deciding to use a convenience dessert, food service managers must evaluate the cost of the convenience item compared with the cost of ingredients and labor for in-house preparation. In addition, the product's quality should be evaluated objectively to determine which approach will yield the most flavorful, attractive product.

Few institutions use convenience desserts exclusively. For high-quality preparation in the facility, standardized recipes, appropriate tools, scales, and standard-size pans are needed. As always, employees should be trained in the correct use of recipes and equipment. Cooks and bakers need to understand the preparation principles for different kinds of desserts and the functional properties of the various ingredients.

Cakes

Cakes are flour-mixture desserts that contain a leavening agent to incorporate air into their structure. In butter cakes, the shortening, sugar, and eggs are creamed to incorporate air. Pound cakes are leavened almost completely by creaming. Angel food and sponge cakes are leavened by egg white foam. Air is also incorporated by sifting ingredients and beating or manipulating the batter.

Butter Cakes

Four common mixing methods are used for butter cakes. One is the *conventional method,* in which the thorough creaming of the fat and sugar is the first step. Eggs or egg yolks are added next. All dry ingredients are sifted together and added alternately with the liquid. If only egg yolks are used, beaten whites may be folded in last. Although more time-consuming and complicated than the others, this method is widely used because it produces very good cakes, with a light, fine, velvety texture.

The *muffin method* is quick and easy. In this method, dry ingredients are weighed, sifted, and mixed together. All the wet ingredients—liquid, eggs, and melted shortening—are stirred into the dry ingredients. Although the muffin method is easy and fast, it tends to produce a coarse-textured cake that quickly becomes stale.

The *quick,* or *one-bowl, method* is sometimes called the *high-ratio method* because it has increased proportions of both sugar and fat. The dry ingredients, shortening, and part of the milk are combined and beaten at medium speed for two minutes. The rest of the milk and the eggs are blended into this mixture for another two minutes. High-ratio cakes have good volume, are tender, and have a moist and flavorful texture.

Many commercial bakers use a fourth method, known as the *pastry-blend method.* In this method, fat and flour are blended before other ingredients are added in two stages. First, half the milk and all the sugar and baking powder are combined and blended into the fat–flour mixture, after which the eggs and remaining milk are added.

All four methods are suitable for quantity recipes. As new recipes are tried and evaluated, it is helpful to see which method is specified. The method will determine the characteristics of the end product.

Panning is an important aspect of making cakes. Uniform and appropriate amounts of batter per pan are essential to produce uniform portions. If possible, the batter that goes into each pan should be weighed. If there is no scale available for this purpose, the same amount of batter should be measured into each pan by using a measuring cup or similar item. Butter cakes are baked in greased and floured pans, either in the standard 12-by-20-by-2-inch pan or in an 18-by-26-by-2-inch pan for sheet cakes. More variety is possible when the shape of the baking pan is varied. Layer cakes are easy to make by stacking two 12-by-20-inch cakes or by stacking quarters of a sheet cake baked in an 18-by-26-inch pan.

The oven temperature specified in the cake recipe should usually be used. Baking temperatures for conventional ovens should be lowered by 25°F (14°C) for convection ovens. Excessive temperatures cause cakes to peak and crack on top; deficient temperatures cause them to fall. Cakes should be cooled before frosting. Staleness will occur more rapidly if the cake is refrigerated, but some frostings make refrigeration necessary. Freezing retains quality in cakes for a long time and allows advance production for service on days when production loads are heavy. Cakes should be frozen unfrosted.

Foam Cakes

Angel food cakes, leavened by egg white foam, contain no shortening. Excellent ready-made mixes have almost eliminated traditional methods of producing angel food cakes. However, if they are to be produced from a recipe, the use of the frozen or dry egg white products that have added ingredients to produce better foaming properties should be considered. Batch size should not be so large that uniform mixing is impossible. Combining dry ingredients with egg white foam may be done by hand using a wire whip; machine blending can be done at low speed just until all ingredients are combined.

Sponge Cakes

Sponge cakes are similar to angel food cakes except that whole egg foam is used, with lemon juice added to stabilize the foam. In either type of cake, overbeating must be avoided. Superfine granulated sugar will produce a cake with a finer grain. Accurate time and temperature control is needed to produce a light brown crust. Cakes should be cooled thoroughly in pans before they are removed for icing and portioning.

Cookies

The methods of cookie preparation are similar to those used for butter cakes: sugar, shortening, and eggs are creamed; any other liquids are added; and dry ingredients are blended in last. Labor time for portioning cookies is greater than for cakes but can be decreased by using scoops to portion, by avoiding cookies that have to be rolled and cut, and by making larger cookies. Bar cookies cut labor time significantly.

Cookies should be baked on bright aluminum baking sheets or pans with low sides. Pans should be oiled with unsalted fat unless the cookies are very rich in fat and the recipe specifies no pan greasing. Baking sheets should be cooled between each use. Most cookies freeze well after they are cooled. When time permits, several varieties should be baked at once to handle the projected needs over several weeks or months.

Pies and Pastries

Pie-crust pastry has very few ingredients but must be in just the right proportion to produce a tender, flaky, and flavorful crust. Pies can be made in round pans or, for greater simplicity, in 12-by-20-inch or 18-by-26-inch pans. If large pans are used, making a single-top crust makes handling easier during service. These pies save assembly time and baking space. If individual round pans are used, pie making can be handled in an assembly line process.

Pastry dough should be weighed before rolling to achieve uniform crusts with minimum waste. Various kinds of pastry rolling or forming machines can be used to eliminate hand labor. If hand rolling is necessary, a lightly floured board should be used, and the dough should be rolled evenly. Pie dough should not be stretched to fit the pan; some slack should be provided to offset shrinkage during baking. Shells baked unfilled should be pricked with a fork and chilled before baking to cut down on shrinkage. Double-crust pies should have cuts in the top crust to allow steam to escape during baking. Brushing the top crust with milk or beaten egg produces a golden brown color.

A wide variety of pie fillings can be made from traditional recipes or from prepared mixes and canned fillings. Broken or irregular pieces of fruit of good quality and flavor can be added to prepared pie fillings to give them a fresher taste.

Pastry and pies can be frozen. The quality of most pies will be better if the pie is frozen unbaked. Most custard- or pudding-filled pies should not be frozen unless special starches for thickening have been used in the fillings.

Fruit Desserts

Fruits make an excellent dessert offering. Cut fresh fruits can be combined in almost endless variations to produce fresh-fruit desserts. They can also be combined with canned fruits. Varied shapes and sizes of fruits and complementary flavors and colors should be used. Fresh-fruit desserts should be garnished attractively, and the fruits should be kept chilled until service.

Canned fruits served as a dessert should be chilled thoroughly. Adding a garnish can dispel the "right-out-of-the-can" look. Frozen fruits should be thawed in the refrigerator before serving.

Canned or frozen fruits can be used in crisps (that is, with crumb topping) or served warm with whipped topping or a hard sauce. A fruit cobbler can be made by spreading a sweetened biscuit dough over layers of canned or fresh fruit and baking until the top is browned. Shortcakes are another simple yet attractive fruit dessert, made in the same way as baking-powder biscuits but using a richer and sweeter dough. Preparation can be streamlined by rolling the dough directly onto 18-by-26-inch pans, baking, and then cutting into squares. Two squares, with fruit in between and on top, are stacked to build the shortcake.

Other Desserts

Light and nutritious desserts can be made from various egg and milk combinations: puddings, dessert soufflés, and cornstarch puddings. They are easily prepared in quantity and are relatively inexpensive compared with many other desserts. Mixes and frozen egg products can simplify the production of these items. (The principles and techniques for the preparation of these foods are described in the sections on eggs and milk earlier in this chapter.) All desserts in this category should be stored in the refrigerator until they are served.

Fruit-flavored gelatins are the basis for many easy and attractive desserts. For an appealing look, plain gelatin can be congealed in shallow layers and cut into cubes. Cubes of various colors can be combined for serving, with or without the addition of whipped topping. Partially congealed gelatins can be whipped and poured over a layer of clear gelatin for other simple, yet attractive layered desserts.

Beverages

Most customers enjoy a beverage with their meals or to accompany a snack. Two of the most popular beverages for these purposes are coffee and tea.

Coffee

Although making coffee is a relatively simple task, a number of principles apply for producing good coffee. The process must begin with clean brewing equipment. Next, the quality and freshness of the coffee, water, and filters must be considered. Ground coffee must be stored tightly sealed in a cool, dry place; usually regular tap water is preferred. The correct grind, proportion, brewing time, and brewing temperature, as specified by the coffee brewing equipment manufacturer, should be followed. Finally, holding of brewed coffee must be monitored carefully so that it is held at 185° to 190°F (85° to 88°C) for no longer than one hour. Flavored and specialty coffees have become very popular. Some food service directors have found that offering these types of coffees along with espresso and cappuccino from takeout counters can be both popular and profitable.

Tea

Tea is a popular beverage served either hot or iced. A simple beverage, it does not require the equipment or labor needed for coffee service. For hot tea, fresh hot water should be poured directly into a pot and served with an individual tea bag. The customer can then brew the tea to the preferred strength.

Larger tea bags can be used for brewing iced tea. Fresh, hot water is poured over the tea bags and allowed to steep for five minutes. The tea bags should then be removed and cold water added to achieve the correct strength. The tea should be held at room temperature for no more than four hours. Specialty teas, particularly herbal blends, have also become popular as a beverage with dessert or at break time.

☐ Summary

Selection of a food production and forecasting system should be carefully considered because each health care operation presents its own unique demands. A variety of food production equipment and forecasting techniques have been developed to help operations meet their specific needs. The food service director must become familiar with all of these options and their cost and versatility. Selection of a food production and forecasting system appropriate for a particular operation also requires a thorough study before a decision can be made. Patients' food preferences, availability of a skilled work force, quality of food products available, budget resources, and cost of the equipment needed for a food production system must all be analyzed.

In this and preceding chapters, procedures for planning the menu; purchasing, receiving, and issuing the ingredients; and measuring and preparing the ingredients in accordance with standardized recipes for a specific number of portions have been discussed in detail. Now it is time to transform the raw materials into finished products, with the objective of producing high-quality products at allowable costs.

High-quality food production depends on the use of appropriate preparation methods and equipment by skilled food service workers. Fulfilling the objective of destroying harmful microorganisms and at the same time producing nutritious, appealing, and affordable food is the responsibility of the food service director as well as the production workers. The success of every food service department depends on the quality and cost of the food served.

☐ Bibliography

Alexander, J. Cook–chill automation. *Hospital Food Service* 24(3):7–8, 1991.

Bobeng, J. B., and David, B. D. HACCP models for quality control of entree production in foodservice systems. *Journal of Food Protection* 40:632, 1977.

Buchanan, P. W. *Quantity Food Preparation: Standardizing Recipes and Contracting Ingredients.* Chicago: American Dietetic Association, 1983.

Dougherty, D. Expanding the use of convenience products. *Hospital Food & Nutrition Focus* 7(11):2–3, July 1991.

Foodservice Systems: Product Flow and Microbial Quality and Safety of Foods. Columbia, MO: University of Missouri, North Central Regional Research Publication No. 245(RB 1018), 1977.

Freshwater, J. F. *Least-Cost Hospital Food Service Systems.* Washington, DC: U.S. Government Printing Office, USDA-AMS Marketing Research Report No. 1116, 1980.

Gisslen, W. *Advanced Professional Cooking.* New York City: John Wiley and Sons, 1992.

Gisslen, W. *Professional Baking.* 2nd ed. New York City: John Wiley and Sons, 1994.

Gisslen, W. *Professional Cooking.* 2nd ed. New York City: John Wiley and Sons, 1983.

Greathouse, K. R., and Gregroire, M. B. Variables related to selection of conventional, cook–chill, and cook–freeze systems. *Journal of The American Dietetic Association* 88:476–78, 1988.

Greathouse, K. R., Gregroire, M. B., Spears, M. C., Richards, V., and Nassar, R. F. Comparison of conventional, cook–chill, and cook–freeze foodservice systems. *Journal of The American Dietetic Association* 89:1606–11, 1989.

Jones, P., and Heulin, A. Foodservice systems: generic types, alternative technologies and infinite variation. *Journal of Foodservice Systems* 5:299–311, 1990.

Klein, B. P., Matthews, M. E., and Setser, C. S. *Foodservice Systems: Time and Temperature Effects on Food Quality.* Urbana-Champaign, IL: Agricultural Experiment Station, University of Illinois, North Central Regional Research Publication No. 293, Illinois Bulletin 779, 1984.

Knight, J. B., and Kotschevar, L. H. *Quality Food Production, Planning, and Management.* 2nd ed. New York City: Van Nostrand Reinhold, 1988.

Kotschevar, L. H. *Standards, Principles, and Techniques in Quantity Food Production.* 4th ed. New York City: Van Nostrand Reinhold, 1988.

McWilliams, M. *Food Fundamentals.* 5th ed. New York City: Plycon Press, 1992.

Messersmith, A., and Miller, J. L. *Forecasting in Foodservice.* New York City: John Wiley and Sons, 1992.

Mizer, D. A., Porter, M., and Sonnier, B. *Food Preparation for the Professional.* New York City: John Wiley and Sons, 1987.

National Live Stock Board. *Meat in the Foodservice Industry.* Chicago: National Live Stock and Meat Board in association with the National Association of Meat Purveyors, 1975.

National Turkey Federation. *The Turkey Handbook.* Reston, VA: National Turkey Federation, 1975.

Norton, C. What is cook–chill? *Hospital Food Service* 24(2):5–7, 1991.

Peckham, G. C. *Foundations of Food Preparation.* 5th ed. New York City: Macmillan, 1987.

Rose, J. C., editor. *Handbook for Health Care Food Service Management.* Rockville, MD: Aspen, 1984.

Shugart, G. S., Molz, M., and Wilson, M. *Food for Fifty.* 9th ed. New York City: John Wiley and Sons, 1992.

Spears, M. C. *Foodservice Organizations: A Managerial and Systems Approach.* 2nd ed. New York City: Macmillan, 1991.

Terrell, M. E. *Professional Food Preparation.* 2nd ed. New York City: John Wiley and Sons, 1979.

Chapter 20

Meal Service

☐ Introduction

How menu items are presented to its customers has as much, or more, impact on the success of a health care food service operation as the menu itself. The department director may plan and the operation may produce menu items that customers want, but unless items are served in a fashion they find satisfactory, customers will rate the operation as unacceptable.

Advances in technology have provided many options in patient, resident, and nonpatient meal service systems for hospitals and extended care facilities. Several factors affect the design of the system: physical layout of the health care operation; customers' nutrition and social needs; type of food production system used; the operation's standards (for food quality, quality monitoring systems, microbiological controls, for example); the timing of meal service; skill levels of service personnel; and cost of equipment. Most health care meal service systems include tray service to patients' rooms and cafeteria service for visitors, staff, and (in extended care facilities) ambulatory residents. Other services may be offered to meet customer needs.

Generally speaking, meal service systems are designed to satisfy three functions: assembly, delivery, and service. *Assembly* involves portioning and plating menu items for specific customers. The items are then *delivered* to the point of service; *service* is the actual presentation of menu items to customers. Depending on the nature of the operation, the service function may be a simple process (such as providing over-the-counter service) or a complex activity (such as providing patient trays). Because most menu items are at peak quality immediately following food preparation, efficient meal service systems rely on the accessibility of appropriate personnel and suitable equipment. The various components of each meal service system should be considered apart from the production system components because many of the meal service systems can be combined with any or all of the alternative production systems, as illustrated in table 20-1.

This chapter will discuss assembly, delivery, and service of meals to three customer groups: patients, residents in long-term care facilities, and nonpatients. Certain advantages, and in some cases disadvantages, of specific delivery systems will be pointed out. Major delivery systems covered in the chapter include centralized and decentralized tray service, cafeteria service, and table service. Service refinements and expansions such as over-the-counter, catering, vending, and off-site meal service operations will be addressed with a view toward their revenue-generating potential.

Table 20-1. Alternative Systems for Food Service to Patients

Production	Assembly/Distribution	Reheating/Service
Cook–serve Cook–chill Cook–freeze Assemble–serve	Kitchen reheat → Insulated tray (insulated components) Unitized pellet Hot/cold cart Split tray cart Tray heater cart	Not required
Cook–chill Cook–freeze Assemble–freeze	Cold plating → Enclosed cart/galley refrigeration Refrigerated cart Insulated cart Open or enclosed monorail cart	Galley reheat → Convection ovens Microwave ovens Infrared ovens Conduction ovens
	Specialized dish-automated reheat module Insulated tray/refrigerated-reheat cart	

Source: Adapted from M. L. Herz, and others. *Analysis of Alternative Patient Tray Delivery Concepts.* Natick, MA: U.S. Army Natick Research and Development Command, 1977.

☐ Meal Service Systems

As indicated earlier, most health care food service operations serve a variety of markets or customer groups. Typically, these are patients, residents, and nonpatients (staff, visitors, and guests). The wants and needs in terms of meal service characteristics differ for each of these markets. Therefore, the food service director must design a variety of approaches to meal service to meet the various demands of these three groups.

Patient Meal Service

Patients comprise the primary target market of health care food service operations. Because patients are unable to dine in a central location and because they are located on different floors or in different buildings, the director must devise a meal service system that incorporates the three broad functions mentioned earlier. That is, they must devise a system that provides food to patients' rooms by means of assembly of individual trays, delivery of trays to patient locations, and service of trays to patients.

Tray Assembly

Two major systems are used to assemble patient trays. In one, bulk food is distributed to patient areas, where it is then plated (decentralized service). In the other, food is assembled at a central location that uses various delivery methods to transport it to individual patients (centralized service).

Decentralized Systems

In *decentralized assembly systems,* most of the food is prepared in the food production area. Bulk quantities are then conveyed in food trucks with heated and unheated compartments to serving galleys in the patient areas, where individual trays are then assembled. For example, breakfast items (coffee, toast, eggs, and special food items) are prepared in the serving galley, which may be equipped with a hot plate, a microwave or convection oven, a coffee maker, a toaster, a cabinet for heating dishes, and a refrigerator. Trays, dishes, and serviceware are returned to the galleys for cleaning and storage. Alternatively, the dishes and flatware can be washed in either an adjacent area or a central dish-washing room. In either case, they are returned to the serving galleys and stored there until the next meal. Decentralized assembly requires less space in the food service department but more in the patient areas. When compared to centralized systems (discussed below), this approach generally results in less time between assembly and the actual service of trays to patients.

Centralized Systems

Centralized assembly systems are used in most health care food service operations today because they permit better control of food quality, portion size, food temperature, and diet modifications. They also reduce overproduction and waste, require less equipment, and greatly diminish labor time. In a centralized assembly system, foods are plated and trays are made up in a central location, in or near the main kitchen. Because centralized assembly requires more tray preparation time than is the case with decentralized assembly, the department director must give special attention to this function of the meal service system. Centralized assembly usually is accomplished by means of a tray line.

Tray lines are composed of several stations, each of which is supported by equipment and staffed by a food service employee. Most tray lines require at least three types of equipment. Temperature maintenance equipment helps preserve the aesthetic and microbiological quality of menu items. Accessibility of trays, dishes, serviceware, and a variety of condiments requires a variety of dispensing equipment. Finally, moving the trays from one station to the next is usually accomplished by means of a conveyor.

Maximizing tray line efficiency is an important goal for operations that use centralized assembly systems. Although the specific requirements of a tray line vary from operation to operation, several common questions should be considered. These include:

- Is the spacing between menu and tray sufficient to allow tray line employees time to read the menu and place correct items on trays?
- Is the spacing between trays appropriate to achieve proper pacing of the work?
- Is there a smooth work flow in each station?
- Is the menu format consistent so that similar items are always located in the same place on every menu?
- Is the work load balanced between each station so that each employee contributes about the same effort on each tray?
- Is there a means of resupplying food and acquiring missing items (for example, a "floating" employee) so that the tray line is not delayed or stopped?

Observation of each workstation will identify work methods that require improvement. To further enhance productivity of the tray line, the food service director can employ a variety of industrial engineering techniques, such as assembly-line balancing. *Assembly-line balancing* is a technique that reassigns tasks so that tray line work assignments are more evenly distributed in terms of time.

Tray Delivery

Because the point of decentralized tray assembly is in close proximity to the patient, tray delivery normally is accomplished by means of small carts, which are wheeled directly to patient rooms. Temperature maintenance does not pose a particular problem, but food items transported from the tray assembly area should be covered.

If centralized tray assembly is utilized, trays are transported to patient units for service, which depends on some means for serving food at the proper temperature through either temperature maintenance or rethermalization. The first five delivery systems shown in table 20-1 are appropriate for use with any of the food production systems described in the previous chapter. The delivery systems are all designed to maintain the hot and cold temperatures of food cooked or reheated in the kitchen. Each delivery method has different characteristics that must be considered in relation to the physical layout and other features of the facility.

Insulated Tray

The insulated tray system uses a lightweight thermal tray with individual molded compartments that hold both hot and cold foods. Specially designed china or disposable tableware is placed in the tray compartments, and the entire tray is covered with an insulated fitted cover. An insulated cup is used for beverages. No external heat or refrigeration sources are used in delivery or holding, so the foods must be at proper serving temperatures when plated. Food temperatures can be maintained up to 30 minutes by the insulating properties of the tray. Meal trays are delivered to the patient areas, either stacked or individually, on an open cart. No specialized carts are needed. It is somewhat difficult, however, to wash the trays and covers in most conveyor dishwashers, and special racks may be needed. Insulated tray systems can be purchased or leased.

Unitized Pellet

The unitized pellet system calls for the assembly of all hot items in a meal on a preheated plate. The plate is placed on a preheated pellet base and covered with a stainless steel or plastic lid that may also contain a pellet to retain heat and moisture. Cold items are placed on a tray simultaneously with the covered hot foods. The trays are delivered to the floor in an uninsulated cart. Insulated cold ware for beverages, cold salads, and cold desserts also may be used. Maximum holding time is about 45 minutes. Either china or disposable tableware can be used. Careful monitoring of pellet, plate, and lid temperatures is necessary.

Hot/Cold Cart

The hot/cold cart system uses a tray cart with electrically heated and refrigerated compartments to maintain proper food temperatures during transport. Standard trays are assembled with cold food plated and placed in the refrigerated compartment. Simultaneously, hot foods are plated and placed on a separate smaller tray and stored in the hot food compartment. Standard or disposable tableware is used. In another variation of this system, plated hot foods are placed in heated drawer compartments. Both versions require that the tray be reassembled at the point of service. Holding time prior to service can be longer because the temperatures are electronically controlled. These transport carts are very heavy, but they can be motorized for use in large facilities or in facilities with ramps. Considerable cart storage space is required, and more labor time is needed for cleaning and maintaining the carts than in most other systems.

Split Tray Cart

The split tray cart system is similar to the hot/cold cart system, except that hot and cold items are loaded on opposite sections of the same tray. The trays are slotted to allow placement of one side of the tray in a heated compartment and the other side in a refrigerated compartment. Special carts are needed, as are electrical outlets for plugging them in on the patient unit. With this system, tray reassembly is unnecessary.

Tray Heater Cart

The tray heater cart system uses specially designed disposable tableware on which hot and cold foods are placed at serving temperatures. Trays with resistance heaters built in at the dinner plate and bowl locations keep hot foods hot. When the loaded trays are placed into the battery-powered cart, the resistance heaters are activated. The heating of individual food items is regulated by preset push-button controls. The temperatures of cold foods are not affected by the tray heaters, but no refrigeration is provided in the cart. The heaters are automatically disconnected as each tray is removed from the cart. Hot beverages are delivered in insulated containers. The cart's batteries, which provide the electricity for heating and moving the cart, must be recharged between uses. This system is more complex than the others described and may require more maintenance. Because specialized disposable tableware is used, operating costs may be higher than for some of the other heat-maintenance systems.

Chill-Delivery/Floor-Rethermalization Systems

The next four delivery systems illustrated in table 20-1 are available for use with cook–chill, cook–freeze, or assembly–serve production systems in which foods are portioned cold and reheated in galleys in the patient areas. These delivery systems are designed to maximize food quality by reheating the food just prior to service, without extended hot-cold conditions required in the heat-maintenance systems. Labor time and costs may be reduced due to the system's greater scheduling flexibility in food portioning and tray assembly.

The rethermalization of foods held and delivered cold can be accomplished by using a heat-support cart or insulated trays and/or insulated components. The heat-support cart controls the amount of energy needed to rethermalize the food on the plate and in the bowl. However, foods must be plated in a specific way. The cart keeps the food hot until the tray is removed from the cart. Each cart has an insulated drawer for ice cream and other frozen products. However, the temperatures of other cold foods cannot be properly maintained. Insulated trays and tray components may be used for heating dinner plates. Mugs for hot and cold beverages also are available.

The features common to most of these systems include the transport of chilled or frozen foods on fully assembled trays to floor galleys. The types of carts used include enclosed nonrefrigerated, insulated, refrigerated, and carts on monorail. When nonrefrigerated carts are used, refrigeration is provided in the floor galley.

Several types of specialized equipment can be used for the rethermalization of foods: convection ovens, microwave ovens, tunnel microwaves, infrared ovens, and conduction ovens. Microwave ovens currently are the most commonly used rethermalization equipment. Service personnel must be trained in proper reheating procedures to attain the best food quality possible.

Several factors should be evaluated in selecting a tray delivery system. These include:

- The system's ability to maintain the desired level of food quality
- The system's compatibility with the existing production system and facility layout
- The number of work hours and level of skill or training needed to operate the system
- The space requirements and mobility of system equipment
- The initial costs for equipment, maintenance, and leasing
- The costs associated with the purchase of specialized or disposable tableware
- The cost of renovating an existing facility to accommodate the system
- The flexibility of the system to accommodate a change in production system, number of meals served, or menu pattern
- The system's energy requirements

Tray Service

Once a tray has been delivered to the designated location, it must be presented to the patient for whom it was assembled. Traditionally, this has been a function of nursing department employees, but this approach can result in delays in meal service that negatively affect food quality. Many food service directors have investigated the option of tray service by their own department's employees, resulting in a decrease in time between the delivery of the tray to the appropriate patient unit and presentation of the tray to the patient. Regardless of the approach, there must be cooperation between these two departments to minimize delays. Employees charged with presenting trays to patients should be trained in presentation procedures and customer relations, as described in chapter 4.

Special Patient Meal Services

In addition to providing basic meal service to patients, a facility may offer a number of optional patient services that can produce additional revenue. Examples include room service, gourmet meal service, wine service, fruit baskets, or in-room food service for patients' family and guests. For each optional service offered, an efficient delivery method must be developed to ensure customer satisfaction.

Resident Meal Service

In response to the environmental changes described in chapter 1, many hospitals have incorporated skilled nursing units, long-term care facilities, and/or rehabilitation centers into their organizations. One such change relates to the social aspects of group dining areas, of particular importance for residents in such extended care facilities. Also, proper implementation of the Omnibus Budget Reconciliation Act (OBRA) may require new and more flexible and appealing dining facilities. Therefore, the dining areas used by ambulatory persons in these facilities should be comfortable and attractive, and provide enough space for wheelchairs and service personnel to move freely. Having one or several dining rooms may be desirable, depending on the needs and capabilities of residents. Several types of service can be used, each of which has advantages and limitations. Three of these—cafeteria service, table service, and tray service—are briefly described below.

Cafeteria Service

As already mentioned, cafeteria service is common in facilities whose residents are sufficiently ambulatory. Some assistance from food servers may be needed for persons who have difficulty carrying their filled trays to their tables. With cafeteria service, attractive food displays, temperature control, and portion control are possible. Furthermore, diners can make their own food selections. In some situations, buffet service, which has similar benefits, is used when residents are able to serve themselves.

Table Service

Table service, another option for dining room service, presents some difficulties when a selective menu is offered, but restaurant-style menus may be used. Because foods are portioned in the kitchen or service area, residents may not be able to modify their portion sizes or choose sauces, gravies, and condiments as easily as in a cafeteria. Unless portion sizes are carefully tailored to the residents' needs, plate waste may be higher than expected. In facilities where table service is customary, an occasional buffet, such as a Sunday brunch for residents and their families, makes a pleasant change in routine.

Family-style service is rarely used in extended care facilities and is not recommended for several reasons. Portion control is difficult, considerable handling of foods at the table increases microbiological hazards and the danger of burns or spills, and food waste can be significant. More tableware is needed because bulk serving bowls and platters are used, and the amount of dish washing is increased. More labor is needed in the dining room to clear tables than with the other styles of dining room service.

Tray Service

Trays for persons confined to their rooms should be attractively arranged for convenience as well as appeal. For patients who must be fed, sufficient time should be allowed so that the person doing the feeding is not hurried. The staff members who feed patients should be familiar with menu items so that they can answer questions and encourage reluctant eaters to eat at least some of every food item. Persons with limited vision find that eating is more enjoyable when the foods they are eating or being fed are described to them. Regardless of the type of service system used, meals are eagerly awaited by residents, and it is especially important that they be served on time.

Nonpatient Meal Services

In most hospitals and in many extended care facilities, the number of nonpatient customers (visitors, staff, guests) exceeds the number of patients. Therefore, meal service for these customers becomes a significant part of food service. A variety of approaches to meal service may be necessary to meet the wants and needs of this consumer group.

Cafeteria Service

The cafeteria may be designed as a traditional straight-line system or a modified version of a free-flow system, in which employees, staff, visitors, and guests serve some food items themselves. The rate of customer flow in the cafeteria is affected by the number of menu choices, the physical layout of serving equipment, the serving speed, the number of lines, and the number of cashiers. When large numbers of diners are to be served in a limited period, special attention to line speed may necessitate setting up additional lines, offering fewer choices, and adding more cashiers. Business during slow periods, typically in the evening and on weekends, may be increased with strategies such as offering special discount prices for senior citizens' meals.

For many years, limiting the operating hours of the employee cafeteria has been standard practice in most health care operations. However, some food service departments have seen the profit potential in cafeteria operations that provide varied menu choices for employees and visitors over an extended period. The cafeteria should offer high-quality, attractively merchandised items. Special theme days for cafeteria service are usually enjoyed by employees of both the food service department and the health care operation as a whole.

How can the food service department respond appropriately to the trend toward more ambulatory and outpatient care? In reviewing cafeteria operations, it is appropriate to examine the particular dietary needs of these patients. Specifically, the cafeteria's accessibility to ambulatory patients, appropriateness of menu offerings, price range of foods, and hours of operation should be evaluated. If the cafeteria is viewed as a profit center as well as a service center, the needs of all persons using the health care facility, including nonpatients, can be met in a fiscally responsible manner.

Table Service

The service provided by full-service restaurants, referred to as *table service,* may be appropriate for some types of health care food service operations. Table service involves plating of food, as ordered by the customer, in the kitchen. Then, a member of the waitstaff presents each course of the meal to the customer. Other waitstaff services include beverage refills and removal of soiled dishes from the dining table. Table service requires more customer time for dining, more service staff skills, and it generally results in higher service costs. Therefore, full-service amenities should not be provided unless careful marketing research (including customer life-style and economic status, among other factors) supports the venture. Table service also is appropriate for catering functions that require banquet service.

Over-the-Counter Service

Because of the speed of over-the-counter service, these types of operations are popular with several of the customer groups served by the health care food service operation. After placing their orders with service personnel, customers expect quick service. Therefore, careful menu planning is essential to meeting this demand, and only those foods that can be prepared or consumed quickly should be offered. Offering special meals of the day at discounted prices also may speed service.

Once customers receive their orders, several dining options may be available. Most over-the-counter operations have on-site seating and disposable serviceware for on-site dining or carryout service. Counters may be designed to offer take-out services for bakery items and special holiday foods. Other over-the-counter options may include delivery of orders to customers. Kiosks or mobile carts, which can be wheeled to other customer locations such as lobbies or patios, also have proven successful. Because many of the customer groups served by the food service department rely on quick meal service, these types of operations are popular.

Catering Services

In today's competitive environment, more and more health care facilities are seeking ways to expand their service lines and generate additional revenue. Catering is one way to accomplish this goal. Catering may take place on or off the premises (as discussed in chapter 15).

The event may be as simple as a coffee and tea setup for a meeting or as elaborate as a reception or banquet.

Before a full-scale catering program can be implemented, its feasibility should be studied. A number of questions need to be answered and logistics planned. For example:

- What type of catering will be done?
- What kinds of menus will be offered?
- Will table decorations be needed?
- Can the existing staff handle the added work load?
- Does current staff have the necessary skills?
- What will additional equipment, supplies, and labor cost?
- Does the facility have space for this additional activity?
- How will start-up costs be covered?
- How will costs of the program be calculated?
- Will the food service department receive the revenue generated from the program?
- Can the revenue generated significantly enhance existing programs?

The food production system generally can accommodate the demands of catering with minor adjustments in its preparation equipment in terms of both type and capacity or volume. With careful attention to scheduling of food production employees, the impact on production labor requirements (for example, in regard to both regular work hours and overtime) can be minimized. The type of meal service specified for a particular catered event will most certainly vary. For customers on limited budgets, buffets can be suggested. For customers who desire more elegant meal service, full table service with waitstaff can be provided.

Although the activities described above vary from one catered event to another, proper food handling is always critical. To implement the guidelines discussed in chapter 13, the operation must provide transportation and holding equipment to ensure that food remains healthful. A variety of such equipment is available on the market.

Aside from being an excellent means of service expansion, special-events catering helps promote the food service department and enhances the larger facility's image. However, this specialized service requires dedication, creativity, expertise, and savvy marketing research.

Vending Operations

Vending operations are a popular alternative for meeting the needs of employees, guests, residents, and outpatients on a round-the-clock basis in many hospitals and long-term care facilities. Compared to cafeteria service, vending services are less labor-intensive and require very little space for the typical bank of machines. Vending machines maintain chilled food items at more appropriate temperatures than when they are displayed for cafeteria service. Potential customers generally are familiar with operation of the microwave, the primary method for heating food items purchased from vending machines. Wherever chilled or frozen foods are vended, microwave ovens usually are provided. Some machines use debit card systems that eliminate the use of coins and cash.

In planning a vending service, a number of options are available for how to control and operate this type of meal service. The food service director can contract with a vending company to provide selections ranging from snacks and hot and cold beverages to full-scale offerings of hot canned foods, preplated convenience foods, sandwiches, pastries, snacks, and frozen desserts. Vending space can be rented on a per-square-foot basis, for a set amount for each item sold, or as a percentage of gross sales. Another option could allow the food service operation to provide food for the machines and contract with the vending company to provide other items (such as candy and beverages). A number of food service departments establish their own self-operated services. This decision, however, should be based on careful analysis of all capital and operating costs, along with close scrutiny of forecasted revenues.

Regardless of who controls the vending operation, food quality, equipment operation and maintenance, and vending area sanitation are major concerns that mandate attentive planning.

Several factors must be considered, such as electricity sources, ease of restocking (review the security measures covered in chapter 14), environmental amenities (comfortable and aesthetically pleasing furnishings), and waste disposal. If sanitation of the vending area is not a term of a contractual agreement with an outside service, this responsibility must be assigned to an appropriate department, such as maintenance or housekeeping.

Off-Site Meal Service

In addition to providing meal service to patients, residents, and nonpatients, many health care food service operations provide services to market segments in their surrounding communities. For example, off-site meal service to child care and elder care centers and to congregate feeding sites (churches or community centers, for example) are not unusual. Meal service also may be provided to home-confined individuals who require special diets and/or cannot prepare nutritious meals for themselves. Sometimes health care food service operations are perceived throughout the community as the organizations best able to meet this need. As with catering special events, responding to the needs of the community can have a positive impact on the operation's public image as well as that of the health care facility as a whole.

Of course, off-site meal service is another route to service expansion. However, as is true of catering services, meal prices must be determined carefully to cover food, labor, and supply costs and yet remain affordable for the customers. In many communities, additional funding is available from federal, state, or local sources. Prices and the extent of service for government-supported programs are contracted in advance.

Other factors must be considered when studying feasibility of or planning for the implementation of off-site meal service. Appropriate operational standards for each functional area, such as menu planning, production, and sanitation, must be maintained. Therefore, to provide high-quality service to off-site locations, it is necessary to develop policies and procedures specific to this type of service. Many of these will depend on whether the food is to be provided to the customer in bulk quantities or as individual meals.

Quantity Meals

If the operation's menus are carefully integrated, providing bulk food for congregate groups, such as community centers, does not require the preparation of additional menu items, just larger quantities. Next, a means for maintaining food temperature during transport is needed for all systems unless immediate delivery can be ensured. Many operations use insulated carriers or carts. The assembly of meals and the loading of delivery vehicles must be carefully integrated into the department's total work schedule.

The potential problems of providing food in bulk include the failure to return serviceware and the excessive expense of disposable bulk food containers. Portion control at service time is more difficult to achieve, and it may be more difficult to monitor special dietary needs among community center attendees.

Individual Meals

Many communities attempt to provide direct home meal service to individuals who are unable to prepare their own meals. One meal per day, which provides one-half to two-thirds of the adult daily requirements five days a week, is the most common service provided. A cold meal for later consumption also may be delivered at the same time as the hot meal. Mostly, meals are preplated in the food service department on disposable insulated tableware.

Transport and delivery of meals to clients' homes is often provided by volunteers or other community agencies, in which case training for the volunteers is required. They need to understand the policies of the meal service program, details about special diets, food-handling procedures, emergency procedures, and techniques for assessing a client's general physical and mental well-being at the time of meal delivery. Home-delivered meal programs not only provide nutritional benefits for recipients, but they also play an important role in providing social contact for isolated persons and in serving as a check on their well-being.

Another type of individual meal service implemented at some operations is the sale of frozen meals for both normal and modified diets. These meals were originally developed for customers with special nutrition needs, such as weight-control patients, the elderly, or recently discharged patients. Operations that stock the meals for sale have found that they also may appeal to consumers who typically buy microwaveable meals. To provide this service efficiently, food service directors need to help design mechanisms for the sale of these products as part of the meal service system. For instance, sales to nonpatients may require a location in the building with easy access to in-and-out parking. Other issues related to the feasibility of such a venture include estimating consumer demand, determining operational costs and capital requirements, and selecting an appropriate pricing method for the products. These and other related factors should be thoroughly explored prior to the implementation of such a venture.

☐ Enhancing Customer Satisfaction

Whichever meal service system and customer group are targeted, to be truly customer oriented and to operate competitively and cost-effectively the health care food service operation must develop a marketing plan as described in chapter 3 that allows room for customer feedback. As mentioned earlier, distributing customer surveys or conducting focus group meetings on proposed and actual menu items; publishing menus in advance; making questionnaires available; and offering daily specials at reduced prices and with evaluation forms are proven incentives for eliciting satisfactory ratings.

Both the design of a service system and how it is marketed are critical to the success of the food service department and to the larger facility. Both activities define the means by which products and services are presented to customers and how future demand for services is affected. A number of strategies described in chapters 3 and 4 can be implemented to enhance satisfaction and demand.

☐ Summary

Health care meal assembly, delivery, and service to patients, residents, and nonpatients presents a discrete set of demands for food service directors who must design meal service systems. The length of time required for a tray to reach the patient's room from its assembly point is one of the most important factors in determining the selection and quality of food to be served. A wide variety of tray delivery equipment helps maintain the quality of food during this process. Numerous factors (such as the physical layout of the health care facility, the timing of service, and the cost of equipment) must be considered when planning an on-site or off-site meal service system.

Meal service for residents of extended care facilities is usually provided by means of cafeteria, table, or tray service in a setting that takes into account the residents' social needs and ability to participate in group dining. The variety among nonpatient customers in terms of service preferences and expectations necessitate a variety of approaches. These range from cafeteria service to catering services to vending operations.

Many health care food service operations provide off-site meal service to community organizations, which can expand the service line, improve the facility's public image, and generate revenue. Regardless of the targeted customer group, it is important to implement marketing principles and customer relations strategies to enhance customer satisfaction.

☐ Bibliography

Adam, E. E., and Ebert, R. J. *Production and Operations Management.* 4th ed. Englewood Cliffs, NJ: Prentice-Hall, 1989.

Axler, B. H. *Foodservice: A Managerial Approach.* Lexington, MA: D. C. Heath, 1979.

Franzese, R. Food services survey shows delivery shift. *Hospitals* 58(16):61, 64, 1984.

Herz, M. L. *Analysis of Alternative Patient Tray Delivery Concepts.* Natick, MA: U.S. Army Natick Research and Development Command, 1977.

Iwamuro, R. A snapshot of the off-premises market. *Restaurants USA* 12(9):40–43, Oct. 1992.

Kaud, F. A., Miller, R. P., and Underwood, R. F. *Cafeteria Management for Hospitals.* Chicago: American Hospital Association, 1982.

Lieberman, J. S. *The Complete Off-Premise Caterer.* New York City: Van Nostrand Reinhold, 1990.

Lutz, S. Baxter, Kraft seek bigger market share. *Modern Healthcare* 19(24):24, June 1989.

Lutz, S. Pleasing patients' palates. *Modern Healthcare* 19(24):20–23, 25–28, June 1989.

Rose, J. C. *Catering Cost Models.* Rockville, MD: Aspen, 1986.

Salkin, S. To meet OBRA regulations: HPSI launches menu plan. *Foodservice Director* 4(6):53, June 1991.

Sawyer, C. A. Safety issues related to use of take-out food. *Journal of Foodservice Systems* 6:41–59, 1991.

Spears, M. C. *Foodservice Organizations: A Managerial and Systems Approach.* 2nd ed. New York City: Macmillan, 1991.

Splaver, B. *Successful Catering.* New York City: Van Nostrand Reinhold, 1991.

Stephenson, S. Hospital catering: for profit or not for profit? *Restaurants & Institutions* 101(27):83, 86, 88, Oct. 1991.

Underwood, R. F. Merchandising for satisfaction and profit. In: J. C. Rose, editor. *Handbook for Health Care Food Service Management.* Rockville, MD: Aspen, 1984.

West, B. B., and Wood, L. (Revised by Harger, V. F., Shugart, G. S., and Payne-Palacio, J.) *Foodservice in Institutions.* 6th ed. New York City: Macmillan, 1988.

Facility Design
and Equipment Selection

☐ Introduction

The unique nature of individual health care organizations presents a challenge in planning and equipping a food service operation that is both functional and efficient in physical design. Several common problems plague some departments: wasted or underused space, inadequate or improper storage facilities, inflexible equipment arrangements, energy-wasting equipment, inappropriate equipment capacity or type, excessive cross-traffic, labor-intensive layout, and inadequate ventilation or lighting. The application of a systematic approach to facility planning and equipment selection can improve existing health care food service operations and guide the design of new ones.

This chapter will explain some of the activities involved when health care food service directors are confronted with providing input on renovating current facilities or constructing new ones, and with helping select the right equipment to do their facilities' work. Depending on the mission, goals, and objectives involved, any number of activities go into the major task of project design. These include appointing a planning team to study project feasibility, gathering retrospective data, and writing a purchase contract and advising buyers on what to look for in a food service equipment vendor.

How the roles of the food service director and the design consultant complement one another, how the team performs its initial research, and how layout plans for various department and work areas are conceived are only some of the topics discussed. Others include how the planning team, of which the director is a member, arrives at a proposed layout for the operation's physical plant and facilities. The implications of the Americans with Disabilities Act (ADA) on facility design also will be discussed.

Guidelines will be given for how to arrive at equipment specifications for purchase contracts. Guidelines also will direct purchasers in buying items, from construction materials to security systems, that ensure that the food preparation equipment received is of the quality ordered. Then an extensive list of food-processing equipment and devices will be described. Some of these include ovens and ranges, refrigerators and freezers, compactors, mixers, dispensing equipment, and coffee makers.

☐ Facility Planning and Design

Planning and design of food service facilities is a complicated process because, generally speaking, no one individual has all the necessary data and information needed to produce an effective and efficient plan. Therefore, most organizations (whether renovating or constructing anew) form a facility planning team to carry out this function. The team should meet routinely to discuss project status, changes in the plan, time lines for activities, and the like. The viewpoint of each team member should be carefully considered prior to making decisions regarding the project. Ample time should be allocated for team meetings and the overall planning process.

Composition of the Planning Team

Composition of the facility planning team varies according to scope of project, availability of specialists, and expertise of the food service director. Depending on the individual organization and its resources, members of the team may include the food service director, an outside food facilities design consultant, a food equipment representative, an architect, a builder, and an interior designer (for decor and furnishings). The director's role and the consultant's role are summarized in the following subsections.

Food Service Director

Food service directors are not expected to be experts in design and construction. Rather, their role is to represent the interests of the operation by developing the operational standards to be supported by the project, providing critical information to other team members, contributing to planning decisions, and evaluating the plans that emerge for the food service operation.

For new construction or major renovations, decisions to be made and conveyed to other team members include identification of the food service operation's target markets, the volume requirements for each market, and the quality standards for food production and service. The director participates in the development of the overall concept, which specifies the type of production and meal service systems to be implemented. A critical function of the director is to evaluate proposed designs in terms of spatial allocation, layout of work areas and their relationship to one another, and the equipment proposed. The planning process is time-consuming, but the director's careful study of each aspect of the operation is critical to successful project outcome.

Food Facilities Design Consultant

If the budget allows, the services of a food facilities design consultant should be considered for major changes in food service production or tray service, major renovations in the kitchen or cafeteria, or construction of a new food service department. The consultant's role varies depending on the director's own level of design expertise. Ideally, the design consultant should specialize in food facility design, construction, and food service equipment selection and be expected to make significant contributions during all phases of the project. Typical contributions to a construction or remodeling project include developing work flow schemes, preparing drawings of equipment layouts, writing equipment specifications, and following up with the builder to ensure that all items on the punch list are resolved. The design consultant should have a thorough knowledge of current laws and regulations (such as the ADA) that may affect the project.

One expert quoted in the *FoodService Director* indicates that a food facilities design consultant should provide expertise, objectivity, creative solutions, a return on investment, and project management. Despite these contributions, the food service director must become as knowledgeable as possible about these issues so as to fulfill his or her responsibility for the project.

In 1977, a joint committee of the American Hospital Association and The American Dietetic Association, recognizing the importance of optimizing capital expenditures while controlling daily operating costs of the food service department, developed guidelines for selecting consultants in hospital food service system management, design, and equipment. The guidelines include information about the planning process, the functions of consultants, appropriate criteria for selecting a qualified consultant, and methods for determining consulting fees.

The Planning Process

A systematic approach to the food facility planning process should be established by the planning team. Typically, this process is initiated by collecting background information from internal and external sources and analyzing operational factors for the specific operation. Then the work areas can be planned and the flow of work between areas considered. At this point, a scale drawing or layout of the operation should be developed and evaluated. The team also should provide input regarding general building features and materials.

Collecting Background Information

Before a layout is designed, the team must gather background information about the proposed operation. For example:

- Mission, goals, and objectives of the health care operation and the food service department
- Long-range plans and philosophy of the parent organization
- Number of beds and spatial configuration of the health care operation
- Number of daily meals served to patients
- Extent of services provided to nonpatients by the food service department
- Availability of labor and skill levels required

Such information is important because these factors affect the type of production and meal service systems to be used by the food service department. The optimum system should be compatible with the mission, goals, and objectives of the operation, with the final decision based on projected capital costs, operating costs, ease of administration, and subjective comparisons (such as the aesthetic characteristics of public dining areas).

In addition to internal background information, external sources of information also must be considered. Key among these are the local, state, and federal laws and regulations that apply to facility design and equipment selection. (To assess the impact of laws and regulations related to environmental, sanitation, and safety issues on facility design and equipment selection, refer to chapters 12, 13, and 14.) The ADA, which guarantees civil rights protection for persons with disabilities, also must be considered.

When planning a renovation or new building project, the food service director should contact the human resource department staff member who manages compliance with the ADA. This individual can assist the planning team in determining appropriate accommodations for persons (both customers and employees) with disabilities. In addition, the facility design consultant should have a working knowledge of this law so that its requirements can be incorporated into the facility plans.

The food service director also should be familiar with this law. In its publication, *Americans with Disabilities Act: Answers for Foodservice Operators,* the National Restaurant Association outlines the steps necessary to accommodate persons with disabilities in eating establishments. These include:

1. Understanding the intent of the law
2. Evaluating employment practices, customer service policies, and facilities to ensure that they are accessible and usable
3. Implementing changes primarily through employee training and removal of barriers
4. Continuing attention to accessibility when planning renovation and new construction

The book focuses on identifying barriers (by means of an easy-to-use checklist), removing common barriers and implementing low-cost solutions, and providing quality service to all customers. The appendixes detail ADA design requirements for restaurants, illustrate accessible design features, and provide references for technical assistance.

Analyzing Operational Factors

Other operational factors, past and future, also must be considered. The food service director can provide information about menu items and menu patterns, the department's production and meal service procedures, and its purchasing policies and practices.

Menu Information

Because the menu determines the equipment needed and the space required in the production area, further analysis should include the following information about each of the operation's menus:

- Menu pattern and number of selections within the pattern for each course or category of food served
- Complexity of menu items served
- Type and number of modified diet menu items served
- Type and number of meals prepared

Type of Production and Meal Service Systems

The type of production system planned affects what equipment, space, and personnel are required in the central kitchen. (Food production systems—cook–serve, cook–chill, cook–freeze, and assembly–serve—were described in chapter 19. The meal service systems described in chapter 20 also must be taken into consideration.) The advance planning process must weigh the following factors:

- Total quantity of each menu item needed to yield the required number of portions
- Batch size preferred
- Amount of time required vis-à-vis amount of time available for production
- Assembly, delivery, and service systems used

Certainly this list is not all-inclusive, and similar information must be gathered for other subsystems (such as receiving, storage, and ware washing) of the operation. An operational plan that states organizational constraints and projected needs can then be developed and used as a basis for designing functional work areas.

Purchasing Policies

The department's purchasing policies and practices determine the type of equipment and the amount of space needed for low-temperature and dry storage areas and production and meal service facilities. Considerations include:

- What market form in which food supplies are purchased (the amount of processing that has taken place prior to purchase)
- The state of food supplies at delivery time (canned, frozen, chilled, dehydrated, or freeze-dried)
- Frequency of delivery for all categories of food
- The volume purchased and the amount of inventory carryover from one purchase period to the next
- The department's issuing and inventory control procedures

Planning Work Areas

Work areas are the basic functional units of an operation. The specific tasks to be performed in a given work area must be identified so that the amount of space and layout for each one can be determined. In an existing facility, improvements in space use often can be made by identifying points of congestion and rearranging equipment or tasks to alleviate them.

For new construction, basic work method principles as described by Kotschevar and Terrell in *Foodservice Planning: Layout and Equipment* should be implemented. Basic work areas for new facilities include receiving, storage, food production, meal service, and ware washing.

Receiving

The receiving area's location and space requirements depend on the health care operation's purchasing policies. For example, if a materials management department is responsible for procuring all goods used by the facility, a central receiving point should be provided for all deliveries. Because materials used in the food service department account for a large proportion of the total deliveries, a location close to food service is desirable.

In designing a new facility, the traffic flow that surrounds the facility, the space needed for parking delivery trucks, and building constraints should be taken into account. The receiving dock should be covered, if possible, to protect receiving clerks and supplies from inclement weather. The size of the receiving area depends on the delivery schedule, the volume of goods in each shipment, and the time lapse between receipt and storage.

Storage

The storage area should include space for nonperishable food as well as refrigerator and freezer space for storing perishable goods. The dry storage space should be close to the receiving area as well as to the ingredient preparation and control area. Storage space needs are based on procurement policies related to product volume, purchase frequency, inventory level, and delivery schedule. A separate storage area should be provided for cleaning supplies, chemicals, paper goods, and other nonfood materials; space needs, equipment requirements, and sanitary construction features are just as important for these goods as for food supplies.

Space requirements for standard and low-temperature, walk-in units vary considerably among food service operations. Specific needs depend on menu offerings, the amount of preparation done before purchase, and the volume of perishables and frozen foods purchased and delivered at specified times. Analysis of these factors and the usable space provided by stationary or mobile shelving can be used as a guide.

Standard and low-temperature, self-contained refrigerator units provide convenient storage at point of use. Where space is limited and in small facilities, self-contained units should be considered in place of walk-ins. Many options are available, so construction features, size, and where and how the unit will be used should be considered before the purchasing decision is made.

A security sash, screen, or bar should be installed on windows in storerooms located at ground level. Other security measures include provisions for locking doors from the outside but for safety purposes allowing them to open from the inside without a key.

Food Production

The production area should be close to raw ingredient storage areas and on a direct route to assembly and service areas. The size and shape of the area allocated to production influence equipment arrangement and work flow patterns. The shortest possible route from one area to the next with a minimum of backtracking or cross-traffic is preferred. In large rectangular kitchens, work and materials can flow in parallel lines by using an island arrangement for cooking equipment. In square or small kitchens, a U-shaped, L-shaped, or E-shaped arrangement for equipment may be more efficient.

Major cooking equipment such as ranges, ovens, braising pans, and fryers usually are grouped together. Steam-jacketed kettles and compartment steamers are placed close by for convenience. Compact central arrangements of such equipment facilitates construction of effective exhaust hoods over all cooking surfaces and steam equipment. The aisles between equipment should be wide enough to park carts, turn them around, and permit employees to use them without blocking traffic.

Space for vegetable and salad preparation, baking, and food preparation should be allocated within the main production area. Dividing the open space into operational areas by equipment arrangement rather than by partitions is an effective way to create a sense of spaciousness, improve air circulation, simplify cleaning, permit more effective supervision, and allow greater flexibility for equipment additions and use of mobile equipment.

Meal Service

The work space, equipment, and layout needed for the assembly of food for patients or residents requiring tray service all depend on the type of delivery and service systems selected (as detailed in chapter 20). All assembly areas require careful planning to achieve maximum efficiency and to ensure delivery of high-quality meals at a reasonable cost to consumers. In a centralized service system, the assembly area should be close to production areas, storage areas, dish-washing facilities, and tray cart storage areas. Easy access to food and materials and minimization of transportation time greatly improve quality and help control costs. Analysis of the basic functions to be performed and the equipment needed to simplify tasks will help determine space requirements. Factors to consider during the planning stage are the following:

- Number of patients or residents served at each meal
- Menu composition (the number of food components offered and selected for normal and modified diets)
- Type of tray assembly, delivery, and service
- Time limitations for tray assembly
- Amount and dimensions of the space available or planned for tray assembly and support equipment

Some hospitals and most extended care facilities provide dining space for ambulatory patients or residents either within the patient care area or near the central kitchen. Service arrangements and dining room furnishings are affected by the type of service (for example, table or cafeteria); the number of diners served at each meal; menu variety; the location of the dining room; health and mobility factors (for example, residents' disabilities); and the activities other than serving food that take place in the area.

Because of its potential for speedy service and food presentation possibilities, cafeteria service is the most popular way of serving employees, staff, visitors, and guests. Food service managers must bear in mind food quality as well as cost components related to service. Location of the service area, layout of the service line, equipment availability, and the employees' work methods affect consumer satisfaction as well as the efficiency and economy of the food service system.

Locating the cafeteria close to the central kitchen reduces transportation time and can help control food quality. For the sake of preserving quality, batch cooking of vegetables and other foods that suffer from overcooking is recommended, but this technique would be difficult if the service area were too far from the production center. Close access to dish-washing facilities also is preferred.

Service lines can be of various sizes and configurations, depending on the number of people served, the service time allotted for each meal, menu complexity, and the dimensions of the available space. Conventional service lines are straight or L-shaped; variations in new and large facilities include circular, scatter, and open square designs. (See figure 21-1.) The flow of traffic is important in whatever configuration is chosen.

The length of the service counter depends on the size of the menu and the amount of food displayed. Adequate space should be provided for attractive display and preservation of food quality. All hot and cold sections should be protected by sneeze guards that meet local sanitation codes.

Additional space is needed on or near the line for trays, tableware, napkins, beverage containers, and so forth. These materials should be located for easy accessibility by the customer but not where traffic flow will be interrupted or slowed. The same principle applies

Figure 21-1. Cafeteria Service Line Configurations

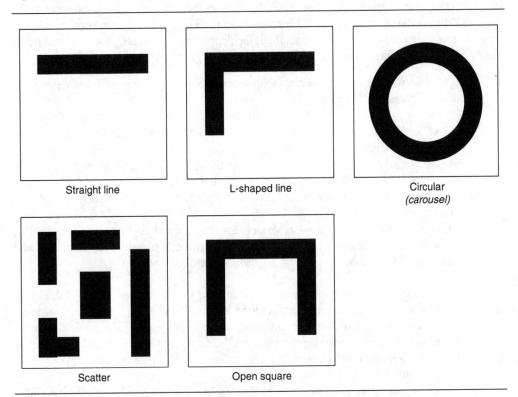

Straight line   L-shaped line   Circular *(carousel)*

Scatter   Open square

to the location of cash registers: A line can form easily when there are not enough cashiers; meanwhile, the customers' food gets cold.

Overall space requirements for the employees' dining area must be carefully analyzed to ensure efficient movement of customers and service workers. Today, more self-service in the cafeteria is preferred by food service directors because labor is saved and by customers because they have more control over the amount and kinds of food they can choose. The space behind the line should be wide enough for transportation equipment and for efficient movement by employees. The customers' side also must be wide enough for bypassing others in the line, if this is allowed, and for easy access to the dining area. A periodic check of waiting times at various stations and customer counts per minute will indicate bottlenecks that can be eliminated by equipment rearrangement or menu changes.

Once customers have been served, adequate space in a pleasant, attractive dining room is needed. Because health care personnel usually have little time to relax at meal breaks, waiting and overcrowding are not conducive to good morale. The size of the dining area should depend on the number of people expected to be seated during a given time and the rate of turnover. Generally, a minimum of 10 to 14 square feet per person is recommended.

Ware Washing

The cost of labor, equipment, and supplies required for sanitizing pots, pans, and serviceware makes the ware-washing facility one of the most important areas of the food service department. Centralized washing, located close to the tray assembly area, cafeteria, dining room, and production areas, eliminates duplication of equipment and personnel. The supervision and control of sanitation can also be more effective when all ware washing is performed in one location.

A location close to the main production and service areas is convenient. The dish room's layout should be planned to provide good work flow, minimize labor time, and ensure efficiency

521

and safety. The arrangement of equipment can take any form: straight-line, L-shaped, oval, square, rectangular, or triangular. The shape depends on the equipment used, the space available, and the methods of soiled dish return and clean dish removal and storage. Before the type and arrangement of equipment is planned, the department's policies, practices, and needs should be analyzed. Factors influencing the space arrangements include:

- *Type of service:* Is it tray, cafeteria, table, or a combination of these? Each style requires different types and quantities of serviceware.
- *Number of persons served:* Are there fluctuations from meal to meal and from day to day? Service demand will affect the type and amount of serviceware used and the space requirements.
- *Type and number of menu items served:* Are there variations among the types of service at one meal as well as from meal to meal? The style and quantity of dishes, trays, and so forth affect the space needed. Storage space for carts and dollies also will vary with these requirements.
- *Length of meal service and time:* Is serviceware used more than once during each meal, or is it stockpiled and washed later? Serviceware inventory, dishwasher capacity, and space requirements vary according to these practices.

Adequate space is needed for scraping, sorting, and racking soiled dishes. Tables that are 2 to 2½ feet wide, the same height as the dishwasher (34 inches high is convenient), and long enough to hold the prewash and waste disposal unit should be provided. Some dish room arrangements include slanted, overhead shelves for holding glass and cup racks while they are being loaded. Convenient placement of these shelves can help to reduce employee fatigue and utilize space efficiently.

Table space for air-drying clean dishes held in racks, carts, and dollies is needed. Table heights and widths should be the same as those mentioned in the preceding paragraph. Length varies according to the type of dishwasher used and the washing load. Flight-type machines require less table space because dishes are removed from the conveyor and placed in storage units almost immediately. Specialized equipment also may be used, such as portable soak sinks, a glasswasher, and a pulper–extractor waste disposer. All these require space and should be carefully planned for in the overall design.

Trends for Work Area Design

The trend to minimize the department's overall dimensions, particularly in the production area but also in other functional areas because of the rising cost of new construction, has been made possible in many operations by changes in the types and forms of food purchased and in the availability of slim-line, modular, and mobile equipment. Once the ideal, or at least the best possible, space relationship and arrangement has been determined, a scale drawing of the work area can be produced.

Planning the Flow of Work

The orderly flow of employees and materials, the work flow, deserves special consideration by the planning team. Therefore, the location of each work area in relation to other areas in the department must be determined to minimize backtracking and cross-traffic. The efficient movement of food, supplies, and people requires consideration of the essential tasks to be performed at each stage of production and meal service (assembly, delivery, and service); the number of employees involved; and the equipment required for the activities. To ensure that the best arrangement of work areas has been planned, a chart that illustrates the work flow can be developed. At this point, the actual amounts of space and equipment are not needed. The chart is merely a diagram showing what happens when food and people travel from the receiving area to the point of service and cleanup area.

Developing the Layout

The next step in the planning process is to draw a schematic plan, based on all the data gathered earlier, that shows work areas, traffic aisles, and the location of specific pieces of equipment. This task is usually performed by the architect in conjunction with the food facilities design consultant. At this point, it is important for the food service director to evaluate the proposed layout. Charting the work flow for typical menu items on the scale diagram is an excellent way to assess the plan's feasibility. A good layout should provide a smooth, orderly flow in as straight, short, and direct a route as possible. It is possible to pinpoint traffic problems that can result from misplaced or inadequate equipment, too little or too much space, and generally poor work flow patterns. The food service director should evaluate the layout before plans are finalized.

The location of the food service department in relation to elevators, other hospital departments, and public areas of the building also must be considered. The distance from the food service department to patient areas is a factor in determining the method of food delivery, but new technology in tray delivery systems has helped reduce temperature control problems.

Specifying General Building Features and Materials

In addition to developing the layout, the planning team must make decisions related to general building features and types of materials to be used in construction. The food service director should be aware of the requirements for interior surfaces, lighting, utilities, and ventilation.

Floors, Walls, and Ceilings

Floors should be durable, easy to clean, nonslippery, nonabsorbent, and resilient. It is difficult to satisfy all these specifications with one material, and the use of the same material throughout all areas is not aesthetically pleasing. For example, a quarry tile floor in the dining area is not conducive to a relaxing atmosphere even though it meets most of the criteria. A hard-surface floor meets the basic requirements, particularly for preparation areas. However, it has two main drawbacks: It may be slippery when wet, and because it lacks resiliency, it tends to increase employee fatigue levels. Quarry or ceramic tile is usually used in kitchens, and vinyl tile or carpeting is used in dining areas. The various types of floor coverings available on the market should be examined before final selections are made because materials are constantly being developed and improved.

Regardless of the floor material chosen for the kitchen, adequate drains installed near steam equipment, food cutters, and ware-washing facilities will help reduce safety hazards and make housekeeping tasks more efficient. All floors should be finished with a baseboard, flush with the wall, for ease in maintaining sanitation.

Walls should be hard, smooth, washable, and impervious to moisture. Glazed tile to the ceiling, or at least to a 5- or 8-foot height (with plaster and washable paint above), is preferred for kitchen and service areas. Pleasing color combinations enhance the area's appearance and can even increase employee morale. Pipes, radiators, and wiring conduits should be placed inside the walls. In the dining area, it may be desirable to have tile wainscoting on the walls and around columns, with corrosion-resistant metal corner guards.

Soundproofing should be considered carefully in planning construction and before selecting equipment. Kitchens can be very noisy, and excessive noise can result in fatigue and low productivity among employees. The use of acoustical materials in ceilings appreciably reduces the noise level. However, selection of ceiling materials should be based on their ease of cleaning as well as their noise-reducing characteristics.

Lighting

The proper amount and kind of lighting in all work areas is important for cleanliness, safety, and efficiency. When energy conservation is the only lighting consideration given, fluorescent lights are used. Because the natural color of foods is enhanced when displayed under incandescent light, however, high-intensity incandescent lighting should be used in display and merchandising areas. Low-intensity incandescent lighting is used in dining areas for mood enhancement. A lighting expert should be consulted for special requirements.

Utilities and Ventilation

In some areas, both natural gas and electricity are available and are used as the power source for various pieces of equipment. Selection of gas as a heat source for cooking equipment should be coordinated with the health care operation's engineering department. Food service directors should be familiar with the power requirements of various pieces of equipment and evaluate the electrical plans to make sure that enough outlets are available and that they are appropriately located.

Proper heat, ventilation, and air-conditioning systems are important for food quality preservation, employee comfort, and building maintenance. The department director should work with the project engineer to identify areas of excessive heat and humidity in order to ensure that space is properly ventilated. Excessive moisture or heat can ruin walls and ceilings as well as employees' dispositions. Therefore, heat must be provided in the winter, and during the summer the air should be cooled and dehumidified to acceptable comfort levels.

☐ Equipment Selection

Many kinds of equipment will be discussed in this chapter to provide some basic information about the types of equipment and arrangements available that help achieve the standards necessary to provide high-quality and healthful food. Because equipment represents a large financial investment, it should be studied carefully before a purchase is made. Well-chosen equipment, used and maintained properly, provides many years of service.

Factors Affecting Equipment Selection

Because of the many variables associated with food service departments, the equipment buyer should fully understand the needs of the department and what equipment would best meet each of those needs. The amount and type of equipment needed depend on the operation's menu pattern, the facility's financial resources, its utility supply, equipment design and construction, and its safety and sanitation features.

Menu Offerings

Because menu offerings influence the choice of equipment, one basic question that should be answered is why a specific piece is needed. If the equipment would save time and money and would improve quality and personnel performance, then further study to justify size, capacity, and space needs can proceed. Analysis of the items listed in the menu, the number of servings needed, the batch size followed, and the production time required provides the background information necessary for making decisions on equipment purchases.

Cost

Another important aspect of the purchase decision is cost, and not just the initial cost. The costs involved with the installation, operation, maintenance, and repair of food service equipment also must be considered.

Utility Supply

Equipment requiring electricity or gas must be compatible with the facility's utility supply unless utilities are so outdated or inadequate that renovation is planned. For example, the facility's wiring and circuits must be able to supply the voltage required for operation of all electrical equipment. A piece of equipment designed for a 230-volt circuit will lose about 20 percent of its efficiency if connected to a 208-volt circuit. A motor designed for

208 volts may burn out at higher voltages. Consequently, the voltage (whether alternating or direct current) and phase (the source of alternating current in the circuit) available in the kitchen must be considered before equipment is ordered. Some equipment items require a single phase of alternating voltage, whereas others require three phases. That is, three separate sources of alternating current are arranged to handle larger power and heating loads. If gas equipment is preferred, an adequate gas supply must be available for peak operating periods, and convenient connections must be provided.

Design and Construction

The importance of design and construction to ensure proper performance without costly repairs cannot be overlooked. Equipment should be functional and durable as well as compatible with other equipment in the facility. The information supplied by manufacturers in catalogs, bulletins, brochures, and specification sheets should be studied carefully. Contact with other food service directors and equipment specialists also is helpful. If standard stock items do not meet the facility's needs, custom-built equipment can be ordered even though it is generally more expensive.

Safety and Sanitation Features

The safety and sanitation features of equipment are critical considerations in the selection process. All equipment should be constructed and installed in a manner that complies with the requirements of the Occupational Safety and Health Act of 1970 and other federal, state, and local regulations and codes. Several national not-for-profit organizations establish standards and controls to ensure the sanitation and safety of food service equipment and of the operating environment. Among them are the National Sanitation Foundation, the Underwriters' Laboratory, the American Gas Association, the National Board of Fire Underwriters, and the American Society of Mechanical Engineers (described in chapters 13 and 14). Choosing equipment bearing the seal of approval of any one or more of these organizations is recommended.

Equipment Specifications

Once the decision to purchase a piece of equipment has been made, information about the type, size, capacity, installation, and conditions of purchase is communicated to the vendor. This communication should be in writing to eliminate any possible misunderstanding of what should be delivered. Specifications can be brief or extended written documents, depending on the facility's procurement policies. The important point is that they be written simply and concisely, giving only those details that are necessary to ensure delivery of the equipment desired.

Some procurement policies prohibit the use of trade names, a proscription usually specified in organizations that use a formal bid system. When this method is used, a great deal of care must be taken to ensure that the equipment ordered actually meets food service requirements. When brand names can be stated on the purchase order but the clause "or approved equal" must be included so that competitive bidding can be undertaken, other manufacturers with reputations for quality, dependability, and service should be listed. Another solution is to require that bidders submit complete, detailed specifications of what they propose to furnish and then compare these statements with the original specifications to be sure that they really are equal. The burden of proof should be placed on the seller. Too often, items are purchased on the basis of price alone. Equipment should be purchased primarily for its quality and performance.

Specifications should spell out who will be responsible for installing and testing the new equipment. Demonstrations of proper equipment use and care also are very important and must be made a term of the written purchase contract. Follow-up on the performance of each piece and appropriate utilization by food service employees is the responsibility of the food service director. A thorough understanding of what is stipulated in the warranty, particularly the warranty period, replacement of parts, and service included will save money in the future.

Receiving Equipment

In the receiving area, accurate scales are needed for weighing all foods purchased by weight. For most operations, platform scales with a maximum capacity of 250 pounds are adequate. A desk or table, clipboards, and file cabinets are additional pieces of equipment that help receiving personnel do their jobs. In addition to the procedures described in chapter 14, closed-circuit television and/or perimeter alarm systems can be installed to increase security in the receiving area.

Heavy-duty two- and four-wheel hand trucks or semilive skids are essential. (*Semilive skids* are low platforms mounted on wheels on which materials can be loaded for handling or moving.) Skids are a good investment when large-quantity deliveries are received and storage space is available. Cases can be loaded on skids, wheeled to the storage area, and dropped in place, thus eliminating excessive handling.

Storage Equipment

The right equipment contributes to maximum use of available space in storage areas. Equipment for dry, refrigerated, and low-temperature storage areas is summarized below.

Dry Storage Equipment

Equipment for dry storage areas may include shelving, metal or plastic containers on wheels or dollies, and mobile platforms. Adjustable metal louvered or wire shelving is recommended to permit air circulation and to allow exact shelf spacing. For safety and convenience, the top shelf should be accessible without the use of a stool or stepladder. Local ordinances may specify at least 6 inches from the floor to the lowest shelf. At least a 2-inch space between the wall and shelf is needed for air circulation and cleaning access.

Shelving may be mobile or stationary. Selecting the right width and length of shelves is important. Widths range from 12 to 27 inches. If space allows, shelves can be placed back to back for easy access from both sides. Widths of 20 to 24 inches can easily accommodate two rows of No. 10 cans on a single shelf. The clearance between shelves should be at least 15 inches to allow the stacking of two No. 10 cans. The length of shelves can vary from 36 to 42 inches or more. Calculations of the dimensions of packaging for each item, the weight per unit, and inventory quantities should be used as a guide to determine the total number of linear feet of shelving needed.

Metal or plastic containers with tight-fitting covers are useful for storing broken lots of flour, cornmeal, other cereals and grains, and sugar. Food from packages that have been opened should be stored in food-grade containers with tight-fitting covers, with the contents clearly marked on the outside. When large amounts of dry food items are stored, mobile platforms and dollies are useful for moving and storing these goods until they are opened.

Refrigerated and Low-Temperature Storage

Standard refrigeration, which operates between 32° and 40°F (0° and 4°C), and low-temperature units, with a temperature range of −10° to 0°F (−24° to 18°C), are needed. Standard refrigerated and low-temperature systems are available in walk-in and self-contained units. Refrigeration systems that can quickly chill, freeze, and thaw foods are needed when a cook–chill or cook–freeze production system is used. Selection should be based primarily on need, flexibility, and convenience.

Walk-In Coolers and Freezers

Important features to consider when assessing cooler and freezer demands include the refrigeration system used, the construction materials and design, optional features, and the amount of usable space inside. In walk-ins, the condenser and motor usually are located in a remote area. They should be built to provide even temperature, balanced humidity, and good air circulation.

The floors, ceilings, walls, and doors of walk-in coolers and freezers should be constructed of durable, vaporproof, and easily cleanable materials. The type and amount of insulation used on all these parts are important. Foamed-in-place or froth-type insulation is used by many cooler manufacturers, but the thickness may vary. Doors should be provided with an effective seal to prevent condensation and loss of energy. Hanging overlapping strips of clear, heavy vinyl inside door openings also reduces energy consumption by keeping cold air in when the door is opened. Locking hardware on the outside is needed for security. An inside safety release prevents entrapment when the door is locked from the outside.

Ideally, the floors of walk-in units should be level with adjacent flooring. However, models are available with built-in interior or exterior ramps. Nonskid strips on an incline are needed for added safety. Automatic audio and visual warning systems outside the unit or in a remote location will indicate significant temperature changes. Built-in thermometers on the outside of the unit should also be checked regularly.

Optional features on some walk-ins include reach-in doors and regular doors with view-through windows. If the walk-in is located in the production area, the reach-in feature could be convenient for in-process holding or obtaining frequently used ingredients. View-through windows should not frost or fog. Walk-in units constructed with modular panels assembled on the premises are recommended over permanently installed models because they allow for future relocation or expansion.

The requirements for walk-in freezers are similar to those for walk-in coolers, except that more insulation is needed. Freezer units installed with the door opening into a walk-in cooler eliminate storage space on one wall of the cooler, and access to the freezer can be very inconvenient.

Self-Contained Refrigerators and Freezers

In self-contained units, the refrigeration system is mounted at the top or bottom. Bottom-mounted models reduce the amount of convenient space available. A compressor, condenser, and evaporator of the right size are needed for uniform temperature control regardless of the load. Foamed-in-place or froth-type urethane insulation of 2½ inches or more thickness is recommended for walls, ceilings, and doors. A one-piece, durable, seamless lining in the interior cabinet is needed to allow for easy cleaning. Exterior finishes vary among manufacturers; vinyl in a choice of colors, stainless steel, and other durable metals are used.

Refrigerators and storage freezers are designed as reach-in or pass-through and roll-in or roll-through units, which are convenient in areas between production and service. Solid or glass doors may be hinged on the right or left. One-piece molded door gaskets that provide a positive seal are recommended to conserve energy. Full- and half-door models with self-closing and safety stop features are available. A system for locking all doors is needed for security. An exterior dial thermometer and audiovisual temperature alarm should be installed in all units. Adjustable legs facilitate leveling of reach-in and pass-through cabinets. Single units may be equipped with casters for mobility. Other design options include provisions for interchangeable interiors that accommodate adjustable rustproof wire shelving; tray or pan slides; roll-out shelves and drawers; and flush-with-floor models for mobile carts and food service racks.

Quick-Chill and Freezing Systems

Refrigeration systems capable of chilling precooked foods to 45°F (7°C) in less than four hours are available in one- or two-section roll-in units. Rapid chilling is accomplished by circulating fans installed within the cabinet. High-velocity air, forced horizontally over the surfaces of the food product, eliminates the formation of layers of warm air that can slow heat transfer.

Self-contained or remote quick-chill models can be purchased. Cabinet finishes, insulation materials and thickness, door gaskets, hinges, locks, and other features are similar to those found in conventional storage refrigerators. One model automatically reverts to a 38°F (3°C) storage refrigerator at the end of the quick-chilling process. Standard equipment includes a chill timer and several temperature probes. An external probe selector switch, temperature indicator, and audiovisual alarms are optional.

Foods can be frozen by blast or cryogenic freezing systems. Self-contained roll-in models or large chambers with a conveyor belt are available. In *blast freezing,* the product's temperature is lowered to 0°F (−18°C) or lower by high-velocity circulating air and a mechanical refrigeration system. In *cryogenic freezing,* liquid nitrogen or carbon dioxide in a liquid or gaseous state and moving air quickly remove heat from the product. The design and construction features of the cabinet are similar to those of other refrigeration systems. Comparisons of the capabilities of the mechanical parts used to lower temperatures and the time required in various models should be made before selecting a freezer.

Tempering Refrigerators

Food service departments that use mostly frozen foods should consider specialized equipment for tempering (thawing) foods rapidly. Conventional refrigeration systems require a great deal of time for this process. Individual units are designed to thaw foods rapidly by using high-velocity airflow and a system of heating and refrigeration. Products are safe throughout the process because the cabinet air temperature never exceeds 45°F (7°C). Upon completion of the tempering process, the cabinet may be operated as a conventional refrigerator. Conventional refrigerator models also are available with accessories designed to convert them to tempering units by using special controls. This type may be more suited to food service departments that use a limited amount of prepared frozen foods.

Food Production Equipment

In modern facilities, the food production center is designed to combine all preparation activities in the same area to save labor time, reduce space needs, and eliminate the potential for duplication of some equipment. Adequate space and equipment are needed for the production and holding of foods prior to assembly, delivery, and service.

Preparation Equipment

The types, styles, capacities, and construction features of various kinds of preparation equipment are chosen according to individual food service policies and standards. The major pieces of preparation equipment commonly used in health care facilities are described in the rest of this section.

Ovens

Oven cooking requires little attention from food service employees, can be energy efficient for large quantities of food, and is the only method efficient enough to achieve the quality desired for some products. New oven designs that incorporate microprocessor controls can be programmed for more carefully controlled cooking times. Some systems enable operators to vary the temperature in different parts of a single oven. More digital readouts indicating things such as elapsed cooking time and interior temperature, push pads rather than dials or buttons, and instruction symbols allow for simpler operation.

The most common method of oven cooking is by radiation or convection. Microwave energy is used primarily for reheating individual portions of ready-prepared foods. Several types of ovens are available.

In small food service operations or those where space is limited, ovens may need to be located below the range top. If range ovens are utilized, doors should be counterbalanced and designed to support at least 200 pounds. Range sections can be joined together with other units in the food preparation work area.

A convection oven is versatile, efficient, compact, and has high-volume output. It has replaced traditional ovens in many food service departments. Because of rapidly moving air, it speeds cooking time and allows for a heavier load than conventional ovens. In addition, the convection oven can operate at lower temperatures because the circulating heat is used more efficiently. Fuel use is lower than with other kinds of ovens for production of an equivalent volume of food.

In some convection ovens, two-speed fans can vary the rate of airflow or can be turned off to convert the oven to a conventional one. Others have a heat source control that regulates the rate at which air is reheated when the oven is partially or fully loaded. This feature affects the amount of fuel used. All of these ovens have thermostatic and timer controls.

Interior capacities are designed for volume production, with five or six shelves considered standard. Two convection ovens can be conveniently stacked to reduce space requirements. The door style can be selected to suit available space. Solid metal doors or doors with tempered glass to permit visual inspection of foods can be purchased.

Other criteria for selection include materials used for interior and exterior surfaces to facilitate cleaning; type and amount of insulation; ignition system for gas models; sturdiness of hinges and door handles; accessibility of components for inspection, adjustment, repair, and replacement; and temperature distribution throughout the oven cavity. Optional features of some large and compact models include provisions for roll-in mobile racks and baskets to minimize food handling.

Deck ovens require more space than other ovens but can be stacked in double or triple units. However, convenient and safe working heights should be maintained so that the top and bottom units are easily accessible without excessive reaching or stooping. Various oven widths and cavity heights are available to accommodate sheet pans, standard-size pans, and roasting pans. Individual thermostatic controls for each compartment are recommended. Heat balance within the oven is improved by having top and bottom heating units for each deck. Thermostats should be sensitive enough to provide quick recovery of the preset temperature. Interior and exterior finishes must be durable and easily cleaned. Gas ovens of all types should have ignition systems that eliminate the need for a constantly burning pilot light.

Rotary and reel ovens may be suited to facilities that produce large volumes of baked goods. Flat shelves are rotated horizontally in a rotary oven; in reel ovens, shelves rotate on a vertical axis. The conventional system of radiant heat transfer is used. Door openings are located at a convenient height for product removal. Various sizes and capacities are available to fit the needs of users. Careful analysis of energy requirements, space, projected utilization, and cost versus other types of ovens is necessary before this type of equipment is chosen.

High-volume food service operations may wish to consider ovens that accept one or more upright mobile racks of food products. These units combine the features of a convection oven with enhanced labor savings made possible by loading and unloading in rack-sized batches. The basic versions accept one rack (2 by 2 feet, 5 feet high), which remains stationary in the oven cavity. Other units accept a full rack and slowly rotate it in the oven cavity so that the food bakes more evenly. Larger units that accept two racks or four racks are available.

Infrared and microwave ovens are considered radiation ovens, in which energy waves are transferred from the source to the food. Infrared ovens are used for broiling. High-density infrared ovens cook food very rapidly. Infrared heating lamps are used to keep food hot once it has been prepared. Microwave ovens are rarely used for cooking foods but are frequently used to reheat foods in vending areas and in galleys in patient areas.

Ranges

Traditionally, designers of food service facilities planned the layout of the food preparation center to include several utility ranges. With the choices of cooking equipment available today, a limited number of surface cooking units are used in renovated and new facilities. However, if space is needed for preparation of small batches of food for modified diets or ingredients used in some recipes, modular units, either gas or electric, should be considered. Modular ranges in 12- to 36-inch widths mounted on casters can be placed side by side or used alone. In addition, they can be relocated easily.

Electric utility ranges are available in two styles: solid tops that are heated uniformly and tops that have round heating elements with individual controls. Combinations of solid tops or round units with griddles or broilers also are available. On a solid-top range, it should be possible to heat only a portion of the top at a time. High-speed heating capacity is important for all types of utility ranges. Heating elements, along with the drip pans underneath them, should be removable for cleaning. As mentioned in the previous section, units may have roasting ovens or pan storage beneath the cooking top. All units should be constructed of durable metals that can be cleaned easily.

The construction of gas ranges is similar to their electric counterparts: solid tops, open burners, and combinations of the two are available. The solid top should be capable of heating the entire surface uniformly, whereas the open burner directs the flame to the bottom of the cooking utensils. In selecting gas ranges, construction materials, ignition systems, thermostatic controls, safety features, and ease of cleaning should be evaluated.

Induction heating, widely used in Europe, is available for cooking surfaces. This systems uses magnetic fields to heat the food in the pan without heating the pan or the air it. According to operators, induction heating is faster and more even than traditional approaches. In addition, the surface of an induction heat range is flat and therefore easier to clean.

Tilting Braising Pans or Skillets

The tilting braising pan is one of the most versatile pieces of cooking equipment. Braising pans replaced or reduced the need for ovens, range tops, grills, and other surface cooking equipment in many facilities because they are designed to grill, fry, sauté, stew, simmer, bake, boil, or just warm an endless variety of foods. The rectangular, shallow, flat-bottomed vessel, made of heavy-duty stainless steel with welded seam construction, may be heated by electricity or gas. Pans are designed with a contoured pouring lip, and most models have a self-locking tilt mechanism to facilitate removal of cooked products and cleaning. Units range in capacity from 10 to 40 gallons. Small units may be table mounted, whereas larger sizes can be wall mounted or supported by tubular legs with or without casters. Braising pans are energy efficient, reducing cooking time by as much as 25 percent on many combination food items. Human energy also can be conserved because a significant volume of pot and pan washing is eliminated.

Steam Equipment

Energy-conscious food service directors have found that steam equipment, properly used, results in significant fuel savings as compared with surface or oven cooking. Equipment operated by steam includes low-pressure, high-pressure, or no-pressure (convection) compartment steamers and steam-jacketed kettles. Any of the compartment steamers may be purchased as individual units, as combination units, or with steam-jacketed kettles. Each classification is discussed separately.

In most models, steam is injected into the compartment at 5 to 7 pounds of pressure per square inch (psi). This means that food is cooked at a temperature of 227° to 230°F (108° to 110°C). The models available offer many choices in size, capacity, and special features such as controls, shelving, and heat source. One-, two-, or three-compartment steamers are available as self-contained units or for connection to a remote steam source. Self-contained units generate their own steam through the use of a boiler powered by gas or electricity. Selection should be based on energy sources available in the operation. Self-contained units do have the advantage of greater mobility if rearrangement of the layout becomes desirable. However, a self-generating unit should be limited to two compartments for ease of handling cooked products. The height of a three-compartment steamer makes it inconvenient and unsafe to use for most employees.

Steamers are equipped with either metal grate shelves or multipan supports to hold standard full-size, half-size, or smaller pans in each compartment. Manual or automatic timers for each compartment are needed. An automatic timer cuts off the steam supply at the end of the preset cooking period, and the steam and condensate are then exhausted. If a manual timer is selected, the bell or buzzer should be loud enough and sound long enough to be easily heard in a busy kitchen. Doors should be equipped with one-piece, easily replaceable gaskets. Self-engaging latches are needed for ease of opening and closing doors. Interiors should be of stainless steel and exterior finishes of baked enamel or other durable material for ease of sanitation.

High-pressure steamers are suitable for cooking small batches of fresh or frozen foods. Energy is conserved because cooking time is reduced by forcing steam directly into foods at a high velocity. High-pressure steamers operate at 15 psi and at a temperature of 250°F (121°C). Sizes and capacities range from compact countertop or freestanding single units to multiunit combinations of large, medium, and small compartments for large-volume operations. Like low-pressure steamers, they can be purchased as self-generating units or units that require a direct steam source. All models come equipped with automatic timers and shutoff valves and safety features that prevent personnel from opening the door before the interior pressure is reduced to zero. Other features to consider before purchasing a high-pressure steamer include doors that can be opened easily, replaceable gaskets, removable or easily cleaned pan holders, and finishes that are durable and easily sanitized.

A convection steamer forces unpressurized steam around the food, vents out, and then replaces it continuously with freshly heated steam. Because a layer of cold air is not allowed to form above the food product, rapid and uniform cooking takes place. The general design features are similar to those for compartment steamers. The steam supply may be generated in self-contained units by gas or electricity or come from a remote source. Single- or two-compartment units and countertop or freestanding models are available. Some are convertible to low-pressure cooking units. Overall dimensions, capacity, pan racks, slides, timers, and construction materials are other features to be considered before purchasing.

Steam-jacketed kettles are suitable for most food service operations because they can be used for browning, simmering, braising, and boiling—just about any type of cooking except frying and baking. Stainless steel double walls through which the steam flows may extend to the full height (fully jacketed) or to a partial height (partially jacketed) of the kettle.

Steam-jacketed kettles are of two types: stationary kettles, from which food must be ladled or drawn off through a valve at the base of the kettle, and tilting kettles, from which food can be poured. Tilting or trunnion kettles can be manually operated or they can have a power-tilting mechanism, which is especially useful for large-capacity models. Capacities range from 2½ to 120 gallons. The depths of the kettles also vary. In larger sizes, such as 40 and 60 gallons, broader, shallower depths may make the kettles easier to use and clean. The smaller sizes, up to 10 gallons, are very convenient for use in vegetable and bakery preparation units and in small operations. In general, the capacity that best suits the batch sizes needed in the food service operation should be selected.

Manufacturers offer many optional features, such as removable or counterbalanced lids, automatic stirrers and mixers (20- to 80-gallon sizes), basket inserts for cooking several different products at the same time, and pan holders for ease of removing products for service. Steam-jacketed kettles may be purchased as self-contained or direct-connect steam models, individually or in combination with other steam equipment.

In some kettles, foods can be cooled after cooking. A cold-water line is connected to the kettle, and when the steam is turned off, water circulates in the jacket. Food service operations using a cook–chill system may want to consider making use of this feature to reduce microbiological hazards. A steam-jacketed kettle that has this feature along with a mixer can lower the product temperature from the cooking zone to a chilled state in one to two hours, thus shortening the product's exposure to temperatures at which rapid bacteriological growth occurs.

Deep-Fat Fryers

Properly prepared deep-fried foods provide menu variety and can increase volume in non-patient cafeterias and snack bars. Several kinds of gas-fired or electric fryers are available with a wide range of capacities and features. Freestanding counter models or built-in single or multiple units are available. Capacities range from 15 to 130 pounds. The type of fat—solid or liquid—that may be used varies in each.

Accurate thermostats and fast heat recovery features are essential for product quality and prevention of fat deterioration. Some models provide a cool zone at the bottom of the kettle where crumbs and other sediment can collect, thus prolonging the life of the fat. An easily accessible drain for removing and filtering the fat and cleaning the fryer also is an important feature. Other features are automatic timers and basket lifts.

Specialty fryers are available for more rapid cooking of foods accomplished by frying under pressure. Pressure fryers are equipped with tightly sealed lids. The moisture given off by the food or steam under pressure is retained during the cooking process to yield a tender yet crispy product in less time than in conventional fryers.

Mixers

The time-saving and labor-saving attributes of mixers make them essential pieces of equipment for producing baked goods, desserts, and some entrees. Mixer sizes range from 5- to 20-quart bowls in bench models to 140-quart bowls in floor models. Capacity should be selected on the basis of volume needs, handling convenience, and product quality level. Bowls are raised or lowered by hand lifts on small-capacity mixers or by power lifts on larger ones. Timed mixing controls with automatic shutoffs are available. Some models have transmissions that allow speed changes while the mixer is in operation. Speed controls range from three to four or more changes in large models.

Standard equipment with most mixers includes one bowl (either heavily tinned or stainless steel), one flat beater, and one wire whip. Optional accessories include bowl adapters to accommodate smaller bowl sizes, splash covers, bowl extenders, bowl dollies, and mixer agitators such as dough hooks, pastry knives, and other specialty whips and beaters. To make this equipment even more versatile, mixers are constructed with a hub on the front of the machine. Attachments such as a slicer, dicer, grinder, chopper, strainer, and shredder can be purchased to increase productivity and reduce human labor. When purchasing more than one mixer or kitchen machine, the same hub size should be selected so that attachments are interchangeable.

Food Cutters

Various types of specialized food cutters and choppers can supplement mixer attachments or perform functions not otherwise possible. High-speed vertical cutter-mixers perform cutting, blending, whipping, mixing, and kneading functions. The capacities of these floor machines range from 25 to 130 quarts. The unit can be mounted on locking casters or permanently installed. Various cutting and mixing blades are available. One model is equipped with an easily removable plastic bowl inserted into the outer metal bowl to facilitate removal of food. The metal bowl also tilts for easy emptying. Bowl covers can be made of solid metal or transparent plastic. Counterbalanced bowl covers interlock with the motor for safety. Because of the extremely high speed of the knife blades, large amounts of food can be prepared in seconds. Vertical cutter-mixers should be located near a hot and cold water supply and convenient floor drain for cleaning.

Several other types of food cutters are available to make production jobs more efficient. Careful study of the construction features and the functions that can be performed by each must be undertaken before a selection is made. Capacities vary considerably, so food-processing requirements must be analyzed carefully. Food cutters can be obtained in table or pedestal models. Attachments for grating, dicing, slicing, and shredding also are available for some brands. Good safety features are built into every reputable manufacturer's models. However, this does not eliminate the need for the continuous training and supervision of personnel.

Food Slicers

Food slicers are machines designed to slice meats and other foods uniformly. Manual or automatic models are available with gravity or pressure feeds. In gravity-feed machines, the food carriage is slanted, and the weight of the food pushes it against the blade. Most automatic machines have more than one carriage speed and can be operated manually. A dial for adjusting cut thickness is standard on slicers. Optional features include chutes for such foods as celery and carrots that are to be cut crosswise or fences for the carriage that allow placement of two or three rows of similar items for simultaneous slicing.

The machine's safety features and ease of operating and cleaning should be checked before a slicer is purchased. Safety features should ensure maximum protection against contact with the knife when the slicer is in use and when the blade is being sharpened. Food slicers should be easy to disassemble for cleaning.

Baking Equipment

A separate baking unit may not be necessary in small facilities or in large operations where most bread and pastry items are purchased ready to serve. However, if any baked goods are produced on-site, some basic equipment is needed, including portable bins, scales, mixers, and other appropriate small equipment, as well as cooling racks and equipment storage space. Whether specialized bakery equipment is needed depends on the type and volume of goods produced. If a great deal of baking is done, the purchase of such labor-saving devices as a dough divider-rounder, electric dough rollers, and sheeters that can handle various types of doughs should be considered. Also, proofing cabinets are available in various sizes. Units may be manually or automatically controlled to maintain proper temperature, humidity, and air movement around the dough.

Ventilation Equipment

A good ventilation system is essential for maintaining a clean, comfortable, and safe working environment. Any equipment that produces heat, odor, smoke, steam, or grease-laden vapor should be vented through an overhead hood with a blower (fan) to move air through exhaust ducts that lead to an area outside the food service facility. Fire protection equipment also is essential.

Hoods are made in canopy or back-shelf styles. Canopy hoods are either wall mounted or hung from the ceiling over a battery of equipment. They extend only partway over the surface rather than over the entire piece. Careful design and placement of either type are important for convenience and safety as well as operating efficiency.

The size of a canopy hood is determined by the overall dimensions of the equipment to be covered and by local health and fire safety code requirements. A 6-inch overhang is adequate. A practical rule of thumb is 2 inches of overhang for each foot of hood clearance. The clearance between the surface of the equipment and the lower edge of the hood must be sufficient for employee safety and yet exhaust air effectively. A minimum of 6 feet 3 inches and a maximum of 7 feet is recommended for the distance between the floor and lower edge of the hood.

The back-shelf hood does not require an overhang. It extends the width of the equipment and is about 18 to 22 inches in depth as measured from the back of each piece. Clearance above the work surface varies according to the type of equipment needing ventilation, the hood design, and the exhaust air volume. Because this type of hood is smaller in size and closer to the cooking equipment, fire hazards may be reduced and maintenance made easier. Both styles of hood are built with a filtering or extracting system to prevent grease deposits and other suspended particles from accumulating and creating a fire and health hazard.

The design and construction of exhaust fans and ducts are extremely important in energy conservation. To maintain a balanced ventilation system, proper air movement is necessary. A continuous supply of makeup air must replace any that is expelled through the system for comfort, cleanliness, and preservation of equipment. However, if makeup air is withdrawn too rapidly, drafts can occur and energy usage increases.

Technological advances in system design for reduction of energy consumption continue to be made. The basic premise behind these energy savers is to reduce the amount of air drawn from the kitchen. Separate air supply ducts and exhaust ducts are placed in the hood; untempered air flows down the ducts, draws off heat and fumes under the hood, and is expelled. Some air from the kitchen is used, but much less than by conventional methods. A design specialist should be consulted so that the most economical, efficient, and safe ventilating and heat recovery system can be selected for the operation.

Worktables

The types and sizes of worktables needed in the food production center are based on the specific tasks to be performed, the number of employees using the space available, optional work heights, and the amount of storage needed for small equipment or food supplies. Well-planned and properly located tables can save time and reduce employee fatigue. A 12- to 14-gauge stainless steel work surface is preferred, because lighter weights are not as durable.

Tables equipped with locking heavy-duty casters provide greater flexibility for rearranging the work center and facilitate cleaning. In determining the length and width of tables needed, the employees' normal reach and need for space in which to arrange supplies or pans should be considered. Tables 6 feet long or shorter are recommended if they are to be on wheels. Standard 30-inch widths accommodate most preparation tasks. Tables with straight 90-degree turned-down edges can be placed together without gaps that collect food particles and fit tightly into corners. For wall arrangements, tables are available with a 2-inch turnup on the back. Adjustable feet, undershelves, tray slides, roller-bearing drawers that self-close, sink bowls, and overhead shelves or pot racks can be selected as optional features. Undershelves and drawers may be made of galvanized metal, painted or anodized metal, or stainless steel. Because of the high cost of specially designed tables, the many options available in standard models should be thoroughly investigated.

Portable stainless steel or less expensive but durable plastic or fiberglass bins are convenient for bulk storage in food production centers. Worktable designs should be planned so that bins can be rolled beneath work surfaces where needed. Also available are portable drawer units that offer convenient storage for small utensils and tools.

Sinks

The exact number of compartment and hand sinks needed in the food service department depends on the extent and complexity of the kitchen layout and local health code requirements. Several recommended construction features include:

- Stainless steel sinks (14-gauge) with coved corners in each compartment and integral drainboards on each side
- Ten-inch splashboards over drainboards and sinks
- Hot and cold faucets for each compartment unless a swing faucet is provided
- Separate drain systems for each compartment, with an exterior activated lever drain control and a recessed basket strainer for the drain
- Variable compartment size (but pot and pan sinks should be at least 11 to 14 inches deep and capable of accommodating 18-by-25-inch pans)
- Approximate sink height of 34 to 36 inches to the top of the rolled rim for convenience
- Rear or side overflows for each compartment
- Garbage disposer in one compartment or on adjacent drainboard for sinks used in preparation or ware-washing area (the drainboard location is more desirable for pot and pan sinks to avoid loss of one compartment for waste disposal)

- Tubular legs with adjustable bullet feet
- Rack or undershelf if space permits

The number and location of hand sinks depend on the size and shape of the kitchen as well as the number of employees. The sinks should be conveniently located near entrances to production and service areas and within work centers to help prevent employees from using sinks in the preparation and ware-washing areas for washing their hands. The sink size should be small enough to discourage use for cleaning small food service equipment. Foot- or knee-operated controls are recommended and may be required by local health codes.

Waste-Handling Equipment

An efficient method for disposing of waste materials is needed for economic and sanitary purposes in any food service operation. The equipment available to simplify cleanup tasks includes mechanical waste disposers, pulper–extractors, and trash compactors. The type or types selected depend on the volume of waste materials generated and local codes and ordinances. For example, mechanical disposers that grind and flush solid waste through drain lines into the sewage system are prohibited in some communities. The number of disposer units needed and their placement should be considered carefully before they are purchased. Operations that produce large quantities of food in an extensive amount of space may need disposers in several work areas such as preparation, salad, cooking, and ware washing. Small facilities can get by with one located in ware washing and another in some other production area.

Mechanical Disposers

Heavy-duty disposers range in size from ½ to 5 horsepower or more; the size selected should be based on the intended use. A 1½- to 3-horsepower unit is recommended for the dish-washing center; smaller units may be acceptable in other areas where the load is smaller. However, horsepower is not the only factor to consider when purchasing a new unit. Because disposers can jam, one that has a reversible rotor turntable that can be operated by a manual switch is recommended to increase the life and efficiency of the grinding elements. Easy-access cutter blocks and replaceable cutter blocks also are desirable features.

Disposers can be table mounted with cones or installed in sinks or trough arrangements as in dish-washing areas. Sink installation is the least desirable option, particularly when sink space is at a minimum. Resilient mountings between the disposer and the cone are needed to prevent vibration and reduce noise. In all disposers, an adequate water supply is necessary to flush waste. Some models feature a dual directional water inlet for this purpose. Accessory components that may be desirable include a silver saver splash guard and an overhead prerinse spray.

Pulper–Extractors

A pulper–extractor is designed to reduce the volume of solid waste and trim handling costs. Food scraps and disposable materials, excluding glass and metal, are pulped by rotating discs and shearing blades in a wet-processing unit. The pulp slurry is picked up by a mechanical steel screw that extracts the water. Waste material is forced into a discharge chute and dropped into waste containers. The water used to wash waste is recycled through the pulping unit. An automatic water level control allows replacement of the small amount lost in the operation. This type of waste system may be used in combination with or instead of other disposers in situations in which sewage and refuse disposer systems are inadequate. Some models are freestanding and others can be installed under counters. Capacities, in terms of pounds of waste handled per hour, vary by manufacturer and should be studied before a selection is made.

Compactors

Another type of waste disposer used in some facilities is the compactor. Solid waste, including paper, glass, and metal containers, is reduced in size by crushing under pressure.

Compression ratios vary from 4 to 1 to 20 to 1. However, the type and density of waste materials affect the actual amount of reduction. The volume of trash generated in a facility should be determined before capacity is selected because several sizes are available in either portable or stationary units. Whatever type of unit is used, trained employees who follow written instructions are the best insurance that the unit will be operated safely.

Meal Service Equipment

Equipment should be provided for the service areas of the food service operation to maintain the quality of the finished products. The type of equipment required to accomplish this goal depends on the type of production and service systems in place. Additionally, the location of the meal service areas and dining facilities should be considered when selecting meal service equipment.

Assembly Equipment

To ensure that each tray is properly prepared, the components of a centralized assembly line should include a conveyor or tray makeup table; hot and/or cold food serving carts for temperature maintenance; and equipment for holding and dispensing trays, dishes, utensils, covers, and condiments. In some cases, preparation equipment for hot beverages is needed. Individual equipment needs vary, of course, from one facility to another. Mobile units are recommended for easy rearrangement and cleaning.

Conveyors

Conveyors are either powered or gravity operated. Small hospitals and extended care facilities may find gravity-operated conveyors adequate. Powered conveyors have a continuous solid or slatted belt made of sturdy material that is resistant to animal fats, oils, and acids. An adjustable speed control and an automatic shutoff are used at the checker's end of the conveyor to prevent trays from piling up. Gravity conveyors are available with skate wheels or rollers in a variety of lengths. Conveyors must be easily cleanable. Heavy-duty, noncorroding, removable scrap pans make cleaning easier, and some conveyors are equipped with a built-in wash system.

Single- or double-stationary or movable overhead shelves can be added to some tray lines to reduce the floor space required for peripheral equipment. Side work shelves of various lengths also can be added. Individual tray carriers attached to a continuous-drive chain mechanism revolve around a rectangular table. The number of tray holders varies according to tray size and length of the assembly system. Flat or sloped shelves placed above the revolving trays hold the food to be assembled within easy reach of personnel and reduce the needed floor space.

Temperature Maintenance Equipment

Temperature maintenance equipment is required to maintain both the microbiological and aesthetic quality of the food served to patients and residents. Serving tables or carts for hot food with heated pan wells, necessary for optimum performance, may be placed at right angles or parallel to the conveyor. Electric outlets on the conveyor should be conveniently placed and wired to accept the voltage, cycle, and phase of the support equipment. Slim-line units that are easy to reach over are better for the parallel arrangement. All wells should be sized to hold standard 12-by-20-by-2-inch or deeper pans and should be designed to hold inserts for smaller pans needed for a variety of modified diet foods. Mobile units with two, three, or more wells are available. Each well should have its own temperature control to keep each type of food at the proper serving temperature and to eliminate energy waste if all the units are not needed at each meal. Wells should be of the dry-heat type for better control. The size and number of units purchased should be based on menu requirements, such as the meal at which the most hot food items will be held, easy reach for placement of food by personnel, and balanced work load by servers.

Backup equipment for keeping hot foods is also needed in most facilities because batch cooking of all foods is not possible or practical. Some units are enclosed with heated compartments underneath. If space permits, hot-holding cabinets placed directly behind the service line are more convenient. All hot-holding equipment must be well insulated and have accurate temperature controls. The employees responsible for turning on the units should know the preheat time and follow good practices to reduce energy waste. Too often, hot food wells are preheated far in advance and left uncovered, resulting in heat loss in the unit and higher temperatures in the kitchen.

Cold-holding equipment is just as necessary as hot-holding equipment. In fact, cook–chill food service systems require only cold-holding equipment to keep foods microbiologically safe. Although the same principles of construction and arrangement previously mentioned apply to chill systems, the type and style may vary according to menu requirements. Some food service departments may use carts with refrigerated wells, chest coolers for beverages and frozen desserts, or portable tables for holding cold preplated salads and other foods placed on 18-by-26-inch trays. Reach-in or roll-in refrigerators located close to the serving line help keep cold foods cold and reduce labor.

Dispensing Equipment

The type and arrangement of dispensing and support equipment affects the efficiency of the tray line. For the tray line starter position, equipment for holding such items as trays, paper supplies, eating utensils, menus, and condiments should be within easy reach if a continuous supply of trays is to advance. Various starter units are made up of several component parts. Self-leveling tray dispensers and mobile carts or stand-type stations for holding flatware and condiments are helpful. The configurations of these stations can be adapted to a variety of requirements. These units should be the right height for visual control of the line.

Other support equipment used in food assembly includes units for holding cups, saucers, glasses, dishes, and covers, if these are necessary for the delivery system. Open and enclosed carts or self-leveling enclosed dispensers are available in various sizes and capacities. Heated units are recommended for dinnerware used for hot foods; unheated carts are suitable for dish storage at room temperature. Heated units equipped with a separate thermostatic control for each section are energy efficient. When all dishes in a unit are not needed in a meal, they do not have to be heated. The control mechanism should be capable of warming dinnerware to a minimum of 165°F (74°C) or higher depending on the type of material used. Access to the thermostat and temperature controls should be convenient for regulating and repairing the equipment. The electric supply cords on mobile dispensers should be retractable for safety. Polyurethane tires are best for equipment carrying heavy loads.

Self-leveling plate units should be equipped with springs adjustable to the weight of the dinnerware. A manual control on top of the units makes adjustment easier, although some models are difficult to adjust. Strong guideposts at the top help prevent dish breakage when dispensers are moved.

Unheated open carts are practical and less expensive for dishes used in the salad and dessert portioning area. Single or double carts, with or without plastic-coated dividers, accommodate various sizes and shapes of tableware. If open carts are used, plastic covers should be provided to keep dishes sanitary when not in use. Cups and glasses can be stored on mobile carts or dollies that hold the racks in which they were washed. Self-leveling units are more convenient for employees, but they are also more expensive.

The principles for equipment selection and efficient use of space in a centralized tray assembly area also apply to a decentralized system. Variations in the type and capacity of equipment vary with the service system selected and the number of patients or residents served from a floor galley. Space for storage of food trucks, tray carts, dinnerware, trays, and the other equipment needed for limited preparation or service must be planned for efficient use of personnel and for quality assurance.

Service and Dining Area Equipment

Dining areas in health care operations should provide an attractive, relaxing atmosphere. Selection of colors for walls, window treatments, lighting, floors, tables, and chairs can set the tone for the dining area—bright and stimulating or subdued and restful. Extended care facilities and rehabilitation centers usually have patient dining areas. The designs for these areas should incorporate the special needs of the customers who will dine there.

Patients and Residents

Regardless of the type of service system used for patient and resident dining room service, mobile hot- and cold-holding carts or tables are more versatile and flexible than stationary equipment. Adequate space is needed for holding trays, dishes, utensils, and beverage containers. Having some on-site preparation equipment—toasters, beverage makers, egg cookers, and so forth—may be desirable for quality control. If cafeteria service is used, height and width of the counter and tray slides affect the convenience and safety of the diners. Residents confined to wheelchairs will need a low tray slide if a self-service system is used.

Attractive, colorful furnishings help boost patient and resident morale. Tables suitable for seating two, four, or more persons are suggested. The space between the tables should allow easy movement of people and cleanup equipment. The height of the tables should be comfortable and yet suitable for wheelchairs. Chairs should be comfortable and sturdy but not too heavy for diners to move.

Employees and Visitors

Mobile hot and cold food holding units lend themselves to the service areas for employees and guests because they can be rearranged when greater efficiency and speed are needed. Whether stationary or mobile, the hot food holding section should contain an adequate number of wells to receive 12-by-20-inch pans to a depth of 6 inches. Dry-heat wells provide superior control. Individual, accurate temperature controls for each unit also help to conserve energy.

The cold food section should provide appropriate storage bins or dispensers for salads, desserts, bread, butter, condiments, and beverages. Mechanical refrigeration may or may not be needed in this section. For example, if the facility is small and a small number of people are served in a short time, a service refrigerator nearby could provide adequate sanitary conditions for holding foods at the proper temperature up to serving time.

Mobile self-leveling dispenser units for dishes help reduce labor, handling, and breakage. Some units should have the capability of being heated; others are merely dish storage units. Hot food holding cabinets or drawers within easy reach of servers save time and help maintain the quality of foods held for short periods. Pass-through units from the kitchen are convenient. Likewise, pass-through, reach-in, or roll-in refrigerators are needed for cold foods.

In facilities serving fast-food items, grills and griddles are available for short-order cooking. Short-order cooking requires more labor, but its benefits are better food quality and customer satisfaction. If this type of service causes delays in the main service line, a separate station could be set up away from the general traffic flow, or fast-food production methods could be instituted.

Also, the type of furnishings should be considered. Tables usually accommodate two, four, or more persons. Attractive booths similar to those used in commercial establishments can add to the decor and provide good space utilization. Instead of being completely open, the room can be divided by partitions, sliding or accordion doors, or large healthy plants or dwarf trees to create an atmosphere of seclusion and relaxation. Wall color and flooring materials also are important. Professional interior decorators are other good sources for decorating ideas.

Beverage Equipment

Beverage-making equipment for dispensing hot beverages, carbonated beverages, juice, and other noncarbonated drinks such as tea along with ice makers are important because these products are popular with customers and are among the highest profit generators on the menu. These machines may be located near the end of the assembly line or in the cafeteria, dining room, or floor galleys. For serving beverages, the main feature needed is temperature control. Therefore, beverages should be served last, in insulated servers or cups.

Coffee makers are available in a wide variety of makes, models, and sizes. An important consideration in selecting a coffee maker is the amount of coffee needed within a certain period. If all coffee is made in a central location, one or more urns with a capacity of several gallons may be needed. When a small quantity of fresh coffee is called for in continuous or intermittent service, half-gallon batch brewers are ideal. Other key factors in balancing equipment and demand are the personnel available to make coffee, the physical dimensions of existing facilities, and the capital allocated to initial investment.

Coffee urns come in three basic types: manual, semiautomatic, and fully automatic. The more sophisticated models help control quality by eliminating human error and reducing personnel time. However, trained personnel can produce good coffee with less expensive equipment. Precision controls that regulate brewing time as well as brewing and holding temperatures are important features.

In semiautomatic models, the water that is siphoned and sprayed over the coffee grounds and the replacement water for the urn jacket are controlled automatically. Timing of the brewing cycle and drawing off and repouring of a portion of the brewed coffee for proper blending must be done manually. Fully automatic urns control the entire process. Water spray, water refill, brew time, temperature, and agitation are accomplished through a simple push-button action.

Urn capacities range from 3 to 10 gallons in single or twin units with a hot water faucet for making tea. Faucets may be placed on one side or both sides of urns or even on the ends to accommodate any serving arrangement. Urns can be permanently installed either above or below the counter, or mobile units may be selected. The source of heat can be gas, electricity, or steam, depending on the make and model of the urn.

Batch brewers are capable of making superb coffee in a short time through automatic controls that accurately measure both the time and the temperature of the brewing cycles. Some models require both water and electric connections; others are the simple pour-over type that require manual addition of water above the coffee grounds. These drip brewers are made in single units that hold a decanter on the base or have modular add-on warmer units beside, above, or as part of the base. Whatever type of coffee maker is chosen, high-quality construction is necessary for ease of cleaning and maintenance.

Postmix, carbonated beverage dispensers come in wide variety of sizes and configurations. Common features include a storage vessel for flavored syrup, a source of chilled water, the carbonation element, and a dispensing head. Dispensers are available with different types of control units. The type appropriate for use on the cafeteria line is simply a mechanical lever that releases the flow of water and syrup when a cup is pressed against it. Control systems that activate the dispensing head at the touch of a button also are available.

For dispensing noncarbonated drinks, such as juice and iced tea, premix and postmix systems are available. Premix systems have the advantage of displaying the product in a clear tank but require more labor because the tank must be refilled frequently. Several postmix dispensing systems for noncarbonated beverages are available. In some machines, the concentrate must be placed in a tank. Other machines are designed to draw the concentration from the concentrate directly from the container in which it is delivered. Some bag-in-box systems offer added convenience, reduce labor, and positively affect product quality.

Many of the beverages described above are served over ice. Ice makers should be selected on the basis of the purity of ice produced, sanitation features, insulation, volume of the storage bin, and capacity to produce ice. Capacities range from 40 to 4,000 pounds per day. Cube ice is the most appropriate format for beverages, but flake machines produce more ice per day. Ice dispensers in the service area should be located before the beverage dispensing equipment.

Ware-Washing Equipment

The production and service of meals to customer groups of the typical health care food service operation requires a large number of utensils and serviceware. After production and service is completed, these items must be washed and sanitized. A variety of equipment is available to make this process more efficient and effective.

Equipment for Washing Cooking Utensils

Basic equipment for washing cooking utensils includes a three-compartment sink with drainboards on each side, a waste disposer, an electric or mechanical pot scraper, and portable carts or racks to hold soiled and clean ware. Providing adequate space will promote good work flow.

As mentioned earlier in this chapter, the sink compartments must be large enough for washing, rinsing, and sanitizing utensils and equipment. However, some equipment is just too large to fit into any sink. In this case, provisions should be made for cleaning through pressure spray methods. All equipment washed manually must be allowed to air dry. Stainless steel wire racks with adjustable shelves are ideal for this use. Mobile racks and carts are recommended for transporting clean ware to the point of use when storage space is not available or when it is more convenient to store clean ware elsewhere.

Large facilities serving many meals a day may find that a mechanical unit capable of washing and sanitizing production equipment is valuable. Such equipment is available in single-tank, stationary, and moving rack models. The necessity of purchasing such a machine should be carefully scrutinized because of the space it requires and the initial cost involved.

Equipment for Washing Serviceware

Many kinds and sizes of dish-washing machines are manufactured to meet the varying volume, labor, and space demands of food service departments. Most machines use hot water for sanitizing. Models designed to reduce energy consumption use chemical sanitizers. Spray dishwashers are classified as single-tank stationary rack, single-tank conveyor, and multitank conveyor units.

Single-Tank Stationary Rack Machines

Single-tank stationary rack machines have revolving wash arms above and below the wash racks to distribute water thoroughly over, under, and around every dish. Separate rinse sprayers above and revolving rinse arms below are available in some models. Others that use the same nozzles for the wash and rinse cycle are known as single-temperature washers. Wash water and rinse water are dumped after each cycle. Chemical sanitizing machines are single-tank models that use approved chemicals in the rinse water rather than 180°F (82°C) hot water. Wash and rinse cycles for single-tank machines may be automatically or manually controlled. Standard equipment includes easily monitored dial thermometers for wash and rinse. Doors may be located on both sides for straight-through operation or on the front and one side for corner installations. Many other standard and optional features are available. Because of their limited capacity, single-tank models are suitable only for very small operations.

Single-Tank Conveyor Machines

Single-tank conveyor machines are similar to the stationary variety except that a drive mechanism carries the tray rack over the sprays and through the machine at a timed rate. Left-to-right or right-to-left operation can be specified, and an integral prewash unit can be included.

Multitank Conveyor Machines

Multitank conveyor units have two or more tanks for prewash, wash, and rinse cycles. They can be built to receive dish racks, or a continuous conveyor with pegs or rods can be used to hold dishes upright as they travel through the machine. Racks may also be used for cups, bowls, and tableware to reduce labor time. Each tank increases the length of the unit. Flight-type dishwashers are the longest because of the space needed at the loading end of the machine for soiled dishes and at the drying end for clean ones. Larger units also include a final rinse as well as a power rinse. Some models have drying mechanisms at the exit. As with single-tank machines, many additional features are included as standard or optional equipment. Most multitank conveyor dish machines are large enough to handle most cooking utensils and other equipment and thus can reduce labor costs and ensure sanitary conditions.

For both single-tank and multitank machines, a booster heater usually is necessary to generate the required final rinse water temperature. The energy supply may be gas, water, or steam. Placing the booster heater as close to the machine as possible and insulating water lines help to eliminate line temperature loss. All machines have an attached data plate indicating the temperatures required for wash and rinse water and the water pressure to be maintained at the manifold of the final rinse. Frequent checks of temperature and pressure gauges are necessary to keep dishwashers in good operating condition. (Minimum temperature requirements for clean wash water and pumped rinse water in spray machines are discussed in chapter 13.)

All dish-washing machines should carry the approval of the National Sanitation Foundation. Once they are installed and in operation, preventive maintenance is necessary to continue to meet federal, state, and local codes and regulations.

A great deal more information than can be presented here is needed before a decision on purchasing a dishwasher can be made. Although equipment experts can help with the technical aspects and preferred features of dish-washing machines, food service directors also must be fully familiar with the department's needs and space requirements in order to make the best selection.

Cart-Washing Equipment

The growing use of mobile equipment has created the need for space and cleaning devices to ensure compliance with the sanitation standards for this class of equipment. An area near the dish room usually is convenient for washing carts. Space is needed for easy access to all sides of carts, food trucks, and other delivery equipment. Hot and cold water connections and a steam supply for sanitizing the equipment are needed. The area should be provided with adequate drains and with walls and floors impervious to cleaning compounds and water. The employees assigned to this job require training and supervision in order to prevent damage to electrical equipment, to maintain a sanitary environment, and, especially, to ensure safety.

Housekeeping Equipment

Trash collection and removal, floor sweeping, mopping, waxing, sealing, and numerous other tasks must be carried out continuously to keep the food service department environment in acceptable condition. Adequate space for cleaning supplies and equipment, close to or within the immediate kitchen vicinity, makes the job easier. A sink for washing mops and a separate area for air-drying mops should be provided. The same area can be used for cleaning trash containers. A separate room may be better when cans are used to collect garbage. Mechanical can washers make sanitizing cans easier.

Equipment Maintenance and Record Keeping

Each piece of major equipment needs preventive maintenance from the time it arrives. When new equipment is purchased, the manufacturer must provide an operator's manual. The information contained in this manual should include the principles of operation; instructions for cleaning and maintenance; long-term preventive maintenance procedures and schedules; descriptions of problems that may occur, with suggestions for solving them; and a parts list with the location of service centers where replacements can be obtained. A second responsibility of the manufacturer is to see that a qualified representative explains and demonstrates the proper operation and care of the equipment to the manager, maintenance personnel, and employees when the equipment is installed. As mentioned in the preceding section, the buyer should specify these obligations in the purchase contract.

The responsibilities of food service directors include keeping equipment records, establishing preventive maintenance procedures and schedules, assigning and training employees to perform activities according to directions, and supervising inspection and follow-up procedures. Setting up a preventive maintenance program includes the following steps:

1. Record pertinent information related to the equipment purchased on a permanent record form, as shown in figure 21-2. When this record is complete, accurate, and up-to-date, it will prove invaluable in ordering new parts, having repairs made, checking warranties, making the decision to replace the equipment, and performing equipment inventories.

2. Study thoroughly the instruction manual on the operation and care of the equipment.

3. Written operating instructions are developed for the employees who will be using the equipment. The instructions should be written simply and easy to understand. Instructions for cleaning the equipment and the supplies to be used also should be included. After employees are trained, these instructions should be posted near the equipment for easy reference.

4. Develop a maintenance and inspection schedule. Instructions should be explicit and complete and should include diagrams that indicate the location of key points or parts. The schedule also should indicate what, when, and how activities are to be performed.

5. Ensure training of those employees responsible for performing maintenance tasks. It is important that the employees understand the instructions and time schedules.

6. Develop a follow-up method of inspection. A master checkoff sheet that lists the equipment, the activities to be performed, and the employees responsible is useful. However, other types of systems also work well. The key is to devise a system that works best for the institution.

7. Review records periodically and take action before a malfunction occurs. If service is required too frequently for any piece of equipment, the records should be checked. Repair costs may far exceed replacement costs in the long run. Accurate records provide management with data that can be presented to administrators in requesting new equipment.

8. File manuals and other information received from the manufacturer in a location convenient to the food service director and maintenance department personnel. Such materials should be part of the permanent equipment file for the life of the equipment. If the maintenance department is in charge of routine inspection and care, an up-to-date file may also be located in that department. Files should be reviewed periodically and outdated materials discarded.

Preventive maintenance circumvents the effects of equipment breakdowns, and employees trained properly in the operation and care of equipment can be a valuable asset to management in this respect. The malfunctioning of equipment not only can damage product quality, but it also is frustrating and possibly unsafe for employees. After training, many employees can practice preventive maintenance on the equipment they use. All employees should learn to report suspected malfunctions, unusual noises, and any other problems with equipment to the food service director.

In many health care institutions, maintenance department personnel are trained for routine inspection, care, and minor repairs. Large institutions may have a staff member who is specially trained to perform these duties. Enhanced diagnostics permit operators to more easily locate the source of equipment problems and begin repairs.

Having skilled personnel within the organization helps equipment repair times. However, additional salaries are involved, and money and storage space may be tied up in an inventory

Figure 21-2. Equipment Record Card

```
                        EQUIPMENT RECORD CARD


Item of Equipment: _____


Trade Name: _____  Manufacturer: _____


Model No.: _____  Serial No.: _____  Motor No.: _____


Capacity: _____  Attachments: _____


Operation: [   ] Electric    [   ] Gas    [   ] Steam    [   ] Hand


Purchased from: _____  [   ] New    [   ] Used    Cost: $ _____


Purchase Date: _____  Guarantee: _____  Free Service Period: _____


_____

     Date                Description of Repairs                    Cost
_____


_____     _____     _____


_____     _____     _____


_____     _____     _____
```

of spare parts. Alternative methods for equipment maintenance and repair are contract service agreements with the equipment manufacturer or vendor or informal agreements with a local repair service. Whatever the arrangement, it is important that factory-trained repair people and spare parts be available within a reasonable distance of the food service operation to eliminate lengthy delays in equipment repair. The cost, convenience, and delay time for each service should be evaluated before a maintenance decision is made.

☐ Summary

Well-planned and efficiently designed receiving, storage, food production, meal service, and ware-washing areas for the food service department are essential for ensuring a smooth work flow and controlling labor costs. The planning stage requires a great deal of time and investigation of the many options in systems and equipment in order to make the best decision for the institution. When faced with the task of renovating or planning for a new facility, the food service director should consider using a food facilities design consultant. Professional design consultants are familiar with the various food service systems and equipment, work flow, and design of work units as well as space requirements. In addition, they can help the food service director develop basic objectives and cost estimates.

☐ Bibliography

Adam, E. E., and Ebert, R. J. *Production and Operations Management.* Englewood Cliffs, NJ: Prentice-Hall, 1989.

American Hospital Association. *Selection of a Consultant for Hospital Food Service Systems Design and Equipment.* Chicago: AHA, 1977. [Out of print.]

American Hospital Association. *Workshop on Planning for Design and Renovation of Health Care Food Service Departments.* Tampa, FL, Jan. 1980.

Avery, A. *A Modern Guide to Foodservice Equipment.* New York City: Van Nostrand Reinhold, 1985.

Casper, C. Beverage systems. *Restaurant Business* 90(9): 182, 184, 186, June 1991.

Current and future application of microwave cooking and reheating. *Journal of The American Dietetic Association* 85:929, Aug. 1985.

For your next renovation: how to take charge. *Foodservice Director* 5(8):152, Aug. 1992.

Hysen, P. Equipment selection. In: J. C. Rose, editor. *Handbook for Health Care Food Service Management.* Rockville, MD: Aspen, 1984.

Hysen, P., and Harrison, J. Facilities design. In: J. C. Rose, editor. *Handbook for Health Care Food Service Management.* Rockville, MD: Aspen, 1984.

Jernigan, H. A., and Ross, L. N. *Food Service Equipment.* 2nd ed. Ames, IA: Iowa State University Press, 1980.

Kotschevar, L. H., and Terrell, M. E. *Foodservice Planning: Layout and Equipment.* 3rd ed. New York City: John Wiley and Sons, 1985.

National Restaurant Association. *Americans with Disabilities Act: Answers for Foodservice Operators.* Chicago: NRA, 1992.

Riell, H. Equipment's cutting edge. *Restaurants USA* 12(4):22–23, Apr. 1992.

Rose, J. C., editor. *Handbook for Health Care Food Service Management.* Rockville, MD: Aspen, 1984.

Spears, M. C. *Foodservice Organizations: A Managerial and Systems Approach.* New York City: John Wiley and Sons, 1990.

Stevens, J., and Scriven, C. *Food Equipment Facts.* Valley Falls, NY: Scriven Duplicating Service, 1980.

Weinstein, J. The secure restaurant. *Restaurants & Institutions* 102(27):122–23, 126, 128, 130, 132, 134, Nov. 1992.

Index

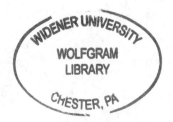

Additional Books of Interest